ENDOCRINE
SECRETS

ENDOCRINE SECRETS

Michael T. McDermott, M.D.
Professor of Medicine and Clinical Pharmacy
University of Colorado Denver Health Sciences Center
Director, Endocrinology and Diabetes Practice
University of Colorado Hospital
Aurora, Colorado

MOSBY

ELSEVIER

1600 John F. Kennedy Blvd.
Ste 1800
Philadelphia, PA 19103-2899

ENDOCRINE SECRETS   ISBN: 978-0-323-05885-8

NOTICE

Knowledge and best practice in this field are constantly changing. As new research and experience broaden our knowledge, changes in practice, treatment and drug therapy may become necessary or appropriate. Readers are advised to check the most current information provided (i) on procedures featured or (ii) by the manufacturer of each product to be administered, to verify the recommended dose or formula, the method and duration of administration, and contraindications. It is the responsibility of the practitioner, relying on their own experience and knowledge of the patient, to make diagnoses, to determine dosages and the best treatment for each individual patient, and to take all appropriate safety precautions. To the fullest extent of the law, neither the Publisher nor the Authors assumes any liability for any injury and/or damage to persons or property arising out of or related to any use of the material contained in this book.

The Publisher

Library of Congress Cataloging-in-Publication Data

Endocrine secrets / [edited by] Michael T. McDermott. – – 5th ed.
      p. ; cm. – – (Secrets series)
   Includes bibliographical references and index.
   ISBN 978-0-323-05885-8
   1. Endocrinology– –Examinations, questions, etc. 2. Endocrine
glands– –Diseases– –Examinations, questions, etc. I. McDermott, Michael
T., 1952- II. Series: Secrets series.
      [DNLM: 1. Endocrine System Diseases– –physiopathology– –Examination
Questions. WK 18.2 E56 2010]
   RC649.M36 2010
   616.40076– –dc22

2008053212

Acquisitions Editor: Jim Merritt
Developmental Editor: Nicole DiCicco
Project Manager: Mary Stermel
Marketing Manager: Allan McKeown

Working together to grow
libraries in developing countries

www.elsevier.com | www.bookaid.org | www.sabre.org

ELSEVIER   BOOK AID
            International   Sabre Foundation

Printed in China

Last digit is the print number: 9 8 7 6 5 4 3 2 1

DEDICATION

I dedicate this book to Emily and Jennifer Cohen, who have inspired us all with their courage and strength.

CONTENTS

III. PITUITARY AND HYPOTHALAMIC DISORDERS

IV. ADRENAL DISORDERS

V. THYROID DISORDERS

VI. REPRODUCTIVE ENDOCRINOLOGY

VII. MISCELLANEOUS TOPICS

[†] Deceased

PREFACE

Completing the fifth edition of *Endocrine Secrets* is immensely satisfying to me. Most of the authors in this edition are the same individuals who wrote these chapters for the first edition in 1995. Their clinical experience, teaching expertise, and sage advice have grown so much richer over these years; this is reflected very clearly in the depth and quality of these present chapters. I am deeply grateful to them for contributing so much time, energy, and talent to the many students, house staff, fellows, and lifelong learners who have benefited from their efforts over the years. I have also celebrated the opportunity to welcome new authors with each successive edition, ensuring that the tradition of teaching excellence will be passed on to new generations of equally talented and dedicated professionals. I am equally indebted to them for their generous efforts and valuable contributions. I hope once again that this book not only will instruct us and help us to take better care of our patients but will also highlight for us the privilege it is to provide healthcare to our patients, the honor it is to teach our colleagues-in-training, and the adventure it is to discover new findings that can make life better for us all.

Michael T. McDermott

CONTRIBUTING AUTHORS

Brian T. Allenbrand, M.D.
Endocrinology and Metabolism, Wilford Hall Medical Center, San Antonio, Texas

Arnold A. Asp, M.D.
Chief, Endocrinology Service, Gundersen Lutheran, La Crosse, Wisconsin

Jeannie A. Baquero, M.D.
Endocrinology and Metabolism, Wilford Hall Medical Center, San Antonio, Texas

Linda A. Barbour, M.D.
Professor of Medicine and Obstetrics and Gynecology, Divisions of Endocrinology, Metabolism and Diabetes and Maternal-Fetal Medicine, University of Colorado at Denver and Health Sciences Center, Aurora, Colorado

Amanda M. Bell, M.D.
Staff Endocrinologist, Keesler Air Force Base, Biloxi, Mississippi

Brenda K. Bell, M.D.
Lincoln, Nebraska

Daniel H. Bessessen, M.D.
Professor or Medicine, University of Colorado at Denver, School of Medicine, Denver, Colorado; Chief of Endocrinology, Denver Health Medical Center, Denver, Colorado

Tamis M. Bright, M.D.
Associate Professor of Medicine, Texas Tech University Health Sciences Center, El Paso, Texas; Internal Medicine Faculty, R.E. Thomason General Hospital, El Paso, Texas

Heather E. Brooks, M.D.
Instructor/Fellow, Division of Endocrinology, Metabolism and Diabetes, University of Colorado at Denver, Aurora, Colorado

Sarah V. Bull, M.D.
Staff Endocrinologist, Presbyterian/St. Lukes Hospital, Denver, Colorado; Assistant Clinical Professor of Medicine, Division of Endocrinology, Metabolism and Diabetes, University of Colorado at Denver, Aurora, Colorado

Henry B. Burch
Walter Reed Army Medical Center, Washington, D.C.

Reed S. Christensen, M.D.
Assistant Professor of Clinical Medicine, Uniformed Services University, Bethesda, Maryland; Endocrinologist, Assistant Chief for Outcomes, Department of Medicine, Madigan Army Medical Center, Tacoma, Washington

William E. Duncan, M.D., Ph.D., MACP
Associate Deputy Under Secretary for Health for Quality and Safety, Department of Veterans Affairs, Veterans Health Administration, Washington, D.C.; Professor of Medicine, Uniformed Services, University of the Health Sciences, Washington, D.C.

William C. Frey, M.D., FACP, FCCP, DABSM
Program Director, SAUSHEC Sleep Medicine Program, Brooke Army Medical Center, San Antonio, Texas

James E. Fitzpatrick, M.D.
Professor, Vice Chair, Department of Dermatology, University of Colorado at Denver, Aurora, Colorado

Christina M. Gerhardt, M.D.
Fellow, Pediatric Endocrinology, University of Colorado Health Science Center, Aurora, Colorado

William J. Georgitis, M.D.
Chief and Regional Director, Endocrinology and Diabetes, Colorado Permanante Medical Group, P.C., Denver, Colorado; Endocrine Department Section Chair, Exempla Saint Joseph Hospital, Denver, Colorado; Clinical Professor, University of Colorado Health Sciences Center, Denver, Colorado

Gary Goldenberg, M.D.
Assistant Professor of Dermatology, Director, Dermatopathology Laboratory, University of Maryland School of Medicine, College Park, Maryland

Marissa Grotzke, M.D.
Fellow, Division of Endocrinology, Metabolism, and Diabetes, University of Utah, Salt Lake City, Utah

Kristin A. Harmon, M.D.
Fellow, Division of Endocrinology, Metabolism, and Diabetes, University of Colorado at Denver, Aurora, Colorado

Bryan R. Haugen, M.D.
Professor of Medicine and Pathology, University of Colorado at Denver, School of Medicine; Head, Division of Endocrinology, Metabolism and Diabetes, Aurora, Colorado

James V. Hennessey, M.D.
Associate Professor of Medicine, Harvard Medical School, Boston, Massachusetts; Director of Clinical Endocrinology, Beth Israel Deaconess Medical Center, Boston, Massachusetts

Robert E. Jones, M.D., FACP
Professor of Medicine, University of Utah School of Medicine, Salt Lake City, Utah; Medical Director, Utah Diabetes Center, University of Utah, Salt Lake City, Utah

Wendy M. Kohrt, Ph.D.
Professor of Medicine, Division of Geriatric Medicine, University of Colorado at Denver, Aurora, Colorado

Homer J. LeMar, Jr., M.D.
Assistant Professor of Medicine, Uniformed University of the Health Sciences, School of Medicine, Bethesda, Maryland; Deputy Commander for Clinical Services, William Beaumont Army Medical Center, El Paso, Texas

Elliot Levy, M.D.
Aventura, Florida

Michael T. McDermott, M.D.
Professor of Medicine and Clinical Pharmacy, University of Colorado Denver Health Sciences Center, Director, Endocrinology and Diabetes Practice, University of Colorado Hospital, Aurora, Colorado

Robert C. McIntyre Jr., M.D.
Professor of Surgery, University of Colorado School of Medicine, Aurora, Colorado; Professor of Surgery, University of Colorado Hospital, Aurora, Colorado

Roger A. Piepenbrink, DO, MPH, FACP
Fellow, Endocrinology and Metabolism, Wilford Hall Medical Center, San Antonio, Texas

Christopher D. Raeburn, M.D.
Assistant Professor of Surgery, University of Colorado School of Medicine, Aurora, Colorado; Assistant Professor of Surgery, University of Colorado Hospital, Aurora, Colorado

Kurt J. Reyes, M.D.
Resident, William Beaumont Army Medical Center, El Paso, Texas

Micol S. Rothman, M.D.
Assistant Professor of Medicine, Department of Medicine, Division of Endocrinology, Diabetes and Metabolism, University of Colorado at Denver, Aurora, Colorado

Jenny L. Ryan, M.D.
Internal Medicine Resident, Madigan Army Medical Center, Tacoma, Washington

Terri Ryan, RD, CDE
Diabetes and Nutrition Consultant, Kailua-Kona, Hawaii

Mary H. Samuels, M.D.
Professor of Medicine, Division of Endocrinology, Diabetes and Clinical Nutrition, Oregon Health and Sciences University, Portland, Oregon

Leonard R. Sanders, M.D.
Outpatient and Dialysis Medical Director, HuHuKam Memorial Hospital, Sacaton, Arizona

Virginia Sarapura, M.D.
Associate Professor of Medicine, University of Colorado at Denver, Anschutz Medical Campus, Aurora, Colorado

Jonathan A. Schoen M.D.
Assistant Professor of Surgery, Director, Surgical Weight Loss Center, University of Colorado Hospital, Denver, Colorado

Robert S. Schwartz, M.D.
University of Colorado at Denver, Aurora, Colorado; Goodstein Professor of Medicine/Geriatrics, Director, Center on Aging, University of Colorado Hospital, Aurora, Colorado

Kenneth J. Simcic, M.D.[†]
San Antonio, Texas

Robert H. Slover, M.D.
Barbara Davis Center for Childhood Diabetes, Aurora, Colorado

Robert C. Smallridge, M.D.
Chair, Division of Endocrinology and Metabolism, Professor of Medicine, Mayo Clinic College of Medicine, Jacksonville, Florida

Elizabeth A. Stephens, M.D.
Endocrinology Faculty, Providence Portland Medical Center, Portland, Oregon

Derek J. Stocker, M.D., FACE
Nuclear Medicine and Endocrinology Services, Walter Reed Army Medical Center, Washington, D.C.

Raul E. Storey, M.D.
Internal Medicine Department, Texas Tech University Health Sciences Center, El Paso, Texas

Craig E. Taplin, MBBS, FRACP
Henry Silver Pediatric Endocrine and Growth Center, The Children's Hospital, University of Colorado, Denver, Denver, Colorado

[†] Deceased

Sharon H. Travers, M.D.
Department of Endocrinology, The Children's Hospital, Aurora, Colorado

Robert A. Vigersky, B.A., M.D.
Professor of Medicine, Uniformed Services University of the Health Sciences, Bethesda, Maryland; Director, Diabetes Institute, Walter Reed Health Care System, Washington, D.C.

Cecilia C. L. Wang, M.D.
Assistant Professor of Medicine, Division of Endocrinology, Metabolism and Diabetes, University of Colorado at Denver School of Medicine, Aurora, Colorado; Staff Physician, Denver VA Medical Center, Denver, Colorado

Katherine Weber, M.D.
Division of Endocrinology, Kaiser Permanente, Denver, Colorado

Margaret E. Wierman, M.D.
University of Colorado at Denver Health Sciences Center, Division of Endocrinology, Metabolism and Diabetes, Aurora, Colorado

Philip S. Zeitler, M.D.
Professor of Pediatrics, Division of Endocrinology, School of Medicine, University of Colorado at Denver, Aurora, Colorado; Pediatric Endocrinologist, Division of Endocrinology, The Children's Hospital, Aurora, Colorado

TOP 100 SECRETS

These secrets are 100 of the top board alerts. They summarize the concepts, principles, and most salient details of pathology.

1. Type 1 diabetes is caused by the autoimmune destruction of pancreatic beta cells resulting in an absolute deficiency of insulin; type 2 diabetes is the consequence of a combination of insulin resistance and progressive beta cell failure.

2. Diabetic patients should be treated to standards that are based upon scientific evidence: hemoglobin $A_{1C} < 7\%$, LDL cholesterol < 100 mg/dL, blood pressure $< 130/80$ mm Hg.

3. Microvascular complications of diabetes mellitus are directly related to hyperglycemia and result from the formation of advanced glycation end products, polyol accumulation, protein kinase C activation, accrual of intracellular glucosamine, and oxidative stress.

4. The propensity for developing vascular disease in type 2 diabetes is likely related to insulin resistance and the pathological clustering of dyslipidemia and hypertension inherent in this condition.

5. Intensive insulin therapy, or basal/bolus therapy, mimics normal pancreatic insulin secretion; basal insulin is the amount required to regulate hepatic glucose production between meals, while bolus insulin is given to match mealtime carbohydrate intake, using a carbohydrate to insulin ratio and a hyperglycemic correction factor with each meal.

6. Insulin is the best medication for managing hyperglycemia in hospitalized patients; in intensive care patients, intravenous insulin infusions are superior to subcutaneous insulin regimens in achieving quick and appropriate glycemic control.

7. Sliding scale regular insulin regimens in hospitalized patients cause more hyperglycemia and hypoglycemia than do scheduled target-based regimens of basal insulin and short acting insulin analogs; sliding scale regular insulin regimens should be abandoned.

8. Women who develop gestational diabetes have approximately a 50% risk of developing type 2 diabetes mellitus within 5 to 10 years.

9. Normalizing the A_{1C} in diabetic women prior to pregnancy and during the first 10 weeks of organogenesis can reduce the fetal major malformation rate from 25% to 2–3%.

10. Elevated LDL cholesterol and low HDL cholesterol are major risk factors for coronary artery disease (CAD); serum triglyceride levels over 150 mg/dl also promote CAD, while levels greater than 1000 mg/dl increase the risk of developing acute pancreatitis.

11. Metabolic syndrome is a major CAD risk factor complex, consisting of any 3 of the following: abdominal obesity, hypertension, hypertriglyceridemia, low HDL cholesterol, and hyperglycemia.

12. Obesity, defined as a body mass index (BMI) > 30 kg/m^2, is associated with an increased risk of developing related medical illnesses, including diabetes mellitus, hypertension, coronary artery disease, pulmonary emboli, sleep apnea, and osteoarthritis.

13. Diet and exercise to alter energy balance are the mainstays of obesity management, but sibutramine, orlistat and phentermine are currently FDA approved medications that can be used to help overweight and obese patients lose weight.

14. Adequate intake of calcium (1000–1500 mg/day) and vitamin D (800–1200 units/day), regular exercise, smoking cessation, and limitation of alcohol and caffeine consumption should be advised for all people who want to prevent osteoporosis and for all patients who are being treated with medications for osteoporosis.

15. Medical therapy for osteoporosis should be given to all patients who have sustained a fragility fracture and to all patients who have a ≥ 30% risk of having a hip fracture or ≥ 20% risk of any major fracture according to the World Health Organization (WHO) fracture risk assessment tool (FRAX).

16. Medications that have been shown to significantly reduce the risk of osteoporotic fractures fall into two main categories: anti-resorptive agents and anabolic agents.

17. Glucocorticoid induced-osteoporosis results from both suppressed bone formation and enhanced bone resorption, accounting for the rapid bone loss often seen in glucocorticoid treated patients.

18. Treatment is recommended for all postmenopausal women regardless of initial BMD and for men or premenopausal women with a BMD T-score ≤ −1.0 when they are being treated or will be treated with ≥ 5 mg/day of prednisone (or equivalent) for ≥ 3 months.

19. The forearm is the most important site for bone mass measurement in patients with hyperparathyroidism.

20. Osteomalacia and rickets result from inadequate or delayed mineralization of bone.

21. The causes of osteomalacia and rickets fall into 3 categories: 1) abnormal vitamin D supply, metabolism or action; 2) abnormal phosphate supply or metabolism; and 3) a small group of disorders in which there is normal vitamin D and mineral metabolism.

22. Paget's disease is characterized by abnormal bone architecture resulting from an imbalance between osteoclastic bone resorption and osteoblastic bone formation.

23. Bisphosphonates are the most effective treatment for Paget's disease of bone.

24. Although there are over 30 major causes of hypercalcemia, hyperparathyroidism and hypercalcemia of malignancy account for > 90%; measuring a serum parathyroid hormone (PTH) level will reliably differentiate these two disorders.

25. Calcimimetics are medications that bind to the calcium sensor-receptor and suppress the secretion of PTH; cinacalcet is FDA approved for the treatment of secondary hyperparathyroidism and parathyroid carcinoma and, though not FDA approved in primary hyperparathyroidism, has been shown to significantly lower serum calcium and PTH levels in patients with this condition.

26. Primary hyperparathyroidism is associated with hypercalcemia, osteoporosis, nephrolithiasis, and symptoms associated with these conditions.

27. The recommendations for surgery in patients with asymptomatic hyperparathyroidism are as follows: serum calcium > 1 mg/dl above the upper normal limit, hypercalciuria > 400 mg per 24 hours, decreased creatinine clearance < 70% of age matched normal persons, reduced bone density with T-Score < −2.5, age < 50 years, and calcium nephrolithiasis.

28. Hypercalcemia of malignancy is most often due to tumor production of parathyroid hormone–related peptide (PTHrp), which binds to PTH/PTHrp receptors to stimulate bone resorption and inhibit renal calcium excretion, causing hypercalcemia.

29. Hypocalcemia is a frequent problem in intensive care settings and is often a result of intravenous medications and/or transfusions.

30. Calcitriol (1,25-dihydroxyvitamin D) is the treatment choice for hypocalcemia in patients with hypoparathyroidism or renal failure.

31. Kidney stones form because of supersaturation of urinary stone precursors (such as calcium and oxalate), insufficient stone inhibitors (such as citrate), abnormal urine pH, or insufficient urine volume.

32. Therapy of kidney stones includes daily intake of 2 liters of fluid, increased intake of citrate containing drinks, 1000 to 1200 mg of calcium, and no more than 2300 mg of sodium and 1g/kg ideal body weight protein; excessive calcium, oxalate, vitamin D and grapefruit juice should also be avoided.

33. Replacement with thyroid hormone alone in a hypothyroid patient with coexistent primary or secondary adrenal deficiency may precipitate an acute adrenal crisis.

34. Aldosterone deficiency generally does not occur in hypopituitarism because the principal physiologic regulator of aldosterone secretion is the renin-angiotensin system, not ACTH from the hypothalamic-pituitary system.

35. Non-functioning pituitary tumors produce symptoms primarily by mass effects, resulting in compression of the optic chiasm, invasion of the cavernous sinuses, erosion into the bony sella turcica, and compression or destruction of the pituitary stalk or gland causing hypopituitarism.

36. Treatment for non-functioning pituitary tumors ≥1.0 cm in size is transphenoidal surgery with subsequent close monitoring for recurrence or regrowth; radiation therapy may be a useful adjunctive therapy for incompletely resected tumors.

37. A prolactin level over 200 ng/ml is almost always indicative of a prolactin-secreting tumor, except when found during late pregnancy.

38. Prolactin elevation often causes galactorrhea and amenorrhea in women and hypogonadism in men; another important consequence of elevated prolactin is decreased bone mineral density, which is not always completely reversible.

39. Acromegaly is caused by a pituitary tumor that secretes excess growth hormone, which causes damage to bones, joints, the heart, and other organs, and is associated with considerable morbidity and excess mortality.

40. The best screening test for acromegaly is a serum IGF-1 level.

41. Glycoprotein-secreting pituitary tumors include gonadotropinomas (LH or FSH secreting) and TSHomas (TSH secreting); these tumors are frequently quite large.

42. Hyperthyroid patients with detectable serum TSH levels should always be evaluated for inappropriate TSH secretion (either a TSHoma or thyroid hormone resistance).

43. Cushing's syndrome screening tests (urinary cortisol, salivary cortisol, overnight 1 mg dexamethasone suppression test) can be misleading, and repeated testing or more extensive confirmatory testing is often needed.

44. Most patients with Cushing's syndrome have a small pituitary tumor producing ACTH.

45. Rapid changes in body water or distribution can cause severe neurological dysfunction and are reflected clinically by hyponatremia or hypernatremia; treatment requires a clear understanding of changes in plasma sodium, plasma osmolality, and effective circulating volume.

46. Identification of growth abnormalities in children requires accurate height measurements and plotting against appropriate standards.

47. Growth abnormalities in children are most commonly due to normal growth variants or chronic medical problems; hormonal abnormalities are less common causes.

48. Chronic abuse of supraphysiologic growth hormone doses may lead to features of acromegaly: osteoarthritis, irreversible bone and joint deformities, increased vascular, respiratory and cardiac abnormalities, hypogonadism, diabetes mellitus and abnormal lipid metabolism.

49. Spontaneous or easily-provoked hypokalemia in a hypertensive patient should suggest the possibility of primary hyperaldosteronism.

50. The best screen for primary hyperaldosteronism is a plasma aldosterone / plasma renin activity (PA/PRA) ratio > 20; most cases of primary hyperaldosteronism are due to bilateral adrenal hyperplasia (idiopathic hyperaldosteronism).

51. Episodic headache, diaphoresis and palpitations in a hypertensive patient suggest pheochromocytoma.

52. Pheochromocytomas are 10% bilateral, 10% extra-adrenal, 10% familial, 10% malignant.

53. Features suggesting that an adrenal tumor is malignant are size > 6 cm, evidence of local invasion or metastases to the liver or lung, and high levels of urinary 17 ketosteroids, homovanillic acid, or plasma dopamine.

54. Incidentally discovered adrenal masses should be evaluated for evidence of malignancy (size >6 cm or progressive growth) and excess hormone secretion (cortisol, aldosterone, androgens, catecholamines).

55. Adrenal insufficiency should be suspected in outpatients who have received supraphysiologic doses of glucocorticoids for > 1 month, ICU patients who are hemodynamically unstable despite aggressive fluid resuscitation or have septic shock, or any patient with signs or symptoms suggesting adrenal insufficiency.

56. Adrenal crisis should be treated aggressively using normal saline with 5% dextrose, intravenous glucocorticoids (dexamethasone if treating before drawing random cortisol and ACTH, hydrocortisone afterwards), other supportive care, and a search for the precipitating illness.

57. Congenital adrenal hyperplasia (CAH), the most common inherited disease, is a group of autosomal recessive disorders, the most frequent of which is 21-hydroxylase deficiency; the most serious consequences of CAH are ambiguous genitalia in females at birth, neonatal salt-wasting, premature puberty and short stature as an adult.

58. The radioactive iodine uptake (RAIU) is used primarily to determine whether patients with thyrotoxicosis have a high RAIU disorder or a low RAIU disorder.

59. A thyroid scan is used to distinguish among the 3 types of high RAIU thyrotoxicosis (Graves' disease, toxic multinodular goiter, toxic nodule) and to determine whether thyroid nodules are non-functioning (cold), eufunctioning (warm), or hyperfunctioning (hot).

60. Older patients with thyrotoxicosis may not have classical hyperadrenergic symptoms and signs, but may instead present with weight loss, depression, or heart disease (worsening angina pectoris, atrial fibrillation, congestive heart failure); this picture is often referred to as apathetic thyrotoxicosis.

61. Radioiodine treatment may worsen eye disease in patients with significant proptosis or periorbital inflammation due to Graves' ophthalmopathy; if radioiodine is used, patients should stop smoking and should take a course of oral corticosteroids immediately after the radioiodine treatment.

62. Levothyroxine is the preferred initial treatment for hypothyroidism; healthy young patients can be started at a dose of 1.6 ug/kg/day but in patients over age 60 and in those with coronary artery disease, a starting dose of 25 ug a day is preferable.

63. The goal TSH for treatment of primary hypothyroidism is between 0.5 and 2.0 mU/L.

64. Amiodarone-induced thyroid disease (AITD) may be due to iodine-induced hyperthyroidism (Type 1 AITD) or destruction-induced thyroiditis (Type 2 AITD).

65. Women with Type 1 diabetes mellitus have a threefold greater risk of developing postpartum thyroid disorders than do non-diabetic TPO antibody positive women.

66. Fine needle aspiration (FNA) of thyroid nodules is a safe outpatient procedure with an accuracy of 90% to 95% in determining malignancy.

67. Toxic thyroid adenomas are almost never cancerous.

68. Thyroglobulin is the best tumor marker for monitoring differentiated thyroid cancer.

69. Suppression of TSH, a thyroid cancer growth factor, with levothyroxine is an important therapeutic intervention in patients with differentiated thyroid cancer.

70. Thyroid storm is treated with anti-thyroid drugs, cold iodine, beta blockers, stress glucocorticoid doses, and management of any precipitating factors.

71. Myxedema coma is treated with rapid repletion of the thyroid hormone deficit with levothyroxine +/− liothyronine, glucocorticoids and treatment of any precipitating causes.

72. The euthyroid sick syndrome is not a thyroid disorder, but is instead a group of changes in serum thyroid hormone and TSH levels that result from cytokines and inflammatory mediators produced in patients with non-thyroidal illnesses.

73. The euthyroid sick syndrome appears to be an adaptive response to reduce tissue metabolism and preserve energy during systemic illnesses and therefore treatment with thyroid hormone is not currently recommended for this condition.

74. Postpartum thyroiditis occurs in ∼5% of normal women and ∼25% of women with Type 1 diabetes mellitus.

75. On average, a women's thyroid hormone replacement dose for hypothyroidism will increase by 25 to 50 μg per day during pregnancy, often during the first trimester.

76. The symptoms of hypothyroidism often mimic those of depression, while those of hyperthyroidism may be confused with mania or depression.

77. About 20% of patients admitted to the hospital with acute psychiatric presentations, including schizophrenia and major affective disorders, but rarely dementia or alcoholism, may have mild elevations in their serum T_4 levels, and less often their T_3 levels.

78. Central precocious puberty occurs more frequently in girls than boys; the condition is often idiopathic in girls while boys with central precocity have a much higher incidence of underlying CNS pathology.

79. Hypogonadism should be characterized as primary (a disorder of the testes) or secondary (a disorder of the hypothalamic-pituitary unit); a reduction in testicular volume (<20 ml) is the most common manifestation of hypogonadism and is seen in nearly all cases of long-standing hypogonadism.

80. The diagnosis of hypogonadism is confirmed with a correctly-obtained serum testosterone measurement or semen analysis; measurement of serum LH and FSH levels then helps to determine whether the hypogonadism is primary (testicular) or secondary (pituitary or hypothalamic).

81. The specific cause of impotence can be diagnosed in 85% of men.

82. The anti-hypertensive medications that are least likely to cause impotence are ACE inhibitors, angiotensin receptor blockers, and calcium channel blockers.

83. Cysts on ovarian ultrasound do not always signify a diagnosis of PCOS.

84. A serum testosterone > 200 ng/dl or a DHEAS > 1000 ng/ml in a hirsute patient suggests the presence of an androgen producing ovarian or adrenal tumor.

85. Primary hypothyroidism can cause amenorrhea, galactorrhea, pituitary enlargement and mildly elevated serum prolactin levels, and thus can mimic a prolactinoma.

86. Many medications and painful lesions of the chest wall can cause galactorrhea.

87. The common causes of hirsutism are PCOS, CAH, idiopathic/familial hirsutism, and medications.

88. The common causes of virilization are androgen secreting ovarian or adrenal tumors and CAH.

89. Side effects of anabolic-androgenic steroid abuse include fluid retention, testicular atrophy, oligospermia, azoospermia, gynecomastia, cholestatic hepatitis, pelioses hepatis, benign and malignant hepatic tumors as well as reduced HDL and higher LDL cholesterol levels.

90. MEN 1, which consists of hyperplasia and/or tumors of the pituitary gland, pancreatic islets and parathyroid glands, results from a mutation inactivating the Menin tumor suppressor gene on chromosome 11.

91. The MEN 2 syndromes, which consist of pheochromocytomas and medullary thyroid carcinoma associated with hyperparathyroidism (MEN 2A) or mucosal neuromas (MEN 2B), result from mutations in the Ret tumor suppressor gene; genetic testing for these conditions is now clinically available.

92. Autoimmune polyendocrine syndrome type 1 (APS-1) is a syndrome marked by hypoparathyroidism, adrenal insufficiency and mucocutaneous candidiasis.

93. Autoimmune polyendocrine syndrome type 2 (APS-2) consists of adrenal insufficiency, thyroid dysfunction and diabetes mellitus type 1.

94. Fasting hypoglycemia often produces neuroglycopenic symptoms and is frequently due to an organic disorder or surreptitious use of insulin or oral hypoglycemic medications.

95. Insulinomas most often cause fasting hypoglycemia with neuroglycopenic symptoms.

96. Most patients with carcinoid syndrome have extensive liver metastases that either impair the metabolic clearance of mediators secreted by the primary tumor or that secrete the mediators directly into the hepatic vein.

97. A carcinoid crisis can be precipitated when a patient with a carcinoid tumor is given an adrenergic medication or a monoamine oxidase inhibitor; effective treatment is available.

98. Mucormycosis is more common during diabetic ketoacidosis because the fungi are thermotolerant, grow well in an acid pH, grow rapidly in the presence of high glucose, and are one of the few types of fungi that can utilize ketones as a food substrate.

99. The most common cause of acanthosis nigricans is diabetes mellitus associated with insulin resistance and obesity.

100. Aging is associated with losses of muscle mass and bone mass and with increases in fat mass, which may be associated with parallel age-related declines in the production of growth hormone and sex steroid hormones and increased cortisol secretion.

I. FUEL METABOLISM

DIABETES MELLITUS

Marissa Grotzke and Robert E. Jones

1. What is diabetes mellitus?

A group of chronic metabolic disorders characterized by abnormalities in insulin secretion or action (or both). The resulting hyperglycemia is associated with disordered carbohydrate, fat, and protein metabolism and can lead to long-term organ dysfunction. The types of diabetes are summarized in Table 1-1.

TABLE 1-1. TYPES OF DIABETES MELLITUS	
Clinical Classes	**Distinguishing Characteristics**
Type 1 diabetes mellitus	Absolute deficiency of insulin secretion due to beta-cell destruction. Beta-cell loss is either immune-mediated (90%) or idiopathic (10%). Patients all require insulin, are typically nonobese, and are prone to ketoacidosis.
Type 2 diabetes mellitus	Combination of insulin resistance and relative insulin deficiency. Often preceded by a period of abnormal carbohydrate metabolism sufficient to cause pathologic changes in target tissues. Patients are typically obese, may not immediately require insulin, and are not prone to ketoacidosis.
Gestational diabetes	Glucose intolerance first recognized during pregnancy.
Secondary to other disorders	Abnormal carbohydrate metabolism caused by other conditions (i.e., acromegaly, hemochromatosis, chronic pancreatitis) or their medications (i.e., glucocorticoids, antipsychotics, antiretrovirals).

2. What is the prevalence of diabetes?

According to 2005 statistics, 20.8 million children and adults, or 7% of the population, have diabetes. Of those, 14.6 million have been diagnosed, and 6.2 million Americans have diabetes but are unaware of it. In individuals 20 years or older, 20.6 million (9.6%) have diabetes. Additionally, an estimated 54 million are classified at prediabetic.

3. Is screening for type 1 diabetes recommended?

No. Because of the acute onset of symptoms, most cases are detected soon after a patient becomes symptomatic. Screening in asymptomatic patients is not recommended because cutoff values for many of the immune marker assays have not been completely established and there is no consensus as to what should be done with positive results. Additionally, because the incidence of type 1 diabetes is low, only a few ($<0.5\%$) patients would be identified with asymptomatic testing.

4. **Who should be screened for type 2 diabetes?**
   The risk of developing type 2 diabetes increases with age, obesity, and sedentary lifestyle. There is an increased risk with a family history of diabetes, in certain ethnic groups, and in women with a history of gestational diabetes. Current recommendations are to screen the general population at 3-year intervals starting at age 45. Earlier or more frequent screening should be performed in individuals with what are considered major risk factors (Table 1-2).

TABLE 1-2. RISK FACTORS FOR DEVELOPING TYPE 2 DIABETES MELLITUS

- Family history of diabetes
- Overweight (BMI $\geq$25 kg/m^2)
- Habitual physical inactivity
- Ethnicity (African American, Hispanic, Native American, Asian American, Pacific Islander)
- History of impaired fasting glucose or impaired glucose tolerance
- History of hypertension ($\geq$140/90)
- History of hyperlipidemia (HDL $\leq$35 mg/dL and/or triglyceride $\geq$250 mg/dL)
- History of gestational diabetes or delivery of a baby weighing more than 9 pounds
- History of polycystic ovarian syndrome

BMI, body mass index; HDL, high-density lipoprotein.

---

5. **How is diabetes diagnosed?**
   Both the fasting plasma glucose (FPG) and 75-g oral glucose tolerance test (OGTT) are acceptable for diagnosis, but the FPG is more convenient and less expensive and therefore preferred. A positive test should be repeated on a different day to confirm the diagnosis. Table 1-3 describes diagnostic criteria.

TABLE 1-3. CRITERIA FOR DIAGNOSING DIABETES MELLITUS

	Normoglycemia	"Prediabetes"	Diabetes
FPG*	110 mg/dL	$\geq$110 but <126 mg/dL (IFG)	<126 mg/dL
OGTT§	2-hr PG <140 mg/dL	2-hr PG $\geq$140 but <200 mg/dL (IGT)	2-hr PG $\geq$200 mg/dL
Casual plasma glucose†			$\geq$200 mg/dL and symptoms‡

FPG, fasting plasma glucose; IFG, impaired fasting glucose; IGT, impaired glucose tolerance; OGTT, oral glucose tolerance test; PG, plasma glucose.
* Fasting defined as no caloric intake for $\geq$8 hours.
§ In nonpregnant individuals, the OGTT should be performed using 75-g anhydrous glucose dissolved in water.
† Casual defined as any time of the day without regard to timing of last meal.
‡ Classic symptoms are polyuria, polydipsia, and unexplained weight loss.

6. **What are the genetics of type 1 diabetes?**
   The exact role of genetics versus environment in the development of type 1 diabetes is unknown. Monozygotic twins have a 20% to 50% concordance for type 1 diabetes. The cumulative risk for siblings of diabetic patients is 6% to 10% versus 0.6% for the general population. Regarding the effect of parental genes, the offspring of women with type 1 diabetes have a lower risk of disease (2.1%) than men with type 1 diabetes (6.1%). The reason for this disparity is unknown. The susceptibility for type 1 diabetes is associated with the genetic expression of certain proteins coded by the human leukocyte antigen (HLA) region of the major histocompatibility complex. These proteins are present on the surface of lymphocytes and macrophages and are considered essential for triggering the autoimmune destruction of beta cells. Although all of the genetic markers (HLA and others) for type 1 diabetes are not known, future progress in this field will allow population screening for genetic susceptibility.

7. **What are the genetics of type 2 diabetes?**
   As with type 1 diabetes, the exact interaction of genetics and environment in developing type 2 diabetes is unclear. However, the familial clustering of type 2 diabetes suggests a strong genetic component. Monozygotic twins have a 60% to 90% concordance for type 2 diabetes. The cumulative risk for type 2 diabetes in siblings of diabetic patients is 10% to 33% versus 5% for the general population. Offspring of women with type 2 diabetes have a two- to threefold greater risk for developing diabetes than do offspring of men with the disease. The exact mode of inheritance for type 2 diabetes is not known but is thought to be polygenic. Specific mutations that are associated with risk for type 2 diabetes have been identified, but many of these genes are widely found in the population at large. Because type 2 diabetes is so commonly associated with obesity, many investigators suspect that genes that predispose to obesity are associated with type 2 diabetes as well. There appears to be a strong interplay between genetic and environmental influences for causing type 2 diabetes. One illustration of this is the demonstration of higher fasting insulin levels for every weight category in offspring of two parents with type 2 diabetes compared with control subjects. High insulin levels are a marker for insulin resistance and are predictive of progression to type 2 diabetes.

8. **Describe the pathogenesis of type 1 diabetes.**
   Type 1 diabetes results from host T-cell destruction of beta cells within the pancreas, causing absolute insulin deficiency. Markers of this autoimmune process include antibodies to islet cells, insulin, and glutamic acid decarboxylase. The autoimmune destruction is believed to be related to genetic predispositions (HLA-DR/DQ alleles) in combination with poorly defined environmental factors. These patients are prone to other autoimmune disorders (Graves' and Hashimoto thyroid diseases, celiac sprue, etc.).

9. **Describe the pathogenesis of type 2 diabetes.**
   The pathogenesis of type 2 diabetes is multifactorial, although specific etiologies are unknown. Autoimmune beta-cell destruction does not occur in this form of diabetes, which accounts for 90% to 95% of all cases of diabetes. Instead, type 2 diabetes is characterized by both a defect in insulin action (known as insulin resistance) and a relative insulin deficiency. Years of hyperglycemia often precede the diagnosis, which typically occurs only after beta-cell failure has begun. Loss of first-phase insulin secretion is the initial defect with resulting elevated postprandial glucose levels. Eventually beta-cell death accelerates, and fasting glucose levels rise. It is estimated that by the time of diagnosis of diabetes, patients have lost nearly 50% of their beta-cell mass.
   With loss of beta-cell mass, insulin secretion is no longer sufficient to compensate for insulin resistance, defined as a subnormal response to a given insulin concentration. Elevated fasting or postprandial insulin levels are the hallmark of insulin resistance, which is often associated with obesity; weight reduction may improve insulin sensitivity.

10. **Can diabetes be prevented?**
    Several recent studies involving individuals at high risk for developing type 2 diabetes have documented potential beneficial effects of thiazolidinediones (TRIPOD study), metformin (Diabetes Prevention Program [DPP]), alpha-glucosidase inhibitors (STOP-NIDDM study), and intestinal lipase inhibitors (XENDOS study) in reducing the rate of progression to overt diabetes. Individuals in the lifestyle modification (diet and exercise) arm of the DPP showed the best results, with a 60% reduction in the risk of developing diabetes. Provocative post hoc analyses of the HOPE and WOSCOPS trials documented an approximately 30% reduction in diabetes risk with ramipril and pravastatin use. However, the American Diabetes Association (ADA) does not currently recommend pharmacotherapy for type 2 diabetes prevention because of a lack of long-term data.
    The lower prevalence of type 1 diabetes has made determining those at risk more difficult. Identifying people in the prediabetic phase of type 1 diabetes requires serial measurements of beta-cell function and close monitoring of immunologic markers, making selection of an appropriate cohort difficult. Two studies, the Diabetes Prevention Trial—Type 1 (DPT-1) and the European Nicotinamide Diabetes Intervention Trial (ENDIT)—overcame this issue and examined the use of insulin and nicotinamide, respectively, in high-risk relatives of type 1 diabetics. However, both failed to demonstrate effective prevention of progression to type 1 diabetes.

11. **What techniques are available to assess insulin resistance?**
    Lack of standardization of insulin assays prevents using a specific insulin concentration to define insulin resistance. The gold standards of defining insulin resistance are the intravenous glucose tolerance test, insulin suppression test, or euglycemic insulin clamp. However, these are research tools and are impractical in a clinical setting. A more clinically applicable tool is the homeostasis model assessment of insulin resistance (HOMA-IR), defined as the product of fasting insulin and fasting plasma glucose concentrations divided by a constant (22.5).

12. **Describe metabolic syndrome.**
    Metabolic syndrome is also known as syndrome X or the insulin-resistance syndrome. In 2001, the National Cholesterol Education Program Adult Treatment Panel III (NCEP ATP III) defined the metabolic syndrome as the presence of three of the five following criteria:
    - Increased waist circumference (>40 inches in men, >35 inches in women)
    - Plasma triglycerides 150 mg/dL or greater
    - Plasma high-density lipoprotein cholesterol less than 40 mg/dL in men, less than 50 mg/dL in women
    - Blood pressure 130/85 mm Hg or greater
    - Fasting plasma glucose 100 mg/dL or greater
    In 2004, the American Heart Association modified this definition to include the use of medications for hypertension or hyperglycemia to the criteria for blood pressure and fasting plasma glucose levels, respectively.

13. **What causes beta-cell failure in type 2 diabetes?**
    It is estimated that at the time of diagnosis, patients with type 2 diabetes have lost nearly 50% of their insulin-producing cells. The system of programmed beta-cell death (apoptosis) occurs progressively over the course of type 2 diabetes and has many potential triggers, although two specific possibilities have been characterized. Elevated levels of glucose and free fatty acids, collectively called glucolipotoxicity, and chronic increases in certain cytokines, notably tumor necrosis factor alpha (TNF-α) and interleukin 1-beta (IL-1β), have been documented to activate "death" genes (caspases) in beta cells. Both of these conditions have been amply described in subjects with either prediabetes or overt diabetes and clearly contribute to the genesis of type 2 diabetes by reducing the amount of functioning beta cells. However, there is considerable excitement over the concept of beta-cell preservation and the possibility that the natural history of type 2 diabetes can be altered. There is emerging data that glucagon-like peptide-1 (GLP-1) may provide either direct or indirect mechanisms to enhance beta-cell survival.

14. **What are the standards of care for management of diabetes mellitus?**
Both the ADA and the American Association of Clinical Endocrinologists (AACE) have published evidence-based minimum standards of diabetes care. Both recommend that patients have a complete history and physical examination at the initial visit. Laboratory testing should include a fasting lipid profile and hemoglobin A_{1C}. Annual surveillance for complications should include an annual physical examination, ophthalmologic examination, and a screen for microalbuminuria. Overall glycemic control (hemoglobin A_{1C}) should be assessed at least semiannually in all patients and quarterly in insulin-treated patients and patients with poorly controlled type 2 diabetes. Published targets include a hemoglobin A_{1C} of under 7.0% (ADA) or 6.5% (AACE), low-density lipoprotein cholesterol less than 100 mg/dL ($<$70 mg/dL in high-risk patients), and blood pressure under 130/80 mm Hg.

15. **Describe the current management approach to type 1 diabetes and the role of intensive therapy modeled by the Diabetes Control and Complications Trial (DCCT).**
Diabetes is a self-management illness and requires that the patient be educated in self-glucose monitoring, nutrition therapy, exercise, and the proper use of medications. Similarly, the patient must be taught how to recognize and treat hypoglycemia. Because patients with type 1 diabetes are completely insulin deficient, the medical regimen is straightforward and centered on insulin replacement. The most physiologic replacement regimen is known as the basal-bolus technique and can be accomplished with either the use of a long-acting (basal) insulin in combination with a rapid-acting (bolus) insulin or a continuous subcutaneous infusion with an insulin pump.
   The DCCT showed a 34% to 76% reduction in clinically significant diabetic microvascular complications (retinopathy, neuropathy, and nephropathy) in subjects randomized to intensive diabetes therapy compared with subjects assigned to standard diabetes management. The only major adverse effect of intensified control was a threefold higher risk of severe hypoglycemia. An intensive therapy regimen requires the monitoring of blood glucose 4 to 8 times daily with multiple daily insulin injections or an insulin pump and is best managed by a team comprising a physician, certified diabetes educator, nurse, and dietitian.

16. **Is intensive diabetes therapy cost-effective?**
The potential reduction in cost for treating diabetic complications (laser photocoagulation, dialysis, hospitalizations and rehabilitation following amputations) has been shown to justify the cost of personnel and supplies for intensive therapy. The risk-to-benefit ratio for intensive therapy may be less favorable for prepubertal children, patients with advanced complications, and patients with coronary or cerebrovascular disease.

17. **What is the United Kingdom Prospective Diabetes Study (UKPDS)?**
The UKPDS is the largest and longest prospective study on type 2 diabetes ever conducted. Investigators recruited 5102 patients with newly diagnosed type 2 diabetes in 23 centers within the United Kingdom between 1977 and 1991. Patients were followed for an average of 10 years to determine the impact of intensive therapy using pharmacologic agents versus dietary therapy alone. The study also tested the efficacy of intensive blood pressure control versus "less tight blood pressure control." The results of the study showed a significant reduction in microvascular complications in patients randomized to the intensive therapy arm. Tight blood pressure was associated with a reduction in both microvascular and macrovascular events. When the entire cohort of patients was studied together, the mean hemoglobin A_{1c} level for the duration of the study was a strong positive predictor of all diabetes-related endpoints, including death, amputation, myocardial infarction, and stroke.

18. **What is the current management approach with type 2 diabetes?**
Because type 2 diabetes is a heterogeneous disorder and patients may have other comorbid illnesses, treatment must be individualized. The most common mistake in management is to label type 2 diabetes as "borderline" or neglect treatment completely. Patients with fasting

glucose levels 126 mg/dL or greater or postprandial glucose levels greater than 200 mg/dL, even of asymptomatic, are at risk for diabetic complications.

19. **Based on the UKPDS and other studies, describe the optimal treatment for type 2 diabetes.**

The optimal treatment strategy for type 2 diabetes is one that normalizes blood glucose levels, blood pressure, and lipids to the aforementioned targets. The lifestyle interventions of diet and exercise can dramatically enhance insulin sensitivity and should be included in any treatment program.

Pharmacologically, because of the dual defects (insulin resistance and insulin deficiency) and the progressive nature of beta-cell failure in type 2 diabetes, management is different from that for type 1 diabetes. Several factors may influence initial treatment. Patients who present with profound hyperglycemia (glucose >300 mg/dL) will respond quickly to insulin therapy, and, after the effects of acute glucotoxicity have been resolved, they may often be managed with oral agents alone. Metformin is the initial drug of choice for obese patients, whereas lean patients may benefit more from sulfonylureas. Because of the progressive nature of type 2 diabetes, these patients will eventually fail initial therapy and require a second agent. If the patient has been on an insulin sensitizer, such as metformin or a thiazolidinedione, an insulin secretagogue should be added. Conversely, if the patient has failed a secretagogue, adding an insulin sensitizer is appropriate. Fixed-dose combination medications are available; however, their use as initial therapy can hinder the titration of the individual components. Most patients will ultimately fail dual therapy and require the addition of a third agent or initiation of insulin.

20. **What are insulin analogs?**

Insulin analogs are recombinant proteins that are based on the structure of insulin but have undergone selected amino acid substitutions or additions. These amino acid alterations are designed either to enhance or protract the subcutaneous absorption of the molecule without altering its biologic properties. Native human insulin (regular) exists as a molecular hexamer that must be progressively broken down into dimers and then monomers before absorption. Amino acid substitutions in the carboxy-terminal region of the beta-chain of insulin tend to destabilize hexamer formation and speed the rate of absorption. Examples of these analogs are the insulins lispro (Humalog), aspart (NovoLog), and glulisine (Apidra). These insulins are excellent for premeal use, and because they also have a shorter duration of action in comparison to native human insulin (regular), they provide better mealtime coverage with a lower risk of postmeal hypoglycemia.

Conversely, basal insulin should have both a peakless action profile and a prolonged duration of action. This is achieved by amino acid additions that shift the isoelectric point to promote hexamer formation. After it is injected, these insulins are buffered to a physiologic pH and form a microprecipitate that is then slowly absorbed. Insulin glargine (Lantus), which uses two arginine additions at the carboxy terminus of the beta chain to lower the isoelectric point to 4, is generally used as a once-daily injection in people with either type 1 or type 2 diabetes. On occasion, the dose of glargine may need to be split into two injections in extremely insulin-sensitive type 1 diabetics. The protraction of insulin detemir (Levemir) is due to fatty acylation fo the insulin molecule which results in albumin binding. Detemir can be used as once- or twice- daily insulin injections in type 2 diabetes, whereas most type 1 diabetics require twice-daily dosing.

21. **What is inhaled insulin?**

A new insulin formulation inhaled insulin is a recombinant human insulin delivered by an inhaler and absorbed through the lungs. The only available formulation, Exubera, is used as a prandial insulin and still requires the use of an injectable basal insulin. Use of inhaled insulin is contraindicated in smokers. Production of this insulin formulation, however, has recently been stopped and availability at this time is limited.

22. **What is amylin?**

Amylin is a beta-cell hormone that is cosecreted with but structurally distinct from insulin. Under normal circumstances, amylin acts to reduce postprandial glucose excursions by reducing the gastric emptying rate and suppressing glucagon production, thereby reducing postprandial hepatic glucose production. It is also believed to inhibit the stomach hormone ghrelin, resulting in appetite suppression. In addition to an absolute insulin deficiency, patients with type 1 diabetes also have a complete deficiency of amylin, and patients with type 2 diabetes taking insulin have clearly reduced amylin responses to meals. Mealtime replacement of amylin in subjects who required insulin was shown to reduce hemoglobin A_{1C} levels modestly while promoting weight loss. Currently available as the synthetic analog pramlintide, amylin is approved for use in type 1 and type 2 diabetics as an injection before meals.

23. What are incretins?

The incretin effect refers to the enhanced insulin secretory response observed after an oral glucose load when compared with an intravenous or parenteral glucose load. After eating, the cells of the distal small intestine release incretins such as GLP-1 into the blood. GLP-1 secretion is under neurogenic control. It acts to increase glucose-dependent insulin secretion, suppress glucagon release, delay gastric emptying, enhance satiety through a direct effect on the central nervous system, and possibly stimulate pancreatic islet growth.

24. How are incretins used to treat type 2 diabetes?

There are currently two types of incretin-based drugs available. The incretin mimetic, exenatide, imitates the actions of endogenous GLP-1. It is currently available only as injection. Its use has been associated with moderate weight loss in addition to modest hemoglobin A_{1C} lowering. The second type of drug, the dipeptidyl peptidase-IV (DPP-IV) inhibitors (sitagliptin), blocks the enzyme that breaks down GLP-1. The same degree of weight loss is not seen with use of sitagliptin; however, it is administered in tablet form. Both types of incretins can be used as monotherapy or in combination with other available hyperglycemic agents.

25. What are the classes of oral diabetes medications? How do they work?

In addition to the earlier-mentioned DPP-IV inhibitors, several classes of diabetes medications are available for optimizing glycemic control in people with type 2 diabetes. Sulfonylureas (glyburide, glipizide, and glimepiride) and meglitinides (repaglinide and nateglinide) enhance the secretion of endogenous insulin through membrane-associated receptors. Metformin, the only biguanide available, reduces hepatic gluconeogenesis, thereby indirectly increasing peripheral insulin sensitivity. The alpha-glucosidase inhibitors (miglitol and acarbose) slow the absorption of dietary carbohydrates by inhibiting the intestinal brush border enzymes (Table 1-4) that break down polysaccharides into absorbable monosaccharides. The thiazolidinediones (pioglitazone and rosiglitazone) act by binding nuclear peroxisome proliferator-activated receptor gamma to increase insulin sensitivity and directly enhance insulin action in muscle and fat cells. Controversy has

TABLE 1-4. SITE OF ACTION OF ORAL DIABETIC MEDICATIONS

Drug	Pancreas	Liver	Muscle/Fat	GI Tract
Sulfonylureas	X			
Meglitinides	X			
Metformin		X		
Thiazolidinediones		X	X	
Alpha-glucosidase inhibitors				X
Dipeptidyl peptidase-IV inhibitors	X			X

GI, gastrointestinal.

arisen recently regarding the potential negative cardiovascular effects of these drugs (particularly rosiglitazone), and their role in the treatment of type 2 diabetes is currently under scrutiny.

BIBLIOGRAPHY

1. American Diabetes Association: Diagnosis and classification of diabetes mellitus. Diabetes Care 31:S12–54, 2008.

2. American Diabetes Association: Screening for diabetes. Diabetes Care 25:S21–24, 2002.

3. Chandra J, Zhivostovsky B, Zaitsev S, et al: Role of apoptosis in pancreatic β-cell death in diabetes. Diabetes 50(Suppl 1):S44–S47, 2000.

4. DeFronzo RA: Pharmacologic therapy for type 2 diabetes mellitus. Ann Intern Med 131:281–303, 1999.

5. Diabetes Control and Complications Trial Research Group: The effect of intensive treatment of diabetes on the development and progression of long-term complications in insulin-dependent diabetes mellitus. N Engl J Med 329:977–986, 1993.

6. Diabetes Prevention Trial—Type 1 Diabetes Study group: Effects of insulin in relatives of patients with type 1 diabetes mellitus. N Engl J Med 346:1685–1691, 2002.

7. Edelman SV, Weyer C: Unresolved challenges with insulin therapy in type 1 diabetes: potential benefit of replacing amylin, a second β-cell hormone. Diabetes Technol Therapeut 4:175–189, 2002.

8. Egan JM, Bulotta A, Hui H, Perfetti R: GLP-1 receptor agonists are growth and differentiation factors for pancreatic islet beta cells. Diabetes Metab Res Rev 19:114–123, 2003.

9. Expert Committee on the Diagnosis and Classification of Diabetes Mellitus: Report of the expert committee on the diagnosis and classification of diabetes mellitus. Diabetes Care 20:1183–1196, 1997.

10. Gale EA. European Nicotinamide Diabetes Intervention Trial (ENDIT): a randomized controlled trial of intervention before the onset of type 1 diabetes. Lancet 363:925–931, 2004.

11. Garber AJ: Benefits of combination therapy of insulin and oral hypoglycemic agents. Arch Intern Med 163:1781–1782, 2003.

12. Grundy SM, Brewer HB, Cleeman JI, et al, for the Conference Participants: Definition of metabolic syndrome: report of the National Heart, Lung, and Blood Institute/American Heart Association conference on scientific issues related to definition. Circulation 109:433–438, 2004.

13. Knowler WC, Barrett-Conner E, Fowler SE, et al: Reduction in the incidence of type 2 diabetes with lifestyle intervention or metformin. N Engl J Med 346:393–403, 2002.

14. Molitch ME: Diabetes and incretin-based therapy. J Clin Endocrinol Metab 92;15A–16A, 2007.

15. Nissen SE: Effect of rosiglitazone on the risk of myocardial infarction and death from cardiovascular causes. N Engl J Med 356:2457–2471, 2007.

16. Pimenta W, Korytkowski M, Mitrakou A, et al: Pancreatic beta-cell dysfunction as the primary genetic lesion in NIDDM: evidence from studies in normal glucose-tolerant individuals with a first-degree NIDDM relative. JAMA 273:1855–1861, 1995.

17. Reaven G: Role of insulin resistance in human disease. Diabetes 37:1595–1607, 1988.

18. Riddle MC: Timely initiation of basal insulin. Am J Med 116:3S–9S, 2004.

19. Saydah SH, Fradkin J, Cowie CC: Poor control of risk factors for vascular disease among adults with previously diagnosed diabetes. JAMA 291:335–342, 2004.

20. Tuomilehto J, Lindstrom J, Eriksson JG, et al: Prevention of type 2 diabetes by changes in lifestyle among subjects with impaired glucose tolerance. N Engl J Med 344:1343–1350, 2001.

21. UK Prospective Diabetes Study (UKPDS) Group: Intensive blood-glucose control with sulphonylureas or insulin compared with conventional treatment and risk of complications in patients with type 2 diabetes (UKPDS 33). Lancet 352:857–858, 1998.

22. Uwaifo GI: Novel pharmacologic agents for type 2 diabetes. Endocrinol Metab Clin North Am 34:155–197, 2005.

23. Vajo Z, Fawcett J, Duckworth WC: Recombinant DNA technology in the treatment of diabetes: insulin analogs. Endocr Rev 22:706–717, 2001.

CHAPTER 2

ACUTE AND CHRONIC COMPLICATIONS OF DIABETES

Marissa Grotzke and Robert E. Jones

1. **What are the acute complications of diabetes?**
   Hyperglycemia and hypoglycemia, which are both the result of an imbalance between medications (insulin or oral diabetic agents) and the patient's food intake and exercise.

2. **Describe the symptoms of hyperglycemia.**
   Initial symptoms are increased thirst (polydipsia), increased urination (polyuria), fatigue, and blurry vision. If uncorrected, hyperglycemia may eventually lead to diabetic ketoacidosis (DKA) or hyperosmolar hyperglycemic syndrome (HHS). Rather than distinct entities, DKA and HHS represent a spectrum of a disease process characterized by varying degrees of insulin deficiency, overproduction of counterregulatory hormones, and dehydration. In some situations, features of both DKA and HHS may occur concurrently.

3. **What is DKA?**
   DKA is a state of uncontrolled catabolism triggered by a relative or absolute deficiency in circulating insulin. The triad of DKA is metabolic acidosis (pH <7.35), hyperglycemia (blood glucose usually >250 mg/dL), and ketonuria. Insulin deficiency is accompanied by a reciprocal elevation in counterregulatory hormones (glucagon, epinephrine, growth hormone, and cortisol), causing increased glucose production by the liver (gluconeogenesis) and catabolism of fat (lipolysis). Lipolysis provides the substrate (free fatty acids) for the uncontrolled production of ketones by the liver. The production of ketones then leads to a metabolic acidosis.

4. **What causes DKA?**
   Any disorder that alters the balance between insulin and counterregulatory hormones can precipitate DKA. A minority of cases occurs in people not previously diagnosed with diabetes, but most cases (up to 80%) occur in people with a previous diagnosis. DKA is most often associated with type 1 diabetes; however, it may also occur in older patients with type 2 diabetes, particularly when associated with a major intercurrent illness.

5. **What illnesses may trigger DKA?**
   Infection and myocardial infarction are the illnesses most commonly known to trigger DKA. Even localized infections, such as urinary tract infections or prostatitis, have precipitated DKA. Other triggers include severe emotional stress, trauma, medications (i.e., corticosteroids), or hormonal changes (i.e., preovulation) in women.

6. **How can deficiencies in education trigger DKA?**
   Many patients with recurrent episodes of DKA have deficient knowledge about their insulin regimen or have not been taught how to test their urine for ketones or how to handle diabetes during times of illness.

7. **What are the signs and symptoms of DKA?**
   Nausea and vomiting, generalized abdominal pain, dehydration, rapid (Kussmaul) respirations, and a sweet (acetone) odor on the breath. Other important features are the pattern of insulin use and symptoms of infection, acute coronary syndrome, or other possible precipitating illnesses.

8. **How is DKA diagnosed?**
   All dehydrated patients should be asked about symptoms of diabetes and have serum electrolytes and glucose checked before initiation of intravenous hydration.
   DKA should be suspected if the patient presents with marked hyperglycemia (glucose >300 mg/dL) and metabolic acidosis. An elevated anion gap (>13 mEq/L) is usually, but not always, present. The finding of elevated ketones in the blood or urine confirms the diagnosis.

9. **Is ketone testing always positive with DKA?**
   No. If blood or urine ketones are negative and DKA is strongly suspected, treatment with fluids and insulin should still be initiated. During the course of treatment, the blood and urine ketones tests will become positive. This "delay" in positivity for measured ketones is due to a limitation of the laboratory test for ketones, which detects only acetoacetate. The predominant ketone in untreated DKA is beta-hydroxybutyrate. As DKA is treated, acetoacetate becomes the predominant ketone, causing the test for ketones to turn positive.

10. **What lab tests are recommended in the first hour of treatment for DKA?**
    - Baseline electrolytes, blood urea nitrogen (BUN), creatinine, glucose, anion gap, urinalysis, urine and blood ketones, and electrocardiogram (ECG) should be performed.
    - An arterial blood gas (ABG) should be obtained if the patient appears ill or tachypneic or if the serum bicarbonate is low (<10 mEq/L).
    - Fluid intake, urine output, and progression of laboratory changes should be recorded.
    - Further lab testing should be based on findings of suspected triggers (i.e., infection, myocardial infarction).

11. **Summarize the strategy for fluid and potassium administration in the first hour.**
    - Fluids: normal saline should be at 15 mL/kg/h (~1 L/h for 70 kg).
    - Potassium: if the T waves on the ECG are peaked or normal, no potassium replacement is initially necessary. If T waves are low or U waves are seen, 40 mEq potassium chloride (KCl) should be added to each liter of intravenous (IV) fluids.

12. **How should insulin treatment be started with DKA?**
    An initial IV bolus of 10 to 20 units regular insulin should be followed by a continuous infusion of 0.5 units/mL of regular insulin mixed in normal saline at a rate of 5 to 10 units per hour (0.1 unit/kg/h).

13. **What assessments should be made in the second hour of treatment?**
    - Vital signs (including respiratory rate), level of consciousness, hydration status, and urine output.
    - Repeat electrolytes, blood glucose, and urine and blood ketones. Calculate anion gap.

14. **Summarize the strategy for fluid and potassium administration in the second hour of treatment.**
    - Fluids: continue normal saline at approximately 1 L/h.
    - Potassium: adjust or add KCl to IV fluids to maintain serum potassium at 4 to 5 mEq/L.

15. **How should insulin be adjusted during treatment?**
    If the serum glucose drops to less than 250 mg/dL, fluids should be changed to 5% to 10% dextrose in saline. The insulin infusion rate may be doubled if the serum glucose does not decline after the first hour. The optimal rate of glucose decline is 100 mg/dL/h. The glucose level should not be allowed to fall to <250 mg/dL during the first 4 to 5 hours of treatment.

16. **Summarize the basic strategy after the second hour of treatment.**
    - Assess the patient and repeat previously discussed lab tests hourly.
    - Fluids: adjust rate of infusion based on level of hydration. Consider changing to 0.45% normal saline if the patient is euvolemic and hypernatremic.
    - Potassium: continue to adjust to a goal serum value of 4 to 5 mEq/L.
    - Insulin: continue IV infusion as long as acidosis is present; supplement with dextrose as necessary.

17. **When can the insulin infusion be discontinued?**
    When the anion gap corrects to normal, the pH is 7.3 or greater, or the serum bicarbonate is 18 mEq/L or greater, the patient can be given a subcutaneous dose of regular insulin or a short-acting insulin analog (lispro, aspart, glulisine) to cover a meal. The infusion should be stopped 30 minutes after the subcutaneous insulin is given. If the patient is unable to eat, give 5 units of regular or a short-acting insulin analog, continue the IV dextrose solution, and give supplemental short-acting insulin every 4 hours on the basis of the glucose level.

18. **What other interventions may be necessary in the treatment of DKA?**
    If the initial serum phosphorus is less than 1.0 mg/dL, consider giving 10 to 20 mEq/h potassium phosphate in the IV fluids.
    Bicarbonate (in the form of sodium bicarbonate) replacement is not recommended unless other causes of severe acidosis are present (e.g., sepsis, lactic acidosis) or the arterial pH is less than 6.9. If used, sodium bicarbonate should be diluted in the IV fluids and given over 1 hour.

19. **What is a possible complication of DKA? How should it be treated?**
    Cerebral edema can be a complication of the DKA itself or of too rapid fluid replacement during treatment. New diabetics or pediatric patients are particularly at risk. If the patient suddenly develops a headache or becomes confused during therapy, give mannitol, 1 mg/kg, immediately.

20. **What is hyperosmolar hyperglycemic syndrome?**
    Formerly known as hyperosmolar hyperglycemic nonketotic syndrome or coma and described first in 1957 by Sument and Schwarts, hyperosmolar hyperglycemic syndrome (HHS) is a constellation of hyperglycemia, hyperosmolarity, and altered level of consciousness, most typically in the absence of acidosis.

21. **Who is at risk for HHS and why?**
    Elderly patients, with or without a history of type 2 diabetes, are at particular risk for HHS because of a higher rate of impaired thirst perception and increased prevalence of impaired renal function. Possible precipitating factors, such as infection, myocardial infarction, cerebrovascular events, pancreatitis, gastrointestinal hemorrhage, or use of exogenous medications, may also be present.

22. **What are the signs of HHS?**
    - Marked hyperglycemia (serum glucose >600 mg/dL)
    - Hyperosmolarity (serum Osm >320 mOsm/L)
    - Arterial pH greater than 7.3
    - Hyperglycemia, once triggered, leads to glycosuria, osmotic diuresis, hyperosmolarity, cellular dehydration, hypovolemia, shock, coma, and, if untreated, death.

23. **Why is metabolic acidosis typically not seen in HHS?**
    Although glucose concentrations are generally higher than with diabetic ketoacidosis, the residual insulin secretory capacity of type 2 diabetics likely prevents severe acidosis and ketosis. The presence of circulating insulin or lower levels of counterregulatory hormones (or both) prevents lipolysis and significant ketone production.

24. **What are the symptoms of HHS?**
    Polyuria and polydipsia often occur days to weeks before presentation of the syndrome. Patients are unable to drink enough to match a brisk osmotic diuresis, exacerbating the hyperglycemia.

The imbalance of fluid intake and output eventually results in impaired renal function, decreasing glucose excretion and further worsening hyperglycemia. Profound dehydration is typical. Fever is not part of the syndrome and, if present, suggests an infectious component.

25. **What is the most common presenting symptom of HHS?**
Altered mental status occurs in approximately 90% of cases and is the most common reason that patients are brought to the hospital. An effective osmolarity greater than 340 mOsm/L is required for coma to be attributed to HHS and is present in 10% of patients on presentation. Effective osmolarity refers to the true osmolarity seen by the cells and is calculated using the following equation:

$$\text{Effective osmolarity(mOsm/L)} = 2[\text{measured Na} + (\text{mEq/L})] + [\text{glucose(mg/dL)}/18]$$

26. **List other possible causes of impaired mental status.**
If the degree of mental status changes is out of proportion to the effective osmolarity, other etiologies should be considered. The mnemonic AEIOU TIPSS is helpful to remember the differential of mental status changes:

A = Alcohol	T = Trauma/Tumor
E = Encephalopathy	I = Insulin
I = Infection	P = Psychosis
O = Overdose	S = Syncope
U = Uremia	S = Seizures

27. **What other neurologic signs may be associated with HHS?**
Bilateral or unilateral hyporeflexia or hyperreflexia, seizures, hemiparesis, aphasia, positive Babinski sign, hemianopsia, nystagmus, visual hallucinations, acute quadriplegia, and dysphagia.

28. **What is the hallmark laboratory finding in patients with HHS?**
   ▪ Marked hyperglycemia (>600 mg/dL and often >1000 mg/dL): the serum sodium is often factitiously low. To correct for the hyperglycemia, the following formula is used:

$$\text{Corrected Na}^+ = \text{serum Na}^{++}[1.6(\text{serum glucose} - 100)]/100$$

   ▪ Other laboratory abnormalities include elevated BUN and creatinine, hypertriglyceridemia, and leukocytosis.

30. **What is the first step in treating HHS?**
Aggressive volume resuscitation is imperative and should be addressed before insulin administration to avoid intracellular fluid shifts (from falling glucose levels) that may worsen systemic perfusion. The fluid deficit is typically severe—on the order of 9 to 12 L. In patients with renal insufficiency or cardiac disease, central venous access may be necessary to monitor response to therapy, and patients with altered mental status may require an indwelling urinary catheter.

31. **Should isotonic or hypotonic fluids be used?**
There is controversy regarding this issue; however, isotonic (0.9%) saline at a rate of approximately 1 to 2 L over the first hour is generally recommended. After the first hour, fluids may be changed on the basis of the serum sodium concentration: if between 145 and 165 mEq/L, a change

to half normal saline may be considered; if lower than 145 mEq/L, isotonic saline should be continued. Replacement of one half of the calculated fluid deficit over the initial 5 to 12 hours is recommended, with the balance of the deficit replaced over the subsequent 12 hours.

32. Summarize the management of electrolytes in HHS.
The replacement of electrolytes other than sodium is identical to the previously outlined protocol for DKA.

33. What role does insulin play in the treatment of HHS?
Continuous IV insulin infusion, as previously described for DKA, is helpful to reduce glucose levels at a predictable rate. Because of the absence of significant acidosis, there is no need for dextrose infusion as there is with DKA. Patients may be transitioned directly from IV to subcutaneous insulin as described for DKA. Because the presence of HHS suggests a significant insulin deficiency, most patients require discharge on an insulin regimen, with the appropriateness of oral agents determined in the outpatient setting.

34. Describe the signs and symptoms of hypoglycemia.
To be defined as hypoglycemia-induced symptoms, Whipple's triad (low blood glucose, symptoms consistent with hypoglycemia, and resolution of symptoms by raising blood glucose) must be fulfilled. Symptoms can be divided into adrenergic and neuroglycopenic symptoms (Table 2-1), with different symptoms presenting at progressively lower blood glucose levels. Adrenergic symptoms originate with the autonomic nervous system and include norepinephrine-mediated palpitations, tremor, anxiety and acetylcholine-mediated sweating, hunger, and paresthesias. Neuroglycopenic symptoms can include weakness, visual changes, behavior changes, confusion, seizure, loss of consciousness, and, if untreated, death; these symptoms represent the effects of low glucose levels on the central nervous system. Typical signs are pallor, diaphoresis, and tremor.

TABLE 2-1. CLINICAL MANIFESTATIONS OF HYPOGLYCEMIA	
Adrenergic	**Neuroglycopenic**
Diaphoresis	Cognitive impairment
Palpitations	Fatigue
Tremor	Dizziness/faintness
Arousal/anxiety	Visual changes
Pallor	Paresthesias
Hypertension	Hunger
	Inappropriate behavior
	Focal neurologic deficits
	Seizures
	Loss of consciousness
	Death

Adapted from Cryer PE, Gerich JE: Hypoglycemia in insulin-dependent diabetes mellitus: insulin excess and defective glucose counterregulation. In Rifkin H, Porte E, editors: *Ellenberg and Rifkin's diabetes mellitus: theory and practice*, ed. 4. New York, Elsevier, 1990, pp. 526–546.

35. **Discuss therapy-related causes of hypoglycemia in diabetes.**
It is impossible to mimic the peaks and troughs of a normal insulin secretory pattern with subcutaneous insulin injections, and even a perfectly designed insulin regimen can lead to hypoglycemia when the patient decreases food intake, delays a meal, or exercises even slightly more than usual. Menstruating women can experience hypoglycemia at the time of menses because of a rapid fall in estrogen and progesterone. Elderly patients given a sulfonylurea for the first time may respond with severe hypoglycemia.

36. **What other factors may contribute to the development of hypoglycemia?**
In addition to therapy-related factors, disorders such as those listed in Table 2-2 may precipitate hypoglycemia.

TABLE 2-2. CAUSES OF FASTING (POSTABSORPTIVE) HYPOGLYCEMIA

1. Drugs: insulin, sulfonylureas, alcohol
2. Critical organ failure: renal, hepatic, cardiac failure; sepsis; inanition
3. Hormonal deficiencies: cortisol and/or growth hormone; glucagon + epinephrine
4. Non-beta-cell tumor
5. Endogenous hyperinsulinism: beta-cell tumor (insulinoma); functional beta-cell hypersecretion; autoimmune hypoglycemia; ? ectopic insulin secretion
6. Hypoglycemias of infancy and childhood

From Cryer PE, Gerich JE: Hypoglycemia in insulin-dependent diabetes mellitus: insulin excess and defective glucose counterregulation. In Rifkin H, Porte E editors: *Ellenberg and Rifkin's diabetes mellitus: theory and practice,* ed. 4. New York, Elsevier, 1990, pp. 526–546.

---

37. **Are some diabetic patients more susceptible to hypoglycemia than others?**
Yes. Some type 1 diabetics have a defect in glucose counterregulation that blunts the normal release of counterregulatory hormones in response to hypoglycemia. These hormones (epinephrine, glucagon, cortisol, and growth hormone) stimulate glycogenolysis and gluconeogenesis by the liver, resulting in a reversal of hypoglycemia. Blunting their normal release leads to severe hypoglycemia or delayed recovery from hypoglycemia.

38. **What is "hypoglycemia unawareness"?**
Defective counterregulation is often associated with hypoglycemia unawareness, in which the patient reports an absence of the normal adrenergic warning symptoms of hypoglycemia. In contrast, the predominant signs and symptoms are due to decreased delivery of glucose to the brain (neuroglycopenic symptoms). The cognitive impairment associated with neuroglycopenia may prevent the patient from responding appropriately to self-treat the hypoglycemia. The result may be a traumatic automobile accident, seizure, coma, or death.

39. **Can hypoglycemia unawareness be prevented?**
Studies suggest that this disorder may be the body's maladaptation to previous episodes of hypoglycemia. A single episode of hypoglycemia has been shown to reduce autonomic and symptomatic responses to hypoglycemia on the following day in normal subjects and in patients with type 1 diabetes. In contrast, meticulous prevention of hypoglycemia has been shown to reverse the defective counterregulation and reestablish the adrenergic symptoms after 3 months. Thus meticulous attention to prevent hypoglycemia in patients without established autonomic neuropathy may be beneficial in reversing hypoglycemic unawareness.

40. How is hypoglycemia treated?

Mild hypoglycemia (blood glucose 50–60 mg/dL) should be treated with 15 g of simple carbohydrate, such as 4 oz of unsweetened fruit juice or nondietetic soft drink. For more profound hypoglycemia, 15 to 20 g of simple carbohydrate should be ingested quickly, followed by 15 to 20 g of a complex carbohydrate, such as crackers or bread. All diabetic patients should be taught how to self-treat hypoglycemia appropriately.

41. What should be done if the patient is unconscious?

Patients who are unconscious should not be given liquids. More viscous sources of sugar (e.g., honey, glucose gels, cake icing in a tube) can be carefully placed inside the cheek or under the tongue. Alternatively, 1 mg of glucagon may be injected intramuscularly. Glucagon indirectly causes the blood glucose level to increase through its effect on the liver. In the hospital setting, IV dextrose (D-50) is probably more accessible than glucagon and results in a prompt return of consciousness.

42. Discuss the role of education in treating hypoglycemia.

Instruction in the use of glucose gels and glucagon should be an essential part of training for all individuals living with insulin-treated diabetic patients. Patients and family members should be instructed not to overtreat hypoglycemia, particularly if it is mild. Overtreatment leads to subsequent hyperglycemia. Patients should also be instructed to test the blood glucose level when symptoms occur to confirm hypoglycemia whenever feasible. If testing is not possible, it is best to treat first. Patients on medication should be instructed to test their glucose level before driving a vehicle. If the glucose level is lower than a preset level (e.g., <125 mg/dL), the patient should be instructed to ingest a small source of carbohydrate before driving.

43. Summarize the common long-term complications of diabetes mellitus.

The complications of diabetes can be divided into the two broad categories of microvascular complications and macrovascular complications. Microvascular complications are considered relatively specific to diabetes; are associated with pathologic endothelial changes, such as basement membrane thickening and increased vascular permeability; and can involve damage to the eye (retinopathy), kidney (nephropathy), and peripheral nerves (neuropathy). The category of macrovascular complications encompasses an increased susceptibility to blood vessel damage (atherosclerosis) and its ensuing complications.

44. What basic mechanism underlies the development of long-term diabetic complications?

Hyperglycemia is the major force underlying the microvascular complications of diabetes and has been implicated in the excessive risk of atherosclerosis seen in patients with insulin resistance. However, it is difficult to ascribe all of these observations to glucotoxicity alone.

45. What other mechanisms may be involved?

- Mass-action-nonenzymatic glycation of proteins: these proteins ultimately form advanced glycosylation end products (AGEs), which are associated with altered protein function. AGEs have been found in the connective tissue of blood vessels and in the renal glomerular matrix and have been shown to modify low-density lipoprotein (LDL) composition.
- Enzymatic conversion of glucose to sorbitol by the enzyme aldose reductase in the eyes and peripheral nerves: because the cellular clearance of sorbitol is extremely slow, it accumulates as an osmotically active molecule. This accumulation is also associated with neuronal myoinositol depletion.
- Excess of intracellular glucosamine: another product of glucose, intracellular glucosamine has been linked to endothelial dysfunction and to impaired insulin action.

- Activation of protein kinase C (PKC) by glucose: thought to be due to depressed nitric oxide production and increased endothelin-1 activity, activation of PKC has been shown to mediate retinal and renal blood flow abnormalities and increase endothelial cell permeability.
- Hyperglycemia-driven oxidative stress: the resulting activation of poly(ADP-ribose) polymerase (PARP) has been tied to glycemic injury and may serve, in part, to increase substrate flux into glucosamine, polyol, and AGE formation, as well as to promote PKC activation.

46. **Describe the characteristics of nonproliferative diabetic retinopathy.**
Significant diabetic retinopathy may progress without symptoms. The initial visible lesions are microaneurysms that form on the terminal capillaries of the retina. Increased permeability of the capillaries is manifested by the leaking of proteinaceous fluid, causing hard exudates. Dot-and-blot hemorrhages result from leaking of red blood cells. These findings by themselves do not lead to visual loss and are categorized as nonproliferative retinopathy (Table 2-3).

TABLE 2-3. CLINICAL MANIFESTATIONS OF DIABETIC EYE DISEASE

Nonproliferative diabetic retinopathy
- Retinal microaneurysms
- Occasional blot hemorrhages
- Hard exudates
- One or two soft exudates

Preproliferative diabetic retinopathy
- Presence of venous beading
- Significant areas of large retinal blot hemorrhages
- Multiple cotton-wool spots (nerve fiber infarcts)
- Multiple intraretinal microvascular abnormalities

Proliferative diabetic retinopathy
- New vessels on the optic disc (NVD)
- New vessels elsewhere on the retina (NVE)
- Preretinal or vitreous hemorrhage
- Fibrous tissue proliferation

High-risk proliferative diabetic retinopathy
- NVD with or without preretinal or vitreous hemorrhage
- NVE with preretinal or vitreous hemorrhage

Diabetic macular edema
- Any thickening of retina <2 disc diameters from center of macula
- Any hard exudates <2 disc diameters from center of macula with associated thickening of the retina
- Any nonperfused retina inside the temporal vessel arcades
- Any combination of the above

From Centers for Disease Control: *The prevention and treatment of complications of diabetes mellitus.* Division of Diabetes Translation, Department of Health and Human Services, Atlanta, 1991.

47. **Describe the characteristics of proliferative retinopathy.**
Proliferative retinopathy (see Table 2-3) develops when the retinal vessels are further damaged, causing retinal ischemia. The ischemia triggers new, fragile vessels to develop, a process termed neovascularization. These vessels may grow into the vitreous cavity and may bleed into preretinal areas or vitreous, causing significant vision loss. Loss of vision also may result from retinal detachment secondary to the contraction of fibrous tissue, which often accompanies neovascularization. Diabetic macular edema occurs when fluid from abnormal vessels leaks into the macula. It is detected with indirect funduscopy by the finding of a thickened retina near the macula and is commonly associated with the presence of hard exudates.

48. **How common is diabetic retinopathy?**
Up to 70% of type 1 diabetics may develop proliferative retinopathy over their lifetime. Among type 2 diabetics, 2% of patients may have significant nonproliferative and even proliferative retinopathy or macular edema at the time of diagnosis. This may be due to the long undiagnosed period of hyperglycemia that often occurs in people with type 2 diabetes.

49. **What are the risk factors for development of diabetic retinopathy?**
   - Duration of diabetes
   - Level of glycemic control
   - Presence of hypertension
   - Diabetic nephropathy is strongly associated with proliferative retinopathy in type 1 diabetes and insulin-treated type 2 diabetes.

50. **List the other ophthalmologic complications of diabetes.**
Cataracts and open-angle glaucoma.

51. **How serious a problem is diabetic nephropathy?**
Diabetic nephropathy is the leading cause of end-stage renal disease in the United States. Its progression follows a predictable pattern characterized into stages I through V (Table 2-4).

TABLE 2-4.	STAGING OF CHRONIC KIDNEY DISEASE.	
Stage	Estimated GFR (mL/min)	Findings
1	$\geq$90	Asymptomatic, $\pm$ HTN, renal hypertrophy, possible increase in GFR (GFR >125 mL/min confers high risk of progression)
2	60–89	$\pm$ Edema, $\pm$ HTN, glomerular histologic changes
3	30–59	Edema, HTN, anemia, microalbuminuria (urinary albumin excretion 30–300 mg/day)
4	15–29	Edema, fatigue, dyspnea, HTN, electrolyte abnormalities, proteinuria (urinary albumin excretion >300 mg/day or total protein excretion >500 mg/day)
5	<15	Anorexia, dyspnea, HTN, encephalopathy, end-stage renal disease

GFR, glomerular filtration rate; HTN, hypertension.

52. **What is the risk that a diabetic person will develop nephropathy?**
Type 1 diabetics are at highest risk for nephropathy, which affects 30% of these patients. The risk of nephropathy is about 10 times less for type 2 patients, but because of the prevalence of type 2 diabetes, this group currently outnumbers type 1 patients with end-stage renal disease.

53. **What factors affect the development of diabetic nephropathy?**
In addition to glycemic control, genetic factors play a key role in determining risk for diabetic nephropathy. Genes coding for essential hypertension appear to increase the risk. Known risk factors for diabetic nephropathy are as follows:
- Family history of hypertension (relative risk [RR] ≥ 3.7).
- Sibling with diabetic nephropathy (RR >4.0).
- Black race (RR ≥ 2.6 vs. white race).
- Smoking history (RR ≥ 2.0).
- History of poor glycemic control (RR ≥ 1.3–2.0).

54. **Name the most common type of diabetic neuropathy.**
Distal symmetric polyneuropathy.

55. **Summarize the symptoms of distal symmetric polyneuropathy.**
The disorder is usually discovered on routine physical examination by the finding of loss of vibratory sense in the toes and loss of ankle reflexes. Light touch and pinprick sensation are subsequently lost. Common associated symptoms are numbness and paresthesias of the feet, especially at night. The paresthesias may evolve to severe knifelike or burning pain, which can be disabling.

56. **Explain the basic pathophysiology of distal symmetric polyneuropathy.**
Pathologically, the nerves show axonal degeneration. Sensory loss or pain in the hands may also occur, but more commonly it is a manifestation of entrapment neuropathy, such as carpal tunnel syndrome. Entrapment neuropathies are common in patients with diabetes and may result from increased susceptibility of these nerves to external pressure.

57. **What causes the foot problems in patients with diabetes?**
Loss of nerve fibers for proprioception can result in an abnormal gait, leading to "pressure spots" on the foot that are signaled by the presence of a thick callus. If untreated, the callus may ulcerate and become infected. Neuropathy, vascular disease, and predisposition to infection are the primary pathogenic components for the increased incidence of foot injury and amputation in patients with diabetes.

58. **How are foot problems treated surgically?**
Revascularization of the foot using distally placed in situ saphenous bypass grafts often results in healing of limb-threatening foot infections or gangrene.

59. **How common is diabetic autonomic neuropathy? How does it affect survival rates?**
Depending on the sophistication of testing used, up to 90% of people with diabetes have some degree of autonomic dysfunction. However, less than 50% of affected people are symptomatic. Patients with clinically significant autonomic neuropathy have a less than 50% 10-year survival rate. Both the sympathetic and parasympathetic nervous systems may be affected by diabetic neuropathy, and because these neuropathies initially damage nerves with the longest axons, patients with diabetic autonomic neuropathy also have readily apparent peripheral neuropathy.

60. **Describe the classic signs of diabetic autonomic neuropathy.**
Unexplained resting tachycardia and postural hypotension (with absence of fever, hypoglycemia, hyperthyroidism, etc.). Gastrointestinal symptoms are due to a lack of peristalsis in the stomach

(gastroparesis) or intestine and include early satiety, bloating, nausea, belching, abdominal distension, constipation, or diarrhea. Urinary retention or overflow incontinence may indicate autonomic neuropathy involving the urinary bladder. Erectile dysfunction is also a frequent symptom of autonomic neuropathy in a diabetic man.

61. How is diabetic autonomic neuropathy diagnosed?

A lack of R-R variation on an electrocardiogram during deep breathing or the Valsalva maneuver can be used to confirm the diagnosis. Postural hypotension can be diagnosed by documenting a fall in upright blood pressure without a concurrent increase in pulse rate. Gastroparesis is diagnosed by demonstrating prolonged gastric emptying using standardized radiolabeled meals; however, even mild hyperglycemia (blood glucose >150 mg/dL) at the time of the test may functionally slow gastric emptying. Urinary and erectile problems are diagnosed by careful history taking.

62. Describe the treatment for diabetic retinopathy.

Early detection is essential for successful treatment of diabetic complications. For retinopathy, this requires annual examination with funduscopic dilatation by an ophthalmologist. If preproliferative or proliferative retinopathy or significant macular edema is seen, laser therapy may be indicated to prevent significant vision loss. Vitrectomy or retinal surgery may be required for restoration of vision loss due to vitreous hemorrhage or retinal detachment.

63. How is diabetic nephropathy managed?

Progression can be slowed by aggressive treatment of hypertension. Angiotensin-converting enzyme (ACE) inhibitors or angiotensin receptor blockers (ARBs) are the agents of choice because they have been shown to have beneficial effects independent of blood pressure control. Other antihypertensive agents are also beneficial, but their effects appear to be more closely mediated by the degree of blood pressure control. The recommended goal is treatment to a blood pressure under 130/80 mm Hg. ACE inhibitors and ARBs have also been shown to attenuate the decline in renal function in normotensive, normoalbuminemic type 2 diabetic patients. Current research supports this as a cost-effective treatment strategy. Additionally, studies such as the Modification of Diet in Renal Disease Study suggest that adoption of a low-protein diet (<0.6 g/kg/day) can reduce progression of disease in patients with established nephropathy.

64. Discuss the management of postural hypotension.

Postural hypotension due to autonomic neuropathy improves with the use of compression stockings that prevent venous pooling in the legs. Fludrocortisone is effective but must be used cautiously to prevent worsening of hypertension or edema. Other drugs with a demonstrated benefit include clonidine, octreotide, and midodrine.

65. What treatments are effective for sensory loss due to diabetic neuropathy?

There is no known treatment for sensory loss from diabetic neuropathy. Educational programs addressing proper foot care and prevention of foot injury have been shown to reduce the incidence of serious foot lesions. Routine foot examination and early referral to a podiatrist or vascular surgeon for patients with foot lesions are considered essential to prevent limb loss.

66. How is painful diabetic neuropathy treated?

Multiple medications have been tried, with mixed success. These include nonsteroidal anti-inflammatory drugs, tricyclic antidepressants, anticonvulsants, opioids, and the serotonin-noradrenaline reuptake inhibitors (SNRIs). The most effective medications among those currently available appear to be pregabalin (Lyrica; starting dose 50 mg three times daily [TID] with titration to 100 mg TID, if tolerated), gabapentin (Neurontin; starting dose 300 mg twice daily with titration to 600 mg TID, as necessary), and the SNRI duloxetine (Cymbalta; dose 60 mg daily).

67. **How are the symptoms of gastroparesis treated?**
    Reducing dietary fiber and fat, decreasing meal size, and increasing exercise may all improve symptoms. The prokinetic drugs metoclopramide and erythromycin have been shown to reduce symptoms in patients with diabetic gastroparesis; however, serious side effects can occur with both drugs and should be discussed with the patient before use.

68. **What are the risks associated with macrovascular disease in diabetes?**
    Patients with diabetes are at a twofold to fourfold increased risk for both cardiovascular disease (CVD) and peripheral vascular disease compared with the nondiabetic population. Women with diabetes have as high a risk for CVD as men. The commonly identified risk factors for CVD—smoking, hypercholesterolemia, and hypertension—also adversely affect CVD risk in diabetic persons.

69. **Which factors specific to diabetes increase the risk for CVD?**
    The blood of diabetics has been found to have increased platelet aggregation, decreased red cell deformability, and reduced fibrinolytic activity. The glycation of lipoproteins may lead to decreased clearance by the liver and increased atherosclerosis. The blood vessels themselves have distinct abnormalities. Long-standing diabetes predisposes the arteries to calcification.

70. **How can macrovascular disease be prevented in the diabetic population?**
    Cardiovascular risk factor reduction should be initiated at the first visit and pursued as aggressively in diabetic patients as in patients with known coronary artery disease. Aggressive blood pressure control is strongly supported by recent randomized controlled trials, with a target blood pressure under 130/80 mm Hg. ACE inhibitors have been reported to be more effective than other antihypertensive agents in preventing CVD events and are currently the antihypertensive agents of choice. Control of hyperlipidemia should be pursued just as aggressively; the recommended goal for LDL cholesterol is less than 100 mg/dL (<70 mg/dL in high-risk patients). Improving glycemic control typically causes a significant reduction in triglyceride levels and modest reduction in LDL cholesterol. If goals for lipids are not achieved through glycemic control, diet, and exercise, then antihyperlipidemic drug therapy should be considered. The HMG-CoA reductase inhibitors (statins) are the drug class of choice for this. Smoking cessation should be strongly encouraged, as should exercise and weight loss (if overweight). Low-dose aspirin therapy is also recommended.

71. **Does aggressive lipid-lowering therapy improve cardiac outcomes in diabetic patients?**
    Yes. The Scandinavian Simvastatin Survival Study compared the outcome of 4242 patients with history of myocardial infarction or angina pectoris and elevated total cholesterol. Patients were randomized to aggressive lipid-lowering therapy with simvastatin or placebo. A post hoc subgroup analysis of the 202 diabetic participants showed a 55% reduction in major coronary events, including myocardial infarction, in the simvastatin-treated group. At 5.4 years, total mortality was reduced 43%. Statistically significant beneficial results were also reported with pravastatin in the Cholesterol and Recurrent Events (CARE) study and Long-term Intervention with Pravastatin in Ischemic Disease (LIPID) trial. On the basis of these reports, aggressive lipid-lowering therapy should be advocated in all diabetic patients, particularly those with known coronary artery disease.

72. **How important is glycemic control in preventing the chronic complications of diabetes mellitus?**
    As discussed in Chapter 1, the Diabetes Control and Complications Trial, Kumamoto study, and United Kingdom Prospective Diabetes Study (UKPDS) have established that improving glycemic control effectively reduces the risk of developing microvascular complications (retinopathy, nephropathy, and neuropathy) in patients with type 1 and type 2 diabetes. The UKPDS also

demonstrated that glycemic control with metformin reduced the risk of macrovascular disease (coronary artery and cerebrovascular disease) and that control with either sulfonylureas or insulin produced a similar, although not statistically significant, trend for coronary artery disease reduction. On the basis of these data, the American Diabetes Association recommends that glycemic control be sufficient to maintain the fasting blood glucose level below 120 mg/dL and the hemoglobin A_{1C} below 7% (the American Association of Clinical Endocrinologists recommends a hemoglobin A_{1C} below 6.5%).

73. Does improved glycemic control in hospitalized patients affect outcome?
Adults with diabetes are 6 times more likely to be hospitalized than those without diabetes and have a 30% longer length of stay. Under any circumstances, poorly controlled diabetes is a catabolic condition, and in hospitalized patients with diabetes who are under physiologic stress, catabolism is certainly detrimental. In addition, leukocytes and immune function are impaired by hyperglycemia. A recent randomized prospective study designed to assess whether lowering blood glucose levels to 80 to 110 mg/dL in patients admitted to an intensive care unit (ICU) using insulin influenced outcomes. In-hospital mortality was reduced 34%; sepsis was reduced 46%; hemodialysis rate was reduced 44%; transfusions were reduced 50%; and critical-illness-related polyneuropathy was reduced 44%. A separate study demonstrated the cost-effectiveness of intensive glycemic management in the ICU setting. Another study showed a reduction in the rate of deep sternal infections in diabetics undergoing open-heart surgery, and the Diabetes and Insulin-Glucose Infusion in Acute Myocardial Infarction (DIGAMI) study demonstrated significant reductions in mortality in diabetic patients treated with insulin during and after hospitalization for acute myocardial infarction.

BIBLIOGRAPHY

1. American Diabetes Association: Dyslipidemia management in adults with diabetes. Diabetes Care 27(Suppl 1): S68–S71, 2004.
2. American Diabetes Association: Hyperglycemic crises in diabetes. Diabetes Care 27(Suppl 1):S94–S102, 2004.
3. American Diabetes Association: Hypertension management in adults with diabetes. Diabetes Care 27(Suppl 1): S65–S67, 2004.
4. American Diabetes Association: Nephropathy in diabetes. Diabetes Care 27(Suppl 1):S79–S83, 2004.
5. American Diabetes Association: Retinopathy in diabetes. Diabetes Care 27(Suppl 1):S84–S87, 2004.
6. CDC Cost-effectiveness Group: Cost-effectiveness of intensive glycemic control, intensified hypertension control, and serum cholesterol level reduction from type 2 diabetes. JAMA 287:2542–2551, 2002.
7. Chong MS, Hester J: Diabetic painful neuropathy: current and future treatment options. Drugs 67:569–585, 2007.
8. Chrysant SG: The ALLHAT study: results and clinical implications. Q J Med 96:771–772, 2003.
9. Clement S, Braithwaite SS, Magee MG, et al: Management of diabetes and hyperglycemia in hospitals. Diabetes Care 27:553–591, 2004.
10. Collins R, Armitage J, Parish S, et al: MRC/BHF heart protection study of cholesterol-lowering with simvastatin in 5963 people with diabetes: a randomized placebo-controlled trial. Lancet 361:2005–2016, 2003.
11. Folwaczny C, Wawarta R, Otto B, et al: Gastric emptying of solid and liquid meals in healthy controls compared with long-term type-1 diabetes mellitus under optimal glucose control. Exp Clin Endocrinol Diabetes 111: 223–229, 2003.
12. Fritsche A, Stefan N, Häring H, et al: Avoidance of hypoglycemia restores hypoglycemia awareness by increasing β-adrenergic sensitivity in type 1 diabetes. Ann Intern Med 134:729–736, 2001.
13. Haffner SM, Lehto S, Ronnemaa T, et al: Mortality from coronary heart disease in subjects with type 2 diabetes and in nondiabetic subjects with and without prior myocardial infarction. N Engl J Med 339:229–234, 1998.
14. Hasler WL: Gastroparesis: symptoms, evaluation, and treatment. Gastroenterol Clin North Am 36:619–647, 2007.
15. Hollenberg NK: Treatment of the patient with diabetes mellitus and risk of nephropathy. Arch Intern Med 164:125–130, 2004.

16. Kitabchi A, Wall BM: Management of diabetic ketoacidosis. Diabetic ketoacidosis and hyperglycemic hyperosmolar syndrome. Crit Care Clin 17:75–106, 2001.

17. Krinsley JS: Cost analysis of intensive glycemic control in critically ill adult patients. Chest 129:644–650, 2006.

18. Pyörälä K, Pederson TR, Kjekshus J, et al: Cholesterol lowering with simvastatin improves prognosis of diabetic patients with coronary heart disease: a subgroup analysis of the Scandinavian Simvastatin Survival Study (4S). Diabetes Care 20:614–620, 1997.

19. Reusch JEB: Diabetes, microvascular complications, and cardiovascular complications: what is it about glucose? J Clin Invest 112:986–988, 2003.

20. Ritz E, Orth SR: Nephropathy in patients with type 2 diabetes mellitus. N Engl J Med 341:1127–1133, 1999.

21. Sarafidis PA: Antihypertensive therapy in the presence of proteinuria. Am J Kidney Dis 49:12–26, 2007.

22. Van den Berghe G, Wouters P, Weekers F, et al: Intensive insulin therapy in the surgical intensive care unit. N Engl J Med 342:1301–1308, 2000.

23. Vinik AI, Mehrabyan A: Diagnosis and management of diabetic autonomic neuropathy. Compr Ther 29:130–145, 2003.

CHAPTER 3

INTENSIVE INSULIN THERAPY

Elizabeth A. Stephens and Terri Ryan

1. **What is intensive insulin therapy?**
   Intensive insulin therapy (IIT), or basal-bolus therapy, is the use of an insulin pump or multiple daily injections (MDIs) of insulin (both long- and rapid-acting formulations) in an effort to mimic normal pancreatic insulin secretion. IIT is complex because it often requires 3 to 6 injections per day but is only one aspect of intensive therapy.

2. **List the other critical components of intensive therapy.**
   - Frequent self-monitored blood glucose (SMBG)
   - Establishment of targeted blood glucose (BG) levels
   - Understanding of diet composition, specifically carbohydrate content
   - Use of carbohydrate-to-insulin ratios according to food intake
   - Use of correction factors (CFs) for the adjustment of insulin according to glucose levels

3. **Summarize studies that support optimal diabetes management to decrease chronic complications from diabetes mellitus.**
   The Diabetes Control and Complications Trial (DCCT), evaluating patients with type 1 diabetes, and the United Kingdom Prospective Diabetes Study (UKPDS), evaluating patients with type 2 diabetes, documented that intensive glycemic control leads to significantly reduced rates of complications, including progression of retinopathy, nephropathy, and neuropathy. The UKPDS trial also evaluated blood pressure control using angiotensin-converting enzyme (ACE) inhibitors and beta-blockers in patients with type 2 diabetes and found that both agents effectively improve cardiovascular outcomes.

4. **Which patients are candidates for IIT?**
   All people with diabetes should be considered as potential candidates for IIT. However, the degree of intensification must be based on each patient's personal situation and abilities. Patient characteristics that predict greater success with IIT include motivation, willingness to perform frequent SMBG (up to 6–10 times/day) and record results, time to spend with the diabetes educator, the ability to recognize and treat hypoglycemia, sick days, and a supportive network of family or friends. In addition, implementation of IIT requires a cohesive diabetes team that is available for frequent interaction and discussion about results from monitoring, insulin adjustments, and other issues.

5. **Explain the difference between basal and bolus insulin coverage.**
   Basal insulin coverage is the insulin required to manage BG fluctuations due to hepatic glucose production overnight or between meals. Basal coverage is usually accomplished with injections of long-acting insulin preparations or with the basal infusion function on the insulin pump. Bolus insulin coverage is the insulin required to manage glucose excursions following meals, accomplished by injections of rapid-acting, or short-acting insulin preparations or using the bolus function on the insulin pump. Bolus insulin doses are estimated for each meal on basis of the amount of insulin required to cover the carbohydrate in the meal, as well as a high BG CF.

6. **What are the currently available long-acting insulins?**
   - Long-acting analogs: insulin glargine (Lantus) and insulin detemir (Levemir)
   - Intermediate-acting insulin: neutral protamine Hagedorn (NPH)
   - Premixed biphasic insulin analogs: Humalog Mix 75/25, Humalog Mix 50/50, and NovoLog Mix 70/30
   - Premixed biphasic human insulins: Humulin 70/30, Novolin 70/30, and Humulin 50/50

7. **How are long-acting insulins used with an MDI regimen?**
   Ideally, basal insulin should cover background insulin needs only, independent of food intake and exercise. Basal insulin is approximately 40% to 60% of a patient's total daily dose (TDD) of insulin. Premixed "biphasic" insulin preparations combine either a rapid-acting insulin analog or regular human insulin with a crystalline protaminated form of the analog or regular human insulin in an attempt to imitate basal and bolus therapy with fewer injections.

8. **What are the currently available bolus insulins?**
   - Rapid-acting analogs: insulin lispro (Humalog), insulin aspart (NovoLog), and insulin glulisine (Apidra)
   - Short-acting human insulin: regular human insulin (Humulin R or Novolin R)

9. **Describe the pharmacodynamics of the bolus and basal insulins.**
   See Table 3-1.

TABLE 3-1. THE PHARMACODYNAMICS OF BOLUS AND BASAL INSULINS			
	Insulin Onset	Peak	Duration*
Humalog, NovoLog, Apidra	5–30 min.	1–2 hours	4–6 hours
Regular	30–60 min.	2–3 hours	8–10 hours
Lantus or Levemir	2–4 hours	6–16 hours	18–24 hours
NPH	2–4 hours	4–12 hours	12–20 hours

NPH, neutral protamine Hagedorn.
* The peak and duration of insulin action are variable, depending on the injection site, duration of diabetes, renal function, smoking status, and other factors.

10. **When should bolus insulin be taken?**
    - Five to ten minutes before meals and snacks when glucose is in the normal range (90–130 mg/dL)
    - Fifteen to thirty minutes before meals if the premeal BG is higher than 130 mg/dL (Supplemental bolus insulin [CF] is added to meal insulin when the BG is elevated.)
    - Immediately after eating, if gastroparesis or an intercurrent illness is present
    - Upon arrival of food, if unfamiliar with meal size, content, or timing (i.e., in restaurant or hospital)

11. **When should basal insulin be taken?**
    - Insulin glargine or detemir should be taken at bedtime if a dawn phenomenon is present or at any consistent time, approximately every 24 hours. (Insulin glargine or detemir cannot be mixed with other insulins.)

- If nocturnal hypoglycemia results from taking a full dose of glargine or detemir at bedtime, an option would be to split the dose so that 50% is taken in the morning and the other 50% is taken in the evening, approximately 12 hours apart.
- NPH insulin is given in the morning and at bedtime to avoid nocturnal hypoglycemia.

12. **What is pramlintide (Symlin)?**
Pramlintide is an injectable analog of amylin, which lowers postprandial glucose levels by suppressing glucagon secretion and slowing gastric emptying, thus reducing the rate of glucose absorption from the gastrointestinal tract. Studies in patients with type 1 diabetes suggest that adding pramlintide to insulin can blunt glycemic excursions after meals, reduce hemoglobin A1C, improve satiety, and control weight. When initiating pramlintide, mealtime insulin doses are initially decreased by 30% to 50% to avoid hypoglycemia. Pramlintide must be taken as a separate injection with the doses titrated depending on whether a patient has type 1 or type 2 diabetes. Side effects, including nausea, vomiting, and anorexia, may be expected but generally resolve within the first few weeks of treatment.

13. **What is an insulin pump?**
An insulin pump is a battery-operated device composed of a pump reservoir (which holds the insulin) connected to an infusion set, which ends in a cannula that is inserted into the skin and changed every 2 to 3 days to prevent infection. Insulin is delivered through this system in microliter amounts continuously over 24 hours. The user is responsible for setting basal rates and determining bolus doses, depending on the meal ingested and the results of SMBG. Currently, five companies offer insulin pumps in the United States. Each pump has special features and functions that are unique and help with the flexibility of pump use. To learn more about each of these pumps, contact the companies listed in Table 3-2.

TABLE 3-2. COMPANIES OFFERING INSULIN PUMPS

Company Name	Phone	Website
Animas	1-877-937-7867	www.animascorp.com
Dana-Diabecare	1-866-342-2322	www.theinsulinpump.com
Deltec/Smith Medical	1-800-826-9703	www.cozmore.com
Disetronic	1-800-280-7801	www.disetronic-usa.com
Insulet Corporation	1-800-591-3455	www.insulet.com
Medtronic/MiniMed	1-800-646-4633	www.minimed.com

14. **What are the patient's responsibilities before insulin pump therapy can be initiated?**
- Commitment to devote at least 2 to 3 months to pump initiation, including multiple meetings with the diabetes team before, during, and after the pump is initiated.
- Monitoring of SMBG values at least 4 to 10 times per day, keeping logs of readings, insulin doses and food consumed, and faxing or mailing information to the team.
- Watching the pump training video and practicing pump functions at least 2 to 3 times before wearing the pump.
- Willingness to perform verifications to ensure that basal rates are set appropriately.

15. **Describe the benefits of insulin pump therapy.**
Benefits include a reduction in frequency of hypoglycemia because of the more predictable absorption of insulin, ability to compensate for the dawn phenomenon by adjustment in the basal rate, improved flexibility of lifestyle, ability to administer small amounts of insulin (as little

as 0.05 units), improved accuracy of dosing with current software on pumps and reduced risk of "stacking" with active insulin features.

16. **What risks are associated with pump use?**
Risks associated with pump use, including weight gain and hypoglycemia, are similar to any therapy that results in an overall lowering of BG values. A unique risk to pump therapy is for diabetic ketoacidosis. This can occur with interruption of insulin delivery because pumps only provide rapid-acting insulin.

17. **What is a glucose sensor?**
Currently there are glucose-sensing devices available for purchase, the Continuous Glucose Monitoring System or free-standing Guardian RealTime by Medtronic MiniMed, the Dexcom sensor and the Abbott Navigator. The sensing-system consists of a monitor that collects the data and a sensor that is placed temporarily under the skin, generating an electrical signal that is proportional to the amount of glucose present in the interstitial fluid. The interstitial values are calibrated with finger-stick readings that must be entered into the system at least three times per day. These devices provide values every 5 minutes within a range of 40 to 400 mg/dL that are available to the wearer and feature alarms that will sound if the values fall out of the target ranges that are programmed. Because systems measure interstitial fluid glucose versus blood glucose (from the fingerstick readings) and lag behind glucose values by approximately 20 minutes, the sensor values cannot be used to determine bolus amounts. However, sensor information can be helpful to follow blood glucose trends and patterns as well as pick up on unexpected hypoglycemia, especially nocturnal episodes. Currently there is limited insurance coverage for these devices.

18. **Define carbohydrate counting. How is it used with IIT?**
Carbohydrate counting is a tool used to match bolus insulin doses to food intake because carbohydrates have the greatest effect on BG levels. The peak of bolus insulin analogs should match the peak of BG following carbohydrate digestion and absorption (~1–3 hours, depending on the fat and fiber content of the meal).

19. **List common foods that contain dietary carbohydrates.**
   - Starch: cereals, grains, beans, bread, rice, pasta, and starchy vegetables
   - Sugar: lactose (milk and yogurt), fructose (fruit, juice, and honey), and sucrose (table sugar and desserts)
   - Fiber: cellulose and hemicellulose, lignins, gums, or pectins found in fruits, vegetables, legumes, and whole grains

20. **How are carbohydrates counted?**
Calculating the number of carbohydrates may initially require measuring and weighing commonly eaten foods. Nutrition labels on the package (Table 3-3) state the number of grams of carbohydrates based on the serving size. Carbohydrate reference books are available at bookstores or through the American Dietetic Association (http://www.eatright.org) or the American Diabetes Association (ADA; http://www.diabetes.org). Software programs are available for PDAs or online. Many restaurant chains provide nutrition brochures.

21. **Explain the carbohydrate-to-insulin (C:I) ratio.**
The C:I ratio is used to estimate how many grams of carbohydrate each unit of rapid-acting insulin will cover (e.g., 20:1 = 20 g of carbohydrate consumed requires 1 unit of meal insulin).

TABLE 3-3. NUTRITION FACTS ON LABELS	
Serving size: 10 crackers (30 g)	Dietary fiber: 1 g
Servings per container: 8	Sugars: 3 g
Calories: 140	Protein: 2 g
Total fat: 6 g	Vitamin A: 0%
Saturated fat: 1 g	Vitamin C: 0%
Cholesterol: 0 mg	Calcium: 2%
Sodium: 260 mg	Iron: 6%
Total carbohydrate: 20 g	

22. **How do you determine an initial C:I ratio?**
Ratios are based on a patient's weight and TDD of insulin, which usually indicates the patient's sensitivity to insulin. An MDI regimen of basal insulin and premeal injections of rapid-acting insulin must be previously (or concurrently) implemented before establishing a C:I ratio. A person must be taught to count carbohydrates before using a C:I ratio safely.
   1. Add up the patient's TDD of insulin on current therapy.
   2. Consider the hemoglobin A1C value (ADA target is <7%), frequency of hypoglycemia, and comorbidities.
   3. Divide the TDD of insulin into 500. Example 500 ÷ 25 units = 20:1 C:I ratio
   It is important to state that all carbohydrate ratios are starting points and must be individually fine-tuned on the basis of a patient's blood glucose records.

23. **Give an example of an initial C:I ratio when changing to basal and bolus insulins.**
   - 35 units of Humulin 70/30 premixed insulin in the morning
   - 15 units of Humulin 70/30 premixed insulin before the evening meal
   - TDD = 50 units (hemoglobin A1C of 8.5% with 2–3 nocturnal hypoglycemic episodes per week)
   - 500/50 = 10
   - C:I = 10:1
   In this example, 1 unit of rapid-acting insulin will be given for every 10 g of carbohydrate eaten.

24. **How do you adjust the C:I ratio once the initial ratio has been established?**
Fine-tuning of a C:I ratio is based on BG records before meals and 2 hours after meals. The desired premeal BG is 90 to 130 mg/dL for most patients using IIT. A C:I ratio is correct if the BG increases by approximately 30 to 50 mg/dL over the premeal value at the 2-hour postprandial reading and returns to the range of 90 to 130 mg/dL by about 5 hours after the bolus insulin is given (Fig. 3-1).

25. **What are common causes of high BG?**
   - Missing an injection of insulin
   - Menstrual cycle
   - Decreased activity
   - Stress, illness, or infection
   - Underestimating carbohydrates
   - Steroids or other medications

2 hours after meal
110–170 mg/dL

3 hours after meal
120–140 mg/dL

4 hours after meal
110–130 mg/dL

BG before meal
90–130 mg/dL

5 hours after meal
80–120 mg/dL

Figure 3-1. Expected postprandial blood glucose (BG) range with rapid-acting bolus insulin.

26. **What are the mysterious or random causes of high BG readings?**
    - Dawn phenomenon: a rise in BG occurs in predawn hours because of increased growth hormone and cortisol production.
    - Shower or nap phenomenon: and unexplained increase in BG occurs when tested before and after a shower or nap.
    - Bad insulin phenomenon: high BG occurs when insulin denatures if exposed to moderate-to-extreme temperatures or agitation (i.e., using a mail-order pharmacy, traveling with insulin, leaving it in a hot car)
    - Bubble-in-the-infusion-set-tubing phenomenon: air bubbles in the tubing of an insulin pump infusion set should be removed by disconnecting and priming the air out. In addition, when the infusion set is disconnected for showering or other purposes, gravity may cause the insulin to back up into the tubing, leaving a bubble. Holding the pump higher than the infusion site when reconnecting or repriming the tubing will avoid these bubbles.

27. **What causes high postprandial BG readings that are difficult to explain?**
    - Coffee phenomenon (caffeine): rise in BG after drinking coffee (including drinking it black, without cream or sugar) is seen in many patients' records and is likely due to increases in epinephrine or free fatty acid mobilization and subsequent worsening insulin resistance.
    - Cereal phenomenon: a rise in BG is seen by patients consuming cereal, which requires a lower C:I (more insulin) and may be related to the glycemic index of most cereals combined with greater insulin resistance in the morning.
    - Food-on-the-fingers phenomenon: high BG occurs from residual food or dextrose on fingers when testing (patient must wash hands or wipe off first drop of blood).
    - Restaurant meal phenomenon: Chinese food, Mexican food, pizza, and fried foods are high in fat and may require more insulin because of insulin resistance. A delay in digestion following a high-fat meal may require a split dose.

28. **How is supplemental insulin added for high BG before meals?**
    Supplemental insulin (high BG correction factor or CF) is used to reduce a high BG detected before meals. A high blood glucose CF is a formula based on the person's insulin sensitivity. A CF estimates the "expected" decrease in BG per unit of administered insulin under normal

circumstances. Davidson et al. introduced a deductive framework to aid in calculating a high BG CF, derived using data from more than 1800 pump patients with well-controlled glucose levels. The initial CF may be estimated by dividing 1700 by the TDD. The CF must then be adjusted on the basis of each patient's records and is therefore only a starting point.

29. **Give an example of determining an initial CF.**
    - Fourteen units of insulin glargine at 12 noon and 5 units Humalog before each meal
    - TDD = 29 units (hemoglobin A1C of 7.2% with 1–2 hypoglycemic episodes per week)
    - 1700/29 = 59
    - Begin with a CF of 60:1

    In this example, 1 unit of rapid-acting insulin will lower the BG about 60 mg/dL; therefore, 1 extra unit will be taken (in addition to the meal insulin dose) for each 60 mg/dL that the premeal BG is over the premeal goal of 100 mg/dL.

30. **Give an example of CF usage.**
    To determine the amount of extra insulin needed if the BG is out of the target range before a meal, subtract the goal BG (100 mg/dL) from the actual BG and divide by the CF.
    - CF is 60:1
    - Preprandial BG is 220 mg/dL
    - Calculation: 220 − 100 mg/dL = 120 mg/dL above target
    - Calculation: 120 (mg/dL)/60 = 2 units of insulin

    In this example, 2 units of rapid-acting insulin will be added to the meal bolus to return the BG to the target range.

31. **When is a CF used?**
    - It is recommended that high BG corrections be taken before meals or at least 5 hours after the last bolus because of the duration of action of the bolus insulin analogs.
    - Hypoglycemia may occur from the accumulation of active insulin if BG corrections are performed too frequently.
    - A CF is more effective if it is taken 15 to 30 minutes before eating. This time frame allows the insulin to begin working before the BG rises further because of the meal.

32. **What can be done for a high postprandial BG reading?**
    - If a postprandial BG is dangerously high (i.e., >300 mg/dL) or a patient insists on making high BG corrections less than 5 hours since the last bolus or during the night, he or she should be instructed in how to take a partial correction for safety.
    - Using one half of the usual premeal CF to lower the BG to the target level is safest between meals.
    - A target level of 150 mg/dL (expected BG level 2 hours postprandial) rather than a target BG of 100 mg/dL is used in the correction calculation between meals.

33. **Provide an example of using a 1/2 CF.**
    - BG before dinner = 100 mg/dL
    - BG 2 hours after dinner = 300 mg/dL
    - "Expected" BG 2 hours after dinner = ~130 to 150 mg/dL
    - Calculation: 300 − 150 mg/dL = 150 mg/dL above target
    - CF is 60:1
    - Calculation: 150/60 = 2.5 units (full CF)
    - The premeal insulin is still active for about 3 more hours; therefore, use half CF
    - Calculation of half CF: 2.5 (units) / 2 = 1.3 units

    In this example, 1.3 units with an insulin pump or 1 unit with a syringe or insulin pen should be given 2 hours after the meal to bring the postprandial BG into the target range. BG should be rechecked within 2 hours to avoid a severe low glucose.

KEY POINTS: INTENSIVE INSULIN THERAPY

1. Studies have clearly demonstrated that optimal diabetes management decreases chronic complications.
2. Intensive insulin therapy, or basal-bolus therapy, is required to mimic normal pancreatic insulin secretion.
3. Basal insulin is physiologic insulin required to manage blood glucose (BG) fluctuations due to hepatic glucose production.
4. Bolus insulin is matched to carbohydrates using a carbohydrate-to-insulin ratio.
5. Supplemental bolus insulin reduces the BG to within normal limits when a high glucose correction factor is used.

34. **Calculate an initial basal rate for insulin pump therapy.**
    - An established C:I ratio and CF on MDI is critical for a smooth transition to pump therapy.
    - To calculate an initial basal rate, take the current TDD of insulin on MDI and reduce it by 25% (or other appropriate reduction, depending on current hemoglobin A1C and number of hypoglycemic episodes).
    - Use 50% of the reduced dose as the total basal dose to be given over 24 hours.
    - Start with one basal rate for 24 hours (divide the total basal dose by 24). [Initial basal rate per hour = (TDD × .75) / (2 × 24).]
    - The remaining 50% will be used as bolus doses for meals on the basis of carbohydrate counting.

35. **Calculate an example of an initial basal rate for insulin pump therapy.**
    1. Current TDD of insulin is: 50 units
       25% reduction of TDD = 37.5 or
       10% reduction of TDD = _____ or
       ____ reduction of TDD = _____
    2. Reduced dose = 37.5 / 2 = 18.75 units as total basal
    3. Total basal insulin = 18.75 / 24 = 0.78 U/h
    In this example, the initial basal rate will be 0.8 U/h. Basal rate adjustments will then be made on the basis of testing and recording BG profiles throughout the day.

36. **When are nighttime basal rate adjustments made?**
    Nighttime basal rates should be adjusted before the daytime basal rates are verified. Testing is typically performed during the first week of insulin pump therapy. Be aware that patients transitioning from Lantus or Levemir may have overlapping insulin, causing hypoglycemia during the first week. Testing is then repeated if a significant weight change occurs, if an exercise routine is begun or altered, following hormonal changes (i.e., puberty, menopause), or as needed.

37. **List recommendations to follow during the nighttime basal rate verification process.**
    - Assess basal rate accuracy on three nights.
    - Eat evening meal early, preferably before 7 p.m. (or begin the test period ~5 hours after eating).

- For patients who typically eat high-fat meals or are unsure of their carbohydrate counting skills, choose a meal that they frequently eat or one for which they are confident of the carbohydrate amount.
- Avoid meals with more than 15 to 20 g of fat, 10 g of fiber, and alcohol on testing nights.
- Avoid any food or insulin bolus after the evening meal.
- Avoid exercise other than typical activity.
- Monitor BG before and 2 hours after the evening meal, at 12 midnight, at 3 a.m., and at 6 a.m.
- Stop the test if BG is less than 70 mg/dL or greater than 250 mg/dL during the basal test and treat the abnormal BG.

38. How are nighttime basal rate adjustments made?

- If BG levels change by more than 20 to 30 mg/dL during overnight monitoring, adjust the basal rate for the next night by 0.1 U/h, starting 1 to 3 hours before the BG change was seen.
- Changes are made until the fasting BG in the morning is within the target range (90–130 mg/dL).
- Daytime basal rates are verified next, usually 1 to 2 weeks after pump initiation or as necessary.

39. Describe the procedure for making daytime basal rate adjustments.

- Have patients skip breakfast and check their BG levels every hour from 7 am to 12 noon to verify the morning basal rate.
- If BG levels change by more than 20 to 30 mg/dL during this time, adjust the basal rate for the next day by 0.1 U/h, starting 1 to 3 hours before the glucose change was seen.
- After the morning basal rate is set, have patients skip their other meals (on separate days) and follow the same monitoring and adjustment procedures to confirm the afternoon and evening basal rate(s).

40. What is the recommended carbohydrate for the treatment of hypoglycemia?
Dextrose should be taken for a BG of less than 70 mg/dL. Dextrose is the first ingredient in the following products: glucose tablets and gel, candies (SweetTarts, Smarties, Sprees, Pixie Stix, and Runts).

41. How does the use of rapid-acting insulin impact the treatment of hypoglycemia with MDI and pump therapy?
With a shorter duration of effect, rapid-acting insulin analogs require less dextrose to raise BG than was previously necessary with regular insulin.

- If the last rapid-acting insulin dose was 1 to 3 hours earlier, 15 g dextrose should be taken.
- If the last rapid-acting insulin dose was more than 4 hours earlier, only 5 to 10 g dextrose may be required.
- After 15 to 20 minutes, the patients should wash their hands and test their BG again.
- If the repeat BG is less than 70 mg/dL, additional dextrose should be taken.

42. Why does rebound hyperglycemia occur after hypoglycemia?

- Overtreatment with an inappropriate amount of carbohydrate may occur.
- No treatment (i.e., sleeping through a low glucose episode) may result in counterregulatory hormone release and increased hepatic glycogenolysis.
- Treatment with a food that contains fat will delay digestion and absorption, thereby prolonging hypoglycemia and causing counterregulatory hormone release with subsequent hepatic glycogenolysis.

43. Discuss the use of glucagon to treat severe hypoglycemia.
All patients using MDI or pump therapy should be given a glucagon emergency kit prescription and a demonstration. Glucagon is used to raise BG when a person is unable to swallow. This may occur either as a result of a seizure or unconsciousness. Family members should receive instruction, and the patient should be able to demonstrate the procedure to a third party (coworker or neighbor).

BIBLIOGRAPHY

1. American Diabetes Association: Implications of the United Kingdom Prospective Diabetes Study. Diabetes Care 23(Suppl 1):S28–S32, 2003.
2. Diabetes Control and Complications Trial Research Group: The effect of intensive treatment of diabetes on the development and progression of long-term complications in insulin-dependent diabetes mellitus. N Engl J Med 329:977–986, 1993.
3. Hirsch IB: Intensive treatment of type 1 diabetes. Med Clin North Am 82:689, 1998.
4. Shichiri M, Kishikawa H: Long-term results of the Kumamoto study of optimal diabetes control in type 2 diabetic patients. Diabetes Care 23(Suppl 2):B21, 2000.

RECOMMENDED PATIENT READING

1. Walsh J, Roberts R: Pumping Insulin. San Diego, Torrey Pines Press, 2006.
2. Walsh J, Roberts R: Using Insulin. San Diego, Torrey Pines Press, 2003.

CHAPTER 4

INPATIENT MANAGEMENT OF DIABETES AND HYPERGLYCEMIA

Sarah V. Bull

1. Does evidence support intensive management of blood glucose in the hospital setting?

The correlation between hyperglycemia and adverse outcomes in hospital inpatients has been well demonstrated. Although somewhat controversial, the data suggest that elevated blood glucose (BG) levels in general medicine and surgical patients, cardiac patients, and critically ill patients lead to an increase in mortality and morbidity. Prolonged intensive care unit (ICU) and hospital stays, sepsis, increased infection rates, and increased rates of reinfarction are examples of the morbidity seen.

2. What are the glycemic targets for the critically ill patient population? How "low" should we go?

In critically ill patients, there is fairly strong evidence that a target BG under 110 mg/dL leads to improved outcomes; however, the concern for risk of hypoglycemia with tight control is valid. Van den Berghe's 2006 MICU study showed a much higher rate of hypoglycemia (18.7%) compared with her previous SICU study (5.1%), and hypoglycemia was identified as an independent risk factor for death. That said, the 80 to 110 mg/dL range should be targeted only if it can be achieved safely.

3. What are the glycemic targets for the general medical-surgical patients?

There is less definitive evidence for this population, and one must take into account various factors such as unpredictable nutritional intake, stress hyperglycemia, and so on; in general, however, lower BG levels are associated with improved outcomes. The American Diabetes Association current recommendations are to maintain fasting BG under 126 mg/dL and all random glucose values under 180 to 200 mg/dL.

4. What are the glycemic targets for pregnant patients?

The goals for BG control during pregnancy are even stricter because hyperglycemia is associated with macrosomia, congenital anomalies, miscarriage, neonatal morbidity, and fetal death. The American College of Obstetricians recommends a fasting glucose less than 95 mg/dL and 2-hour postprandial glucose less than 120 mg/dL.

5. Why is poor glycemic control so common in hospitalized patients?

Many patient factors, such as infection, fever, steroids, stress, and inactivity, exacerbate hyperglycemia in the hospital setting. In addition, three major physician issues should be acknowledged: (1) fear of hypoglycemia, (2) lack of understanding of how to use insulin appropriately, and (3) underappreciation of the importance of glycemic control.

6. **What can we do to help prevent hypoglycemia in the hospital setting?**
   - Use physiologic (basal-bolus) insulin regimens.
   - Avoid the use of sliding-scale regular insulin. This leads to "insulin stacking" and subsequent hypoglycemia.
   - Avoid using oral hypoglycemic agents, especially metformin and sulfonylureas.
   - Review the chart daily for changes such as nutritional status and medication dose. (An NPO [non per os] status or decrease in prednisone dose may significantly effect glycemia.)

7. **What is the best agent available for inpatient management of diabetes?**
   Insulin, given physiologically as an intravenous infusion or subcutaneously with basal and nutritional coverage, is clearly the best and most appropriate medication. Many insulin infusion protocols have been published.

8. **Are oral agents appropriate to use in hospitalized patients?**
   Rarely. In the inpatient setting, oral agents should be limited to patients who took them before admission, who are eating consistently, and who do not have contraindications. If fasting blood glucose levels are greater than 180 mg/dL, oral agents are unlikely to control hyperglycemia.

9. **Discuss the use of the various oral agents in the hospital setting.**
   - Sulfonylureas: These drugs are long-acting medications metabolized by the kidney and liver that have significant potential for causing hypoglycemia in hospitalized patients who are eating erratically. Of note, glipizide is associated with less hypoglycemia than glyburide in patients with renal insufficiency.
   - Metformin: There is a risk of lactic acidosis when this agent is used in patients with hypoperfusion, renal insufficiency, congestive heart failure, hypoxemia, or chronic lung diseases. This medication should also be discontinued in anticipation of a procedure requiring intravenous (IV) contrast and held for 48 hours or until renal function is considered normal.
   - Thiazolidinediones: These medications are slow-acting and not appropriate for acute glycemic control. In addition, the known side effect of fluid retention is inappropriate for hospitalized patients with underlying heart failure, liver failure, and renal insufficiency.

10. **List the indications for intravenous insulin therapy.**
    - Diabetic ketoacidosis (DKA)
    - Nonketotic hyperosmolar state
    - Critical illness
    - Prolonged NPO status
    - Perioperative period
    - Acute myocardial infarction
    - Coronary artery bypass surgery
    - Stroke
    - Labor and delivery
    - Total parental nutrition
    - Uncontrolled hyperglycemia exacerbated by illness or steroids
    - Any illness requiring prompt glucose control
    - Dose-finding strategy

11. **Why is the intravenous route superior to the subcutaneous route for insulin?**
    Although there is frequent resistance to using IV insulin over subcutaneous (SC) insulin, this route of delivery is safer in appropriately monitored conditions. IV insulin has a more rapid onset, enhanced flexibility and is more efficient in achieving glycemic control.

KEY POINTS: TARGET GLUCOSE LEVELS FOR HOSPITALIZED PATIENTS

1. Intensive care unit: 80–110 mg/dL
2. General medicine and surgical units: preprandial 90–126 mg/dL; postprandial 180 mg/dL
3. Pregnancy: preprandial <95 mg/dL; 2 hours postprandial <120 mg/dL

12. **At what rate should an insulin infusion be started?**
    For an unstressed, normoglycemic adult of average body mass index (BMI), an insulin infusion using regular insulin is commonly initiated at 1 to 2 U/hr and adjusted as necessary. Alternatively, a weight-based dose may be calculated using 0.02 U/kg/hr as a starting rate, or one may calculate a predicted rate using approximately 50% of the previous day's total daily dose (TDD) divided by 24 hours. Certain conditions such as DKA and steroid-induced hyperglycemia may require much higher infusion rates.

13. **How should the IV insulin infusion rate be adjusted?**
    Adjustments should be made based on the BG level as well as the rate of change. An appropriate rate of change is 80 to 100 mg/dL/hr. If the BG does not change by at least 60 mg/dL after 1 hour, the rate should be increased. Conversely, if the BG drops by more than 100 mg/dL, the rate should be decreased. Insulin action lasts approximately 1 hour. Many hospitals have existing insulin infusion protocols in place; when this is not the case, numerous algorithms have been published and are easily accessible. Frequent bedside glucose testing is essential.

14. **Discuss the treatment of hypoglycemia (BG <60 mg/dL).**
    - Discontinue insulin drip
    - Give D50W IV:
        - 25 mL ({½} ampule) for a patient who is awake
        - 50 mL (1 ampule) for a patient who is not awake
    - Recheck BG every 20 minutes and repeat 25 mL of D50W IV if BG less than 60 mg/dL
    - Restart drip at a lower rate once BG is greater than 70 mg/dL for two checks

15. **When should the physician be notified?**
    - For any BG change greater than 100 mg/dL within 1 hour
    - For any BG greater than 360 mg/dL
    - For hypoglycemia that has not resolved within 20 minutes of D50W IV administration and insulin infusion discontinuation

16. **How do I transition a patient off an insulin drip?**
    To maintain glycemic control, it is imperative to give SC long- or intermediate-acting insulin 2 to 3 hours before or rapid-acting insulin 1 to 2 hours before stopping the infusion. A combination of long- and rapid-acting insulin is preferred. An SC dosing strategy may be calculated, estimating the total daily dose to be 4 times the IV insulin required over the previous 6 hours. This dose should be divided into a 50% basal and 50% bolus regimen.

17. **What is a "sliding-scale," and how does it differ from correction-dose insulin?**
    Sliding-scale insulin refers to a set amount of insulin administered for hyperglycemia without regard to the timing of food, preexisting dosing or individual insulin sensitivity. These scales are not typically modified throughout the hospital stay and are not useful in preventing hyperglycemia because insulin is given in response to an elevated glucose. Hypoglycemia due to

"insulin stacking" is a common problem, especially with regular insulin. However, correction-dose or "supplemental" insulin, using a short-acting insulin analog, is an important adjunct to scheduled mealtime insulin and should be given at the same time. Dosing is variable and depends on the level of insulin resistance and glucose level in the individual.

KEY POINTS: INPATIENT MANAGEMENT OF DIABETES AND HYPERGLYCEMIA

1. Evidence shows that glycemic control in hospitalized patients improves outcomes.

2. Insulin is the best agent for management of hyperglycemia in hospital patients.

3. Physiologic (basal-bolus) dosing is the preferred approach in this population.

4. Use of sliding-scale insulin alone to control blood sugars should be avoided.

18. **How do I write admit orders if I do not know whether the patient will require insulin?**
    Because the prevalence of hyperglycemia is reported to be more than 25% in hospitalized adults, all patients should have either a plasma or capillary BG determination as part of their initial assessment. If the BG is high, scheduled BG checks should be ordered. If the patient is critically ill, an insulin infusion may be started if two BG checks are greater than 110 mg/dL. If the patient is on the general medical ward, SC insulin should be initiated if two BGs greater than 170 mg/dL or a single BG greater than 300 mg/dL is documented.

19. **What is considered effective insulin therapy in the hospital?**
    Effective insulin therapy must provide both basal and nutritional coverage, as well as correction-dose insulin. Daily review of BG values and review of the correction doses required is essential when modifying the insulin regimen. Those patients who were on insulin pumps or who were taking insulin before admission may self-manage as long as they have adequate oral intake and are cognitively intact.

20. **How should you select a basal insulin dose?**
    Long-acting insulin (glargine, detemir) given once or twice a day or intermediate-acting insulin (neutral protamine Hagedorn; NPH) given twice a day will usually provide adequate basal coverage. NPH causes more glucose variability and more hypoglycemia due to unpredictable insulin peaks and therefore most providers prefer to use glargine or detemir. The basal dose should be approximately 50% of the total daily insulin dose required.

21. **How should you select a prandial dose for patients on insulin?**
    Prandial insulin is best provided by giving a rapid-acting insulin analog 0 to 15 minutes before a meal or regular insulin 30 to 60 minutes before a meal. Rapid-acting insulins (Lispro, Aspart, glulisine) allow more flexible dosing and are less likely to cause hypoglycemia because the duration of action is shorter (4–5 hours) than with regular insulin (5–8 hours). In the outpatient setting, the total daily prandial dose is calculated as approximately 50% of the total daily insulin dose; however, because intake is more erratic in the hospital, one may want to start with 20% to 40% of the total daily dose divided among meals.

22. **How should you choose the correction dose of insulin?**
    Ideally, correction-dose insulin should be given using a rapid-acting insulin and in conjunction with the mealtime insulin dose. The goal is to determine how much supplemental insulin

has been used so that scheduled insulin doses can be up-titrated. For most insulin-sensitive patients with type 1 diabetes, a safe starting point is to correct by giving 1 unit of insulin to lower a BG by 50 mg/dL if BG is above 150 mg/dL. For more insulin-resistant type 2 diabetic patients, one can estimate that 1 unit of insulin will lower BG by approximately 25 mg/dL.

23. **How should you deal with diabetic patients undergoing surgery or hospital procedures?**
There is significant risk for both hypoglycemia and hyperglycemia because patients are typically made NPO before their procedure; medication orders are adjusted, and time to recovery is variable. In general, routine insulin and oral agents may be taken up until the evening before the procedure (except metformin, which should be discontinued ∼48 hours earlier). It is essential to determine what level of insulin deficiency the patient has and plan accordingly. A type 1 or insulin-deficient diabetic will need basal insulin at all times, and only the mealtime insulin should be withheld. Type 1 patients using pumps or long-acting basal insulin may continue with their regular doses. For patients on intermediate-acting insulin (NPH) with some postprandial effect, the dose should be reduced by one third to one half. Correction-dose insulin may be used every 4 to 6 hours as necessary, and an insulin infusion is recommended if a prolonged NPO status is anticipated.

24. **Characterize steroid-induced hyperglycemia and describe how it is best treated.**
Glucocorticoids exaggerate postprandial BG excursions and increase insulin resistance. Patients can often be treated with supplemental prandial insulin alone; however, if basal insulin is necessary, a 12-hour insulin such as NPH (∼70% prandial, 30% basal) given in the morning works well. Uncontrolled patients on high doses of steroids may require an insulin infusion. Many of these patients are discharged on steroid tapers, and thus close follow-up to adjust doses and prevent hypoglycemia is critical.

25. **How should hyperglycemic patients on Total Parenteral Nutrition or enteral feedings be treated?**
A variable-rate insulin infusion is the quickest way to achieve BG stabilization. After the total parenteral nutrition (TPN) infusion is constant, 70% to 100% of the total insulin units infused over the previous 24 hours may be added to the subsequent TPN bag. One may also consider SC basal insulin to match the timing of the TPN infusion. We have found 70/30 insulin given twice daily to be particularly helpful in patients on continuous or intermittent tube feedings.

26. **How should daily insulin doses be adjusted?**
Assessing daily BG trends and adjusting scheduled insulin doses are the keys to better glucose control. The fasting BG is affected mainly by the basal insulin, whereas prelunch and predinner BGs are affected by both prandial and basal insulins. To assess prandial insulin doses, check BG 2 hours after eating; postprandial BG values should be 30 to 50 mg/dL above the preprandial BG values and less than 180 mg/dL.

27. **How do I decide what to order when the patient is sent home?**
As previously stated, it is more effective to manage the inpatient with basal-bolus therapy. After the patient is stable for discharge, the physician, with the help of a diabetes educator, can reassess the regimen. Factors such as cost of medications, the patient's ability to monitor and self-manage, previous control of diabetes, and contraindications to medications must be evaluated. One can also use the calculated inpatient TDD to change insulin back to a split mix if necessary, but once- and twice-daily insulin regimens are no longer suitable for type 1 patients. Type 2 diabetic patients with TDD requirements under 0.3 U/kg per day can be considered for transition to an oral regimen.

28. **How can the hospital system work to improve glycemic outcomes?**
    A team approach, including physicians, nurses, pharmacists, and diabetes educators, has been shown to decrease length of stay and cost of care. In the hospital system, patients with new-onset diabetes or insulin resistance can be identified for appropriate follow-up and education. In one study, 60% of patients with a random BG greater than 126 mg/dL during hospitalization were found to have diabetes at follow-up testing. During the hospital stay, home regimens can be reassessed and improved. Most important, the patients are watching how physicians manage their blood sugars. It is extremely significant for patients to see that the physician can control the blood sugar and that the physician considers control   important.

BIBLIOGRAPHY

1. American College of Obstetricians: Pregestational diabetes mellitus. Obstet Gynecol 105:675, 2005.

2. American Diabetes Association: Standards of medical care in diabetes—2008. Diabetes Care S36–40, 2008.

3. American Diabetes Association: Summary and recommendations of the fifth international workshop-conference on gestational diabetes mellitus. Diabetes Care 30:S251–260, 2007.

4. McCulloch D, Inzucchi SE, et al: Management of diabetes in the acute care setting. UptoDate ONLINE 16.1.

5. Schmeltz LR, DeSantis AJ, et al: Conversion of intravenous insulin infusions to subcutaneously administered insulin glargine in patients with hyperglycemia. Endocr Pract 12:641–650, 2006.

6. Van den Berghe G, Wilmer A, et al: Intensive insulin therapy in the medical ICU. N Engl J Med: 354:449–446, 2006.

7. Wilson M, Weinreb J, Hoo GW. Intensive insulin therapy in critical care: a review of 12 protocols. Diabetes Care 30:1005–1011, 2007.

CHAPTER 5

DIABETES IN PREGNANCY

Linda A. Barbour

1. **How does normal pregnancy affect fuel metabolism?**

   Pregnancy is a complex metabolic state that involves dramatic alterations in the hormonal milieu (increases in estrogen, progesterone, prolactin, cortisol, human chorionic gonadotropin, placental growth hormone, and human placental lactogen), inflammatory cytokines (tumor necrosis factor alpha [TNF-α], C-reactive protein), and adipokines (leptin and adiponectin) to increase maternal insulin resistance so that the mother can provide the necessary nutrients for the growing fetal-placental unit.

2. **Summarize the changes in the first trimester of pregnancy.**

   Pregnancy is characterized by profound changes in metabolism that promote adipose tissue accretion in early gestation, and many women show an increase in insulin sensitivity in the first trimester. Fasting insulin levels and glucoses are lower, and women are prone to nocturnal hypoglycemia and ketogenesis, especially if they suffer from nausea and vomiting during pregnancy.

   Metabolically, the first trimester is characterized by increased insulin sensitivity and accelerated starvation with an increased turnover of maternal metabolic fuels and an earlier transition from carbohydrate to fat utilization in the fasting state. Pregnant women deplete their glycogen stores quickly and switch from carbohydrate to fat metabolism within 12 hours, often becoming ketonemic.

3. **Summarize the changes in the second and third trimesters and immediate postpartum period.**

   The second and third trimesters, in contrast, are characterized by insulin resistance, with a nearly 50% decrease in insulin-mediated glucose disposal (assessed by the hyperinsulinemic-euglycemic clamp technique) and a 200% to 300% increase in insulin secretion in late pregnancy. These changes shunt necessary fuels to meet the metabolic demands of the placenta and growing fetus, which requires 80% of its energy as glucose, while maintaining euglycemia in the mother. Women usually have lower fasting levels of plasma glucose and fasting hypoinsulinemia because of continued shunting of carbohydrate to the placental-fetal unit in the unfed state. This results in an increase in maternal free fatty acids (FFAs) and ketones. Because of the increasing placental-fetal glucose demands, glycogen stores are depleted rapidly, and pregnant women must transition from carbohydrate to fat metabolism earlier in the fasting state, a phenomenon called "accelerated starvation." There is dramatic insulin resistance in skeletal muscle as well as at the level of the liver, which results in increased hepatic gluconeogenesis to ensure adequate substrate to the fetus. The ability of insulin to suppress whole body lipolysis is also reduced during late pregnancy, and FFA levels increase. However, due to the placental hormone-mediated increased insulin resistance in the fed state, pregnant women demonstrate modestly elevated postprandial glucose excursions associated with maternal hyperinsulinemia. Immediately after delivery, insulin sensitivity returns, at which time all diabetic women should have their insulin doses at least halved. The immediate postpartum period is often one of extreme insulin sensitivity, especially if mothers are breast-feeding, and a subgroup of women require almost no insulin for several days.

4. **Is glucose the only fuel altered in normal pregnancy?**
No. Amino acids, triglycerides, cholesterol, and FFAs are also increased; the increase in FFAs may further accentuate the insulin resistance of pregnancy.

5. **Explain the effect of the metabolic changes in pregnancy on diabetes management in the first trimester.**
Diabetes should optimally be under tight control before conception. During the first trimester, nausea, accelerated starvation, and increased insulin sensitivity may place the mother at risk for hypoglycemia. This risk is especially high at night because of prolonged fasting and continuous fetal-placental glucose utilization. Women with type 1 diabetes mellitus must have a bedtime snack and usually need to have their basal insulin or evening dose of neutral protamine Hagedorn (NPH) insulin lowered and moved from suppertime to bedtime to avoid early-morning hypoglycemia. Severe hypoglycemia occurs in 30% to 40% of pregnant women with type 1 diabetes in the first 20 weeks of pregnancy, most often between midnight and 8:00 a.m. Diabetic women who have gastroparesis or hyperemesis gravidarum are at the greatest risk for daytime hypoglycemia. During the first trimester, glycemic control just above the normal range (hemoglobin A_{1C} [HbA_{1C}] $<7.0\%$) may thus be safer than "normal" and may decrease the risk of both maternal and fetal hypoglycemia.

6. **How do metabolic changes in pregnancy affect the management of diabetes in the second and third trimesters?**
After 20 weeks, peripheral insulin resistance increases insulin requirements. It is not unusual for a pregnant woman to require 2 to 3 times as much insulin as she did before pregnancy. Postprandial hyperglycemia is the strongest risk factor for macrosomia. Therefore, tight glucose control in women with preexisting diabetes usually requires short-acting insulin with each meal with frequent monitoring to allow appropriate insulin dosage adjustments.

7. **What is the most important preconception recommendation in counseling a diabetic woman who wants to become pregnant?**
The most important recommendation in preconception counseling is the need for optimal glucose control before conception. Unplanned pregnancies occur in about two thirds of women with diabetes, making it critical that the primary care physician, endocrinologist, or obstetrician-gynecologist address preconception care in women of childbearing age. In a retrospective study, only 25% of women of childbearing age with preexisting diabetes had preconception counseling of any kind. Four times as many fetal and neonatal deaths and congenital abnormalities occurred in a group of women who did not receive prenatal counseling compared with those who did. In all series, preconception counseling significantly improved glycemic control, lowered major malformations, and reduced major adverse pregnancy outcomes including very premature delivery, stillbirth, and neonatal death.

8. **Why is maintenance of glucose control essential for the well-being of the fetus?**
The maintenance of normal glucose control is the key to prevention of complications, such as fetal malformations in the first trimester, macrosomia in the second and third trimesters, and neonatal metabolic abnormalities. Hyperglycemia modulates the expression of an apoptosis regulatory gene as early as the preimplantation blastocyst stage in the mouse, resulting in fetal wastage that can be prevented by treating with insulin. This finding may account for the high risk of first-trimester loss in pregnant women with poor glycemic control.

9. **Describe the relationship among HbA$_{1C}$, the teratogenic effects of hyperglycemia, and abnormal fetal growth.**

Epidemiologic and prospective studies have shown that the level of HbA$_{1C}$ in the 6 months before conception and during the first trimester correlates with the incidence of major malformations, such as neural tube and cardiac defects. The neural tube is completely formed by 4 weeks and the heart by 6 weeks after conception. This underscores the need for preconception counseling to achieve these goals because many women do not even know that they are pregnant at these times. It has been demonstrated that women with a normal HbA$_{1C}$ at conception and during the first trimester have no increased risk, whereas women with a HbA$_{1C}$ of greater than 12% have up to a 25% risk of major malformations. Excess fetal growth has been associated with an abnormal A$_{1C}$ in the first trimester but is probably most strongly associated with a higher A$_{1C}$ in the second and third trimesters in women with preexisting diabetes. Postprandial hyperglycemia appears to be the more important risk factor.

10. **How has the incidence of congenital abnormalities in the offspring of diabetic mothers changed over the past decade?**

The incidence of congenital abnormalities in the offspring of diabetic mothers in the early era of insulin use was 33%. Since the mid-1990s, with the advent of home glucose monitoring and more rigid objectives, this percentage has fallen to less than 10% of offspring. The randomized prospective Diabetes Control and Complications Trial has shown that timely institution of intensive therapy for blood glucose is associated with rates of spontaneous abortion and congenital malformations that are similar to those in the nondiabetic population.

11. **What are the risks if a woman conceives while taking an oral hypoglycemic agent?**

Oral hypoglycemic agents, such as sulfonylureas and metformin, do not appear to be teratogenic. A retrospective series of 332 women with type 2 diabetes treated with diet, insulin, or oral sulfonylureas during the first 8 weeks of gestation found no significant adverse effects. Women who are actively trying to become pregnant should be switched to insulin during the preconception period because it may take some time to determine the ideal insulin dose before the critical time of embryogenesis. There are few data on the risk of thiazolidinediones in the first trimester and these agents should definitely be stopped before a women actively tries to become pregnant.

12. **How is glyburide different from the other sulfonylureas?**

Glyburide is the only sulfonylurea shown not to cross the placenta or significantly to affect fetal insulin levels. In the only large randomized prospective trial, however, it was not given until after 24 weeks to women with gestational diabetes. Since that time, five more nonrandomized trials have demonstrated its relative safety in treating women with gestational diabetes, for which therapy is usually started in the late second or early trimester. The Fifth International Workshop approved the use of glyburide as an alternative treatment in a subset of gestational diabetes mellitus (GDM) women.

13. **Can oral hypoglycemic agents be continued in pregnancy?**

It is recommended that oral hypoglycemic agents be avoided during pregnancy, with the possible exception of glyburide and metformin which have been used to treat GDM in the late 2nd and 3rd trimester. At this time, there is a fair amount of data using metformin throughout the first trimester of pregnancy in women with polycystic ovarian disease (PCOS) and a single recent trial in which it was used to treat GDM (Rowan et al.). Metformin, unlike glyburide, crosses the placenta. The results of a large randomized controlled trial comparing metformin to insulin was recently published and demonstrated the relative safety of Metformin in pregnancy to treat GDM, although 46% of women required that insulin be added to the Metformin to achieve adequate glycemic control. (Metformin in Gestation, or MIG, trial).

14. **Summarize the evidence related to the role of metformin during pregnancy.**
Metformin has been continued during the first trimester in nonrandomized studies of women with polycystic ovary syndrome (PCOS) and spontaneous fetal loss. It may decrease first-trimester loss in patients with PCOS. In one small trial that continued its use throughout pregnancy, it was shown to decrease the incidence of gestational diabetes. However, in a retrospective series in which 50 pregnant women were treated with metformin, 68 women with a sulfonylurea, and 42 with insulin, there was a higher incidence of preeclampsia in the metformin group, as well as an increase in perinatal mortality.

15. **How should hypertensive women who take angiotensin-converting enzyme inhibitors or have risk factors for coronary artery disease be counseled in the preconception period?**
Women should be counseled that angiotensin-converting enzyme (ACE) inhibitors are contraindicated in the second and third trimesters of pregnancy because of the risk of fetal anuria. A recent report described increased cardiac and central nervous system malformations in fetuses exposed in the first trimester. Therefore it is now recommended that women who are actively trying to conceive and who have no history of infertility should probably be switched to a safer agent before pregnancy (calcium channel blocker, methyldopa, hydralazine). A woman who receives treatment with an ACE inhibitor for significant diabetic nephropathy and is not actively trying to conceive should be told to perform home pregnancy tests if she misses a period and to immediately stop her ACE inhibitor if there is any suspicion of pregnancy. At that time, she can be switched safely to an alternative agent.

16. **How does pregnancy affect the morbidity and mortality of coronary artery disease in diabetic women?**
The morbidity and mortality rates of coronary artery disease are high in pregnant women with diabetes. Cardiac status should be assessed with functional testing before conception in women possessing any additional cardiac risk factors, such as hyperlipidemia, hypertension, smoking, advanced maternal age (>35 years), or a strong family history. Pregnancy causes a 25% increase in cardiac output, a significant decrease in systemic vascular resistance (which can shunt blood away from the coronary arteries), and an increase in oxygen consumption, all of which decrease the ability of maternal coronary blood flow to meet the demands of the myocardium. Myocardial demands are even higher at labor and delivery, and activation of catecholamines can cause myocardial ischemia.

17. **Should statins be discontinued before conception?**
Yes. Data about their safety during human pregnancy are inadequate, and animal data are concerning. However, if a woman has severe hypertriglyceridemia, which places her at high risk for pancreatitis, it may be necessary to continue fibrate therapy, which has not been associated with malformations, if a low-fat diet and fish oils are not effective or tolerated.

18. **Should diabetic women take folic acid supplements before conception?**
All women should take folic acid supplements (1 mg/day) before conception.

19. **Summarize the effect of smoking during pregnancy.**
Smoking continues to be the leading cause of low-birth-weight infants in patients with and without diabetes and places the infant at increased risk for respiratory infections, reactive airway disease, and sudden infant death syndrome. Smoking cessation efforts need to be intensified

before conception, because agents, such as the nicotine patch and Wellbutrin, are not approved for use during pregnancy.

20. **How does pregnancy affect diabetic nephropathy?**

    Proteinuria increases in pregnancy, and women with proteinuria often become nephrotic because of the increased glomerular filtration rate (GFR) of protein during pregnancy. In some patients, the proteinuria can become massive and results in significant edema, hypoalbuminemia, and a hypercoagulable state. Although women with mild renal insufficiency are not at an appreciable risk for irreversible progression of their nephropathy, those with more severe renal insufficiency (creatinine >2.5 mg/dL) have a 30% to 50% risk of a permanent pregnancy-related decline in GFR.

21. **Does nephropathy increase the risk of preeclampsia?**

    Preeclampsia complicates approximately 20% of pregnancies in women with preexisting diabetes, and the risk is much higher in women with hypertension or renal disease. The risk of developing preeclampsia in women with nephropathy is greater than 50%. The preeclampsia may be severe, especially in women who are hypertensive and have decreased renal function. Women with significant nephropathy are also at higher risk of having preterm and low-birth-weight infants. Therefore women with diabetic nephropathy should be counseled to have children when their diabetes is optimally controlled and preferably early in the course of their nephropathy.

22. **How does renal transplantation affect the outcome in pregnant women?**

    Women who have had a successful renal transplant at least 1 to 2 years before the pregnancy and who have good renal function, adequate blood pressure control, and a low requirement for antirejection medications have a much more favorable outcome than women with severe renal disease who have not received a transplant.

23. **Summarize the effects of pregnancy on diabetic retinopathy.**

    Proliferative retinopathy may progress during pregnancy either from the institution of tight control or because of increases in growth factors, blood volume, cardiac output, the hypercoagulable state of pregnancy, and anemia. Women with proliferative retinopathy are at the highest risk of progression, and in one series, retinopathy worsened in more than 50% of the women. It is therefore imperative that retinopathy be optimally treated with laser therapy before pregnancy, although laser therapy can be instituted in pregnancy. It is less likely for women with only background retinopathy to progress significantly during pregnancy, although there are reports that as many as 20% of women may progress. Baseline and follow-up ophthalmologic examinations are recommended for all diabetic pregnant women at risk for retinopathy.

24. **What is the White Classification of diabetes in pregnancy?**

    Priscilla White observed that the patient's age at onset of diabetes, duration of diabetes, and severity of complications, including vascular disease, nephropathy, and retinopathy, significantly influenced maternal and perinatal outcomes. In 1949, she developed a classification scheme based on these parameters. The initial scheme was developed for women with type 1 diabetes; there is no separate classification for type 2 diabetes.

25. **Why is the White Classification used by obstetricians?**

    Its predictive value allows identification of patients at greatest risk for obstetric complications during pregnancy so that physicians can intensify management and fetal surveillance. In the updated classification (Table 5-1), pregestational diabetic women are designated by the letters B, C, D, F, R, T, and H according to duration of diabetes and complications.

| | | | Type of | |
| | Age at Onset | Duration | Vascular | |
Class	(Years)	(Years)	Disease	Medication
Gestational Diabetes				
A1	Any	Pregnancy	None	None
A2	Any	Pregnancy	None	Yes
Pregestational Diabetes				
B	≥20	<10	None	Yes
C	10–19 or	10–19	None	Yes
D	<10 or	>20	Benign retinopathy	Yes
F	Any	Any	Nephropathy	Yes
R	Any	Any	Proliferative retinopathy	Yes
T	Any	Any	Renal transplant	Yes
H	Any	Any	Coronary artery disease	Yes

TABLE 5-1. MODIFIED WHITE CLASSIFICATION OF PREGNANT DIABETIC WOMEN

26. **What are the goals of glucose control for pregnant women with diabetes?**
    The goals of blood glucose control during pregnancy are rigorous. Optimally, the premeal whole blood glucose should be less than 95 mg/dL, the 1-hour postprandial glucose less than 140 mg/dL, and the 2-hour postprandial glucose less than 120 mg/dL. However, new data suggest that these goals may need to be intensified further. Continuous glucose monitoring system data suggest that the mean fasting glucose in normal pregnancy is only approximately 75 mg/dL and that peak postprandial values may be closer to 110 mg/dL at 70 to 90 minutes after eating. The results from the multicenter HAPO trial (Hyperglycemia and Adverse Pregnancy Outcomes), which studied 25,000 pregnant women in nine countries, suggest that abnormal fetal growth occurs along a continuum and at lower glucose values than previously recognized and a 2.7-fold risk of LGA (large for gestational age) infants occurs at a FBG of ≥ 90. Given that macrosomia is more strongly related to both fasting and the postprandial glucose excursions, pregnant diabetic women need to monitor premeal and postprandial glucose values regularly. Type 1 and Type 2 diabetic patients usually require 3 to 4 injections per day or an insulin pump to achieve adequate control during pregnancy. Short-acting insulins, such as lispro or aspart, may be especially helpful in women with hyperemesis or gastroparesis because they can be dosed after a successful meal and still be effective.

27. **What is the role of continuous glucose monitoring system in pregnancy?**
    A continuous glucose monitoring system (CGMS) can be helpful, especially in type 1 patients who are having frequent hypoglycemic episodes and suffer from hypoglycemic unawareness, allowing better delineation of glucose patterns so that basal or bolus insulin can appropriately be adjusted. It has also been shown to reveal postprandial hyperglycemia that might be otherwise unrecognized and that is strongly associated with excess fetal growth. In one series, a mother had to check her glucoses a minimum of 10 times per day to give an indication of the glucose patterns obtained during CGMS.

28. **Discuss the role of the insulin pump during pregnancy.**
    Experience using the insulin pump in the treatment of type 1 diabetes in pregnancy is increasing. Most trials have found that continuous subcutaneous insulin infusion is equivalent to multiple daily injections using basal and bolus insulin. It may be advantageous in women with recurrent

hypoglycemia, especially at night, because different basal rates can be programmed. However, there are reports of women who began using the pump in pregnancy and developed ketoacidosis from pump failure. Therefore it may be optimal to begin pump therapy before pregnancy, given the steep learning curve involved in its use and the continuous changes that must be made in dosing basal and bolus insulins because of the changing insulin resistance throughout pregnancy.

29. Discuss the role of glargine during pregnancy.

Experience with insulin glargine (Lantus) is increasing in pregnancy with several case series reporting use in nearly 200 patients. However, there are still some concerns about its potential mitogenic effects and higher affinity for the IGF-1 receptor, especially in women with proliferative retinopathy. It does not cross the placenta, and no evidence indicates reproductive toxicity or embryotoxicity. Similar pregnancy outcomes have been reported in women taking glargine compared with women taking NPH. If a patient without proliferative retinopathy is doing well on insulin glargine, it is probably not necessary to switch her to another insulin during pregnancy. It may also be useful in women with recurrent hypoglycemia on NPH. However, the absence of a peak with glargine can sometimes result in inadequate fasting glucose control in pregnancy, and a small dose of NPH may need to be added before bedtime.

30. What is the role of short-acting insulin analogs in pregnancy?

Both Humalog (lispro) and Novolog (aspart) have been used in pregnancy and have been shown to be safe and effective. The largest randomized controlled trial of 322 women confirmed that Aspart reduces postprandial hyperglycemia and the risk of hypoglycemia compared with regular insulin in type 1 patients. It may be especially helpful in type 1 women with gastroparesis because it can be dosed 20 minutes after eating to ensure that food is not immediately vomited after a full bolus is given. Both short-acting insulins have been used in type 2 and GDM women and appear to be superior to regular insulin in reducing postprandial glucose excursions.

31. How common is hypoglycemia in pregnant women with type 1 diabetes?

Maternal hypoglycemia is common and often severe in pregnant women with type 1 diabetes. In one series, hypoglycemia requiring assistance occurred in 71% of patients, with a peak incidence at 10 to 15 weeks. One third of the women had at least one episode resulting in seizures, loss of consciousness, or injury, any of which may have long-term effects on the offspring, including neuropsychological defects. Current data suggest that the counterregulatory hormonal response to hypoglycemia is diminished in pregnancy. The physician must have a low threshold for bringing the expectant mother into the hospital to optimize education and glycemic control. Occasional monitoring in the middle of the night is recommended in women with type 1 diabetes because of the increased risk of nocturnal hypoglycemia, especially if the woman has hypoglycemia unawareness.

32. Discuss special concerns in pregnant women with type 2 diabetes as compared with type 1 diabetes.

Women with type 2 diabetes are at least as high a risk of pregnancy complications as women with type 1 diabetes, especially if they have hypertension, obesity, or are in poor glycemic control. Many series, in fact, show that pregnancy outcome may be less favorable in women with type 2 compared with type 1 diabetes, including a higher perinatality rate. The reasons for this may include older age, a lower rate of preconception counseling, a higher incidence of poor glycemic control in the first trimester, and the coexistence of the metabolic syndrome (hypertension and obesity), all of which are significant risk factors for pregnancy complications. Failure to achieve optimal control in early pregnancy in women with any type of preexisting diabetes may have teratogenic effects or lead to early fetal loss. Poor control later in pregnancy increases the risk of intrauterine fetal demise, macrosomia, and metabolic complications in the newborn. As in the case with type 1 diabetes, an early dating ultrasound is necessary to determine the gestational age of the fetus, and a formal anatomy scan at 18 to 20 weeks should be performed to evaluate for fetal anomalies. A fetal echocardiogram should be offered at 20 to 22 weeks if the HbA_{1C} was elevated during the first trimester with any type of preexisting diabetes. Women with either type 1 or type 2 DM should be offered fetal surveillance beginning at approximately 32 weeks gestation with fetal movement monitoring and twice weekly NSTs (non-stress tests). A fetal ultrasound for growth should be considered at 28-32 weeks and before term. An earlier delivery should be offered to women with pre-existing diabetes of longer duration, especially if glucose control is suboptimal, after an amniocentesis confirms fetal lung maturity.

33. **What is the risk of diabetic ketoacidosis in pregnancy?**
Pregnancy predisposes to accelerated starvation, which can result in ketonuria after an overnight fast. Diabetic ketoacidosis (DKA) may thus occur at lower glucose levels (often referred to as "euglycemic DKA") because of the increased glomerular glucose filtration, continuous glucose utilization by the fetal-placental unit, and increased volume of distribution of glucose due to a 30% to 40% expansion of plasma volume. Women also have a lower buffering capacity because of progesterone-induced respiratory alkalosis, which results in a compensatory metabolic acidosis. A rapid switch from carbohydrate metabolism to lipolysis occurs in pregnant women who have depleted their glycogen stores after a 12-hour fast, resulting in a starvation ketoacidosis.

34. **How should the risk of DKA be managed?**
Any pregnant women with type 1 diabetes who is unable to keep down food or fluids should check urine ketones at home; if the results are positive, a chemistry panel should be ordered to rule out an anion gap, even if the maternal glucose is less than 200 mg/dL. Often the only precipitant for DKA in pregnancy is nausea and vomiting, but the possibility of an infection, particularly urinary tract infections, should be aggressively investigated. Women with type 2 diabetes and even women with gestational diabetes can also develop DKA, especially in the context of prolonged fasting, infections, use of beta-agonists for preterm labor, or steroids to promote fetal lung maturity.

35. **How does maternal DKA affect the fetus?**
In a study of 20 consecutive cases of DKA, only 65% of the fetuses were alive on admission to the hospital. Risk factors for fetal loss included DKA presenting later in pregnancy (32 weeks vs. 24 weeks), high insulin requirements, and longer duration of DKA. Electrolyte disturbances and fetal hypoxemia are additional risk factors for fetal death. The fetal heart rate must therefore be monitored continuously until the acidosis has resolved.

36. **What must the physician remember about DKA in pregnant women?**
Pregnant women unable to take oral nutrients require an additional 100 to 150 g/day of intravenous glucose to meet the metabolic demands of the fetal-placental unit. Without adequate carbohydrate (often a D10 glucose solution is necessary), fat will be burned for fuel, and the patient in DKA will remain ketotic.

KEY POINTS: DIABETES IN PREGNANCY

1. Although hyperglycemia is a major teratogen, the fetal malformation rate can be decreased from 25% to the normal baseline risk with optimal glycemic control before pregnancy and during the first 10 weeks of gestation.

2. Diabetic ketoacidosis may occur at glucose levels less than 200 mg/dL in pregnancy and may also occur in women with gestational diabetes.

3. Inadequately controlled diabetes may place the fetus at risk for developing childhood obesity and glucose intolerance.

4. Women who develop gestational diabetes have an approximate 50% risk of developing type 2 diabetes within 5 to 10 years.

5. Pregnancy does not usually accelerate the progression of diabetic nephropathy unless severe; however, proteinuria, diabetic retinopathy, and autonomic neuropathy may worsen.

6. Insulin requirements often decrease in the first trimester placing the mother at high risk of severe hypoglycemia, but requirements may double or triple in the late second and third trimesters due to the insulin resistance of pregnancy.

37. What is gestational diabetes mellitus?

GDM is a glucose-intolerant state with onset or first recognition during pregnancy. The incidence of GDM ranges from 3% to 14% of pregnancies throughout the world and is highest in ethnic groups that have a higher incidence of type 2 diabetes (Hispanic Americans, African Americans, Native Americans, and Pacific Islanders). The prevalence has doubled in the past 10 years, in large part secondary to the obesity epidemic, and may be a high as 1 in 10 in high-risk populations.

38. How is GDM diagnosed?

The criteria for diagnosis in the United States have recently changed. The Carpenter and Coustan criteria have been adopted by the American Diabetes Association (ADA) and the Fourth International Workshop-Conference on Gestational Diabetes. The criteria may be further modified in the near future given the preliminary data from the HAPO trial, suggesting that diagnostic and therapeutic glucose targets be lowered to prevent fetal overgrowth. In fact, the HAPO trial demonstrated that a FBG $\geq$ 90 or a 1-hour value $\geq$ 172 or a 2-hour value of $\geq$ 140 after a 75gm glucose load increases the risk of an LGA infant by more than 2-fold. Screening recommendations have been stratified according to low-risk, average-risk, and high-risk status of GDM. Most obstetricians employ universal screening of all women at 24 to 28 weeks, which is a reasonable approach, especially in a population that contains ethnic groups with a higher prevalence of GDM. An increasing number of women make criteria for early screening. Some of these women who meet diagnostic criteria in the first trimester will be found to have elevated A_{1Cs}, suggesting preexisting diabetes or hyperglycemia during embryogenesis, which could result in an increased risk of major malformations.

39. Summarize the recommendations for low-risk status.

Low-risk status requires no glucose testing, but this category is limited to women meeting ALL of the following criteria: age under 25 years, normal weight before pregnancy, member of an ethnic group with a low prevalence of GDM, no known diabetes in first-degree relatives, no history of abnormal glucose tolerance, and no history of poor obstetric outcome or macrosomic infant.

40. What are the recommendations for high-risk status?

High-risk status requires glucose testing as soon as pregnancy is diagnosed and again at 24 to 28 weeks if the early testing is normal. Women meeting ANY of the following criteria should be tested early: obesity, personal history of GDM or previous macrosomic infant, glycosuria, family history of diabetes in a first degree relative, or polycystic ovary syndrome (PCOS). Women with a fasting blood glucose greater than 125 mg/dL or a random or postprandial glucose greater than 200 mg/dL meet the criteria for diabetes, and this diagnosis precludes the need for any glucose challenge. All other high-risk women should be given a 50-g glucose challenge (glucola test) or proceed directly to a 100-g oral glucose tolerance test (OGTT) as soon as they establish prenatal care. If initial testing is normal, repeat testing should be performed at 24 to 28 weeks gestation.

41. **How should women of average risk be approached?**
    Women who do not fall in the low-or high-risk categories should receive a 50-g glucose
    challenge at 24 to 28 weeks. If the results are positive, they should undergo diagnostic testing
    with a 100-g, 3-hour OGTT.

42. **Describe the 50-g glucose challenge.**
    At this time, the 50-g glucose challenge is the accepted screen for the presence of GDM in the United
    States, but a positive result must be followed by a diagnostic 100-g, 3-hour OGTT. A positive screen
    is in the range of 130 to 140 mg/dL. The sensitivity and specificity of the test depend on what
    threshold value is chosen, and the cutoff may be selected according to the prevalence of GDM in the
    population being screened. The test does not have to be performed during a fasting state but a
    serum sample must be drawn exactly 1 hour after administering the oral glucose.

43. **Describe the 100-g, 3-hour OGTT.**
    The 100-g, 3-hour test must be performed after 3 days of an unrestricted carbohydrate diet and
    while the patient is fasting. A positive test requires that two values be met or exceeded. One
    abnormal value should be followed with a repeated 3-hour test 1 month later because a single
    elevated value increases the risk of macrosomia, and one third of patients ultimately meet
    the diagnostic criteria for GDM (Table 5-2). A lowering of these diagnostic criteria may be
    anticipated in the future because of the findings from the HAPO study that fetal overgrowth is
    associated with lower glucose levels than previously recognized. Furthermore, the HAPO trial
    used a 75 gm, not 100 gm, 2 hr OGTT and for the first time demonstrated that fetal overgrowth
    and high cord blood insulin levels were associated with lower values than are currently defined
    as abnormal on the 100 gm OGTT.

TABLE 5-2. CRITERIA FOR A POSITIVE 100–G ORAL GLUCOSE TOLERANCE TEST	
Fasting glucose	95 mg/dL
1-hour glucose	180 mg/dL
2-hour glucose	155 mg/dL
3-hour glucose	140 mg/dL

44. **Summarize the risks to the mother with GDM.**
    The immediate risks to the mother with GDM are an increased incidence of cesarean section
    ($\approx$30%), preeclampsia ($\approx$20%–30%), and polyhydramnios ($\approx$20%), which can result in
    preterm labor. The long-term risks to the mother are related to recurrent GDM pregnancies
    and the substantial risk of developing type 2 diabetes mellitus.

45. **What factors increase the risk of subsequently developing type 2 diabetes?**
    Women with GDM have an extremely high risk ($\approx$50%) of developing type 2 diabetes in the
    subsequent 5 to 10 years. Risk factors include fasting hyperglycemia, an insulin requirement,
    GDM diagnosed before 24 weeks of gestation (preexisting glucose intolerance), obesity,
    membership in an ethnic group with a high prevalence of type 2 diabetes, and impaired
    glucose tolerance at 6 weeks postpartum. Women with GDM who have multiple
    pregnancies also have a higher risk of developing type 2 diabetes.

46. **What factors may reduce the risk of developing type 2 diabetes?**
    Counseling with regard to diet, weight loss, and exercise is essential and is likely to improve
    insulin sensitivity, given the findings of the Diabetes Prevention Program (DPP) Trial (DPT). A
    subgroup analysis examining women in the DPP with a history of GDM showed that they had a

much higher risk of developing type 2 DM (17% per year) compared with women with IGT but without a history of GDM. This risk could be halved to approximately 8% per year with diet and exercise or metformin. Such dietary modifications should be adopted by the family, because the infant is also at risk for developing obesity and the metabolic syndrome. One trial also demonstrated that the use of a thiazolidinedione versus placebo postpartum decreased the rate of developing type 2 diabetes in 30 months from 12.1% to 5.4% in the 133 women randomized, apparently by decreasing insulin secretion and preserving beta-cell function. At this time, it is recommended that intensified efforts through diet and exercise be made to help women return to their prepregnancy weight and to lose additional weight if their body mass index (BMI) is still elevated. If diet and exercise are unsuccessful or do not normalize glucose tolerance, metformin may be a consideration.

47. What is the incidence of complications in the infant of a mother with GDM?
Even with the advent of screening and aggressive management of GDM, the incidence of neonatal complications ranges from 12% to 28%.

48. Summarize the basic mechanism behind complications related to GDM.
Excessive transfer of glucose, amino acids, FFA, and triglycerides from mother to fetus induces fetal hyperglycemia, which results in fetal pancreatic islet hypertrophy and beta-cell hyperplasia with consequent fetal hyperinsulinemia. Fetal insulin is a potent growth hormone.

49. What is the most common complication of GDM?
The most common complication is macrosomia (Fig. 5-1). Increased fat synthesis by the fetus leads to adiposity and visceromegaly (especially heart, liver, and pancreas), which places the mother at increased risk of requiring a cesarean section and the infant at risk for shoulder dystocia. The excessive supply of nutrients causes an increase in fetal abdominal girth disproportionate to other body measurements, resulting in a difficult delivery.

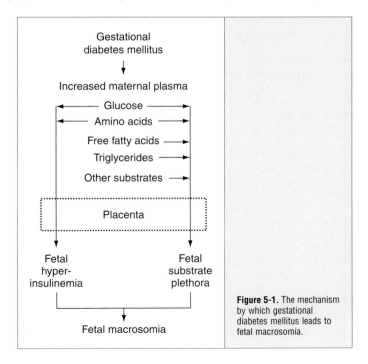

Figure 5-1. The mechanism by which gestational diabetes mellitus leads to fetal macrosomia.

50. **What other complications may result from GDM or pre-existing diabetes?**
    - Shoulder dystocia can result in Erb's palsy, clavicular fractures, fetal distress, low APGAR scores, as well as birth asphyxia when unrecognized.
    - If mothers have poor glycemic control, respiratory distress syndrome may occur in up to 30% of infants because of decreased lung surfactant synthesis.
    - Cardiac septal hypertrophy may be seen in 35% to 40%.
    - With extremely poor glucose control, there is also an increased risk of fetal mortality as a result of fetal acidemia and hypoxia.
    - Common metabolic abnormalities in the infant of a mother with DM include neonatal hypoglycemia from sustained hyperinsulinemia, as well as hypocalcemia, polycythemia, and hyperbilirubinemia.
    - Excess FFA and triglycerides delivered to the fetus may also contribute to excess fetal growth and is now the subject of increased research to discern whether these substrates may need to be targeted for lowering as well as glucose.

51. **Explain the fetoplacental glucose steal phenomenon.**
    Fetal hyperinsulinemia may cause exaggerated fetal siphoning of glucose from the mother, which blunts the maternal postload glucose peaks. This fetoplacental glucose steal phenomenon can actually decrease maternal glucose concentrations on an OGTT, leading to an illusion of improved maternal glucose control. Maternal glucose monitoring alone may not accurately reflect the fetal metabolic situation when fetal hyperinsulinemia is present.

52. **Describe the fetal-based strategy to manage GDM.**
    Five randomized controlled trials have demonstrated that using fetal overgrowth as an indicator of optimal diabetes management is beneficial. Because maternal glucose measurements may be deceptive and other nutrients such as excess lipids may also contribute to fetal fat accretion, assessing fetal growth as a gauge for the adequacy of treatment is now recommended. Amniotic fetal insulin levels, a marker of fetal hyperinsulinemia (given maternal insulin does not cross in appreciable quantities) correlates strongly with the fetal abdominal circumference at 28 to 32 weeks. These randomized controlled trials support intensifying maternal medical therapy for fetuses whose abdominal circumference is above the 70th percentile, which is associated with increased abdominal and visceral fat accretion. Women with GDM who require medical therapy or with suboptimal glycemic control should undergo fetal surveillance at ~32 weeks' gestation. Delivery should be considered at around 39 weeks if the woman has good dating criteria and a favorable cervix. An estimated fetal weight of greater than 4500 g carries such a high risk of shoulder dystocia that an elective cesarean section is usually recommended in women with GDm or pre-existing diabetes.

53. **Discuss the long-term sequelae of GDM or pre-existing diabetes in offspring of affected mothers.**
    The long-term sequelae of DM for offspring are concerning. Proliferation of fetal adipocytes and pancreatic beta cells may be responsible for "fetal programming" the later development of obesity and the metabolic syndrome. Reports of an increased risk of adolescent obesity and type 2 diabetes are compelling. The incidence of childhood type 2 diabetes was approximately 10-fold higher in Pima Indian offspring born to mothers with diabetes compared with offspring whose mothers did not develop diabetes until after pregnancy. Furthermore, despite a similar incidence of obesity at 20 years of age between the two groups of offspring, the incidence of type 2 diabetes was approximately 70% at age 25 to 29 years in the offspring of diabetic mothers compared with approximately 10% in the offspring of prediabetic mothers (mothers who did not develop diabetes until after the pregnancy).

54. How does in utero hyperglycemia affect the long-term sequelae of infants born to diabetic mothers?

In utero hyperglycemia appears to be an independent risk factor for the development of childhood glucose intolerance. Elevated insulin levels in amniotic fluid (owing to fetal hyperinsulinemia as a result of maternal hyperglycemia) predicted teenage obesity in one study, independently of fetal weight, and approximately 30% of these offspring had impaired glucose tolerance by 17 years of age. Fetal programming or epigenetic influences appears to occur in this intrauterine environment of nutrient excess and may contribute to the growing incidence of type 2 diabetes as children with impaired glucose tolerance become mothers themselves, perpetuating the cycle.

55. What causes women to get GDM?

GDM is caused by abnormalities in at least three aspects of fuel metabolism: insulin resistance, increased hepatic glucose production, and impaired insulin secretion. The increased insulin resistance of pregnancy cannot be compensated because of impaired beta-cell function, resulting in inadequate insulin secretion. The insulin resistance is thought to be due primarily to the effects of increased production of human placental lactogen, placental growth hormone, and TNFα, and inflammatory cytokines. Women developing GDM have a lower pregravid insulin sensitivity compared with matched control groups, and some abnormalities may persist after delivery. The vast majority of these women are overweight, and many have characteristics of the metabolic syndrome before pregnancy. Thin or normal weight women who develop GDM are in the minority and may display a MODY gene or, more commonly, be at risk of developing latent autoimmune diabetes. Many of these unusual cases are found to be GAD-antibody positive and have low C-peptide levels, placing them at increased risk for manifesting type 1 DM.

56. What causes increased hepatic glucose production?

Increased hepatic glucose production results from inadequate insulin suppression of excessive hepatic gluconeogenesis. Beta-cell sensing of glucose is also abnormal and is manifested as an inadequate insulin response for a given degree of hyperglycemia.

57. Summarize the role of impaired insulin secretion.

Impaired insulin secretion renders the woman unable to meet the requirement for greater insulin production necessitated by the insulin resistance and increased hepatic glucose production. These same pathophysiologic disorders, which are in large part genetically determined, make the patient with GDM more likely to develop type 2 diabetes mellitus later in life when weight gain and aging often contribute further to insulin resistance and impaired insulin secretion. Pregnancy can be thought of as a "stress test" for the development of type 2 diabetes, because the marked insulin resistance of pregnancy necessitates a two- to threefold increase in insulin secretion that the beta cell may not be able to achieve, resulting in a clinically evident abnormality in glucose metabolism.

58. What is the best therapy for women with GDM?

Women with GDM should be taught home glucose monitoring to ensure that glycemic goals are met throughout the duration of pregnancy. The best therapy for GDM depends entirely on the extent of the glucose intolerance and on the mother's response. In at least half of cases, diet alone maintains the postprandial blood glucose values within the target range but is more likely to fail if fasting hyperglycemia exists. Because postprandial glucose levels have been most strongly associated with the risk of macrosomia, restriction of simple carbohydrates may be helpful to blunt the postprandial glucose excursions, and saturated fats should be limited because of their effect on worsening insulin resistance. Women with a BMI greater than 30 kg/m^2 may benefit from a 30% to 33% caloric restriction to approximately 20 to 25 kcal/kg or approximately 1800 calories per day, which has been shown to reduce hyperglycemia and plasma triglycerides with no increase in ketonuria.

59. **Discuss the role of oral diabetes medication in the management of GDM.**
    The only oral hypoglycemic drugs approved for use in GDM women by the Fifth International Workshop on Gestational Diabetes are glyburide and acarbose, but the latter is usually problematic because of gastrointestinal side effects. None of the other insulin secretagogues are approved, nor is metformin or thiazolidinediones. In a landmark multicenter trial, 400 women with GDM were randomized to receive either insulin or glyburide after 24 weeks gestation. Maternal glycemic control, macrosomia, neonatal hypoglycemia, and neonatal outcomes were not different between groups. Most important, the cord serum insulin concentrations were similar between the two groups, and glyburide was not detected in the cord serum of any infant tested. However, subsequent studies suggest that approximately 20% of GDM women will fail glyburide and require insulin treatment to achieve adequate glycemic control. Risk factors associated with glyburide failure include diagnosis of GDM before 24 weeks, fasting hyperglycemia, recurrent pregnancies, and more severe hyperglycemia. Recently, the MIG trial was published which was an RCT of 751 women with GDM randomized to Metformin or insulin. Due to concerns about the possible risk of fetal lactic acidosis, women with a contraindication to Metformin, fetal anomalies, gestational hypertension, preeclampsia, fetal growth restriction, and ruptured membranes were excluded. Women with pre-existing diabetes were also excluded. Metformin did not apear to increase any adverse outcomes, although it was associated with a slight increase in preterm birth and 46% of women in the Metformin group required supplemental insulin. The offspring are being followed for evidence of any long-term effects. Given this single RCT is so recent, Metformin has not yet been approved in pregnancy for the treatment of GDM, and it appears to have a higher failure rate than Glyburide. There are no studies published as yet exploring the combination of Glyburide and Metformin to treat GDM.

60. **When should insulin be used to treat GDM?**
    Women who have fasting blood glucose levels greater than 95 mg/dL, 1-hour postprandial glucose levels greater than 140 mg/dL, or 2-hour postprandial glucose levels greater than 120 mg/dL should be started on insulin therapy. Those who are unwilling to start insulin, who exhibit mild hyperglycemia without a significant elevation in fasting blood glucose, and who were not diagnosed before 24 weeks gestation may be candidates for glyburide therapy or possibly Metformin, although the latter is not yet approved. Women with a fetus that is large for gestational age, as demonstrated by ultrasound, are also candidates for medical management. Often GDM can be treated with twice-daily injections of NPH and regular insulin, but occasionally postprandial glycemic excursions are so excessive that mealtime injections of a short-acting insulin analog are necessary. Serious hypoglycemia tends to be an infrequent occurrence in such patients because of their underlying insulin resistance and symptomatic awareness of hypoglycemia.

61. **What is the role of exercise in patients with GDM or pre-existing diabetes?**
    Moderate exercise is well tolerated in pregnancy, and the Fifth International Workshop on Gestational Diabetes advises that pregnant women adopt the national guidelines of exercising 30 minutes daily as long as there is not an obstetric contraindication. Exercise also improves insulin sensitivity in women with type 2 diabetes and may limit excess weight gain. Fetal safety has been established if the maternal heart rate is maintained under 140 beats/minute in women who are not well-conditioned or < 160 beats/min in women with higher exercise capacity at durations of 30 minutes and if the mother is well hydrated and does not get overheated. Two of three trials in GDM pregnancies have shown that exercise three times a week can achieve glycemic control and infant birth weights that are similar to those seen in women who are treated with insulin. Establishing a regular routine of modest exercise during pregnancy may also have long-lasting benefits for the mother with GDM, who clearly has an appreciable risk of developing type 2 diabetes in the future. Home glucose monitoring must be continued throughout pregnancy to determine whether insulin therapy is necessary.

62. **When is a controlled exercise program contraindicated?**
Women at risk for preterm labor, vaginal bleeding, or conditions predisposing to growth restriction are not candidates for a controlled exercise program. Women with poorly controlled hypertension and preeclampsia are usually advised to adhere to bed rest. Somen women, especially with longstanding type 1 DM, may be at risk for placental insufficiency or growth restriction and may not be candidates.

63. **What important postpartum management issues should be addressed in women with pregestational or gestational diabetes?**
Critical issues in the postpartum period include maintenance of glycemic control, diet, exercise, weight loss, blood pressure and renal protection management, breast-feeding, and contraception. Breastfeeding has been shown to be advantageous to mothers with type 2 diabetes and GDM by facilitating weight loss. Women with type 1 diabetes should be checked for TPO antibodies and, if positive, may have up to a 50% risk of postpartum thyroiditis. The majority of women with pregestational diabetes, even those who have been extremely compliant and have had optimal glycemic control during pregnancy, experience a dramatic worsening of glucose control after delivery. Furthermore, many quit seeking medical care for their diabetes. The postpartum period is relatively neglected as both the new mother and her physician relax their vigilance. However, this period offers a unique opportunity to institute health habits that can have highly beneficial effects on the quality of life of both the mother and her infant. The importance of effective contraception cannot be overstated given 50% of pregnancies are unplanned and each subsequent pregnancy in a woman with GDM increases her risk for the development of type 2 diabetes.

64. **Explain the value of diet and exercise in the postpartum period.**
A weight loss program consisting of diet and exercise should be instituted for women with GDM to improve insulin sensitivity and prevent the development of type 2 diabetes. It has been shown that most women with GDM or type 2 diabetes do not lose their pregnancy weight gain and often enter a subsequent pregnancy at an even higher weight. Diet and exercise reduced the development of type 2 diabetes by approximately 50% in the subgroup of women with GDM in the DPP trial, and every effort must be made to try to intervene in this exceedingly high-risk population.

65. **Discuss the importance of monitoring during the postpartum period.**
Home glucose monitoring should be continued in the postpartum period in women with pregestational diabetes because insulin requirements drop almost immediately and often dramatically at this time, increasing the risk of hypoglycemia. In women with a history of GDM, glycemic status should be reassessed 6 weeks after delivery. Hyperglycemia generally resolves in the majority of GDM patients during this interval but may persist in up to 10%. At the minimum, a fasting blood glucose should be performed to determine whether the woman has persistent diabetes (glucose >125 mg/dL) or impaired fasting glucose (glucose of at least 100 mg/dL). A 75-g, 2-hour glucose tolerance test is recommended by the ADA, ACOG, and Fifth International Workshop on Gestational Diabetes because a 2-hour value of at least 200 mg/dL establishes a diagnosis of diabetes and a 2-hour value of at least 140 mg/dL but less than 200 mg/dL makes the diagnosis of impaired glucose tolerance. The majority of women with persistent impaired glucose tolerance will be missed if only a fasting blood glucose level is checked.

66. **Why is a diagnosis of impaired glucose tolerance or "prediabetes" of critical importance?**
The importance of diagnosing impaired glucose intolerance or prediabetes lies in its value in predicting the future development of type 2 diabetes. In one series, a diagnosis of impaired glucose tolerance was the most potent predictor of the development of type 2 diabetes in Latino women with a history of GDM; 80% of such women developed diabetes in the subsequent

5 to 7 years. Intensified efforts promoting diet, exercise, and weight loss, and possibly metformin if lifestyle changes fail, should be instituted in this extraordinarily high-risk group of women.

67. Summarize the role of ACE inhibitors in the postpartum period.

Women who are candidates for an ACE inhibitor can be started on enalapril, which has not been shown to appear in breast milk at appreciable concentrations.

68. Should women with GDM breast-feed their infants?

Women should be encouraged to breast-feed unless difficulties in glycemic control arise. There are small reports suggesting that modest doses of glyburide and metformin can be used in breast-feeding mothers, but the sample sizes are small, and the pediatrician should be notified. Insulin is still preferred in women who breast-feed due to the long-term safety data in nursing infants. Women with a history of GDM who breast-feed appear to have a lower incidence of developing type 2 diabetes, partly because of enhanced weight loss given that breast-feeding requires approximately 300 to 400 calories per day. Breast-feeding also appears to decrease the risk of childhood obesity and impaired glucose tolerance in offspring of GDM women. The mother must also ensure that her calcium intake is at least 1500 mg/day.

69. How common is postpartum thyroiditis in women with type 1 diabetes? When does it appear?

Women with type 1 diabetes have been reported to have a 20–25% incidence of postpartum thyroiditis, the risk being highest in women with positive TPO antibodies. Hyperthyroidism can occur in the 2- to 4-month postpartum period, and hypothyroidism may present in the subsequent 4- to 8-month period. Given the significance of this disorder, measurement of thyroid-stimulating hormone (TSH) is recommended in type 1 patients with positive TPO antibodies at 3 and 6 months after delivery or with any suggestive symptoms.

70. Summarize the long-term follow-up of nondiabetic women with a history of GDM.

Women with a history of GDM should receive a 75-g OGTT at approximately 6 weeks postpartum to make the diagnosis of normal versus impaired glucose tolerance ("prediabetes" or diabetes). The Fifth International Workshop recommends a second 75-g OGTT 1 year postpartum, fasting blood glucoses annually, and then 75-g OGTTs every third year.

71. Which contraceptive agents can be used by women with diabetes or a history of GDM?

It should be documented at every visit that women are using or have been offered an effective birth control method. The vast majority of contraceptive methods are relatively safe in women with diabetes, including combined oral contraceptives, unless women have poorly controlled hypertension, hypertriglyceridemia, or are at risk for thromboembolic disease. Triglycerides should be measured after the initiation of oral contraceptives in all women with diabetes or a history of GDM because of the significant incidence of hypertriglyceridemia and the associated risk of pancreatitis with oral estrogen use.

72. Summarize the role of low-dose combined oral contraceptives.

Low-dose combined oral contraceptives have been shown to be effective and have minimal metabolic effects in women with diabetes. The Ortho Evra patch and Nuva Ring are also options, but have not been studied to determine whether they offer fewer metabolic side effects. In a retrospective cohort of 904 women with GDM, combined oral contraceptives did not influence the development of type 2 diabetes.

73. What other contraceptive options are appropriate?

Progestational agents, such as Depo-Provera or norethindrone, are also alternatives, although they may slightly affect carbohydrate tolerance and Depo-Provera has been associated with an increased risk of type 2 diabetes in nursing mothers with a history of GDM, primarily because of excess weight gain. There is no increase in pelvic inflammatory disease with the use of intrauterine devices in women with well-controlled type 1 or type 2 diabetes after the postinsertion period. Therefore this may be an attractive choice in older women who do not desire future pregnancies. The Nuva Ring also does not appear to be associated with any increased risks. Nearly any contraceptive method is superior to an unwanted pregnancy given the maternal risks to the mother with pregestational diabetes and the increased risk of developing type 2 DM in mothers with a history GDM.

BIBLIOGRAPHY

1. Pregestational diabetes mellitus. ACOG Practice Bull 60:675–85, 2005.

2. American Diabetes Association: Preconception care of women with diabetes (Position Statement). Diabetes Care 30(Suppl 1):S26, 2007.

3. Barbour LA: Gestational diabetes. In Rosene Montella K, Keely E, Barbour L, Lee RV, editors: *Medical care of the pregnant patient*, Philadelphia, 2007, American College of Physicians.

4. Barbour LA: New concepts in insulin resistance of pregnancy and gestational diabetes: long-term implications for mother and offspring. J Obstet Gynaecol 24:545–549, 2003.

5. Barbour LA, McCundy CE, Hernandez TL, et al: Cellular mechanisms in gestational diabetes. Diabetes Care 30 (Suppl 2):S112–119, 2007.

6. Buchanan TA, Xiang A, Kjos SL, Watanabe R: What is gestational diabetes? Diabetes Care 30(Suppl 2): S105–111, 2007.

7. Catalano PM, Thomas A, Huston-Presley L, Amini SB: Phenotype of infants of mothers with gestational diabetes. Diabetes Care 30(Suppl 2):S156–160, 2007.

8. Clausen TD, Mathiesen E, Ekbom P, et al: Poor pregnancy outcome in women with type 2 diabetes. Diabetes Care 28:323–328, 2005.

9. Conway DL, Obstetric management in gestational diabetes. Diabetes Care 30(Suppl 2):S175–179, 2007.

10. Cooper WO, Hernandez-Diaz S, Arbogast PG, et al: Major congenital malformations after first-trimester exposure to ACE Inhibitors. N Engl J Med 354:2443–2451, 2006.

11. Coustan DR: Pharmacologic management of gestational diabetes. Diabetes Care 30(Suppl 2):S206–208, 2007.

12. Crowther CA, Hiller JE, Moses JR, et al: for the Australian Carbohydrate Intolerance Study in Pregnant Women (ACHOIS) Trial Group: Effect of treatment of gestational diabetes mellitus on pregnancy outcomes. N Engl J Med 352:2477–2486, 2005.

13. Dabelea D: The predisposition to obesity and diabetes in offspring of diabetic mothers. Diabetes Care 30 (Suppl 2):S169–S174.

14. Dabelea D, Knowler WC, Pettett DJ: Effect of diabetes in pregnancy on offspring: follow-up research in the Pima Indians. J Mat Fet Med9:83–88, 2000.

15. Damm P, Mathiesen ER: Contraception after gestational diabetes. Diabetes Care 30(Suppl 2):S236–241, 2007.

16. DeViciana M, Major CA, Morgan MA, et al: Postprandial versus preprandial blood glucose monitoring in women gestational diabetes requiring insulin therapy. N Engl J Med 333:1237–1241, 1995.

17. Diabetes Control and Complications Research Group: Pregnancy outcomes in the diabetes control and complications trial. Am J Obstet Gynecol 177:1165–1171, 1996.

18. Diabetes Prevention Program Research Group: Reduction in the incidence of type 2 diabetes with lifestyle intervention or metformin. N Engl J Med 346:393–403, 2002.

19. Gimenez M, Conget I, Nicolau J, et al: Outcome of pregnancy in women with type 1 diabetes intensively treated with continuous subcutaneous insulin infusion or conventional therapy. A case-control study. Acta Diabetologica 44:34–37, 2007.

20. Glueck CJ, Wang P, Goldenberg N, Sieve-Smith L: Pregnancy outcomes among women with polycystic ovary syndrome treated with metformin. Human Reprod 17:2858–2864, 2002.

21. The HAPO Study Cooperative Research Group: Hyperglycemia and adverse pregnancy outcmoes. New Engl J Med 358:1991–2002, 2008.

22. Hellmuth E, Damm P, Molsted-Pederson L: Oral hypoglycemic agents in 118 diabetic pregnancies. Diabetic Med 17:507–511, 2000.

23. Hod M, Yogev Y: Goals of metabolic management of gestational diabetes. Diabetes Care 30(Suppl 2):S180–187, 2007.

24. Jakubowicz DJ, Iuorno MJ, Jakubowicz S, et al: Effects of metformin on early pregnancy loss in the polycystic ovary syndrome. J Clin Endocrinol Metab 87:524–529, 2002.

25. Kahn B, Davies JK, Lynch AM, et al: Predictors of glyburide failure in women with gestational diabetes. Obstet Gynecol 107:1306–1309, 2006.

26. Kerssen A, deValk HW, Visser GHA: Increased second trimester maternal glucose levels are related to extremely large for gestational age infants in women with type 1 diabetes. Diabetes Care 30:1069–1074, 2007.

27. Kitzmiller JL, Dang-Kilduff, Taslimi MM: Gestational diabetes after delivery. Diabetes Care 30(Suppl 2): S225–235, 2007.

28. Kjos SL, Peters RJ, Xiang A, et al: Predicting future diabetes in Latino women with gestational diabetes. Diabetes 44:586–591, 1995.

29. Kjos SL, Schaeffer-Graf UM: Modified therapy for gestational diabetes using high-risk and low-risk fetal abdominal circumference growth to select strict versus relaxed maternal glycemic targets. Diabetes Care 30 (Suppl 2):S200–205, 2007.

30. Langer O, Conway DL, Berkus MD, et al: A comparison of glyburide and insulin in women with gestational diabetes. N Engl J Med 343:1134–1138, 2000.

31. Mathiesen E, Kinsley B, Amiel SA, et al: The Insulin Aspart Pregnancy Study Group: Maternal glycemic control and hypoglycemia in type 1 diabetes pregnancy: a randomized trial of insulin aspart versus human insulin in 322 pregnant women. Diabetes Care 30:771–776, 2007.

32. Metzger BE, Buchanan TA, Coustan DR, et al: Summary and recommendations of the Fifth International Workshop-Conference on Gestational Diabetes Mellitus. Diabetes Care 30 (Suppl 2):S251–260, 2007.

33. Nielsen GL, Moller M, Sorenson HT, HbA$_{1C}$ in early diabetic pregnancy and pregnancy outcomes: a Danish population-based cohort study of 573 pregnancies in women with type 1 diabetes. Diabetes Care 29:2612–2616, 2006.

34. Price N, Bartlett C, Gillmer M: Use of insulin glargine during pregnancy: a case-control study. BJOG 114:453–457, 2007.

35. Ratner RE: Prevention of type 2 diabetes in women with previous gestational diabetes. Diabetes Care 30 (Suppl 2):S242–245.

36. Reader DM: Medical nutrition therapy and lifestyle interventions. Diabetes Care 30(Suppl 2):S188–913, 2007.

37. Reece EA, Homko CJ: Why do diabetic women deliver malformed infants? Clin Obstet Gynecol 43:32–45, 2000.

38. Roland JM, Murphy HR, Northcote-Wright J, Temple RC: The pregnancies of women with type 2 diabetes: poor outcomes but opportunities for improvement. Diabetes Med 22:1774–1777, 2005.

39. Rossing K, Jacobsen P, Hommel E, et al: Pregnancy and progression of diabetic nephropathy. Diabetologia 45:36–41, 2002.

40. Rowan JA, Hague WM, Gao W, et al: Metformin versus insulin for the treatment of gestational diabetes. New Engl J Med 358:2003–2015, 2008.

41. Sabai BM, Caritis S, Hauth J, et al: Risks of preeclampsia and adverse neonatal outcomes among women with pregestational diabetes mellitus. Am J Obstet Gynecol 182:364–369, 2000.

42. Temple RC, Aldridge VJ, Murphy HR: Prepregnancy care and pregnancy outcomes in women with type 1 diabetes. Diabetes Care 29:1744–1749, 2007.

43. Temple RC, Aldridge VA, Sampson MJ, et al: Impact of pregnancy on the progression of diabetic retinopathy in type 1 diabetes. Diabetic Med 18:573–577, 2001.

44. Xiang AH, Peters RK, Kjos S, et al: Effect of pioglitazone on pancreatic β-cell function and diabetes risk in hispanic women with prior gestational diabetes. Diabetes 55:517–522, 2006.

CHAPTER 6

LIPID DISORDERS

Michael T. McDermott

1. **What are the major lipids in the bloodstream?**
   Cholesterol and triglycerides (TGs) are the major circulating lipids. Cholesterol is used by all cells for the synthesis and repair of membranes and intracellular organelles and by the adrenal glands and gonads as a substrate to synthesize adrenal and gonadal steroid hormones. TGs are an energy source that can be stored as fat in adipose tissue or used as fuel by muscle and other tissues.

2. **What are lipoproteins?**
   Cholesterol and TGs are not water soluble and thus cannot be transported through the circulation as individual molecules. Lipoproteins are large, spherical particles that package these lipids into a core surrounded by a shell of water-soluble proteins and phospholipids. Lipoproteins serve as vehicles that transport cholesterol and TGs from one part of the body to another.

3. **What are the major lipoproteins in the bloodstream?**
   Chylomicrons, very-low-density lipoproteins (VLDL), low-density lipoproteins (LDL), and high-density lipoproteins (HDL) are the major circulating lipoproteins. Their functions are as follows:

Lipoprotein	Function
Chylomicron	Transport exogenous TGs from the gut to adipose tissue and muscle
VLDL	Transport endogenous TGs from the liver to adipose tissue and muscle
LDL	Transport cholesterol from the liver to peripheral tissues
HDL	Transport cholesterol from peripheral tissues to the liver

4. **What are the apoproteins?**
   Apoproteins are located on the surface of the lipoproteins. They function as ligands for binding to lipoprotein receptors and as cofactors for metabolic enzymes. Their functions are as follows:

Apoprotein	Function
Apoprotein A	Ligand for peripheral HDL receptors
Apoprotein B	Ligand for peripheral LDL receptors
Apoprotein E	Ligand for hepatic receptors for remnant particles
Apoprotein C-II	Cofactor for lipoprotein lipase (LPL)

5. **Name other enzymes and transport proteins that are important in lipoprotein metabolism.**
   See Table 6-1 and Fig 6-1.

TABLE 6-1. ENZYMES AND TRANSPORT PROTEINS IMPORTANT IN LIPOPROTEIN METABOLISM

Enzyme/Protein	Function
HMG CoA reductase	The rate-limiting enzyme in hepatic cholesterol synthesis
Lipoprotein lipase	Removes TG from chylomicrons and VLDL in adipose tissue, leaving remnant particles
Hepatic lipase	Removes additional TG from remnant particles in the liver, converting them into LDL
Lecithin cholesterol acyl transferase	Esterifies cholesterol molecules on the surface of HDL, drawing them into the HDL core
Cholesterol ester transfer protein	Shuttles esterified cholesterol back and forth between HDL and LDL

HDL, high-density lipoprotein; LDL, low-density lipoprotein; TG, triglycerides; VLDL, very low-density lipoprotein.

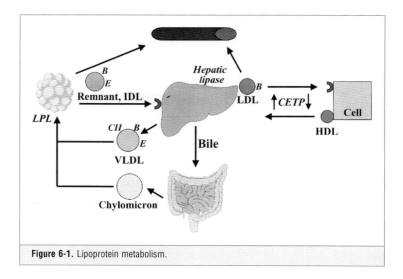

Figure 6-1. Lipoprotein metabolism.

6. **Explain the function and metabolism of TGs.**
   Food and hepatic synthesis are the major sources of TGs. They are transported by chylomicrons (dietary TGs) and VLDL (endogenous TGs) to adipose tissue and muscle, where LPL and cofactor apoprotein C-II break down TGs into fatty acids (FAs) and monoglycerides. FAs enter

adipose cells to be stored as fat or muscle cells to be used as fuel. The chylomicron and VLDL remnant particles return to the liver, where HL converts VLDL remnants into LDL.

7. **Describe the function and metabolism of LDL.**
   LDL transports cholesterol from the liver to peripheral tissues where surface apoprotein B-100 binds to cellular LDL receptors (LDLR). LDLR clustering in clathrin-coated pits on the cell membrane, promoted by LDLR adaptor protein 1 (LDLRAP1), is necessary for efficient LDL uptake. After LDL is internalized, it is degraded to free cholesterol (FC) for intracellular use. Excess LDL is cleared from the circulation by scavenger macrophages.

8. **What is the function of HDL?**
   HDL removes excess cholesterol from cells by 2 mechanisms. Nascent pre-βHDL is made in the liver and intestine. Surface Apo A1 on pre-βHDL acquires free cholesterol (FC) through the ATP-binding cassette transporter A1 (ABCA1) on arterial wall macrophages. Plasma lecithin cholesterol acyl transferase (LCAT) then esterifies the FC to cholesterol ester (CE), forming a mature βHDL particle. Mature βHDL accepts additional FC from arterial macrophages through the ABCG1 transporter and the scavenger receptor, class B, type 1 (SR-B1) receptor. Cholesterol ester transfer protein (CETP) transfers some CE back to LDL particles, and the mature HDL transports the remaining CE to the liver, where transfer occurs through hepatic SR-B1 receptors. In addition to reverse cholesterol transport, HDL also reduces LDL oxidation, inhibits vascular inflammation, and improves endothelial function. All of these functions make HDL a potent antiatherogenic lipoprotein.

9. **Describe the pathogenesis of the atherosclerotic plaque and arterial thrombosis.**
   LDL can be modified by oxidation. Scavenger macrophages located beneath the intimal surface of arteries engulf oxidized LDL, becoming lipid-laden foam cells, which secrete growth factors that stimulate smooth muscle cell proliferation. These developing plaques also secrete cytokines that attract inflammatory cells, which secrete proteolytic enzymes that erode the fibromuscular plaque cap, making it prone to rupture. When rupture occurs, platelets aggregate and release chemicals that promote vasoconstriction and initiate thrombus formation, which may ultimately occlude the artery.

10. **Are elevated serum TG levels harmful?**
    Serum TG levels that exceed 200 mg/dL are associated with atherosclerosis. The mechanism, however, is unclear. High TG levels are often accompanied by low HDL cholesterol levels and by small, dense LDL particles that are more easily oxidized and therefore more atherogenic. Elevated TG levels are also frequently associated with hypertension and insulin resistance. It is unclear whether atherosclerosis results directly from elevated TGs or from the associated metabolic changes that accompany hypertriglyceridemia. TG values greater than 1000 mg/dL significantly increase the risk of developing acute pancreatitis.

11. **What is metabolic syndrome?**
    Metabolic syndrome (MS) is a condition that is diagnosed when a patient has any three of the following: elevated fasting glucose (>100 mg/dL), high TGs (>150 mg/dL), low HDL (<40 mg/dL), hypertension (>140/90), and abdominal obesity (waist >40 inches in men, >35 inches in women). The common thread among the disorders that comprise MS appears to be insulin resistance. MS carries a high risk for atherosclerotic vascular disease.

12. **What is lipoprotein(a)?**
    Apoprotein(a) has approximately 85% amino-acid sequence homology with plasminogen. When an apoprotein(a) molecule attaches to apoprotein B on the surface of an LDL particle, the new particle is referred to as lipoprotein(a). Excessive lipoprotein(a) promotes atherosclerosis,

possibly because it is easily oxidized and engulfed by macrophages, because it inhibits thrombolysis, or both.

13. **What are the primary dyslipidemias?**
Primary dyslipidemias are inherited disorders of lipoprotein metabolism. The major primary dyslipidemias and their lipid phenotypes are as follows:

Primary Dyslipidemia	Phenotype
Familial hypercholesterolemia (FH)	↑↑Cholesterol
Polygenic hypercholesterolemia	↑Cholesterol
Familial combined hyperlipidemia (FCH)	↑Cholesterol and ↑TGs
Familial dysbetalipoproteinemia (FDL)	↑Cholesterol and ↑TGs
Familial hypertriglyceridemia (FHT)	↑TGs
Familial hyperchylomicronemia (FHC)	↑↑TGs

14. **What is familial hypercholesterolemia?**
FH is an inherited disease characterized by extreme elevations of serum cholesterol but normal serum TG levels. The disorder has a population frequency of 1:500 for heterozygotes, who generally have serum cholesterol levels of 300 to 800 mg/dL, and 1:1,000,000 for homozygotes, who have serum cholesterols 800 to 1200 mg/dL. Most patients have genetic mutations resulting in deficient or dysfunctional LDL receptors (LDLR). Other less common monogenic hypercholesterolemic disorders include apoprotein B mutations that produce a defective apo B that cannot bind to LDLR, proprotein convertase subtilisin-like kexin type 9 (PCSK9) mutations that cause accelerated LDLR degradation, LDLR adaptor protein 1 (LDLRAP1) mutations that prevent normal clustering of LDLR in cell surface clathrin-coated pits, and ATP-binding cassette G5 or G8 (ABCG5/8) mutations that cause abnormal cellular transport of cholesterol and plant sterols (sitosterolemia). These disorders are characterized by premature coronary artery disease (CAD), often before the age of 20 in homozygous FH, and tendon xanthomas.

15. **What is familial combined hyperlipidemia?**
FCH is an inherited disorder characterized by variable elevations of both serum cholesterol and TG levels. Affected patients have excessive hepatic apoprotein B synthesis, with increased numbers of apoprotein B–containing VLDL and LDL particles. The genetic basis for the disorder has not yet been determined, but it may be related to mutations of the gene for Upstream Regulatory Factor 1 on chromosome 1q21-23. These patients are prone to develop premature CAD.

16. **What is familial dysbetalipoproteinemia?**
Familial dysbetalipoproteinemia (FDL) is an inherited condition characterized by significant and relatively balanced elevations of both serum cholesterol and TGs. It is also referred to as type III hyperlipidemia. This disorder results from an abnormal apoprotein E phenotype (E2/E2), which binds poorly to hepatic receptors, resulting in impaired clearance of circulating VLDL remnants by the liver. Affected patients often develop premature CAD. Planar xanthomas in the creases of the palms and soles of the feet are a characteristic finding in patients with FDL.

17. **What is polygenic hypercholesterolemia?**
Polygenic hypercholesterolemia, which is characterized by mild-to-moderate elevations of serum cholesterol alone, is the most common type of inherited hypercholesterolemia. This condition generally occurs when one or more mild defects of cholesterol metabolism

combine to elevate the serum cholesterol level. Affected patients have an increased risk of developing CAD.

18. **What are familial hypertriglyceridemia and familial hyperchylomicronemia?**

Familial hypertriglyceridemia (FHT) is an inherited condition featuring moderate-to-severe elevations of serum TGs with normal serum cholesterol levels. Familial hyperchylomicronemia (FHC) is characterized by extremely high serum TG and chylomicron levels. The genetic basis for FHT is unclear, but it may be polygenic or due to milder forms of the mutations that cause FHC. FHC is due to inactivating mutations in the gene for lipoprotein lipase (LPL) or Apo CII. Cases have also been linked to mutations of the apolipoprotein AV (APOA5) gene. Severe hypertriglyceridemia with chylomicronemia may predispose to the development of eruptive xanthomas, lipemia retinalis, hepatosplenomegaly, and acute pancreatitis.

19. **How do you distinguish between familial combined hyperlipidemia and familial dysbetalipoproteinemia?**

Because FCH and FDL are characterized by combined elevations of both cholesterol and TGs, additional tests may be necessary to make the distinction. Patients with FCH have increased serum apoprotein B levels, whereas patients with FDL have an E2/E2 apoprotein E phenotype and a broad beta-band on lipoprotein electrophoresis. Family studies are also helpful.

20. **What causes familial low HDL?**

Familial hypoalphalipoproteinemia (familial low HDL), characterized by extremely low serum HDL levels and premature CAD, is caused by inactivating mutations in the genes that encode apolipoprotein A1 (APOA1), ABCA1, or LCAT.

21. **Name the secondary dyslipidemias.**

The secondary dyslipidemias are serum lipid elevations that result from systemic diseases, such as diabetes mellitus, hypothyroidism, nephrotic syndrome, renal disease, obstructive liver disease, and dysproteinemias. Lipids also may be increased by medications, such as beta-blockers, diuretics, estrogens, progestins, androgens, retinoids, corticosteroids, cyclosporin A, phenothiazines, anticonvulsants, and certain antiviral agents used in the treatment of human immunodeficiency virus (HIV) infection. These disorders usually improve when the primary condition is treated or the offending drugs are discontinued.

KEY POINTS: CAUSES OF LIPID DISORDERS

1. Elevated low-density lipoprotein (LDL) cholesterol is a major risk factor for coronary artery disease (CAD).

2. Low high-density lipoprotein (HDL) cholesterol is also a significant risk factor for CAD.

3. High serum triglycerides (TGs) may not directly cause atherosclerosis but are often associated with an atherosclerotic profile, consisting of low HDL, small dense LDL particles, insulin resistance, hypertension, and abdominal obesity.

4. Serum TG levels greater than 1000 mg/dL significantly increase the risk of developing acute pancreatitis.

5. Inflammation within the atherosclerotic plaque plays a major role in plaque rupture and the occurrence of acute coronary events.

22. **What is the cause of severe elevations of serum TGs?**
TG levels above 1000 mg/dL pose a very high risk for the development of acute pancreatitis, a condition with a mortality rate of up to 10%. Most patients with such severe TG elevations have a primary TG disorder, such as FHT, FCH, or FDL, combined with a secondary disorder, most commonly poorly controlled diabetes mellitus, alcohol abuse, estrogen use, or the use of HIV medications.

23. **Summarize the revised (2004) CAD risk stratification from the Adult Treatment Panel III (ATP III) of the National Cholesterol Education Program (NCEP).**

HIGH RISK

1. Known CAD
2. CAD Risk Equivalents
   a. Peripheral arterial disease
   b. Cerebral arterial disease
   c. Abdominal aortic aneurysm
   d. Diabetes mellitus
   e. 2+ risk factors with CAD 10-year risk >20%

MODERATELY HIGH RISK

2+ risk factors with CAD 10-year risk = 10%–20%

MODERATE RISK

2+ risk factors with CAD 10-year risk <10%

LOW RISK

0–1 risk factors with CAD 10-year risk <10%

Risk factors: smoking; hypertension ($\geq$140/90); HDL <40 mg/dL; age $\geq$45 years (men), >55 years (women); CAD in first-degree relative (<55 years [men], < 65 years [women])

CAD 10-year risk calculation: http://www.nhlbi.nih.gov/guidelines/cholesterol

24. **What are the revised (2004) lipoprotein treatment goals from the ATP III?**

Patient Risk	LDL Cholesterol	Non-HDL
High risk	<70 mg/dL	<100 mg/dL
Moderately high risk	<100 mg/dL	<130 mg/dL
Moderate risk	<130 mg/dL	<160 mg/dL
Low risk	<160 mg/dL	<190 mg/dL

25. What treatment approaches are recommended for lipoprotein levels above these goals?

- LDL cholesterol <30 mg/dL above risk stratified goal: therapeutic lifestyle change (TLC)
- LDL cholesterol >30 mg/dL above risk stratified goal: medications to lower lipids
- Summary of TLC as recommended by the ATP III:

Component	Goals
Total fat	25%–35% of total calories
Saturated fat	<7% of total calories
Polyunsaturated fat	<10% of total calories
Monounsaturated fat	<20% of total calories
Carbohydrate	50%–60% of total calories
Protein	15% of total calories
Total calories	Adjust to achieve and maintain ideal body weight
Dietary fiber	20–30 g/day
Physical activity	Expend at least 200 kcal/day

26. What medications most effectively lower serum LDL cholesterol?

Medication	LDL Reduction (%)
Statins	20–60
Ezetimibe	20–25
Bile acid resins	15–25
Niacin	15–25

27. How do the currently available statin medications differ?

The statins inhibit 3-hydroxy-3-methyl-glutaryl-CoA reductase, the rate-limiting enzyme in cholesterol synthesis. Some statins are "natural" (simvastatin, pravastatin; fungal derived) and the others are synthetic. Some are more hydrophilic (pravastatin, rosuvastatin), whereas the others are more lipophilic. The main differences of clinical interest, however, are their LDL-lowering potencies. A randomized controlled trial involving 2240 patients (STELLAR; Ref. 14) reported the following results for the four most commonly used agents:

Medication	Doses (mg)	LDL Reduction (%)	HDL Increase (%)
Pravastatin	10–40	20–30	3–6
Simvastatin	10–80	28–46	5–7
Atorvastatin	10–80	37–51	2–6
Rosuvastatin	10–40	46–55	8–10

28. **What medications significantly lower TGs?**

Medication	TG Decrease (%)
Fibrates	30–50
Niacin	20–30
Statins	10–20
Fish oils	Up to 45%

29. **What medications most effectively raise serum HDL cholesterol levels?**

Medication	HDL Increase (%)
Niacin	10–25
Fibrates	10–20
Statins	5–10
Fish oils	5–10
CETP Inhibitors	>50

30. **Once a statin is being used, how effective are subsequent dose increments?**
    The initial statin dose will produce the greatest LDL cholesterol reduction. Each subsequent doubling of the statin dose will, on average, result only in an additional 6% decrease in serum LDL cholesterol. This "6% rule" is derived from numerous prospective studies.

31. **How effective and safe are combinations of lipid-lowering medications?**
    For severe cholesterol elevations, the addition of ezetimibe, niacin, or a bile acid resin to a statin will often reduce serum LDL cholesterol by an additional 20%, compared with only 6% when the statin dose is doubled. These combinations are generally safe to use, but side effects can be additive. For elevations of both cholesterol and TGs, adding a fibrate to a statin can lower the serum TG level up to 50%. However, the risk of myositis and frank rhabdomyolysis increases. Fenofibrate appears to be significantly safer than gemfibrozil when combination with a statin is considered necessary.

32. **Does aggressive cholesterol lowering therapy effectively and safely reduce the risk of coronary artery disease?**
    Clinical trials have repeatedly demonstrated the efficacy of aggressive cholesterol lowering in reducing surrogate endpoints, such as c-reactive protein (PROVE IT [Ref. 6], REVERSAL [Ref. 23]) and coronary artery plaque burden as assessed by intravascular ultrasound (REVERSAL) or coronary angiography (FATS [Ref. 4], Post CABG Study [Ref. 25]), and hard cardiovascular endpoints, such as myocardial infarction, strokes, and cardiovascular mortality in patients with (4S [Ref. 29], CARE [Ref. 28], LIPID [Ref. 20], HPS [Ref. 13], TNT [Ref. 19], PROVE IT, AVERT [Ref. 24], ALLIANCE [Ref. 16]) and without (WOSCOPS [Ref. 32], AFCAPS [Ref. 8], HPS, ASCOT-LLA [Ref. 3], CARDS [Ref. 7]) a previous history of CAD. The major safety concerns with statin therapy are hepatotoxicity and myopathy; both of these were relatively rare in the clinical trials, but occur more commonly in clinical practice in patients who require higher doses or take them in combination with other medications that may interfere with statin metabolism.

33. **Do interventions that raise serum HDL cholesterol or lower serum TGs have a significant effect on coronary events?**

HDL levels independently predicted cardiovascular events in atorvastatin-treated patients in the TNT study. A trial of combined gemfibrozil, niacin, and cholestyramine increased HDL by 36%, and decreased LDL by 26% and TGs by 50% and prevented angiographic progression of coronary stenosis, although the benefits of increasing HDL could not be distinguished from the benefits of LDL and TG reduction. Two large randomized controlled trials examined the effects of gemfibrozil in dyslipidemic patients with (VA-HIT [Ref. 27]) and without (HHS [Ref. 21]) known CAD. HDL increased by 6% to 8%, TGs decreased by 30% to 40%, and there was a significant reduction in CAD events in both studies. The FIELD study (Ref. 15) of fenofibrate in patients with type 2 diabetes, in contrast, reported a nonsignificant 11% reduction in cardiovascular events. A large trial examining torcetrapib, which increases HDL more than 50% by inhibiting the enzyme CETP, was terminated because of an increase in coronary events and mortality in treated patients. The reasons for the increase in events and mortality are still being investigated. Other CETP inhibitors are currently in development.

KEY POINTS: TREATMENT OF LIPID DISORDERS

1. Statins are the most effective low-density lipoprotein (LDL) cholesterol–lowering agents, but additional LDL reduction can be achieved by adding ezetimibe, niacin, and bile acid resins.

2. Fibrates are the most effective TG-lowering agents, but additional reductions can be achieved by adding niacin, fish oils, and high-dose statins.

3. Combined statin and fibrate therapy may be necessary when both cholesterol and TGs are significantly elevated; in such patients, it is advisable to use fenofibrate and low statin doses. Creatine kinase (CK) levels should be closely monitored.

4. The Adult Treatment Panel III (ATP III) recommends LDL goals of less than 100 mg/dL for patients with coronary artery disease (CAD) or CAD equivalents, less than 130 mg/dL for patients with two or more CAD risk factors, and less than 160 mg/dL for patients with no or one CAD risk factor. An optional LDL goal of less than 70 mg/dL may be more appropriate for the highest-risk patients.

5. The ATP III recommends non-high-density lipoprotein cholesterol goals of 30 mg/dL above the LDL cholesterol goals in patients whose serum TG levels are greater than 200 mg/dL after the LDL goal has been achieved.

34. **Should all high-risk patients be treated with lipid-lowering therapy regardless of LDL cholesterol level?**

Two large randomized controlled trials, the HPS (simvastatin) and ASCOT (atorvastatin) showed that patients at high risk of CAD events by virtue of a past history of CAD, non-CAD vascular disease, diabetes mellitus, or hypertension had a significant reduction in CAD events in response to statin therapy even when their initial LDL cholesterol levels were not elevated. In the HPS, patients whose initial serum LDL cholesterol level was less than 100 mg/dL had a significant 24% reduction in events. Whether lipid-lowering therapy should be routinely recommended in all such patients is currently a subject of debate.

35. **Is measurement of inflammatory markers a useful tool in CAD risk assessment?**

Inflammation within an atherosclerotic plaque makes the plaque more likely to rupture, precipitating an acute ischemic event. Highly sensitive C-reactive protein (hsCRP), a nonspecific marker of inflammation, appears to predict CAD risk, as do LDL cholesterol levels. Measurement of LDL cholesterol and hsCRP together has even greater predictive value. This information can be useful to providers when making decisions about which patients to treat more aggressively but need not be performed routinely in all patients. Other markers, such as myeloperoxidase (MPO) and glutathione peroxidase 1 (GTX-1), are currently under investigation.

36. **Should we be using measurements of lipoprotein size and number?**
Lipoprotein size and number can now be assessed by a variety of commercially available techniques. These analyses provide additional information about the atherogenicity of a lipoprotein profile. The cost-effectiveness of obtaining this additional information has not yet been demonstrated. Decisions regarding the need for treatment and the choice of agents can be made on the basis of the clinical risk factor profile and standard lipid profile in the majority of patients. Therefore these additional tests should be limited to situations in which they are likely to have a clear impact on the choice and aggressiveness of therapy.

37. **How should the patient with severe hypertriglyceridemia be managed?**
Serum TG levels above 1000 mg/dL must be lowered quickly because of the high risk of precipitating acute pancreatitis. Medications alone are not effective when TG levels are this high. Patients must immediately be placed on a very low fat (less than 5% fat) diet until the TG level is less than 1000 mg/dL. Such a diet lowers serum TGs approximately 20% each day. Contributing factors, most commonly uncontrolled diabetes mellitus, alcohol abuse, estrogen use, and HIV medications, must simultaneously be addressed. After serum TG levels are less than 1000 mg/dL, the most effective medications to reduce serum TGs further are the fibrates. If these medications do not lower serum TG sufficiently, niacin, fish oils, or a statin may be added to the regimen.

BIBLIOGRAPHY

1. Ashen MD, Blumenthal RS: Low HDL cholesterol levels. N Engl J Med 353:1252–1260, 2005.

2. Barter PJ, Caulfield M, Erikssen M, et al: Effects of torcetrapib in patients at high risk for coronary events. N Engl J Med 357:2109–2122, 2007.

3. Barter P, Gotto AM, LaRosa JC, et al: HDL cholesterol, very low levels of LDL cholesterol, and cardiovascular events. N Engl J Med 357:1301–1310, 2007.

4. Brown G, Albers JJ, Fisher LD, et al: Regression of coronary artery disease as a result of lipid-lowering therapy in men with high levels of apolipoprotein B. N Engl J Med 323:1289–1296, 1990. (FATS)

5. Brunzell JD: Hypertriglyceridemia. N Engl J Med 357:1009–1017, 2007.

6. Cannon CP et al: Intensive versus moderate lipid lowering with statins after acute coronary syndromes (Prove It Trial). N Engl J Med 350:1495–1504, 2004. (PROVE IT)

7. Colhoun HM, Betteridge DJ, Durrington PN, et al: Primary prevention of cardiovascular disease with atorvastatin in type 2 diabetes in the Collaborative Atorvastatin Diabetes Study (CARDS): multicentre randomised placebo-controlled trial. Lancet 364:685–696, 2004. (CARDS)

8. Downs JR, Clearfield M, Weis S, et al: Primary prevention of acute coronary events with lovastatin in men and women with average cholesterol levels: Results of AFCAPS/TexCAPS. Air Force/Texas Coronary Atherosclerosis Prevention Study. JAMA 279:1615–1622, 1995. (AFCAPS)

9. Executive Summary of the Third Report of the National Education Program (NCEP) Expert Panel on Detection, Evaluation, and Treatment of High Blood Cholesterol in Adults (Adult Treatment Panel III). JAMA 285:2486–2497, 2001.

10. Ford I, Murray H, Packard CJ, et al. Long-term follow-up of the West of Scotland Coronary Prevention Study. N Engl J Med 357:1477–1486, 2007.

11. Garg A, Simha V: Update on dyslipidemia. J Clin Endocrinol Metab 92:1581–1589, 2007.

12. Grundy SM, Cleeman JI, Merz CN, et al: Implications of recent clinical trials for the National Cholesterol Education Program Adult Treatment Panel III Guidelines. Circulation 110:227–239, 2004.

13. Heart Protection Collaborative Group: MRC/BHF Heart Protection Study of cholesterol lowering with simvastatin in 20,536 high-risk individuals: a randomized placebo-controlled trial. Lancet 360: 7–22, 2002 (HPS).

14. Jones PH, Davidson MH, Stein EA, et al: Comparison of the efficacy and safety of rosuvastatin versus atorvastatin, simvastatin, and pravastatin across doses. Am J Cardiol 93:152–160, 2003. (STELLAR)

15. Keech A, Simes RJ, Barter P, et al: Effects of long-term fenofibrate therapy on cardiovascular events in 9795 people with type 2 diabetes mellitus (the Field Study): randomised controlled trial. Lancet 366:1849–1861, 2005. (FIELD Study)

16. Koren MJ, Hunninghake DB, et al: Clinical outcomes in managed care patients with coronary heart disease treated aggressively in lipid lowering disease management clinics. J Am Coll Cardiol 44:1772–1779, 2004. (ALLIANCE)

17. Kreisberg RA, Oberman A: Medical management of hyperlipidemia/dyslipidemia. J Clin Endocrinol Metab 88:2445–2461, 2003.

18. Laine C, Goldmann D, Kopin LA, Pearson TA. In the clinic: dyslipidemia. Ann Intern Med Sep 4 : ITC9-1–ITC9-14, 2007.

19. LaRosa J, Grundy SM, Waters DD, et al: Intensive lipid lowering with atorvastatin in patients with stable coronary disease. N Engl J Med 352:1425–1435, 2005. (TNT)

20. Lipid Study Group: Prevention of cardiovascular events and death with pravastatin in patients with coronary heart disease and a broad range of initial cholesterol levels. N Engl J Med 339:1349–1357, 1998. (LIPID)

21. Manninen V, Elo MO, Frick MH, et al. Lipid alteration and decline in the incidence of coronary heart disease in the Helsinki Heart Study. JAMA 260:641–651, 1988. (HHS)

22. Navab M, Anantharamaiah GM, Reddy ST, et al: Mechanisms of disease: proatherogenic HDL—an evolving field. Nat Clin Pract Endocrinol Metab 2: 504–511, 2006.

23. Nissen SE et al: Effect of intensive compared with moderate lipid-lowering therapy on progression of coronary atherosclerosis (reversal trial). JAMA 291:1071–1080, 2004. (REVERSAL)

24. Pitt B, Waters D, Brown WV, et al: Aggressive lipid-lowering therapy compared with angioplasty in stable coronary artery disease. N Engl J Med 341:70–76, 1999. (AVERT)

25. Post Coronary Artery Bypass Graft Trial Investigators: The effect of aggressive lowering of low-density lipoprotein cholesterol levels and low-dose anticoagulation on obstructive changes in saphenous-vein coronary-artery bypass grafts. N Engl J Med 336:153–162, 1997.

26. Ridker PM, Hennekens CH, Buring JE, Rifai N: C-reactive protein and other markers of inflammation in the prediction of cardiovascular disease in women. N Engl J Med 342:836–843, 2000.

27. Rubins HB, Robins SJ, Collins D, et al: Gemfibrozil for the secondary prevention of coronary heart disease in men with low levels of high-density lipoprotein cholesterol. N Engl J Med 341:410–418, 1999. (VA-HIT)

28. Sacks FM, Pfeffer MA, Moye LA, et al: The effect of pravastatin on coronary events after myocardial infarction in patients with average cholesterol levels. N Engl J Med 335:1001–1009, 1996. (CARE)

29. Scandinavian Simvastatin Survival Study Group: Randomized trial of cholesterol lowering in 4444 patients with coronary heart disease: The Scandinavian Simvastatin Survival Study (4S). Lancet 344:1383–1389, 1994. (4S)

30. Scanu AM: Lipoprotein(a) and atherosclerosis. Ann Intern Med 115:209–218, 1991.

31. Sever PS, Dahlof B, Poulter NR, et al: Prevention of coronary and stroke events with atorvastatin in hypertensive patients who have average or lower than average cholesterol concentrations, in the Anglo-22. Scandinavian Cardiac Outcomes Trial-Lipid Lowering Arm (ASCOT-LLA): A multicenter randomized controlled trial.Lancet 361:1149–1158, 2003. (ASCOT-LLA)

32. Shepherd J, Cobbe SM, Ford I, et al: Prevention of coronary heart disease with pravastatin in men with hypercholesterolemia. N Engl J Med 333:1301–1307, 1995. (WOSCOPS)

33. Third Report of the National Education Program (NCEP) Expert Panel on Detection, Evaluation, and Treatment of High Blood Cholesterol in Adults (Adult Treatment Panel III) final report. Circulation 106:3143–3421, 2002.

34. Tirosh A, Rudich A, Shochat T, et al: Changes in triglyceride levels and risk for coronary heart disease in young men. Ann Intern Med 147:377–385, 2007.

35. Whitney EJ, Krasuski RA, Personius BE, et al: A randomized trial of a strategy for increasing high density lipoprotein cholesterol levels: effects on progression of coronary heart disease. Ann Intern Med 142:95–104, 2005.

CHAPTER 7

OBESITY

Kristin A. Harmon and Daniel H. Bessesen

1. **Define the terms "overweight" and "obesity."**
   Overweight and obesity are defined as degrees of excess weight that are associated with increases in morbidity and mortality. In 1998, the National Heart, Lung, and Blood Institute of the National Institutes of Health (NIH) published guidelines on the diagnosis and treatment of overweight and obesity. The expert panel advocated using specific body mass index (BMI) cutoff points to diagnose both conditions. The BMI is calculated by dividing a person's weight in kilograms by his or her height in meters squared. A BMI (kg/m^2) of 25 or less is normal; 25 to 29.9, overweight; 30 to 34.9, mild obesity; 35 to 39.9, moderate obesity; and greater than 40, severe or morbid obesity.

2. **Does fat distribution affect the assessment of risk in an overweight or obese patient?**
   Yes. Accumulation of excessive adipose tissue in a central- or upper-body distribution (android or male pattern) is associated with a greater risk of adverse metabolic health consequences than lower-body obesity (gynoid or female pattern). Abdominal adiposity is an independent predictor of risk for diabetes, hypertension, coronary artery disease, and dyslipidemia. It appears that the absolute amount of intra-abdominal or visceral fat is most closely linked to these adverse health risks.

3. **Explain the role of waist circumference in risk stratification.**
   For this reason, the waist circumference is now the favored measure for risk stratification on the basis of fat distribution. Men with a waist circumference greater than 40 inches (>102 cm) and women whose waist circumference is greater than 35 in. (>88 cm) have increased risk. Waist circumference is most useful for risk stratification in people with a BMI between 25 and 30 kg/m^2. In this intermediate-risk group, those with increased waist circumference should undertake greater efforts directed at preventing further weight gain, whereas those with a smaller waist circumference can be reassured that their weight does not pose major health hazards.

4. **How is waist circumference measured?**
   Waist circumference should be measured with a tape measure parallel to the floor at the level of the iliac crest at the end of a relaxed expiration.

5. **What adverse health consequences are associated with obesity?**
   Obesity is clearly associated with diabetes, hypertension, hyperlipidemia, coronary artery disease, degenerative arthritis, gallbladder disease, and cancer of the endometrium, breast, prostate, and colon. It has also been associated with urinary incontinence, gastroesophageal reflux, infertility, congestive heart failure and sleep apnea. The incidence of these conditions rises steadily as body weight increases (Figs. 7-1 and 7-2). Risks increase with even modest weight gain. Health risks are magnified with advancing age and a positive family history of obesity-related diseases.

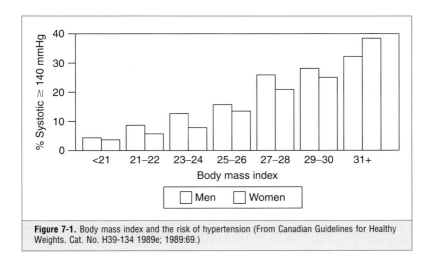

Figure 7-1. Body mass index and the risk of hypertension (From Canadian Guidelines for Healthy Weights. Cat. No. H39-134 1989e; 1989:69.)

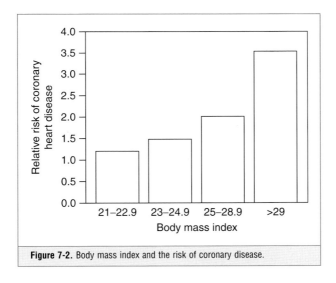

Figure 7-2. Body mass index and the risk of coronary disease.

6. **Summarize the economic consequences of obesity.**
   The total direct and indirect health care costs associated with obesity were estimated to be $117 billion for 2001. These costs represented 9.1% of all medical expenditures in the United States. The costs associated with caring for an obese adult are 37% higher than those for a normal-weight individual. In addition, the NIH estimated that Americans pay $44 billion for weight loss products and services.

7. **What are the psychological complications of obesity?**
   Situational depression and anxiety related to obesity are common. The obese person may suffer from discrimination that contributes further to difficulty with poor self-image and social isolation. Severely obese people may avoid leaving their home for fear of ridicule. It may be difficult in some patients to determine whether depression is accelerating weight gain or

whether weight gain is exacerbating an underlying depression, but treating both conditions may improve quality of life. It may be difficult or impossible for a care provider who has never experienced discrimination based on obesity to understand the scope of these effects.

8. **How common is obesity?**

   Obesity has reached epidemic proportions in the United States. The National Health and Nutrition Examination Survey (NHANES) conducted by the federal government uses direct measures of height and weight in a representative sample of Americans to estimate the prevalence of obesity. The most recent published data from the NHANES showed that in 2003 to 2004, 32.2% of adults were obese as defined by a BMI greater than 30 kg/m^2. The prevalence of overweight was found to be 66.3%. The prevalence of extreme obesity (BMI >40 kg/m^2) was found to be 4.8%. The prevalence of overweight in U.S. children and adolescents aged 2 to 19 years was found to be 17.1%. The prevalence of overweight among children and adolescents and obesity among men increased significantly between 1999 and 2004. However, among adult women, no significant increase in the prevalence of obesity was observed.

9. **What caused the dramatic rise in the prevalence of obesity between 1980 and 2004?**

   The prevalence of obesity has indeed risen over a short period; it seems that the primary culprit is a changing environment that promotes increased food intake and reduced physical activity. This statement should not be taken to mean, however, that body weight is not subject to physiologic regulation. The control of body weight is complex with multiple interrelated systems controlling caloric intake, macronutrient content of the diet, energy expenditure, and fuel metabolism.

10. **Describe the current model for obesity as a chronic disease.**

    Professionals are increasingly viewing obesity as a chronic, often progressive metabolic disease much like diabetes or hypertension. This model requires a conceptual shift from the previous widely held belief that obesity is simply a cosmetic or behavioral problem. Development of obesity requires a period of positive energy balance during which energy intake exceeds energy expenditure. Maintaining energy balance is one of the most important jobs of any organism. Between ages 20 and 60 years, the average human eats more than 32 tons of food. A sustained negative imbalance between energy intake and expenditure is potentially life threatening within a relatively short time. To maintain energy balance, the organism must assess energy stores within the body; assess the nutrient content of the diet; determine whether the body is in negative energy or nutrient balance; and adjust hormone levels, energy expenditure, nutrient movement, and ingestive behavior in response to these assessments.

11. **Do abnormal genes cause obesity?**

    Obesity is clearly more common in people who have family members who are also obese. The problem of human obesity involves an interaction between genetic susceptibility and environmental triggers. The genes that we possess to regulate body weight evolved somewhere between 200,000 and 1 million years ago. The environmental factors controlling nutrient acquisition and habitual physical activity were dramatically different then. Although a few cases of human obesity caused by single gene mutations have been found, most human obesity appears to be polygenic, involving probably 10 to 30 genes in any individual. Genetics appears to be responsible for 20% to 40% of the variance in weight in most populations.

12. **What is leptin?**

    Leptin is a hormone secreted by adipose tissue. It was discovered in 1994. Its name comes from the Greek word *leptos* meaning thin. Leptin was cloned from the ob/ob mouse model of obesity that has a genetic mutation resulting in leptin deficiency. In ob/ob mice, the administration of recombinant leptin produces sustained weight loss through both decreases in food intake and increases in energy expenditure. The weight loss occurs largely from fat mass with little loss in lean body mass.

13. **Does leptin deficiency cause human obesity?**
Although leptin is produced in humans, there are only a handful of cases in which leptin deficiency was identified as the cause of human obesity. In fact, leptin levels are typically increased in obese compared with lean humans in proportion to their increased fat mass. Studies in which recombinant human leptin was administered to obese humans produced minimal weight loss. These findings suggest that common forms of human obesity are associated with leptin resistance, not leptin deficiency.

14. **Explain how the melanocortin system is involved in weight regulation.**
Alpha melanocortin (MSH) is one of the hormone products of the POMC gene. This neuropeptide acts in the hypothalamus on melanocortin receptors, particularly the MC4-R subtype to regulate body weight. By stimulating the MC4-R, Alpha-MSH inhibits food intake, whereas the natural antagonist agouti-related peptide (AGRP), also made in the hypothalamus, stimulates food intake. Several companies now have drugs that interact with the MC4-R as agonists. These drugs decrease food intake in rats and reduce body weight. There is hope that they may be useful in treating human obesity in the future.

15. **What is ghrelin?**
Ghrelin is a hormone produced by the stomach and proximal small intestine that appears to regulate appetite. Ghrelin levels rise before meals and promptly fall following food intake. Self-reported hunger mirrors serum ghrelin levels. Twenty-four-hour ghrelin levels rise when people go on an energy-restricted diet and are dramatically reduced after gastric bypass surgery. Ghrelin has been described as a "hunger hormone" and is another possible target for weight loss drugs.

16. **Does a decrease in energy expenditure play a role in the development of obesity?**
The development of obesity requires an imbalance between caloric intake and caloric expenditure. For fat mass to increase, there must be an imbalance between the amount of fat deposited compared with the amount of fat oxidized. One possibility is that people become obese because of a reduction in their energy expenditure. Despite the common idea that a "low metabolic rate" predisposes to obesity, there is little evidence that this is true.

17. **What are the components of energy expenditure.**
   1. Basal metabolic rate (BMR): The amount of energy necessary to keep sodium and potassium where they belong, to keep the body warm, to pump blood, to breathe, and to perform other basic body functions.
   2. Physical activity energy expenditure (PAEE): This is the most variable component. It can account for as little as 10% to 20% of total energy expenditure in people who are bedridden or as much as 60% to 80% of total energy expenditure in training athletes. PAEE increases with planned physical activity or with activities of daily living, such as stair climbing or even fidgeting. The unconscious component of physical activity has been termed nonexercise activity thermogenesis and may be a regulated parameter.
   3. Thermic effect of food: A relatively small component (5% to 10%) that represents the increase in energy expenditure that occurs after the ingestion of a meal.

18. **Explain the concept of energy balance.**
When an individual is weight stable, total daily energy expenditure equals total daily energy intake. Total energy expenditure is linearly related to lean body mass. Studies using indirect calorimetry have shown that obese people clearly consume more calories than lean people. The obese person who says that he or she eats only a small salad my be telling the truth in the

short term, but over longer periods, high caloric intakes are required to maintain the obese state. Although reduced levels of PAEE may predispose to obesity, BMR is not reduced in obese people. The central cause of obesity is the failure to couple energy intake to energy expenditure accurately over time.

19. **What options are available for treating the obese patient?**
   The treatment options for an overweight or obese patient include diet, exercise, pharmacotherapy, surgery, and combinations of these modalities. The specific modality should be based on the individual's BMI and associated health problems. A more aggressive treatment approach is warranted in those whose BMI is higher and those with adverse health consequences. Behavioral approaches can be advocated for all overweight and obese patients. Pharmacologic treatment should be considered in those whose BMI is greater than 27 kg/m^2 in the presence of medical complications or greater than 30 kg/m^2 in the absence of medical complications. Surgical treatment should be reserved for those with a BMI greater than 40 kg/m^2, or a BMI greater than 35 with comorbidities.

20. **What is the goal of a weight loss program?**
   Before discussing the treatment options with a patient, it is important to decide the goal of the treatment program. Many obese patients have unrealistic expectations about the amount of weight that they might lose through a weight loss program. Most would like to achieve ideal body weight and are disappointed if they lose only 5% to 10% of their initial weight. These desires stand in stark contrast to the magnitude of weight loss that has been seen with all treatment modalities short of bariatric surgery. The most effective diet, exercise, or drug treatment programs available result in roughly a 10% weight loss in most people.

21. **Is a 5% to 10% reduction helpful in terms of health improvement?**
   This degree of weight reduction has been associated with improvements in health-related measures, such as lower blood pressure, reductions in low-density lipoprotein (LDL) cholesterol levels, improved functional capacity, and a markedly reduced risk of developing diabetes. Most experts now believe that a sustained 5% to 10% weight loss (e.g, a weight loss of 11–12 lb for someone who initially weighted 220 lb) is a realistic goal with probable medical benefits. Alternatively, prevention of further weight gain may be a reasonable and attainable goal, or the health care provider may encourage the patient to focus on eating and activity habits and not on a weight goal at all.

22. **How can a patient's readiness to change his or her diet or physical activity be assessed?**
   Stages of change theory can help the clinician focus counseling activities within the context of a brief office visit. Prochazka has hypothesized six predictable stages through which a person passes before he or she is able to change long-standing behaviors, such as diet, physical activity patterns, or smoking: precontemplative, contemplative planning, action, maintenance, and relapse. Identifying the stage that the patient is in and targeting counseling efforts to that stage may improve the effectiveness of the counseling activities.

23. **Define the precontemplative stage.**
   In this stage, people are not even thinking about changing their behavior. The issue is generally lack of perceived benefits to behavior change. For such people, perhaps a simple statement about the association between obesity and adverse health consequences may be appropriate, similar to what would be said about smoking cessation.

24. **What is the contemplative stage?**
   People in this stage acknowledge the potential benefits of behavior change but have not yet decided what they are going to do. They are "thinking about it." The important issues to discuss during this stage are perceived barriers to behavior change. Lack of time, lack of money, or a lack of sense of control may be preventing progress.

25. What happens in the relapse stage?

People in this stage have reverted to a previous pattern of behavior. They may feel like they will always fail. They may say, "I've tried diets. They never work for me." People in the relapse stage feel frustrated and may make the care provider feel frustrated as well. Counseling time should acknowledge and reward previous successes. The discussion should also explore what happened in the previous efforts. Can the patient learn from past efforts? Why did the patient fail? Were expectations too high? Were the changes too great? Where did the patient succeed? What would be reasonable new goals?

26. What is "motivational interviewing," and how is it used in counseling an obese patient?

Motivational interviewing is a counseling style that was developed for use with alcoholics. It is based on the idea that behavior change only occurs when individuals overcome their ambivalence. The method is useful when interacting with patients who are ambivalent about changing their diet or physical activity behaviors. The strategies used focus on resolving this ambivalence by having patients explore reasons why they want to change and reasons why they find their current behavior more comfortable.

27. Discuss the role of diet in the treatment of the obese patient.

The mainstays of dietary modification in weight loss therapy have been diets low in fat and reduced in calories. Compelling evidence in favor of this approach comes from the Diabetes Prevention Project and the Finnish Diabetes Prevention Trial. Whatever changes the person makes must be sustainable to be beneficial. The clinician should assess the current diet with a good nutritional history, which may involve a verbal 24- or 72-hour diet recall. Alternatively, the patient may keep a written 5- to 7-day food diary. Assessing meal pattern is important, because many people skip breakfast and eat lunch erratically. Attention should be paid to how often the person eats out, especially fast food. Small, gradual changes may be more successful than drastic ones.

28. Should patients be encouraged to attend a commercial weight loss program?

Yes. Most people know what they should eat. The problem is that they either do not pay attention to what they eat or do not find a "good diet" palatable. Many of the settings in which care is provided do not allow the teaching of sophisticated behavioral modification techniques. The use of commercial programs, such as Weight Watchers, can provide reasonable nutritional counseling along with social support. Many patients are surprised at the cost of these programs, which may be a deterrent to their continued use. However, this kind of program involves no risk and may be cheaper in the long term than pharmacologic treatment. The scientific literature supports the notion that for many people, commercial weight loss programs are a reasonable option.

29. Are meal replacements useful in a weight loss program?

For some people, it is difficult to control calories through self-selected meals. Often time is not available for food preparation, and convenience overrides health concerns. For such people, meal replacements, which are reduced-calorie, nutritionally complete meals, are a reasonable option with scientifically proven effectiveness if used as a long-term strategy. In fact, this approach is currently used in the NIH-funded Look Ahead Trial, which is examining the health benefits of long-term weight loss.

30. What is a very low-caloric diet? When should its use be considered?

A very low-caloric diet (VLCD) is a nutritionally complete diet of 800 kcal/day that produces rapid weight loss. Commercially available products typically consist of liquid meals that have been supplemented with essential amino acids, essential fatty acids, vitamins, and micronutrients taken 3 to 4 times per day. Experienced medical teams should administer VLCDs, and when used in this manner, complications are rare. Long-term weight loss with VLCDs is no better than with other dietary programs. For this reason, their usefulness is limited. They may be helpful for the patient who needs short-term weight loss for a diagnostic or surgical procedure.

31. What is the Atkins diet? Does it work?
The Atkins diet is a severely carbohydrate-restricted (<20 g/day during the induction phase) diet. The severe carbohydrate restriction produces what Dr. Robert Atkins calls "benign dietary ketosis," which he argues suppresses appetite. The diet has few other restrictions. Several studies support the idea that the Atkins diet produces more weight loss than a low-fat diet over 6 months but that long-term weight loss is no better. The diet can be difficult for people to adhere to long term. These studies have shown no adverse effects on blood lipid levels.

KEY POINTS: OBESITY

1. Obesity is defined as a body mass index greater than 30 kg/m^2.

2. A 5% to 10% weight loss is a good goal with known health benefits.

3. Three randomized controlled clinical trails show that over 6 to 12 months, there are no adverse effects on lipids from the Atkins diet plan.

4. Sibutramine, orlistat, and phentermine are currently Food and Drug Administration–approved medications to help overweight and obese patients lose weight.

5. The average weight loss following gastric bypass surgery is 30%.

32. Describe the Zone Diet.
The Zone Diet contains 30% protein, 30% fat, and 40% carbohydrate. The goal is not weight loss per se but rather "optimizing" health. Dr. Barry Sears's thesis is that foods are like drugs in that they have dose-response curves. Therefore, one can optimize metabolism by eating a diet that has optimal ratios of fat, carbohydrate, and protein. Like Atkins, Sears believes that the excessive emphasis on low-fat, high-carbohydrate diets is partly responsible for the increased prevalence of obesity.

33. Discuss the Ornish diet.
Dr. Dean Ornish was looking for an alternative to bypass surgery for patients with coronary artery disease that was based on nutrition and lifestyle change. His target audience is not obese people but rather those with known coronary artery disease. The Ornish diet is not a weight loss diet. It is a "lifestyle change program" incorporating diet (specifically, a very low-fat [10% fat, 10% protein] vegetarian diet) with group interactions designed to increase physical activity and decrease "type A" behaviors. Group psychological support, smoking cessation, yoga-based physical activities, and meditation are part of this program. As currently practiced, it is a labor intensive program for the care provider and participants.

34. What is the South Beach Diet?
This dietary program was developed by a cardiologist in Florida, who advocates a diet somewhat restricted in carbohydrate, especially refined carbohydrates, but believes that low glycemic index carbohydrate sources are beneficial. He advocates increased consumption of monounsaturated fats, omega-3 fatty acids, and nuts. He gave these principles to several chefs at fashionable restaurants in South Beach. The dietary principles are reasonable; the recipes look quite appetizing; and the program is clearly defined.

35. Which popular diet book is the "best"?
Several recent studies have compared a number of popular diet books with commercial programs and older diet manuals. The results of these studies suggest that there is no

one diet that is best. It appears that the most important factor in the success of a diet is the person's ability to adhere to the diet. Those who can stick to the diet, no matter what the diet is, will have the most weight loss. This means that health care providers should probably not take a rigid view of what constitutes the "best diet." Rather, what is important is to explore what patients are most likely to tolerate—what they feel will work best for them. Good texts include *The LEARN Manual for Weight Control* by Dr. Kelly Brownell. This book represents the best of his behavioral weight loss program. However, many patients find it dull. Two other books address behavioral issues in dieting: *The Personality Type Diet* by Dr. Robert Kushner and *The Ultimate Weight Solution* by Dr. Phil McGraw address these issues in a more reader-friendly manner. Both books give reasonable and readable advice about a variety of important behavioral topics related to diet and exercise and can be recommended to patients.

36. **What drugs are available to treat obesity?**
    - Phentermine (Adipex-P, Fastin, Ionamin)
    - Orlistat (Xenical, Alli)
    - Sibutramine (Meridia)

37. **Are phentermine and amphetamine related?**
    Yes, phentermine is chemically related to amphetamine and works predominantly on the neurotransmitter norepinephrine to reduce appetite. The addictive effects of amphetamine are thought to be due to its actions on the neurotransmitter dopamine. Phentermine has substantially fewer dopaminergic effects than amphetamine and thus has minimal potential for addiction.

38. **Is phentermine effective? How much does it cost?**
    Compared with placebo, it produces roughly a 5% to 8% weight loss in 50% to 60% of those who take it. The average cost is about $35 a month. The dose used ranges from 15 to 37.5 mg/day. It is the most widely prescribed weight loss medication.

39. **Discuss the side effects of phentermine.**
    Phentermine is a central stimulant and can cause hypertension, tachycardia, nervousness, headache, difficulty sleeping, and tremor in some people. It should not be used in people with poorly controlled hypertension. Blood pressure should be monitored closely after initiation of this medicine. There is no evidence that, when used alone (in contrast to the combination of phentermine with fenfluramine), it is associated with cardiac valvular or pulmonary vascular toxicity. Phentermine is only approved by the Food and Drug Administration (FDA) for 3-month use. There are no long-term studies of its safety and efficacy. However, it has been widely prescribed longer than any other weight loss agent, and there has been no evidence of serious side effects.

40. **How does orlistat work? What is the usual dose? How much does it cost?**
    Orlistat is a pancreatic lipase inhibitor. At the prescription strength of 120 mg three times a day with meals, it reduces the absorption of dietary fat by roughly 30% by inhibiting the enzyme responsible for the fat digestion. The average weight loss seen is about 7% to 8%. This medication may be preferred in people currently using a serotonin-specific reuptake inhibitor (SSRI). In spring 2007, a 60-mg strength was approved by the FDA for over-the-counter sale. This strength is less effective than the prescription strength, giving roughly a 2% to 4% weight loss. The average wholesale price for the prescription strength is $120/month. The over the counter strength costs roughly half that amount.

41. **What are the side effects of orlistat?**
    The main side effects are due to the malabsorption of fat. Patients who eat a high-fat meal experience greasy stools and may even have problems with incontinence of stool. If the patient

chooses to skip the medication, he or she can eat a high-fat meal without side effects and without the benefit that the medication would otherwise provide. The FDA has approved orlistat for long-term use, and there is no specific mention in the package insert of when it should be stopped. Because of the potential to cause fat-soluble vitamin deficiencies, patients should be instructed to take a multiple vitamin daily. Orlistat should be used with caution in those taking coumadin (warfarin) and is contraindicated in those on cyclosporin.

42. How does sibutramine work?

Sibutramine is a combination norepinephrine and serotonin reuptake blocker. The effect is to increase satiety, helping the patient "feel the end of the meal." Unlike fenfluramine and dexfenfluramine, it has no serotonin-releasing action and therefore is pharmacologically more like the SSRIs that are widely prescribed for the treatment of depression.

43. How effective is sibutramine? How much does it cost?

Taken at doses ranging from 10 to 15 mg/day, sibutramine produces weight loss in the range of 5% to 8%. Sibutramine is currently available for roughly $100/month.

44. Discuss the side effects of sibutramine.

Sibutramine has been associated with an increase in blood pressure in some people particularly at higher doses. It should not be used in people with poorly controlled hypertension. Blood pressure should be monitored closely after initiation of this medicine. The most common side effects are dry mouth, headache, nervousness, and difficulty falling asleep. However, these side effects are generally well tolerated. Sibutramine has been widely used, and no evidence indicates that its use is associated with serious side effects, such as valvular heart disease or pulmonary hypertension. The FDA has approved it for 1-year treatment, with longer use to be decided by physician and patient. Two-year safety and efficacy data have been published.

45. Discuss the role of bupropion in the treatment of obesity.

A number of studies demonstrate that bupropion can produce gradual weight loss over as long as 1 year in many people. This medication is not FDA approved for weight loss. Bupropion may be useful in obese patients with depression severe enough to warrant pharmacotherapy.

46. Does topiramate have a role in the treatment of obesity?

Topiramate is FDA approved for the treatment of seizure disorder and migraine. It has been associated with weight loss in the range of 8% to 12%. Studies designed to show weight loss benefits were stopped because of neurological side effects (numbness, forgetfulness, difficulty thinking). If a person has a seizure disorder or migraines requiring medication and is also obese, this may be a good alternative. It should not be prescribed for weight loss only.

47. How long will a weight loss medication need to be taken?

Medications used to promote weight loss will work only as long as they are taken. If a patient loses weight while taking a medication and then stops using it, he or she is likely to regain the lost weight. If a physician and a patient decide to try a weight loss medication, it should be taken for a minimum of 3 months to determine whether the patient will lose at least 5% to 8% of his or her weight. Then some form of chronic use should be considered, given the available information about the risks and potential benefits of the medication. There are also data supporting the intermittent use of weight loss medications.

48. Discuss the role of exercise in a weight loss program.

Increased physical activity appears to be a central part of a successful weight loss program. Although exercise does not produce much added weight loss over diet alone in the short run, it appears to be extremely important in maintaining the reduced state. The National Weight Control Registry is a group of 3000 people who were identified because they successfully lost 30 lb and kept it off for a least 1 year. They self-report 2000 calories/week of planned physical activity (60–80 min/day on most days of the week). A discussion of physical activity should begin with a physical activity history. Ask about the frequency of engaging in planned physical activity. Then ask about hours per day of television viewing, computer time, and other sedentary activities. Finally, discuss activities of daily living, including work-related activities. Assess the individual's readiness to change his or her physical activity.

49. **How much physical activity is necessary to lose weight and maintain a reduced weight?**
    The American Heart Association and the American College of Sports Medicine recommend that all healthy Americans accumulate at least 30 minutes of moderate intensity physical activity 5 days per week. This recommendation is not for weight loss but is designed to maintain health and reduce the risk of chronic disease. Increasing evidence suggests that it may take 60 to 90 minutes per day of moderate intensity exercise to promote and maintain weight loss.

50. **What are pedometers? How are they used?**
    Pedometers are small devices that clip to the waistband of clothing. They can be used both to assess usual physical activity and to make and monitor physical activity goals. The usual number of steps taken by an average person is 6000/day. The recommended number of steps to prevent weight gain is 10,000 steps/day. People in the National Weight Control Registry using physical activity to maintain a reduced obese state average 12,000 steps/day.

51. **What are the two categories of weight loss surgeries?**
    Restrictive and restrictive-malabsorptive. Restrictive surgeries limit the amount of food the stomach can hold and slow the rate of gastric emptying. The most commonly performed restrictive operation is the laparoscopic adjustable silicone gastric banding (Lap-Band). The restrictive-malabsorptive bypass procedures combine the elements of gastric restriction and selective malabsorption. The Roux-en-Y gastric bypass (RYGB) is the most commonly performed and accepted bypass procedure and may be performed with an open incision or laparoscopically. The malabsorptive approach produces more rapid and profound weight loss, but it also puts patients at risk of complications, such as vitamin deficiencies and protein-energy malnutrition. Restrictive procedures are considered simpler and safer but may result in less long-term weight loss.

52. **Who are good candidates for surgical treatment of obesity?**
    Patients with a BMI greater than 35 kg/m^2 with comorbidities or BMI greater than 40 kg/m^2 without comorbidities; patients aged 20 to 60; patients with comorbidities such as diabetes, sleep apnea, reflux, hypertension, or degenerative joint disease (DJD); patients with a family history of comorbidities; patients who have failed other forms of therapy; and patients with no serious cardiac, pulmonary, or psychiatric disease.

53. **What are the expected outcomes and health benefits of weight loss surgery?**
    Bariatric surgery is the most effective weight loss treatment available for those with clinically severe obesity. In a meta-analysis by Buchwald et al, the overall percentage of excess weight loss for all surgery types was 61.2%. This translates into roughly a 30% loss compared with preoperative weight. Weight loss is greater after the combined restrictive-malabsorptive procedures compared with the restrictive procedures. In the meta-analysis by Buchwald et al, diabetes completely resolved in 77% of patients and resolved or improved in 86% of patients following bariatric surgery. Two other recently published series by Schauer et al and Sugerman

et al report resolution of diabetes in 83% and 86%, respectively. In the meta-analysis by Buchwald et al, hyperlipidemia improved in 70% or more of the patients, hypertension resolved in 62% and resolved or improved in 79% of the patients, and obstructive sleep apnea resolved in 86% of the patients. Hypertension improves in many patients but is more resistant to improvement than diabetes or sleep apnea.

54. What is the mortality rate associated with bariatric surgery?
The surgical mortality rate associated with bariatric surgery is 0.1% to 2.0%. In the meta-analysis by Buchwald et al, mortality at 30 or less days was 0.1% for the purely restrictive procedures, 0.5% in patients undergoing gastric bypass procedures, and 1.1% in patients undergoing biliopancreatic diversion or duodenal switch procedures. Common causes of death among patients undergoing bariatric surgery include pulmonary embolism and anastomotic leaks. Factors that have been found to contribute to increased mortality include lack of experience on the part of the surgeon or the program, advanced patient age, male sex, severe obesity (BMI $\geq$50), and coexisting conditions. Risk is higher in low-volume programs.

55. What are the most common complications of bariatric surgery?
Nonfatal perioperative complications include venous thromboembolism, anastomotic leaks, wound infections, bleeding, incidental splenectomy, incisional and internal hernias, and early small bowel obstruction. Stomal stenosis or marginal ulcers (occurring in 5% to 15% of patients) present as prolonged nausea and vomiting after eating or inability to advance the diet to solid foods. These complications are treated by endoscopic balloon dilatation and acid suppression therapy, respectively. Abdominal and incisional hernias occur in roughly 30% of patients following open RYGB. Dumping syndrome caused by simple sugar intake, especially added sugars, has been reported in as many as 76% of the RYGB patients. To prevent dumping syndrome, patients should be encouraged to consume frequent, small meals and to avoid fruit juices and added sugars.

56. What is a rare cause of hypoglycemia following RYGB?
Nesidioblastosis, or beta-cell hyperplasia, has been observed as a late complication following gastric bypass operations. Some investigators have hypothesized that changes in gut hormones following gastric bypass may promote beta-cell hyperplasia and predispose to this condition.

57. What vitamin and micronutrient deficiencies are patients at risk for following bariatric surgery?
By bypassing the stomach, duodenum, and varying portions of the jejunum and ileum, malabsorption of thiamine, iron, folate, vitamin B12, calcium, and vitamin D may occur. In general, the greater the malabsorption, the higher the risk of nutritional deficiencies. To prevent deficiency, patients should routinely be discharged from the hospital with daily vitamin and mineral supplementation that contains between 1.5 and 1.8 mg thiamine, 28 and 40 mg elemental iron, 500 µg oral B12, 400 µg folate, 1200 to 1500 mg calcium, and 800 to 1200 IU vitamin D.

58. What laboratory tests should be performed when following a patient who has had weight loss surgery?
The following lab tests should be performed preoperatively and at 6-month intervals for the first 2 years, followed by annual assessments thereafter: complete blood count, comprehensive metabolic panel, lipid panel, hemoglobin A_{1C} (for diabetic patients), ferritin, folate, vitamin B12, 25 Hydroxy vitamin D, and PTH. With more extensive procedures, such as biliopancreatic diversion, protein malnutrition and deficiencies of the fat-soluble vitamins (A, D, E, and K) may occur. Some patients who develop iron deficiency anemia following weight loss surgery require

treatment with parenteral iron. With judicious monitoring and adequate supplementation, all of these deficiencies are largely avoidable and treatable.

WEBSITES

http://www.win.niddk.nih.gov/statistics/index.htm

http://www.acsm.org

http://www.motivationalinterview.org

http://www.niddk.nih.gov/health/nutrit/nutrit.htm

BIBLIOGRAPHY

1. Agastston A: *The South Beach Diet*. New York, 2003, Random House.

2. Brownell KD: *The LEARN Program for Weight Control*, ed 7, Dallas, 1997, American Health.

3. Buchwald H, Avidor Y, Braunwald E, et al: Bariatric surgery: a systematic review and meta-analysis. JAMA 292:1724–1728, 2004.

4. Dansinger ML, Gleason JA, Griffith JL, et al: Comparison of the Atkins, Ornish, Weight Watchers, and Zone diets for weight loss and heart disease risk reduction: a randomized trial. JAMA 293:43–53, 2005.

5. Foster GD, Wyatt HR, Hill JO, et al: A randomized trial of a low-carbohydrate diet for obesity. N Engl J Med 348:2082–2090, 2003.

6. Heymsfield SB, Van Mierlo CA, Van Der Knapp HC, et al: Weight management using a meal replacement strategy: meta and pooling analysis. Int J Obesity Relat Metab Disord 27:537–549, 2003.

7. Knowler WC, Barrett-Conner E, Fowler SE, et al: Reduction in the incidence of type 2 diabetes with lifestyle intervention or metformin. N Engl J Med 393–403, 2002.

8. Kral JG, Naslund E: Surgical treatment of obesity. Nat Clin Pract Endocrinol Metab 3:574–583, 2007.

9. Kushner RF: Obesity management. Gastroenterol Clin North Am 36:191–210, 2007.

10. Kushner RF, Bessesen DH. *Treatment of the obese patient*. Totowa, NJ, 2007, Humana Press.

11. Kushner RF, Kushner N: *Dr. Kushner's Personality Type Diet*. New York, 2003, St. Martin's Press.

12. Li Z, Maglione M, Tu W, et al: Meta-analysis: pharmacologic treatment of obesity. Ann Intern Med 142:532–546, 2005.

13. Maggard MA, Shugarman LR, Suttorp M, et al: Meta-analysis: surgical treatment of obesity. Ann Intern Med 142:547–559, 2005.

14. Maria EJ: Bariatric surgery for morbid obesity. N Engl J M 356:2176–2183, 2007.

15. McGraw P: *The ultimate weight solution*. New York, 2003, Simon & Schuster.

16. McTigue KM, Harris R, Hemphill B, et al: Screening and interventions for obesity in adults: summary of the evidence for the U.S. Preventive Services Task Force. Ann Intern Med 139:933–1049, 2003.

17. National Institutes of Health: The practical guide to the identification, evaluation and treatment of overweight and obesity in adults. Obesity Res 6(Suppl 12), 1998.

18. Ogden CL, Carroll MD, Curtin LR, et al: Prevalence of overweight and obesity in the United States, 1999–2004. JAMA 295:1549–1555, 2006.

19. Ogden CL, Carroll MD, McDowell MA, Flegal KM. Obesity among adults in the United States—no change since 2003–2004. NCHS Data Brief No 1. Hyattsville, MD, 2007, National Center for Health Statistics.

20. Samaha FF, Iqbal N, Seshadri P, et al: A low-carbohydrate as compared with a low-fat diet in severe obesity. N Engl J Med 348:2074–2081, 2003.

21. Service GJ, Thompson GB, Service FJ, et al: Hyperinsulinemic hypoglycemia with nesidioblastosis after gastric-bypass surgery. N Engl J Med 353:249–254, 2005.

22. Shah M, Simha V, Garg A: Review: long-term impact of bariatric surgery on body weight, comorbidities, and nutritional status. J Clin Endocrinol Metab 91:4223–4231, 2006.

23. Snow V, Barry P, Fitterman N, et al: Pharmacologic and surgical management of obesity in primary care: a clinical practice guideline from the American College of Physicians. Ann Intern Med 142:525–531, 2005.

24. Tsai AG, Wadden TA: Systematic review: an evaluation of major commercial weight loss programs in the United States. Ann Intern Med 142:56–66, 2005.

25. Tuomilehto J, Lindstrom J, Eriksson JG, et al: Prevention of type 2 diabetes mellitus by changes in lifestyle among subjects with impaired glucose tolerance. N Engl J Med 344:1343–1350, 2001.

26. Wadden TA, Berkowitz RI, Womble LG, et al: Randomized trial of lifestyle modification and pharmacotherapy for obesity. N Engl J Med 353:2111–2120, 2005.

II. BONE AND MINERAL DISORDERS

OSTEOPOROSIS

Michael T. McDermott

CHAPTER 8

1. **What is osteoporosis?**
   Osteoporosis is a skeletal disorder characterized by compromised bone strength, predisposing to an increased risk for the development of fragility fractures. This definition emphasizes the critical role of bone strength, which is determined by both bone mass and bone quality, and the importance of fractures, which cause the major morbidity and mortality from this condition.

2. **What is a fragility fracture?**
   A fragility fracture is one that occurs spontaneously or following minimal trauma, defined as falling from a standing height or less. Fractures of the vertebrae, hips, and distal radius (Colles fracture) are characteristic, but any fracture may occur. Osteoporosis accounts for approximately 1.5 million fractures in the United States each year.

3. **What are the complications of osteoporotic fractures?**
   Vertebral fractures cause loss of height, anterior kyphosis (dowager's hump), reduced pulmonary function, and an increased mortality rate. Approximately one third of all vertebral fractures are painful, but two thirds are asymptomatic. Hip fractures are associated with permanent disability in nearly 50% of patients and with a 20% excess mortality rate compared with the age-matched nonfracture population.

4. **What factors contribute most to the risk of developing an osteoporotic fracture?**
   - Low bone mass (twofold risk increase for every standard deviation decrease of bone mass)
   - Age (twofold risk increase for every decade above age 60 years at same bone mass level)
   - Previous fragility fracture (fivefold risk increase if there has been a previous fracture)
   - Propensity to fall

5. **What are the currently accepted indications for bone mass measurement?**
   - Age greater than 65 years
   - Estrogen deficiency plus one risk factor for osteoporosis
   - Vertebral deformity, fracture, or osteopenia by x-ray
   - Primary hyperparathyroidism
   - Glucocorticoid therapy, greater than 5 mg/day of prednisone for more than 3 months
   - Monitoring the response to Food and Drug Administration (FDA)-approved osteoporosis medication

6. **How is bone mass currently measured?**
   The most accurate and widely used methods in current practice are dual energy x-ray absorptiometry (DXA), computed tomography (CT), and ultrasound (US). In my opinion, DXA offers the best accuracy and precision with the least radiation exposure in most patients.

Central densitometry measurements (spine and hip) are the best predictors of fracture risk and have the best precision for longitudinal monitoring. Peripheral densitometry measurements (heel, radius, hands), however, are more widely available and less expensive.

7. **How do you read a bone densitometry report?**
   - *T-score:* The number of standard deviations (SDs) the patient is below or above the mean value for young normal subjects (peak bone mass). The T-score is a good predictor of the fracture risk.
   - *Z-score:* The number of SDs the patient is below or above the mean value for age-matched normal subjects. The Z-score indicates whether the patient's bone mass is appropriate for age or whether other factors are likely to account for excessively low bone mass.
   - *Absolute bone mineral density (BMD):* The actual bone density value expressed in g/cm^2. This is the value one should use to calculate percent changes in bone density during longitudinal follow-up.

8. **How is the diagnosis of osteoporosis made?**
   Osteoporosis should be diagnosed or suspected in any patient who sustains a fragility fracture. In the prefracture patient, the World Health Organization currently recommends making the diagnosis based on the BMD value at the lowest skeletal site, using the following criteria:
   - T-score greater than equal to -1 = Normal
   - T-score between -1 and -2.5 = Osteopenia
   - T-score less than or equal to -2.5 = Osteoporosis

9. **What are the major risk factors for developing low bone mass?**

Nonmodifiable	Modifiable
Age	Low calcium intake
Race (Caucasian, Asian)	Low vitamin D intake
Female gender	Estrogen deficiency
Early menopause	Sedentary lifestyle
Slender build	Cigarette smoking
Positive family history	Alcohol excess (>2 drinks/day)
Caffeine excess (>2 servings/day)	
Medications (glucocorticoids, excess thyroxine)	

10. **What other conditions must be considered as causes of low bone mass?**
    - Osteomalacia
    - Celiac disease
    - Osteogenesis imperfecta
    - Idiopathic hypercalciuria
    - Hyperparathyroidism
    - Multiple myeloma
    - Hyperthyroidism
    - Rheumatoid arthritis
    - Hypogonadism
    - Renal failure
    - Cushing's syndrome
    - Mastocytosis

11. **Outline a cost-effective evaluation to rule out these possibilities**
A complete history and physical examination should always be performed. Afterward the following tests should be adequate in most patients:
- Complete blood count with erythrocyte sedimentation rate
- Serum calcium, phosphate, alkaline phosphatase, and creatinine
- Serum 25 (OH) vitamin D
- Serum testosterone (men)
- 24-hour urine calcium and creatinine

12. **What is the best way to determine whether a patient has had a previous vertebral fracture?**
Back pain or tenderness may be absent because two thirds of vertebral fractures are asymptomatic. Height loss of 2 inches or more or dorsal kyphosis on examination are highly suggestive findings. However, lateral spine films or morphometric x-ray absorptiometry (vertebral fracture assessment) are the most accurate ways to detect existing vertebral fractures.

13. **What are the most significant risk factors for sustaining a fall from the upright position?**
- Use of sedatives
- Visual impairment
- Cognitive impairment
- Lower extremity disability
- Obstacles to ambulation in the home

14. **What nonpharmacologic measures are useful for preventing and treating osteoporosis?**
1. Adequate calcium intake (diet plus supplements):
   - 1000 mg/day, premenopausal women and men
   - 1500 mg/day, postmenopausal women and men aged 65 years or older
2. Adequate vitamin D intake: 800 to 1200 U/day (D3 preferred)
3. Regular exercise: aerobic and resistance
4. Limitation of alcohol consumption to less than 2 drinks/day
5. Limitation of caffeine consumption to less than 2 servings/day
6. Smoking cessation
7. Fall prevention

15. **How do you clinically assess a patient's dietary calcium intake?**
The major bioavailable sources are dairy products and calcium-fortified fruit drinks. Ask their daily intake of these products and assign the following approximate calcium contents for their responses:
- Milk: 300 mg/cup
- Cheese: 300 mg/oz
- Yogurt: 300 mg/cup
- Fruit juice with calcium: 300 mg/cup
- Add 300 mg for the general nondairy diet for a reasonable estimate of daily intake

16. **How do you ensure adequate intake of calcium?**
Consumption of low-fat dairy products should be encouraged. Calcium supplements should be added when dietary calcium intake cannot reach the goal levels. Calcium carbonate and calcium citrate are both well absorbed when taken with meals. Because gastric acid is necessary for normal calcium absorption, calcium carbonate absorption can be decreased up to 60% by the concomitant use of proton pump inhibitors (PPIs). Being more acidic, calcium citrate is likely

not affected by PPI use. When doubt exists about the adequacy of calcium intake or absorption, 24-hour urine calcium excretion can be measured and the calcium intake titrated to a target urinary calcium of 100 to 300 mg/day.

17. **How does one best achieve appropriate intake of vitamin D?**
The body acquires vitamin D through dietary intake and sunlight exposure. Because of decreased sun exposure and reduced amounts of cutaneous 7 dehydrocholesterol, the vitamin D precursor, elderly patients must often rely more heavily on dietary sources. The best dietary sources are fatty fish and vitamin D–fortified dairy products and cereals. When these sources are not adequate, supplementation with vitamin D3 (cholecalciferol) is preferred over vitamin D2 (ergocalciferol). The currently recommended intake is 800 to 1200 units/day but up to 2000 units/day is safe in most patients. The goal serum 25 OH vitamin D level is 30 to 100 ng/mL.

18. **When should medical therapy be initiated for the prevention and treatment of osteoporosis?**
Nonpharmacologic measures are appropriate for all individuals who want to reduce their risk of developing osteoporosis. The National Osteoporosis Foundation further recommends that pharmacologic therapy be considered in patients with a T-score of -2.5 or less and in patients with a T-score of -1.0 to -2.5 if their fracture risk is 3% for hip fractures or $\geq$ 20% for other major fractures as assessed by the FRAX assessment tool, available at http://www.shef.ac.uk/FRAX. Patients who have had vertebral, hip, or distal radius fractures should be considered for pharmacologic therapy regardless of their bone density.

19. **Describe bone remodeling.**
Bone remodeling is the process by which old bone is removed and new bone is formed (Fig. 8-1). Osteoclasts are multinucleated giant cells that attach to bone surfaces where they secrete acid and proteolytic enzymes that dissolve underlying bone, leaving a resorption pit. Osteoblasts then move in and secrete osteoid, which is subsequently mineralized with calcium and phosphate crystals (hydroxyapatite), refilling the resorption pit with new bone. Bone remodeling occurs throughout the skeleton as an adaptation to changing mechanical stresses on bone.

Figure 8-1. Bone remodeling.

20. **Explain the roles of Receptor Activator of Nuclear Factor K (RANK), RANK ligand, and osteoprotegerin in normal bone physiology?**
Receptor activator of nuclear factor K (RANK) is a receptor that activates osteoclastic bone resorption. RANK ligand (RANK-L) is the normal ligand that binds to and activates RANK. Osteoprotegerin is a decoy receptor that can bind RANK-L and prevent it from attaching to RANK. RANK-L is therefore a normal endogenous stimulator of osteoclastic bone resorption, and osteoprotegerin is a normal endogenous inhibitor of bone resorption.

21. **How do the pharmacologic agents for the prevention and treatment of osteoporosis work?**
Medications for osteoporosis fall into two main categories: antiresorptive agents (inhibit bone resorption) and anabolic agents (stimulate bone formation).

Antiresorptive Agents	Anabolic Agents
Bisphosphonates	Parathyroid hormone (PTH)
Raloxifene	Growth hormone/growth factors
Calcitonin	Sodium fluoride
Estrogens	Strontium

22. **Which bisphosphonates are available for the treatment of osteoporosis, and how are they used?**
   - Alendronate (Fosamax): 10-mg tablet daily or 70-mg tablet weekly (without or with 2800 or 5600 units D3)
   - Risedronate (Actonel): 5-mg tablet daily, 35-mg tablet weekly, or 150-mg tablet monthly
   - Ibandronate (Boniva): 150-mg tablet monthly
   - Ibandronate (Boniva): 3-mg intravenous (IV) push over 15 seconds every 3 months
   - Pamidronate (Aredia): 30-mg IV in 250 mL NS over 2 to 4 hours every 3 months
   - Zoledronic acid (Reclast): 5-mg IV over 15–30 minutes once a year

   Fosamax, Actonel, Boniva, and Reclast are FDA-approved for the treatment of osteoporosis; pamidronate is not. The oral medications should be taken in the morning on an empty stomach with a full glass of water, and the patient should remain upright and take nothing by mouth for 30 minutes afterward. Renal function should be assessed with a serum creatinine before each dose of an intravenous bisphosphonate.

23. **How effective are the bisphosphonates in reducing the risk of fragility fractures?**
All of the FDA-approved bisphosphonates (Fosamax, Actonel, Boniva, Reclast) have been shown in large randomized controlled trials (RCTs) to reduce vertebral fractures by 50% to 70% in women with postmenopausal osteoporosis (PMO). Fosamax, Actonel, and Reclast have also been demonstrated to reduce hip fractures by 40% to 50% and peripheral fractures by variable amounts. There is no significant fracture reduction data for pamidronate; this is the reason it has not received FDA approval for the treatment of osteoporosis.

24. **Discuss the use of raloxifene in the management of osteoporosis.**
Raloxifene (Evista), a selective estrogen receptor modulator (SERM), is an estrogen agonist in bone and an antagonist in the breast and uterus. It was shown in a large RCT to reduce vertebral fractures by 50% in women with PMO but no previous vertebral fractures and by 30% in those with prior vertebral fractures. The dose is 60 mg once a day. Side effects can include hot flashes, leg cramps, and a twofold increased risk of venous thrombosis. Raloxifene has also been shown to reduce the risk of invasive breast cancer and to have no effects (adverse or beneficial) on the risk of developing coronary artery disease (CAD).

25. **Does calcitonin also reduce osteoporotic fractures?**
Calcitonin nasal spray (Miacalcin) reduced vertebral fractures by 33% in women with PMO in a large RCT. The effective dose is 200 units intranasally every day. Side effects are uncommon, consisting mainly of nasal congestion and skin rashes. Calcitonin may also have modest analgesic effects in some patients with recent vertebral fractures.

26. **Briefly discuss the issues regarding hormone replacement therapy.**

The Women's Health Initiative (WHI) is an RCT investigating the effects of hormone replacement therapy (HRT; Premarin, Provera) and estrogen replacement therapy (ERT; Premarin alone) in women who have an intact uterus (HRT) or a previous hysterectomy (ERT). The HRT arm was stopped after 5 years because of mild increases in the occurrence of CAD events (29%), invasive breast cancer (26%), strokes (41%), and venous thromboembolic events (110%). However, vertebral fractures and hip fractures were both reduced by 34%. As a result of this and other studies, HRT is no longer recommended for the prevention or treatment of osteoporosis. HRT may still be useful for the treatment of hot flashes in the first few years after menopause.

27. **What other antiresorptive medications are being developed?**

Several are being investigated, but the most promising at this time is denosumab. This is a monoclonal antibody that binds to and inactivates RANK-L with high affinity and specificity. Given as a subcutaneous (SQ) injection every 6 months, denosumab has been shown to increase bone mass and to reduce vertebral fractures by 68% and hip fractures by 40% after 3–4 years of use. Working on the same pathway, osteoprotegerin administration is also being actively investigated.

28. **What is osteonecrosis of the jaw, and how common is it in patients using antiresorptive medications?**

Osteonecrosis of the jaw (ONJ) presents as persistently exposed bone due to failure of the gums to heal over necrotic bone following a dental procedure. ONJ occurs most commonly in cancer patients receiving frequent high doses of IV bisphosphonates to treat bone metastases or hypercalcemia of malignancy; many affected patients have also received radiation, steroids or chemotherapy. It occurs rarely in osteoporosis patients taking lower doses of oral or IV bisphosphonates. Good oral hygiene and regular dental care are the best preventive measures. There is no evidence that stopping bisphosphonate therapy before dental procedures prevents ONJ, but there is little harm in stopping bisphosphonate therapy for 3 months if the oral surgeon expresses significant concern.

29. **How could PTH be an anabolic agent for treating osteoporosis?**

Persistently elevated serum PTH levels, as occur in primary hyperparathyroidism, promote osteoclastic bone resorption and bone loss. However, intermittent daily pulses of exogenous PTH actually stimulate new osteoblastic bone formation with a resultant increase in both cortical and trabecular bone mass. Intact PTH is an 84-amino-acid peptide. Because only the first 13 amino acids are necessary for binding to PTH receptors, smaller fragments, such as teriparatide (1–34 PTH), can be injected daily to produce this effect.

30. **Does teriparatide effectively and safely reduce fractures in osteoporotic patients?**

Teriparatide (Forteo), given as 20 mcg SQ daily for 18 months to women with PMO, increased vertebral bone mass by 10% and reduced vertebral fractures by 65% and nonvertebral fractures by 53% in a large multicenter RCT. Significant hypercalcemia did not occur, and side effects were uncommon. Transient orthostatic hypotension sometimes develops but can be minimized by administering the dose at bedtime in affected individuals.

31. **Are other anabolic agents being developed for the treatment of osteoporosis?**

Strontium ranelate was shown in an RCT of 1649 women with PMO to increase bone mass by 14% in the spine and 8% in the hip and to reduce new vertebral fractures by 49% after 1 year and by 41% after 3 years. Low-dose, slow-release sodium fluoride also increases bone mass and has been reported to reduce fractures. Neither strontium nor fluoride is currently FDA approved for use in osteoporosis. Growth hormone and insulin-like growth factor-1 (IGF-1) are agents with potential anabolic bone effects, but neither has been adequately tested for antifracture efficacy or safety in humans.

32. **Are combinations of osteoporosis medications more effective than single agents?**
Combinations of antiresorptive agents increase bone mass more than do single agents used alone. However, fracture data are not yet available for such regimens. Although it may seem intuitive that greater bone mass gains would result in fewer fractures, experts have raised the concern that oversuppression of bone resorption could impair the removal of older bone to such an extent that bone strength might ultimately be reduced. Combinations of anabolic and antiresorptive agents used concurrently have disappointingly shown no greater BMD effects than single agents alone. Additional studies investigating sequential use of various agents are currently in progress.

33. **How should providers interpret serial BMD changes when monitoring patients on osteoporosis therapy?**
BMD monitoring is useful, but providers must be aware of the least significant change (LSC) for BMD and the BMD changes that indicate treatment efficacy. The LSC is the BMD change that must occur to exceed the precision error of the BMD instrument. The LSC in large RCTs has been about 2.7% in the spine and 5.7% in the hip, but the LSC should be calculated for each machine. Equations for the LSC calculation are available on the International Society for Clinical Densitometry Web site (http://www.ISCD.org). BMD tends to increase in the first 2 years of medication use and then stabilizes; this stability indicates continued effectiveness, because fracture protection persists.

34. **What markers are available to assess bone remodeling, and how are they used?**

Bone Formation	Bone Resorption
Serum alkaline phosphatase	Urine or serum N-telopeptides
Serum osteocalcin	Serum C-telopeptides
Serum P1NP	Urine or serum pyridinoline crosslinks

Elevation of one or more biomarkers at baseline predicts an increased risk of future bone loss and fragility fracture development. A 30% reduction of biomarkers 3 to 6 months after therapy is initiated verifies compliance and predicts an increase in bone mass and reduction in fracture risk. However, marked variability in biomarker measurement limits the utility of this tool.

KEY POINTS: PREVENTION AND TREATMENT OF OSTEOPOROSIS

1. Nonpharmacologic measures that are important for both the prevention and treatment of osteoporosis include adequate calcium and vitamin D nutrition, regular exercise, fall prevention, discontinuation of smoking, and limitation of alcohol and caffeine intake.

2. Pharmacologic interventions for osteoporosis fall into two main categories: antiresorptive agents and anabolic agents.

3. The antiresorptive agents approved by the Food and Drug Administration (FDA) increase bone mineral density (BMD) and decrease the risk of vertebral fractures. Three of the bisphosphorates have also been shown to decrease hip fractures.

4. Teriparatide, an FDA-approved anabolic agent, increases BMD and reduces the risk of both vertebral and nonvertebral fractures.

5. Combination therapy with two antiresorptive agents increases BMD to a slightly greater extent than does monotherapy. However, no fracture data exist to verify the overall effectiveness of such regimens.

6. Combination therapy with antiresorptive and anabolic agents does not appear to increase BMD more than either type of agent used alone, but sequential regimens are under investigation and appear promising.

35. **What is the role of vertebroplasty and kyphoplasty following vertebral fractures?**
Vertebroplasty is a procedure in which a trochar is inserted into a collapsed vertebra, and cement (methyl methacrylate) is infused under pressure to reexpand the vertebral body. Kyphoplasty differs in that the vertebra is first expanded with a balloon, and cement is then infused under low pressure to avoid extravertebral extrusion of the cement. These procedures are useful to relieve chronic pain from vertebral fractures and may help to reduce the development of progressive kyphosis.

36. **How common is osteoporosis in men?**
Approximately 1 to 2 million men in the United States have osteoporosis by bone densitometry criteria. Worldwide, approximately 30% of hip fractures occur in men. Men have a substantially higher risk of having a hip fracture than they do of developing prostate cancer and have a higher mortality rate after hip fractures than do women. Elderly men have a 25% lifetime risk of sustaining any type of fragility fracture. BMD screening is recommended for all men who have significant risk factors for osteoporosis and in otherwise healthy men at age 70 years and older.

37. **How is the diagnosis of osteoporosis made in men?**
The presence of a fragility fracture establishes the diagnosis, provided no other metabolic bone disease can be identified as the culprit. However, bone densitometry criteria for the diagnosis of osteoporosis in men without fragility fractures have not been firmly established. Most experts propose that we should use the same criteria as those employed in women (T-score <-2.5) and that a normal male reference database should be used to calculate the T-scores. Better data comparing the fracture risk for the various BMD levels and the cost-to-benefit ratios of treatment at each level are clearly needed.

38. **What are the causes of osteoporosis in men?**
Osteoporosis in men often occurs as a consequence of another condition or disorder. The more common underlying conditions include hypogonadism, alcohol abuse, glucocorticoid use, and idiopathic hypercalciuria. The use of Gonadotropin releasing hormone (GnRH) analogs to lower serum testosterone levels for the treatment of prostate cancer also frequently causes substantial bone loss and increases the risk of fractures in men.

39. **How effective is pharmacologic therapy in men with osteoporosis?**
Bisphosphonates and teriparatide improve BMD in men, as they do in women. Testosterone replacement increases BMD in men with low serum testosterone levels but not in those with normal values and is therefore recommended only in hypogonadal men. Thiazide diuretics improve BMD in men with idiopathic hypercalciuria. Bisphosphonate therapy also prevents bone loss in men taking GnRH analogs for prostate cancer.

40. **How can falls be prevented?**
   - Sedatives should be minimized or discontinued.
   - Visual impairment should be corrected.

- Ambulatory aids should be used when appropriate.
- Make the home "fall-proof": adequate lighting, carpeting, handrails, nonslip surfaces in bathrooms, and removal of clutter and other obstacles to walking.

KEY POINTS: PREVALENCE AND RISK FACTORS FOR OSTEOPOROSIS

1. Approximately 10 million Americans have osteoporosis and are therefore at high risk of developing fragility fractures; this condition affects both women and men.

2. The major risk factors for fragility fractures are low bone mass, advancing age, previous fragility fractures, and the propensity to fall.

3. Secondary disorders causing bone loss are present in approximately 30% of women and 64% of men who have osteoporosis.

4. Patients who have a fragility fracture or low bone mass should have a complete history and physical examination and a limited number of key, cost-effective laboratory tests to identify any underlying responsible disorders.

BIBLIOGRAPHY

1. Adams JS, Song CF, Kantorovich V: Rapid recovery of bone mass in hypercalciuric, osteoporotic men treated with hydrochlorothiazide. Ann Intern Med 130(8):658–660, 1999.

2. Barrett-Connor E, Mosca L, Collins P, et al: Effects of raloxifene on cardiovascular events and breast cancer in postmenopausal women. N Engl J Med 355:125–37, 2006.

3. Black DM, Cummings SR, Karpf DB, et al: Randomized trial of effect of alendronate on risk of fracture in women with existing vertebral fractures. Lancet 348:1535–1541, 1996. (FIT 1)

4. Black DM, Delmas PD, Eastell R, et al: Once yearly zoledronic acid for treatment of postmenopausal osteoporosis. N Engl J Med 356:1809–22, 2007.

5. Black DM, Greenspan SL, Ensrud KE, et al: The effects of parathyroid hormone and alendronate alone or in combination in postmenopausal osteoporosis. N Engl J Med 349:1207–1215, 2003.

6. Black DM, Schwartz AV, Ensrud KE, et al: Effects of continuing or stopping alendronate after 5 years of treatment: the Fracture Intervention Trial Long Term Extension (FLEX), a randomized trial. JAMA 296:2927–2938, 2006.

7. Bonnick S, Johnston CC, Kleerekoper M, et al: Importance of precision in bone density measurements. J Clin Densitom 4:1–6, 2001.

8. Canalis E, Giustina A, Bilezikian JP: Mechanisms of anabolic therapies for osteoporosis. N Engl J Med 357:905–916, 2007.

9. Chesnut CH, Silverman S, Andriano K, et al: A randomized trial of nasal spray salmon calcitonin in postmenopausal women with established osteoporosis: the Prevent Recurrence of Osteoporotic Fractures Study. Am J Med 109:267–276, 2000. (PROOF)

10. Cummings SR, Palermo L, Browner W, et al: Monitoring osteoporosis therapy with bone densitometry. JAMA 283:1318–1321, 2000.

11. Delmas PD, Recker RR, Chesnut CH, et al: Daily and intermittent oral ibandronate normalize bone turnover and provide significant reduction in vertebral fracture risk: results from the BONE study. Osteoporosis Int 15:792–298, 2004.

12. Ettinger B, Black DM, Mitlak BH, et al: Reduction of vertebral fracture risk in postmenopausal women with osteoporosis treated with raloxifene. JAMA 282:637–645, 1999.

13. Faulkner KG, Orwoll E: Implications in the use of T-scores for the diagnosis of osteoporosis in men. J Clin Densitom 5:87–93, 2002.

14. Finkelstein JS, Hayes A, Hunzelman JL, et al: The effects of parathyroid hormone, alendronate or both in men with osteoporosis. N Engl J Med 349:1216–1226, 2003.

15. Garnero P, Hausherr E, Chapuy MC, et al: Markers of bone resorption predict hip fracture in elderly women: the EPIDOS prospective study. J Bone Miner Res 11:1531–1538, 1996.

16. Greenspan SL, Nelson JB, Trump DL: Effect of once-weekly oral alendronate on bone loss in men receiving androgen deprivation therapy for prostate cancer: a randomized trial. Ann Intern Med 146:416–424, 2007.

17. Harris ST, Watts NB, Genant HK, et al: Effects of risedronate treatment on vertebral and nonvertebral fractures in women with postmenopausal osteoporosis. A randomized controlled trial. JAMA 282:1344–1352, 1999. (VERT-NA)

18. Khosla S, Melton LJ: Osteopenia. N Engl J Med 356:2293–2300, 2007.

19. Lindsay R, Cosman F, Lobo RA, et al: Addition of alendronate to ongoing hormone replacement therapy in the treatment of osteoporosis: A randomized, controlled clinical trial. J Clin Endocrinol Metab 84:3076–3081, 1999.

20. Lindsay R, Silverman SL, Cooper C, et al: Risk of new vertebral fracture in the year following a fracture. JAMA 285:320–23, 2001.

21. Lyles KW, Colon-Emeric CS, Magaziner JS, et al: Zoledronic acid and clinical fractures and mortality after hip fracture. N Engl J Med 357:1799–1809, 2007.

22. McClung MR, Geusens P, Miller PD, et al: Effect of risedronate on the risk of hip fracture in elderly women. N Engl J Med 344:333–340, 2001. (HIP)

23. McClung MR, Lewiecki EM, Cohen SB, et al: Denosumab in postmenopausal women with low bone mineral density. N Engl J Med 354:821–831, 2006.

24. Melton LJ III, Orwoll ES, Wasnich RD: Does bone density predict fractures comparably in men and women? Osteoporos Int 12:707–709, 2001.

25. Meunier PJ, Roux C, et al: The effects of strontium ranelate on the risk of vertebral fracture in women with postmenopausal osteoporosis. N Engl J Med 350:459–468, 2004.

26. Neer RM, Arnaud CD, Zanchetta JR, et al: Effect of parathyroid hormone (1–34) on fractures and bone mineral density in postmenopausal women with osteoporosis. N Engl J Med 344:1434–1441, 2001.

27. Orwoll E, Ettinger M, Weiss S, et al: Alendronate for the treatment of osteoporosis in men. N Engl J Med 343:604–610, 2000.

28. Orwoll E, Scheele WH, Paul S, et al: The effect of teriparatide [human parathyroid hormone (1–34)] therapy on bone density in men with osteoporosis. J Bone Miner Res 18:9–17, 2003.

29. Orwoll ES: Osteoporosis in men. Osteoporosis 27:349–367, 1998.

30. Rea JA, Li J, Blake GM, et al: Visual assessment of vertebral deformity by x-ray absorptiometry: a highly predictive method to exclude vertebral deformity. Osteoporos Int 11:660–668, 2000.

31. Rittmaster RS, Bolognese M, Ettinger MP, et al: Enhancement of bone mass in osteoporotic women with parathyroid hormone followed by alendronate. J Clin Endocrinol Metab 85:2129–2134, 2000.

32. Rosen CJ, Rackoff RJ: Emerging anabolic treatments for osteoporosis. Rheum Dis Clin North Am 27:215–233, 2001.

33. Shoback D: Update in osteoporosis and metabolic bone disorders. J Clin Endocrinol Metab 92:747–53, 2007.

34. Snyder PJ, Peachey H, Hannoush P, et al: Effect of testosterone treatment on bone mineral density in men over 65 years of age. J Clin Endocrinol Metab 84:1966–1972, 1999.

35. Tinetti ME, Speechley M, Ginter SF: Risk factors for falls among elderly persons living in the community. N Engl J Med 19:1701–1707, 1998.

36. Vogel VG, Costantino JP, Wickerham DG, et al: Effects of tamoxifen vs raloxifene on the risk of developing invasive breast cancer and other disease outcomes: the NSABP Study of Tamoxifen and Raloxifene (STAR) P-2 trial. JAMA 295:2727–2741, 2006.

37. Writing Group for the Women's Health Initiative Investigators: Risk and benefits of estrogen plus progestin in healthy postmenopausal women. Principle results from the women's health initiative randomized controlled trial. JAMA 288:321–333, 2002. (WHI)

GLUCOCORTICOID-INDUCED OSTEOPOROSIS

Michael T. McDermott

CHAPTER 9

1. **How common is glucocorticoid-induced osteoporosis (GIOP)?**
   Glucocorticoid-induced osteoporosis (GIOP) is currently the most common cause of drug-induced osteoporosis. Significant bone loss and skeletal fractures may occur within 6 months of starting glucocorticoid therapy, and up to 50% of people on chronic glucocorticoid treatment develop osteoporotic fractures.

2. **What are the important determinants of bone loss with glucocorticoid therapy?**
   Bone loss is related mainly to the dose and the duration of glucocorticoid therapy. Glucocorticoid doses of 7.5 mg or higher of prednisone (or equivalent) are associated with the greatest risk. However, a large cohort study showed a significantly increased fracture risk even in those whose median prednisolone doses had been as low as 2.5 mg per day. Decreased bone mass and an increased fracture risk have even been demonstrated in patients using only inhaled glucocorticoids.

3. **Explain the pathogenesis of GIOP.**
   Glucocorticoids adversely affect both phases of bone remodeling. They impair bone formation by promoting cell death (apoptosis) of existing osteoblasts and by reducing the recruitment of new osteoblasts, partly through inhibitory effects on local growth factors such as IGF-1. At the same time, they increase bone resorption through various mechanisms, such as decreasing the production of sex steroids and osteoprotegerin, an endogenous inhibitor of bone resorption (Fig. 9-1).

Figure 9-1. Pathophysiology of glucocorticoid-induced osteoporosis.

4. **What are the BMD criteria for a diagnosis of GIOP?**

The ideal BMD criteria for the diagnosis of GIOP are still being debated, but the best existing evidence suggests that the fracture risk per BMD decrement is higher in GIOP than in primary osteoporosis. The same BMD criteria are currently used to diagnose osteoporosis in these patients as in those who are not taking glucocorticoids, but active treatment should be considered at an earlier stage (T-score ≤ -1.0) because of the rapidity of bone loss in GIOP.

5. **In which patients on glucocorticoids should BMD be tested?**

Patients starting glucocorticoid therapy (prednisone dose ≥ 5 mg/day or equivalent) with planned duration of treatment 3 months or more or on existing treatment for 3 months or more.

6. **When should BMD be tested?**

- BMD (spine and hip) should be measured at initiation of glucocorticoid therapy or as soon as possible thereafter.
- BMD should be repeated every 6 to 12 months as long as glucocorticoid therapy is continued.

7. **What measures should be instituted in all patients on glucocorticoids?**

All glucocorticoid-treated patients should be advised to consume adequate calcium (1500 mg/day; combination of dietary intake plus supplements) and vitamin D (800–1200 U/day), exercise regularly (aerobic and resistance), stop smoking, and limit alcohol and caffeine consumption.

8. **Which medications are effective in preventing and treating GIOP?**

Bisphosphonates and teriparatide have been shown to increase bone mass significantly and to prevent fractures in patients with GIOP. The dose regimens for these agents are discussed in the chapter on osteoporosis (Chapter 8). These are currently the most effective agents for this condition.

9. **Which glucocorticoid-treated patients should receive active intervention?**

- Postmenopausal women (all)
- Men and premenopausal women with T-score ≤ -1.0

10. **When should gonadal steroids be considered?**

Gonadal steroids may be considered, usually in combination with other agents, in postmenopausal women and hypogonadal men (men with low serum testosterone).

11. **List the indications for thiazide diuretics**

- If urine calcium > 300 mg/day in men.
- If urine calcium > 250 mg/day in women.

KEY POINTS: PREVALENCE AND PATHOPHYSIOLOGY OF GIOP

1. Glucocorticoid-induced osteoporosis is the most common type of drug-induced osteoporosis.

2. High doses and prolonged use of glucocorticoids produce greater risk, but all doses of oral glucocorticoids and even inhaled steroids appear to increase the risk of osteoporotic fractures.

3. The pathophysiology of glucocorticoid-induced osteoporosis involves both suppressed bone formation and enhanced bone resorption, which account for the rapid bone loss often seen in glucocorticoid-treated patients.

KEY POINTS: PREVENTION AND TREATMENT OF GIOP

1. Bone mineral density (BMD) testing is recommended before initiation of glucocorticoid therapy in patients who will receive ≥5 mg/day of prednisone (or equivalent) for ≥3 months duration and every 6 to 12 months thereafter as long as glucocorticoid therapy is continued.

2. Treatment is recommended for all postmenopausal women regardless of initial BMD and for men or premenopausal women with a BMD T-score of ≤−1.0 who are treated or will be treated with ≥5 mg/day of prednisone (or equivalent) for 3 months or more.

3. Both antiresorptive and anabolic agents improve BMD in patients with glucocorticoid-induced osteoporosis; alendronate, risedronate, and teriparatide have also been shown to reduce the occurrence of fragility fractures.

BIBLIOGRAPHY

1. Adachi JD, Olszynski WP, Hanley DA, et al: Management of corticosteroid-induced osteoporosis. Semin Arthritis Rheum 29:228–251, 2000.

2. American College of Rheumatology Ad Hoc Committee on Glucocorticoid-induced Osteoporosis: Recommendations for the prevention and treatment of glucocorticoid-induced osteoporosis. 2001 update. Arthritis Rheum 44:1496–1503, 2001.

3. Amin S, LaValley MP, Simms RW, Felson DT: The comparative efficacy of drug therapies used for the management of corticosteroid-induced osteoporosis: A meta-regression. J Bone Miner Res 17:1512–1526, 2002.

4. Canalis E: Glucocorticoid-induced osteoporosis. Curr Opin Endocrinol Diabetes 7:320–324, 2000.

5. Devogelaer JP: Glucocorticoid-induced osteoporosis: mechanisms and therapeutic approach. Rheum Dis Clin North Am 32:733–756, 2006.

6. Gourlay M, Franceschini N, Sheyn Y: Prevention and treatment strategies for glucocorticoid induced osteoporotic fractures. Clin Rheumatol 26:144–153, 2007.

7. Isreal E, Banerjee TR, Fitzmaurice GM, et al: Effects of inhaled glucocorticoids on bone density in premenopausal women. N Engl J Med 345:941–947, 2001.

8. Lane NE, Sanchez S, Modin GW, et al: Parathyroid hormone treatment can reverse corticosteroid-induced osteoporosis. Results of a randomized controlled clinical trial. J Clin Invest 102:1627–1633, 1998.

9. Manolagas SC, Weinstein RS: New developments in the pathogenesis and treatment of steroid-induced osteoporosis. J Bone Miner Res 14:1061–1066, 1999.

10. Reid DM, Hughes RA, Laan RF, et al: Efficacy and safety of daily risedronate in the treatment of corticosteroid-induced osteoporosis in men and women: a randomized trial. European corticosteroid-induced osteoporosis treatment study. J Bone Miner Res 15:1006–1103, 2000.

11. Rubin MR, Bilezikian JP: The role of parathyroid hormone in the pathogenesis of glucocorticoid-induced osteoporosis: a re-examination of the evidence. J Clin Endocrinol Metab 87: 4033–4041, 2002.

12. Saag KG, Emkey R, Schnitzer TJ, et al: Alendronate for the prevention and treatment of glucocorticoid-induced osteoporosis. N Engl J Med 339:292–299, 1998.

13. Sambrook PN: How to prevent steroid induced osteoporosis. Ann Rheum Dis 64:176–178, 2007.

14. Van Staa TP, Leufkens HGM, Abenhaim L, et al: Use of oral corticosteroids and risk of fractures. J Bone Miner Res 15:993–1000, 2000.

15. Van Staa TP, Leufkens HGM, Cooper C: Use of inhaled corticosteroids and risk of fractures. J Bone Miner Res 16:581–588, 2001.

CHAPTER 10

MEASUREMENT OF BONE MASS
William E. Duncan

1. **Why measure bone mass?**
   Bone mass is measured by bone mineral densitometry to establish the diagnosis of osteoporosis, to predict the risk of subsequent fractures, and to monitor changes in bone mass during therapy for osteoporosis. No clinical finding, laboratory test, or other radiographic examination can reliably identify individuals with osteoporosis. Conventional x-ray techniques are not sensitive indicators of bone loss because they do not reliably indicate osteoporosis until 30% to 40% of the bone mineral is lost. Although bone densitometry can determine a low bone mass, it cannot determine its cause. Thus bone densitometry must be used along with a complete clinical evaluation, laboratory testing, and other diagnostic studies to determine the cause of and the most appropriate treatment for osteoporosis.

2. **Is bone mass the only factor that determines whether a bone will fracture?**
   Although a decreased bone mass is the primary determinant of whether a bone will fracture, bone architecture and geometry are also important factors contributing to bone strength. The relationship between bone mass and fracture risk is more powerful than the relationship between serum cholesterol concentration and coronary artery disease. A decrease in bone mass of 1 SD doubles the risk of fracture. In comparison, a decrease in the cholesterol concentration of 1 SD increases the risk of coronary artery disease by only 20% to 30%.

3. **How does bone densitometry measure bone mass?**
   All bone densitometry techniques use an ionizing radiation source (either from a radionuclide or from x-rays) and a radiation detector to measure the amount of calcium present in bone. Bone densitometry is based on the principle that bone will absorb radiation in proportion to its bone mineral content. The bone mineral content of the bone (or a region of interest within a bone) is then divided by the measured area. The result is the bone mineral density in grams per unit area (g/cm^2). This bone mineral density is not a true volumetric density (gm/cm^3) but rather an area density. In this chapter, bone mass and bone density are used interchangeably.

4. **What techniques are available to measure bone mass?**
   The techniques available to measure bone mass include single-photon absorptiometry (SPA), single-energy x-ray absorptiometry, dual-photon absorptiometry (DPA), dual-energy x-ray absorptiometry (DXA), quantitative computed tomography (QCT), and radiographic absorptiometry (RA). Another technique, quantitative ultrasound (QUS), transmits ultrasound waves through the bone. The more complex and dense the bone structure, the greater the attenuation of the ultrasound wave. Thus QUS may determine both density and structure of the bone. Table 10-1 compares several of these bone mass measurement techniques.

5. **What is the preferred method for measuring bone mass?**
   DXA is the preferred method for measuring bone mass in the United States. DXA measures bone mass at the spine, hip, or wrist—the most common sites for osteoporotic fractures.

TABLE 10-1. COMPARISON OF BONE MASS MEASUREMENT TECHNIQUES

Method	Sites Measured	Precision Error* (%)	Accuracy Error† (%)	Radiation Dose (mSV)
Single-photon absorptiometry	Forearm, calcaneus	1–2	2–5	<1
Dual-energy x-ray absorptiometry	PA spine	1	5–8	1
	Proximal femur	1–2	5–8	1
	Total body	1	1–2	3
Quantitative computed tomography	Single-energy (spine)	2–4	5–10	60
	Dual-energy (spine)	4–6	3–6	90
	Peripheral (radius)	0.5–1.0	0.5	<2
Quantitative ultrasound	Calcaneus	0.3–3.8	—	0
	Patella	<2	—	0

* The error around repeated measurements (reproducibility or coefficient of variation).
† A measure of the agreement between the test result and true value (accuracy).

6. **Discuss the advantages and disadvantages of DXA.**
   DXA has the best correlation with fracture risk, requires relatively short scanning times (<5 minutes), determines bone mass in all areas of the skeleton with high accuracy and reproducibility (precision), and is associated with a low radiation exposure. DXA does not require replacement of the radiation source. A drawback of DXA is the initial cost of the equipment.

7. **What are the indications for the measurement of bone mass?**
   Widespread bone density screening for osteoporosis is not recommended at this time. However, individuals at high risk for osteoporosis should be considered for bone mineral density testing. The National Osteoporosis Foundation recommends bone mineral density testing for:
   - Women aged 65 years or older (regardless of risk factors)
   - Postmenopausal women under 65 years of age who have at least one risk factor for osteoporosis other than being Caucasian, postmenopausal, and female
   - Postmenopausal women who present with fractures

   Other indications for measurement of bone mass include x-ray findings suggestive of osteoporosis or vertebral deformity, glucocorticoid therapy for more than 3 months, primary hyperparathyroidism, and monitoring the response to or effectiveness of drug therapy for osteoporosis. DXA is also increasingly being used in the pediatric population and for vertebral fracture assessment (VFA).

8. **What do bone densitometry results mean?**
   The bone densitometry report gives the absolute bone mass measurements (in g/cm^2), which do not provide clinically useful information unless these values are compared with those of reference populations. To do so, the bone mineral density report usually provides two scores: a T-score and a Z-score (Fig. 10-1).

WALTER REED ARMY MEDICAL CENTER

k = 1.229   d0 = 109.2(1.000H)

·Jun 1 14:41 2000   [110 x 112]
Hologic QDR-2000 (S/N 2419)
Right Hip V4.76

H06010017   Thu Jun 1 14:32 2000
Name:
Comment:
I.D.:   Sex:
S.S.#:   Ethnic:
ZIP Code: Height:
Scan Code: Weight:
BirthDate: Age:
Physician: DUNCAN
Image not for diagnostic use
  TOTAL BMD CV 1.0%
  C.F.   1.007   1.083   1.000

Region	Area (cm²)	BMC (grams)	BMD (gms/cm²)
Neck	6.51	4.81	0.738
Troch	15.41	9.70	0.629
Inter	23.85	26.58	1.114
TOTAL	45.78	41.09	0.898
Ward's	1.14	0.64	0.559

Midline (116,136)-(18, 76)
  Neck   58 x 16 at [-27, 6]
  Troch   -8 x 56 at [0, 0]
  Ward's 11 x 11 at [-6, 3]

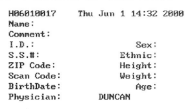

HOLOGIC

WALTER REED ARMY MEDICAL CENTER

Right Hip
Reference Database ◆

BMD(Neck[R]) = 0.738 g/cm²

H06010017   Thu Jun 1 14:32 2000
Name:
Comment:
I.D.:   Sex:
S.S.#:   Ethnic:
ZIP Code: Height:
Scan Code: Weight:
BirthDate: Age:
Physician: DUNCAN

Region	BMD	T	Z
Neck	0.738	-2.19 75% (20.0)	-1.01 87%
Troch	0.629	-1.52 79% (20.0)	-1.03 85%
Inter	1.114	-0.86 90% (20.0)	-0.23 97%
TOTAL	0.898	-1.34 84% (20.0)	-0.67 91%
Ward's	0.559	-2.28 67% (20.0)	-0.68 87%

◆ Age and sex matched
T = peak bone mass
Z = age matched   TK   10/25/91

HOLOGIC

Figure 10-1. Printout of dual-energy x-ray absorptiometry scan of the hip (personal data deleted).

9. **What are T-scores?**

The T-score is the number of standard deviations above or below the mean bone mass of a normal young adult sex-matched population. This population represents the optimal or peak bone mass for the patient. A patient whose bone mass is 1 SD below that of the young reference population has a T-score of -1.0. At the spine, 1 SD represents about 10% of the bone mass. Thus someone with a T-score of -1.0 has lost about 10% of his or her bone mass. Because the T-score is a measure of bone loss, this score is used to diagnose osteoporosis.

10. **What do Z-scores tell us about the patient?**

The Z-score is the number of standard deviations above or below the mean bone mass of an age- and sex-matched reference population. The Z-score compares a patient's bone mass to that of other individuals of the same age. A Z-score less than expected for a given individual (e.g., less than -2.0) indicates that the individual has lost more bone mass than is normal for his or her age. Such a finding should prompt a search for associated medical or lifestyle conditions (either current or in the past) that may have accelerated bone loss or prevented the patient from reaching peak bone mass in early adulthood.

11. **How is bone mass classified?**

In 1994, the World Health Organization (WHO) developed criteria for the diagnosis of osteoporosis and osteopenia in postmenopausal white women using T-scores from any skeletal site. A T-score greater than -1.0 is defined as normal bone mass, a T-score between -1.0 and -2.5 is defined as low bone mass (or osteopenia), and a T-score less than -2.5 is defined as osteoporosis. Established (or severe) osteoporosis is defined as a T-score less than -2.5 with one or more osteoporotic fractures.

12. **How should the WHO classification be used?**

The WHO classification criteria were derived from data from white postmenopausal women. Thus applying these definitions to other ethnic groups or to men should be done with caution. The WHO criteria were not intended to apply to premenopausal women. Also, these criteria were developed from studies using DXA. Therefore applying the WHO criteria to bone mass measurements obtained with other technologies (such as QUS) may be misleading. Finally, WHO definitions for osteopenia and osteoporosis were developed as general guidelines for diagnosis and were not intended to require or restrict therapy for individual patients.

13. **How are bone density measurements interpreted in men and non-Caucasians?**

The criteria by which a densitometric diagnosis of osteoporosis can be made in males and in non-Caucasians is extremely controversial because it is unclear whether fractures occur at the same bone mineral density in men and non-Caucasians as they do in Caucasian women. Pending additional studies, the International Society for Clinical Densitometry has recommended that osteoporosis in these groups be diagnosed at or below a T-score of -2.5 using a sex but not a race-adjusted normative database.

14. **Discuss how bone mass measurements are used to determine the need for treatment of osteoporosis.**

The health care provider should use information from bone mass testing in conjunction with knowledge of the patient's specific medical and personal history to determine the most appropriate treatment. The bone mineral density results should not be used as the sole determinant for treatment decisions. The National Osteoporosis Foundation has proposed that women with T-scores less than -2.0 by hip DXA in the absence of risk factors for osteoporosis, women with T-scores less than -0.5 by hip DXA with one or more risk factors, or women with a prior vertebral or hip fracture should be treated for osteoporosis. The WHO recently released the FRAX Fracture Risk Assessment Tool to evaluate patient fracture risk utilizing clinical factors as well as bone mineral density at the femoral neck (http://www.shef.ac.uk/FRAX). Before entering a patient's T-score into FRAX, it must be converted to a T-score based on the reference values used by FRAX using the FRAX Patch program (available at www.NOF.org). Fracture risk probabilities can then also be used to guide therapeutic decisions (see guidelines at the NOF website).

15. **Which bone(s) should be selected for measurement of bone mass?**
It is possible to measure the bone mass at several sites (Fig. 10-2). Measurement of bone mass at any skeletal site has value in predicting fracture risk. However, the bone density of the hip is the best predictor of hip fractures (the osteoporotic fracture with the greatest mortality and morbidity). The bone mass of the hip also predicts fractures at other sites, as do bone mass measurements at those sites. For these reasons, the hip is the preferred site for measurement of bone mass. Although there is significant concordance between skeletal sites in predicting bone mass, there is still enough discordance in bone mass at various sites not to rely on single bone mass measurements to diagnose osteoporosis. Thus bone mass should be measured at both the hip and the posteroanterior (PA) spine, and the diagnosis of osteoporosis should be based on the lowest T-score.

16. **What is the role for bone mass measurements of the forearm?**
Measurement of peripheral bone mass (e.g., the forearm) generally adds little to the evaluation of an individual with postmenopausal osteoporosis. However, the forearm appears to be the best site to assess the effects on bone of excess parathyroid hormone associated with primary hyperparathyroidism. In addition, measurement of forearm bone mass should be performed when the hip and spine cannot be accurately measured or when a patient is over the weight limit for the DXA table. Peripheral bone mass measurements have not yet been shown to be useful for monitoring the effects of therapy for osteoporosis as changes in bone density occur very slowly at this site.

17. **How often should bone mass measurements be repeated?**
The frequency of bone density measurements is determined, in part, by the precision error (or reproducibility) of the technique. The precision of bone mass measurements by DXA is approximately 1% for spine and 1% to 2% for the femoral neck. This means that the smallest difference between two bone mass measurements that is significant is a change of 2.83% at the spine and 5.66% at the femoral neck. In contrast, the average amount of early postmenopausal bone loss from the spine is 1% to 2% per year. Therefore to obtain statistically meaningful bone density results, postmenopausal women should not undergo routine DXA measurements of spine more often than once every 1.4 years unless accelerated bone loss is suspected. Measurement of bone mass every 6 months is recommended for patients in whom glucocorticoid therapy is being initiated for this reason.

18. **What conditions limit the accuracy of bone mass measurements?**
Several factors may limit the accuracy of PA spine mass measurements: degenerative changes, oral contrast taken for other radiographic studies, and osteophytes artificially elevate the measured bone density. Anatomic distortions that affect the accuracy of these measurements may also result from lumbar disc disease, compression fractures, scoliosis, prior surgical intervention, or vascular calcifications in the overlying aorta, which are common in the elderly. Likewise, previous surgery on the hip may alter bone mass.

19. **Interpret the bone mineral density results from the following four patients**
Each patient is a white postmenopausal woman. The bone mass was measured at any skeletal site.

Patient 1	T-score = −0.9	Z-score = +0.2
Patient 2	T-score = −2.0	Z-score = −0.9
Patient 3	T-score = −3.0	Z-score = −1.4
Patient 4	T-score = −3.0	Z-score = −2.5

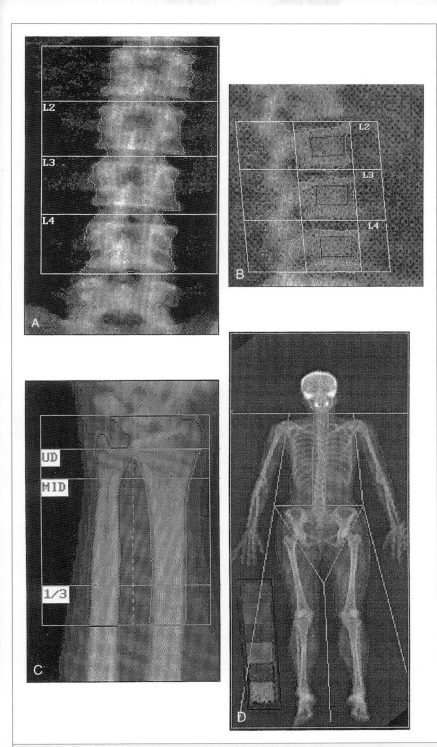

Figure 10-2. Images of several skeletal sites scanned by a dual-energy x-ray absorptiometry bone densitometer. **A,** anteroposterior spine; **B,** lateral spine; **C,** forearm; **D,** whole body.

Interpretation:

Patient 1: This woman has a normal bone mass.

Patient 2: This woman has a low bone mass (osteopenia) that is appropriate for her age (the Z-score is greater than −2.0).

Patient 3: This woman has osteoporosis that is appropriate for her age.

Patient 4: This woman has osteoporosis with bone loss that is greater than expected for her age. This bone density finding should prompt a thorough evaluation to rule out secondary causes of osteoporosis (such as hyperthyroidism, malabsorption, Cushing syndrome, hypogonadism, vitamin D deficiency, excessive alcohol consumption, celiac disease, and use of certain drugs).

KEY POINTS: MEASUREMENT OF BONE MASS

1. Direct measurement of bone mass is the only method to diagnose osteoporosis. No clinical finding, laboratory test, or other radiographic examination can reliably identify people with a low bone mass.

2. The preferred technique for diagnosis of osteoporosis is dual-energy x-ray absorptiometry of the spine and hip.

3. The diagnosis of osteoporosis is made using the World Health Organization criteria of a T-score less than or equal to −2.5.

4. Bone mass measurement of the forearm is the study of choice for patients with hyperparathyroidism.

WEBSITES

1. National Osteoporosis Foundation: http://www.nof.org

2. International Society for Clinical Densitometry: http://www.iscd.org

BIBLIOGRAPHY

1. Binkley N, Schmeer P, Wasnich R, Lenchik L: What are the criteria by which a densitometric diagnosis of osteoporosis can be made in males and noncaucasians? J Clin Densitom 5(Suppl):S19–S27, 2002.

2. Binkovitz LA, Sparke P, Henwood MJ: Pediatric DXA: clinical applications. Pediatr Radiol 37:625–635, 2007.

3. Blake G, Fogelman I: Dual energy x-ray absorptiometry and its clinical applications. Semin Musculoskelet Radiol 6:207–218, 2002.

4. Cummings SR, Bates D, Black D: Clinical use of bone densitometry. Scientific review. JAMA 288:1889–1897, 2002.

5. Hamdy R, Petak S, Lenchik L: Which central dual x-ray absorptiometry skeletal sites and regions of interest should be used to determine the diagnosis of osteoporosis? J Clin Densitrom 5(Suppl):S11–S18, 2002.

6. Lenchik L, Kiebzak G, Blunt B: What is the role of serial bone mineral density measurements in patient management? J Clin Densitrom 5(Suppl):S29–S38, 2002.

7. Lewiecki EM, Laster AJ: Clinical applications of vertebral fracture assessment by dual-energy x-ray absorptiometry. J Clin Endocrinol Metab 91:4215–4222, 2006.

8. Miller P: Bone mineral density-clinical use and application. Endocrinol Metab Clin North Am 32:159–179, 2003.

9. Miller PD, Leonard MB: Clinical use of bone mass measurements in adults for the assessment and management of osteoporosis. In Favus MJ, editor, *Primer on the metabolic bone diseases and disorders of mineral metabolism*, ed 6, New York, 2006, Raven Press, p. 150.

10. Miller PD, Zapalowski C, Kulak CA, Bilezikian JP: Bone densitometry: the best way to detect osteoporosis and to monitor therapy. J Clin Endocrinol Metab 84:1867, 1999.

11. Shagam J: Bone densitometry: an update. Radiol Technol 74:321–338, 2003.

12. WHO Study Group: Assessment of fracture risk and its application to screening for postmenopausal osteoporosis. WHO Tech Rep Ser 843. Geneva, 1994, World Health Organization.

CHAPTER 11

OSTEOMALACIA AND RICKETS

William E. Duncan

1. **What are osteomalacia and rickets?**

   Osteomalacia and rickets are terms that describe the clinical, histologic, and radiologic abnormalities of bone that are associated with more than 50 diseases and conditions. Osteomalacia is a disorder of mature (adult) bone, whereas rickets occurs in growing bone. In both conditions, mineralization of newly formed osteoid (the bone protein matrix) is inadequate or delayed. Thus, in individuals with rickets, defective mineralization occurs in both bones and cartilage of the epiphyseal growth plates and is associated with growth retardation and skeletal deformities that are not typically seen in adults with osteomalacia. Although rickets and osteomalacia were initially viewed as distinct clinical entities, the same pathologic processes may result in either disorder, depending on whether a growing or nongrowing skeleton is involved.

2. **Why is it important to know about osteomalacia and rickets?**

   In the United States at the beginning of the 20th century, rickets was caused by a deficiency of vitamin D that was common in urban areas. In the 1920s, it was virtually eliminated by an appreciation of the antirachitic properties of sunlight and the use of cod liver oil (which contains vitamin D). However, with the development of effective treatments for previously fatal diseases that affect vitamin D metabolism (such as chronic renal failure) and with an improved understanding of both vitamin D and mineral metabolism, many additional syndromes with osteomalacia or rickets as a feature have emerged. Many recent studies have demonstrated that undiagnosed vitamin D deficiency is not uncommon, and for a significant number of adult women with osteoporosis, vitamin D insufficiency may be an unsuspected component of their bone loss.

3. **List the causes of osteomalacia and rickets.**

   The primary abnormality of bone in patients with osteomalacia or rickets is defective mineralization of bone matrix. The major mineral in bone is hydroxyapatite [$Ca_{10}(PO_4)_6(OH)_2$]. Thus any disease that results in decreased availability to bone of either calcium or phosphorus may result in osteomalacia or rickets (Table 11-1). The causes of osteomalacia and rickets fall into three categories: (1) disorders associated with abnormalities of vitamin D metabolism or action that limit the availability of calcium for mineralization of bone, (2) disorders associated with abnormalities of phosphorus metabolism, and (3) a small group of disorders in which there is normal vitamin D and mineral metabolism.

4. **Describe how vitamin D is metabolized.**

   Serum vitamin D comes from two sources: dietary intake and conversion by ultraviolet (UV) irradiation of 7-dehydrocholesterol in the skin. Vitamin D is then transported through the blood to the liver, where it is converted to 25-hydroxyvitamin D by the hepatic 25-hydroxylase enzyme. The 25-hydroxyvitamin D is then converted in the kidney to the active vitamin D hormone, 1,25-dihydroxyvitamin D, by the renal 1-α-hydroxylase. The active vitamin D hormone has effects in many tissues, including the intestine (increases calcium absorption), the kidney (increases calcium reabsorption), and bone (stimulates osteoblast maturation and bone

TABLE 11-1. CONDITIONS ASSOCIATED WITH OSTEOMALACIA AND RICKETS

Condition	Primary Mechanism*
Abnormal Vitamin D Metabolism or Action	
Nutritional deficiency	Vitamin D deficiency
Malabsorption	Vitamin D deficiency
Primary biliary cirrhosis	Malabsorption of vitamin D
Chronic renal disease	Impaired 1α-hydroxylation of 25 hydroxyvitamin D
Chronic liver disease	Impaired 25-hydroxylation of vitamin D
VDDR type I	1α-hydroxylase deficiency
VDDR type II	Overproduction of hormone-responsive-element binding proteins
Drugs (phenytoin, barbiturates, cholestyramine)	Increased catabolism and/or excretion of vitamin D
Phosphate Deficiency or Renal Phosphate Wasting	
Diminished phosphate intake	Phosphate deficiency
Excessive aluminum hydroxide intake	Increasing binding of intestinal phosphate
X-linked hypophosphatemic rickets	Renal phosphate transport defect
Tumor-induced osteomalacia	Renal phosphate transport defect
Miscellaneous renal tubular defects (RTA, FS)	Renal phosphate transport defect
Normal Vitamin D and Phosphate Metabolism	
Hypophosphatasia	Alkaline phosphatase deficiency
Drugs (fluoride, aluminum, high dose etidronate)	Inhibition of mineralization or stimulation of matrix synthesis
Osteogenesis imperfecta	Abnormal bone collagen
Fibrogenesis imperfecta ossium	Defective bone matrix

FS, Fanconi syndrome; RTA, renal tubular acidosis; VDDR, vitamin D dependent rickets.
* Although only one mechanism for osteomalacia or rickets is given, other mechanisms also may contribute to the bone disease.

matrix synthesis) (Fig. 11-1). From an understanding of how vitamin D is metabolized, it is apparent that even when dietary intake and UV-mediated vitamin D synthesis are adequate, malabsorptive, renal, and liver diseases may be associated with vitamin D deficiency.

5. **Discuss the disease processes that interfere with the metabolism of vitamin D.**
   Clinically apparent vitamin D deficiency is rarely seen in the United States except when exposure to sunlight or intake of vitamin D–fortified milk and other dairy products is limited. However, elderly Americans are particularly at risk for occult vitamin D deficiency because of age-related decrease in the dermal synthesis of vitamin D, impaired hepatic and renal hydroxylation of vitamin D, and diminished intestinal responsiveness to 1,25-dihydroxyvitamin D. Celiac disease or sprue, regional enteritis, intestinal bypass surgery, partial gastrectomy, chronic liver disease, primary biliary cirrhosis, pancreatic insufficiency, and chronic renal failure have been associated

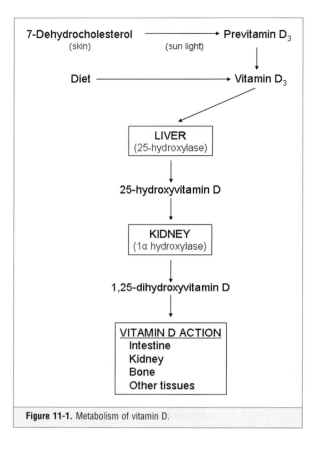

Figure 11-1. Metabolism of vitamin D.

with the development of osteomalacia. Anticonvulsant drugs (e.g., phenytoin, phenobarbital) may interfere with the action of 1,25-dihydroxyvitamin D in the peripheral tissues and accelerate hepatic metabolism of this steroid hormone.

6. **List genetic disorders that interfere with vitamin D synthesis or action.**
   Three extremely rare genetic syndromes are also associated with rickets. Vitamin D–dependent rickets (VDDR) type I (also called pseudovitamin D deficiency rickets) is associated with an almost complete absence of renal 25-hydroxyvitamin D-1α-hydroxylase activity. VDDR type II results from a mutation of the vitamin D receptor gene, and VDDR type III, from an overproduction of hormone-responsive-element binding protein. Both VDDR type II and III cause an end-organ resistance to 1,25-dihydroxyvitamin D and a lack of vitamin D action.

7. **What conditions associated with abnormalities of phosphate metabolism result in osteomalacia or rickets?**
   Nutritional phosphate deficiency, decreased intestinal absorption of phosphate due to ingestion of phosphate binders (such as aluminum hydroxide) or renal phosphate wasting may result in osteomalacia or rickets. Hypophosphatemic rickets (also called vitamin D–resistant rickets) is a syndrome of renal phosphate wasting and decreased renal synthesis of 1,25-dihydroxyvitamin D. Hypophosphatemic rickets is the most common inherited form of rickets. This condition is

transmitted as an X-linked dominant trait. The abnormal gene for this disorder has been localized to the short arm of the X chromosome. Another syndrome, tumor-induced osteomalacia, is observed when usually benign neoplasms of mesenchymal origin produce osteomalacia by secreting fibroblast growth factor 23 or other phosphatonins.

8. **Does chronic renal failure cause osteomalacia and rickets?**
Chronic renal failure is associated with several bone diseases: osteomalacia or rickets, adynamic bone, osteitis fibrosa cystica (due to long-standing secondary hyperparathyroidism), and a combination of both osteomalacia and osteitis fibrosa cystica (termed mixed renal osteodystrophy). Rickets or osteomalacia is usually a late finding in the course of the kidney disease and is rarely seen before patients begin dialysis. Rickets or osteomalacia associated with chronic renal failure is caused by decreased circulating concentrations of 1,25-dihydroxyvitamin D, by aluminum intoxication from aluminum-containing antacids used as phosphate binders or an aluminum-contaminated dialysate, and possibly by the chronic metabolic acidosis associated with the renal failure.

9. **What clinical symptoms and findings are associated with osteomalacia?**
In adults, osteomalacia may be asymptomatic. When symptomatic, osteomalacia may present with diffuse skeletal pain (often aggravated by physical activity or palpation), proximal muscle weakness, and sometimes muscle wasting. The muscle weakness often involves the proximal muscles of the lower extremities and may result in a waddling gait and difficulties rising from a chair or climbing stairs. The bone pain is described as dull and aching and is usually located in the back, hips, knees, legs, and at sites of fractures. Fractures may result from only minor trauma.

10. **Describe the clinical findings in children with rickets.**
Because of the impaired calcification of cartilage at the growth plates in children with rickets, clinical manifestations of rickets are significantly different from those of osteomalacia. Widening of the metaphyses (the growth zones between the epiphysis and diaphysis), slowed growth, and various skeletal deformities are prominent in this condition. The effects of rickets are greatest at sites where the growth of bone is most rapid. Because the rate of growth of the skeleton varies with age, the manifestations of rickets likewise will vary with age. One of the earliest signs of rickets in infants is craniotabes (abnormal softness of the skull). In older infants and young children, thickening of the forearm at the wrist and of the costochondral junctions (also known as the rachitic rosary) and Harrison's groove, a lateral indentation of the chest wall at the site of attachment of the diaphragm, may be present. In older children, bowing of the tibia and fibula may be observed. At any age, if rickets (or osteomalacia) is associated with hypocalcemia, paresthesias of the hands and around the mouth, muscle cramps, positive Chvostek and Trousseau signs, tetany, and seizures may be evident.

11. **What are the biochemical abnormalities associated with osteomalacia and rickets caused by vitamin D deficiency?**
The laboratory abnormalities associated with osteomalacia or rickets depend on the underlying defect or process causing the bone disease. To understand the biochemical abnormalities observed in conditions associated with the abnormal metabolism of vitamin D, an understanding of the body's response to hypocalcemia and knowledge of the vitamin D metabolic pathway is necessary. Thus in patients with nutritional vitamin D deficiency or malabsorption, the low vitamin D concentrations result in a low-to-low normal serum calcium concentration, which serves as a stimulus for increased secretion of parathyroid hormone (secondary hyperparathyroidism). This hyperparathyroid state in turn causes increased renal excretion of phosphate, decreased serum phosphate and elevated alkaline phosphatase concentrations, and a reduced urinary calcium excretion.

12. **What are the vitamin D metabolite concentrations associated with the diseases that interfere with vitamin D metabolism or action?**

    Depending on the abnormality of vitamin D metabolism, different vitamin D metabolite patterns may be observed. In nutritional vitamin D deficiency, the 25-hydroxyvitamin D concentrations are low. In VDDR type I, in which there is a deficiency of the renal 25-hydroxyvitamin D-1α-hydroxylase enzyme, normal or increased serum 25-hydroxyvitamin D and low or undetectable serum 1,25-dihydroxyvitamin D concentrations are observed. In contrast, in VDDR type II and type III, which cause a resistance of target organs to 1,25-dihydroxyvitamin D, the concentrations of both 25-hydroxyvitamin D and 1,25-dihydroxyvitamin D are elevated.

13. **Describe the laboratory finding in disorders associated with the hypophosphatemic osteomalacia syndromes.**

    The hallmarks of the hypophosphatemic osteomalacia syndromes are fasting hypophosphatemia and renal phosphate wasting (as assessed by a decrease in the maximum renal tubular reabsorption of phosphate/glomerular filtration rate [TmP/GFR]). Serum calcium and parathyroid hormone concentrations are usually normal. Inexplicably, serum 1,25-dihydroxyvitamin D concentrations are inappropriately low for the degree of hypophosphatemia, which is normally a stimulus for renal 1α-hydroxylation of 25-hydroxyvitamin D.

14. **What radiographic findings are associated with osteomalacia and rickets?**

    The biochemical abnormalities associated with rickets and osteomalacia are usually evident before radiographic abnormalities are observed. The most common radiographic change in patients with osteomalacia is a reduction in skeletal density (generalized osteopenia or osteoporosis). Pseudofractures (also called Looser zones or Milkman fractures) or complete fractures also may be observed. Pseudofractures are transverse radiolucent bands ranging from a few millimeters to several centimeters in length, usually perpendicular to the surface of the bones. They are most often bilateral and are particularly common in the femur, pelvis, and small bones of the hands and feet.

    Certain radiographic abnormalities are primarily observed in children. These include fraying of the metaphyses of the long bones, widening of the unmineralized epiphyseal growth plates, and bowing of the legs. The skeletal deformities observed in children with rickets may persist into adulthood. Patients with osteomalacia may have additional radiographic findings due to secondary hyperparathyroidism. Such findings may include subperiosteal resorption of the phalanges, loss of the lamina dura of the teeth, widening of the spaces at the symphysis pubis and sacroiliac joints, and presence of brown tumors or bone cysts.

KEY POINTS: OSTEOMALACIA AND RICKETS

1. Osteomalacia and rickets are disorders resulting in inadequate or delayed mineralization of bone.

2. Osteomalacia occurs in mature bone, whereas rickets occurs in growing bone. Thus the clinical and radiographic findings of the two conditions differ.

3. The causes of osteomalacia and rickets fall into three categories: (1) disorders associated with abnormal vitamin D metabolism or action, (2) disorders associated with abnormal phosphate metabolism, and (3) a small group of disorders with normal vitamin D and mineral metabolism.

15. **Discuss the histologic features of osteomalacia.**

    The two diagnostic histologic findings of osteomalacia are the presence of widened osteoid seams and increased mineralization lag time (the time necessary for newly deposited matrix to mineralize). The mineralization lag time is assessed clinically by administration of two short courses of oral tetracycline several weeks apart before the bone biopsy. Because tetracycline is deposited at the mineralization front in newly formed bone, the lag time may be determined by measuring the distance between the two fluorescent tetracycline bands in the biopsied bone. Depending on the cause of the osteomalacia, hyperparathyroid bone changes may also be seen. Because of the varied clinical signs and symptoms, radiographic findings, and biochemical abnormalities associated with osteomalacia and rickets, none of these tests or findings is pathognomonic. The bone biopsy remains the gold standard in establishing the diagnosis of rickets and osteomalacia. The evaluation of a bone biopsy must be performed by personnel specially trained in the interpretation of bone histology.

16. **Describe the therapy for vitamin D deficiency.**
The goal of therapy for patients with osteomalacia and rickets caused by an abnormality of vitamin D metabolism is to correct the hypocalcemia and the deficiency of active vitamin D metabolites by administration of calcium salts and vitamin D preparations. In the United States, vitamin D_2 (ergocalciferol), 1,25-dihydroxyvitamin D (calcitriol), and analogs of calcitriol are available. Each of these preparations has a different half-life and potency. The choice and dose of vitamin D preparation are determined by the underlying pathologic defect of vitamin D metabolism. For patients with vitamin D deficiency, treatment with ergocalciferol along with elemental calcium is often sufficient to heal the osteomalacia.

17. **What are the treatments for osteomalacia and rickets not caused by vitamin D deficiency?**
In contrast to the treatment for vitamin D deficiency, therapy for osteomalacia associated with VDDR type II, which involves profound resistance to the effects of vitamin D, consists of administration of the most potent vitamin D metabolite, 1,25-dihydroxyvitamin D, in doses up to 60 mcg/day (an extraordinarily high dose), along with large doses of oral calcium. In severe cases, high-dose intravenous calcium infusions are required to heal the rickets in patients with VDDR type II. For treatment of hypophosphatemic rickets, both phosphate supplements and calcitriol are necessary to heal the bone disease. Tumor removal or irradiation is required to treat tumor-induced osteomalacia. In chronic renal failure with aluminum-induced osteomalacia, aluminum is removed from the affected bone by treatment with the chelating agent deferoxamine. The osteomalacia can then be treated by calcium together with 1,25-dihydroxyvitamin D. Osteomalacia associated with renal tubular acidosis is treated with vitamin D and bicarbonate to correct the acidosis.

18. **What are the complications of treatment with vitamin D2 or vitamin D metabolites?**
When high doses of vitamin D2 or one of the potent vitamin D metabolites are used, it is important to monitor carefully for the development of hypercalcemia. Mild hypercalcemia may be asymptomatic. However, severely hypercalcemic patients may complain of anorexia, nausea, vomiting, weight loss, headache, constipation, polyuria, polydipsia, and altered mental status. Impaired renal function, nephrocalcinosis, nephrolithiasis, and even death may eventually ensue. If vitamin D intoxication occurs, all calcium supplements and vitamin D preparations must be discontinued immediately and therapy for hypercalcemia instituted.

BIBLIOGRAPHY

1. Alon US: Hypophosphatemic vitamin D-resistant rickets. In Favus MJ, editor, *Primer on the metabolic bone diseases and disorders of mineral metabolism*, ed 6, Washington, DC, 2006, American Society for Bone and Mineral Research, p. 342.
2. Berry JL, Davies M, Mee AP: Vitamin D metabolism, rickets, and osteomalacia. Semin Musculoskelet Radiol 6:173, 2002.

3. Bingham CT, Fitzpatrick LA: Noninvasive testing in the diagnosis of osteomalacia. Am J Med 95:519, 1993.

4. Bliziotes M, Yergey AL, Nanes MS, et al: Absent intestinal response to calciferols in hereditary resistance to 1,25-dihydroxyvitamin D: documentation and effective therapy with high-dose intravenous calcium infusions. J Clin Endocrinol Metab 66:294, 1988.

5. Demay MB: Rickets caused by impaired vitamin D activation and hormone resistance: pseudovitamin D deficiency rickets and hereditary vitamin D resistant rickets. In Favus MJ, editor, *Primer on the metabolic bone diseases and disorders of mineral metabolism*, ed 6, Washington, DC, 2006, American Society for Bone and Mineral Research, p. 338.

6. Drezner MK: Vitamin D-resistant rickets/osteomalacia. Endocrinologist 3:392, 1991.

7. Francis RM, Selby PL: Osteomalacia. Baillieres Clin Endocrinol Metab 11:145, 1997.

8. Harvey JN, Gray C, Belchetz PE: Oncogenous osteomalacia and malignancy. Clin Endocrinol 37:379, 1992.

9. Holick MF: Resurrection of vitamin D deficiency and rickets. J Clin Invest 116:2062, 2006.

10. Holick MF: Vitamin D: a millennium perspective. J Cell Biochem 88:296, 2003.

11. Holick MF: Vitamin D deficiency. N Engl J Med 357:266, 2007.

12. Holick MF, Garabedian M: Vitamin D: photobiology, metabolism, mechanism of action and clinical applications. In Favus MJ, editor, *Primer on the metabolic bone diseases and disorders of mineral metabolism*, ed 6, Washington, DC, 2006, American Society for Bone and Mineral Research, p. 106.

13. Jan de Beur SM: Tumor-induced osteomalacia. In Favus MJ, editor, *Primer on the metabolic bone diseases and disorders of mineral metabolism*, ed 6, Washington, DC, 2006, American Society for Bone and Mineral Research, p. 345.

14. Pettifor JM: Nutritional and drug-induced rickets and osteomalacia. In Favus MJ, editor, *Primer on the metabolic bone diseases and disorders of mineral metabolism*, ed 6, Washington, DC, 2006, American Society for Bone and Mineral Research, p. 330.

15. Pitt MJ: Rickets and osteomalacia are still around. Radiol Clin North Am 29:97, 1991.

16. Wolinsky-Friedland M: Drug-induced metabolic bone disease. Endocrinol Metab Clin North Am 24:395, 1995.

CHAPTER 12

PAGET'S DISEASE OF BONE

William E. Duncan

1. **What is Paget's disease of bone?**

   Paget's disease of bone is characterized by abnormal bone architecture resulting from an imbalance between osteoblastic bone formation and osteoclastic bone resorption. Sir James Paget first described this disease in 1876. Although he called the condition osteitis deformans, we now know that Paget's disease of bone is not an inflammation of bone (osteitis) and only rarely results in deformity.

2. **Discuss how Paget's disease is diagnosed.**

   The diagnosis of Paget's disease is generally based on a combination of clinical manifestations, radiographic signs, and characteristic biochemical changes. Although histologic examination of pagetic bone is diagnostic, a bone biopsy is often unnecessary. Bone biopsy should be performed when the diagnosis of Paget's disease is unclear or when osteogenic sarcoma or metastatic carcinoma must be excluded.

3. **What are the clinical manifestations of Paget's disease?**

   Most patients (70%–80%) with Paget's disease are asymptomatic. This diagnosis is often suspected from radiographs performed for other reasons or from an unexpected elevation of the serum alkaline phosphatase concentration. The most common symptom of Paget's disease is bone or joint pain. The pain is often described as dull and aching. Other manifestations of Paget's disease, such as headache, bone deformity, skull enlargement, fracture, change in skin temperature over an involved bone, high-output congestive heart failure, and entrapment neuropathies that cause loss of hearing or other neurologic deficits, are much less common (Table 12-1). Neurologic deficits may arise from bony impingement on the brain or cranial nerves exiting from the skull, spinal nerve entrapment, or direct pressure of pagetic vertebrae on the spinal cord. Bone deformity is usually seen in patients with long-standing Paget's disease. Most commonly, the skull, clavicles, and long bones are deformed and exhibit both an increase in size and an abnormal contour. There is speculation that Ludwig Von Beethoven's hearing loss, headaches, and progressive hyperostosis frontalis were the results of long-standing Paget's disease of bone.

4. **What disorders are associated with Paget's disease of bone?**

   Several disorders are more prevalent in patients with Paget's disease than in unaffected individuals. These include arthritis, fractures, primary hyperparathyroidism, osteoporosis, thyroid disease, and kidney stones.

5. **What are the three phases of Paget's disease of bone?**

   Paget's disease progresses through three distinct phases. The initial phase is an osteolytic phase which is characterized by predominantly osteoclastic bone resorption. Approximately 1% to 2% of patients exhibit this purely lytic phase. The osteolytic phase evolves into one marked by both osteoclastic and osteoblastic overactivity. This mixed phase is followed by phase characterized by less active bone remodeling and marked sclerosis. In this final phase, excessive osteoblastic bone deposition predominates. Most patients who come to medical attention will exhibit findings compatible with this phase.

TABLE 12-1. COMPLICATIONS ASSOCIATED WITH PAGET'S DISEASE OF BONE

- Bone pain
- Bone deformity and enlargement
- Secondary osteoarthritis adjacent to pagetic bone
- Neurologic abnormalities
  - Spinal stenosis
  - Hearing loss and other cranial nerve palsies
  - Radiculopathy
- Obstructive hydrocephalus
- Cardiovascular complications
  - High-output cardiac failure
  - Vascular and aortic valve calcifications
- Fracture
- Malignant transformation
- Immobilization hypercalcemia

---

6. **Describe the radiographic findings associated with the osteolytic phase of Paget's disease.**

The characteristic radiographic finding found in patients in the initial osteolytic phase of Paget's disease of bone is an advancing wedge-shaped resorption front at either end of long tubular bones. In the skull, this phase is manifested by large circumscribed osteolytic lesions (termed osteoporosis circumscripta).

7. **What are the radiographic findings most commonly found in the osteoblastic phase of the disease?**

Evolution of osteolytic lesions into the osteoblastic phase may require years or even decades, during which the affected bone may become sclerotic and enlarged and demonstrate bowing deformities, incomplete transverse fractures (termed pseudofractures), and even complete fractures. When the skull is involved in the osteoblastic phase, thickening of the calvarium and a patchy increase in bone density may give the skull a "cotton-wool" appearance. In this phase, the sclerotic bone changes may be so extensive that they may be confused with metastatic disease. Both metastatic cancer and Paget's disease are common in the elderly and may coexist in the same patient. Thus the clinician caring for patients with Paget's disease must be alert for evidence of metastatic disease to bone.

8. **What is the best radiographic test to determine the extent of Paget's disease?**

The metabolic activity of osteoblastic pagetic bone lesions is most easily assessed by radionuclide scanning because these lesions avidly take up the technetium-labeled bisphosphonate. Although bone scans are diagnostically less specific than radiographic studies, they will identify approximately 15% to 30% of pagetic lesions not visualized in x-rays. Conversely, when radiographs demonstrate pagetic involvement but the serum alkaline phosphatase concentration is normal and the bone scan reveals little isotope uptake at those sites, the diagnosis of relatively inactive or "burned out" Paget's disease is most likely. Predominantly lytic bone lesions (such as osteoporosis circumscripta) may not be detected on bone scan. Computed tomography (CT) and magnetic resonance imaging (MRI) scans add little to the workup of patients with uncomplicated Paget's disease.

9. **Which bones are involved in Paget's disease?**
Paget's disease is monostotic (i.e., involves only one skeletal site) in about 20% of patients. Polyostotic Paget's disease involves several areas of the skeleton; common sites of pagetic involvement include the pelvis, hip, spine, skull, tibia, and humerus. Less common sites of involvement (<20% of cases) include the forearm, clavicles, scapulae, and ribs.

10. **Discuss the laboratory abnormalities associated with Paget's disease.**
The abnormal laboratory values associated with Paget's disease reflect either increased bone formation or increased bone resorption. Unless a patient with widespread Paget's disease is immobilized, serum calcium and phosphate concentrations should be normal. An elevated serum alkaline phosphatase concentration reflects increased osteoblastic function. Serum osteocalcin, another marker of bone formation, provides little additional information to that supplied by alkaline phosphatase. The serum bone-specific alkaline phosphatase is a more sensitive marker of bone formation than the total alkaline phosphatase concentration and thus may be a useful parameter to follow in the management of monostotic disease. Urinary pyridinium collagen cross-links (pyridinoline) is a better indicator of increased bone resorption than measurement of urinary hydroxyproline.

11. **Which laboratory test should be used to follow patients with Paget's disease?**
When the Paget's disease is primarily lytic, the alkaline phosphatase concentration may be normal. Otherwise, the serum alkaline phosphatase activity generally parallels the chemical indices of bone resorption. Thus the total serum alkaline phosphatase concentration is the simplest and least expensive laboratory test to follow the course and response to treatment of most cases of Paget's disease. Of interest, a markedly elevated alkaline phosphatase concentration (e.g., 10 times the upper limit of normal) is usually associated with pagetic involvement of the skull, whereas widespread disease in the rest of the skeleton without involvement of the skull may be associated with more modest elevations of serum alkaline phosphatase. In patients with increased total alkaline phosphatase concentrations, liver disease should be excluded because this enzyme is abundant in both liver and bone. If liver-specific tests, such as 5'-nucleotidase, gamma-glutamyl transpeptidase, or the liver alkaline phosphatase isoenzyme are normal, it is likely that the elevated alkaline phosphatase originates from bone.

12. **What are the histological findings in bone affected by Paget's disease?**
The early lesions of Paget's disease are characterized by increased numbers of large multinucleated osteoclasts, some containing up to 100 nuclei. In the mixed osteolytic-osteoblastic phase, large numbers of active osteoblasts are seen forming bone at sites of prior osteoclastic bone resorption. In areas of intense osteoblastic activity, bone is deposited in a chaotic fashion (in a mosaic or woven pattern) rather than in the orderly lamellar pattern of normal bone. The woven bone of Paget's disease is structurally weaker than normal lamellar bone and explains the propensity for pagetic bone to fracture or deform.

13. **Which patients are most likely to have Paget's disease?**
The incidence of Paget's disease varies with age, gender, and geographic location. Although Paget's disease may present in younger individuals, the disease is most common in patients older than 50 years. Men are more commonly affected than women. (The male-to-female ratio is approximately 3:2.) Although there is no definite hereditary pattern, between 15% and 40% of affected patients have a first-degree relative with Paget's disease. The disease is more common in the populations of eastern and northern Europe and in areas where Europeans have immigrated (such as the United States, Australia, New Zealand, and South Africa). Paget's disease is uncommon in Scandinavia, Asia, and Africa, as well as in African Americans.

14. **What is the cause of Paget's disease?**

Although the cause of Paget's disease is unknown, both genetic and nongenetic factors have been implicated in the pathogenesis of this disease. Several susceptibility loci for Paget's disease have been identified. However, the finding of monostotic disease, the variable penetrance of Paget's disease in families with a genetic disposition, and the observation that the incidence of Paget's disease has been decreasing over the last 25 years support a role for environmental factors in the etiology of this disease. Reports of structures resembling paramyxovirus nucleocapsids in the osteoclasts of active pagetic bone suggest a viral etiology. The measles virus, respiratory syncytial virus, and canine distemper virus have been suggested as etiologic agents, although to date no virus has ever been cultured from pagetic osteoclasts or osteoclast precursors.

15. **What medications are available to treat Paget's disease?**

Although there is no cure for Paget's disease, several medications are available to control the accelerated osteoclastic bone resorption seen in this disease. The medications used for the treatment of Paget's bone disease include bisphosphonates and calcitonin (Calcimar, Miacalcin injection). At present, there are six bisphosphonates approved for the treatment of Paget's disease of bone: four oral preparations and two intravenous medications. The bisphosphonates available for use in the United States for the treatment of Paget's disease include etidronate (Didronel), alendronate (Fosamax), risedronate (Actonel), tiludronate (Skelid), pamidronate (Aredia), and zoledronic acid (Reclast). Although another bisphosphonate, ibandronate, has been used for treatment of Paget's disease in research studies, this drug (intravenous and oral) has not been approved for the treatment of Paget's disease. Salmon calcitonin is a parenteral preparation requiring intramuscular or subcutaneous injection. Salmon calcitonin nasal spray (Miacalcin) is not effective for treating Paget's disease because of low drug bioavailability.

16. **Which agents are the treatment of choice for Paget's disease of bone?**

Bisphosphonates are the agents of choice for treatment of Paget's disease. Treatment with bisphosphonates often results in suppression of disease activity for prolonged periods, sometimes lasting for several years, whereas the response to calcitonin is generally short-lived after treatment is discontinued.

Etidronate, tiludronate, and calcitonin are rarely used given the availability of more potent medications. A recent study compared a 15-minute infusion of zoledronic acid with 60 days of oral risedronate in patients with Paget's disease. The single infusion of zoledronic acid produced a more rapid, complete, and sustained response than did daily treatment with risedronate. Thus intravenous bisphosphonate therapy may be more appropriate for extensive active disease or for those patients unresponsive to oral bisphosphonate therapy. Treatment of symptomatic patients should also include other therapeutic modalities, such as analgesics, nonsteroidal anti-inflammatory drugs, canes, orthotics, hearing aids, and surgery.

17. **Does resistance to therapy for Paget's disease of bone occur?**

Resistance to both bisphosphonates and calcitonin does occur. Resistance to treatment of Paget's disease with salmon calcitonin is usually associated with neutralizing antibody formation. Development of resistance after therapy with some bisphosphonates has also been reported. However, studies suggest that resistance to one bisphosphonate does not preclude a good response to a second bisphosphonate.

18. **What is osteonecrosis of the jaw, and do patients with Paget's disease treated with bisphosphonates get this disorder?**

Osteonecrosis of the jaw (ONJ) is a rare finding in which an area of exposed bone in the maxillofacial area persists for more than 6 weeks. This condition usually occurs following dental surgery. The symptoms vary from painless exposed bone to severe jaw pain. ONJ has also been described in patients receiving prolonged intravenous bisphosphonates for cancer with bony metastases, although there have been a few reports of this condition occurring in patients with Paget's disease treated with intravenous pamidronate. Thus the risk of ONJ should not preclude the use of bisphosphonates for the treatment of Paget's disease. However, it is recommended that treatment with bisphosphonates be delayed until after planed extensive dental work or oral surgery is completed and that all patients treated with bisphosphonates receive routine dental exams and oral care.

19. **What are the indications for treatment of Paget's disease?**
The primary indication for treatment is the presence of symptoms. However, not all symptoms respond to treatment. Bone pain usually responds, as do certain neurologic compression syndromes. In contrast, hearing loss, bony deformities, and mechanically dysfunctional joints are not likely to improve with therapy. Additional indications for treatment of Paget's disease are the prevention of local progression and future complications (Table 12-2), planned surgery at a pagetic site, and widespread pagetic involvement in patients in whom prolonged immobilization is anticipated, because immobilization increases the risk for hypercalcemia.
   Treatment of asymptomatic patients with Paget's disease is controversial. However, untreated Paget's disease appears to be progressive with time, and not all asymptomatic patients remain asymptomatic. Thus many physicians treat patients with osteolytic Paget's disease or asymptomatic patients with active disease involving weight-bearing bones, vertebral bodies, the skull, or areas adjacent to major joints.

TABLE 12-2. INDICATIONS FOR TREATMENT OF PAGET'S DISEASE OF BONE

- Symptoms (bone pain, headache, and some neurologic abnormalities)
- Osteolytic bone disease
- Active asymptomatic disease in:
  - Weight-bearing bones
  - Areas adjacent to major joints
  - Vertebral bodies
  - Skull
- Young patients
- Before orthopedic surgery on pagetic bone
- Immobilization hypercalcemia

---

20. **In asymptomatic patients with Paget's disease, at what concentration of alkaline phosphatase should treatment begin?**
The answer to this question is controversial. The level of alkaline phosphatase should be viewed in the context of the radiographic picture. A concentration of alkaline phosphatase only 2 to 3 times the upper limit of normal with polyostotic involvement may simply reflect the late "burned-out" phase of the disease. Little benefit results from treatment in these cases. However, the same alkaline phosphatase concentration in a patient with monostotic Paget's disease in a weight-bearing bone or in an area adjacent to a major joint would lead most physicians to consider treatment. In addition, patients with lytic pagetic lesions and normal or near-normal alkaline phosphatase values should also be considered for treatment.

21. **What is the most serious complication of Paget's disease of bone?**
The most serious complication of Paget's disease is the development of malignant sarcomas in pagetic bone. Such tumors are usually isolated, but 20% may be multicentric. Fortunately, this is

a rare complication of Paget's disease, occurring in less than 1% of patients with clinically apparent disease. The tumors are extremely aggressive. Patients with Paget's sarcoma generally survive less than a year. The pelvis and long bones (humerus, femur, and tibia) are the most common sites for sarcomatous transformation. The tumors are usually osteogenic sarcomas, but fibrosarcomas and chondrosarcomas have also been reported in bone affected by Paget's disease. A biopsy of the involved bone is usually diagnostic. Other bone neoplasms, such as benign giant cell tumors, are also associated with Paget's disease, but these tumors do not carry such a grave prognosis.

22. **When should malignant sarcoma in a pagetic bone lesion be suspected?**
Malignant transformation within pagetic bone is usually heralded by the onset of new or worsening bone pain and/or soft tissue swelling. Usually, progressive destruction of pagetic bone is found on radiographs. Less commonly, increasing sclerosis or masses of dense amorphous deposits in bone are suggestive of malignant change. The concentration of serum alkaline phosphatase may rise rapidly in an otherwise previously stable patient. Bone scans usually demonstrate decreased uptake of radionucleotide in the area of the tumor. However, gallium scans show increased uptake in the involved area(s).

KEY POINTS: PAGET'S DISEASE OF BONE

1. Paget's disease is the second most common metabolic bone disease, affecting up to 5% of the Caucasian population over the age of 50.

2. Paget's disease is characterized by abnormal bone architecture resulting from an imbalance between osteoblastic bone formation and osteoclastic bone resorption.

3. Bisphosphonates are the most effective treatment for Paget's disease of bone.

WEBSITE

The Paget Foundation: http://www.paget.org

BIBLIOGRAPHY

1. Ankrom MA, Shapiro JR: Paget's disease of bone (osteitis deformans). J Am Geriatr Soc 46:1025, 1998.

2. Delmas PD, Meunier PJ: The management of Paget's disease of bone. N Engl J Med 336:558, 1997.

3. Drake WM, Kendler DL, Brown JP: Consensus statement on the modern therapy of Paget's disease of bone from a Western Osteoporosis Alliance Symposium. Clin Ther 23:620, 2001.

4. Hadjipavlou A, Lander P, Srolovitz H, Enker IP: Malignant transformation in Paget's disease of bone. Cancer 70:2802, 1992.

5. Hain SF, Fogelman I: Nuclear medicine studies in metabolic bone disease. Semin Muscoskelet Radiol 6:323, 2002.

6. Joshua F, Epstein M, Major G: Bisphosphonate resistance in Paget's disease of bone. Arthritis Rheum 48:2321, 2003.

7. Leach RJ, Singer FR, Roodman GD: The genetics of Paget's disease. J Clin Endocrinol Metab 86:24–28, 2001.

8. Lyles KW, Siris ES, Singer FR, Meunier PH: A clinical approach to diagnosis and management of Paget's disease of bone. J Bone Miner Res 16:1379, 2001.

9. Mills BG: Etiology and pathophysiology of Paget's disease—update. Endocrinologist 7:222, 1997.

10. Papapoulos SE: Paget's disease of bone: clinical, pathogenetic and therapeutic aspects. Baillieres Clin Endocrinol Metab 11:117, 1997.

11. Proceedings of the Third International Symposium on Paget's Disease. J Bone Mineral Res 14(Suppl 2), 1999.

12. Reid IR, Miller P, Lyles K, et al: Comparison of a single infusion of zoledronic acid with risedronate for Paget's disease. N Engl J Med 353:9, 2005.

13. Roodman GD, Windle JJ: Paget disease of bone. J Clin Invest 115:200, 2005.

14. Sawin CT: Historical note: Sir James Paget and osteitis deformans. Endocrinologist 7:205, 1997. (Also see p 255 in the same issue for a reproduction of one of James Paget's original articles on osteitis deformans.)

15. Sellars SL: Beethoven's deafness. S Afr Med J 48:1585, 1974.

16. Siris ES: Clinical review—Paget's disease of bone. J Bone Miner Res 13:1061, 1998.

17. Siris ES, Lyles KW, Singer FR, Meunier PJ: Medical management of Paget's disease of bone: indications for treatment and review of current therapies. J Bone Miner Res 21(Suppl 2):P94, 2006.

18. Siris ES, Roodman GD: Paget's disease of bone. In Favus MJ, editor, *Primer on the metabolic bone diseases and disorders of mineral metabolism*, ed 6, New York, 2006, Raven Press, p. 320.

19. Whyte MP: Paget's disease of bone. N Engl J Med 355:593, 2006.

20. Wimalawansa SJ, Gunasekera RD: Pamidronate is effective for Paget's disease of bone refractory to conventional therapy. Calcif Tissue Int 53:237, 1993.

CHAPTER 13

HYPERCALCEMIA

Leonard R. Sanders

1. **What is hypercalcemia? How does protein binding affect the calcium level?**
   Hypercalcemia is a corrected total serum calcium value above the upper limit of the normal range or elevated ionized calcium. Calcium is 50% free (ionized), 40% protein-bound, and 10% complexed to phosphate, citrate, bicarbonate, sulfate, and lactate. Only elevations in the free calcium are associated with symptoms and signs. Of the protein-bound calcium, about 80% is bound to albumin and 20% to globulins. A decrease or increase in serum albumin of 1 g/dL from 4 g/dL decreases or increases the serum calcium by 0.8 mg/dL. An increase or decrease in serum globulin by 1 g/dL increases or decreases serum calcium by 0.16 mg/dL. Such protein changes do not affect free calcium and do not cause calcium-related symptoms.

2. **How common are hypercalcemia and its main associated conditions?**
   Hypercalcemia affects 0.5% to 1% of the general population. The incidence may increase to 3% among postmenopausal women. Primary hyperparathyroidism causes 70% of outpatient and 20% of inpatient hypercalcemia. Cancer causes 50% of inpatient hypercalcemia. Ten percent of patients with malignancy develop hypercalcemia. Hyperparathyroidism and cancer cause 90% of all hypercalcemia. About 10% of patients with hyperparathyroidism develop nephrolithiasis. Although calcium oxalate stones are most common, calcium phosphate stones are most characteristic of hyperparathyroidism.

3. **How would you classify mild, moderate, and severe hypercalcemia?**
   First, consider the patient's general health, hypercalcemic symptoms, and the normal upper limit for calcium in your laboratory. For example, a patient with renal failure and serum phosphorus of 8.5 mg/dL may have metastatic calcification with serum calcium of 10.5 mg/dL. Then correct the serum calcium for the albumin concentration:

   $$Ca_{corrected} = Ca_{observed} + [(4.0 - albumin) \times 0.8].$$

   With this in mind, serum calcium of 1.5 to 3.5 mg/dL above the upper normal limit defines moderate hypercalcemia. Mild hypercalcemia occurs below this range, and severe hypercalcemia, above. Thus if the upper normal limit for calcium is 10.5 mg/dL, serum calcium of 12 to 14 mg/dL is moderate hypercalcemia. Serum calcium less than 12 mg/dL is mild hypercalcemia and greater than 14 mg/dL severe hypercalcemia.

4. **Discuss the signs and symptoms of hypercalcemia.**
   No symptoms are usually present with mild hypercalcemia (<12 mg/dL). Moderate or severe hypercalcemia and rapidly developing mild hypercalcemia may cause symptoms and signs. Common symptoms and signs involve (1) the central nervous system (lethargy, stupor, coma, mental changes, psychosis), (2) the gastrointestinal tract (anorexia, nausea, constipation, acid peptic disease, pancreatitis), (3) the kidneys (polyuria, nephrolithiasis), (4) the musculoskeletal system (arthralgias, myalgias, weakness), and (5) the vascular system (hypertension). The classic electrocardiographic (ECG) change associated with hypercalcemia is a short Q-T interval. Occasionally severe hypercalcemia also causes dysrhythmias, ST segment depression, sinus arrest, and disturbances in atrioventricular (AV) conduction.

5. **What are the sources of serum calcium?**
   Bone calcium approximates 1 kg and 99% of body calcium. Normal serum calcium is maintained by integrated regulation of calcium absorption, resorption, and reabsorption; these processes occur, respectively, in the gut, bone, and kidney. Of the 1000 mg/day of dietary calcium intake, the gut absorbs 300 mg/day, secretes 100 mg/day, and excretes 800 mg/day. Net absorption averages 200 mg/day. Absorption may vary from 30% to 70% of dietary calcium depending on the amount of 1,25(OH)2D present. The kidney reabsorbs 98% of filtered calcium and excretes 200 mg/day. Bone exchanges about 500 mg of calcium per day with serum (Fig. 13-1).

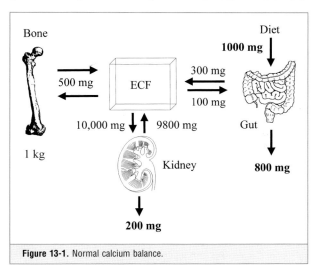

Figure 13-1. Normal calcium balance.

6. **What are the major anatomic and physiologic determinants of vitamin D?**
   Diet, skin, liver, and kidney control the amount, synthesis, and secretion of vitamin D. Dietary sources of vitamin D include liver, fish oils, egg yolks, vitamin D-fortified foods, and vitamin D supplements. Skin exposure to ultraviolet sunlight activates 7-dehydrocholesterol to pre–vitamin D, which subsequently rearranges to form vitamin D. Hepatic 25-hydroxylase then converts vitamin D to 25-hydroxyvitamin D (25-OHD). 25-OHD circulates and interacts with two renal mitochondrial hydroxylases. High parathyroid hormone (PTH), low phosphate, and low calcium stimulate 1-hydroxylase activity to increase conversion of 25-OHD to 1,25(OH)2D (calcitriol)— the most potent metabolite of vitamin D. Low PTH, high phosphate, and high calcium suppress 1-hydroxylase activity and stimulate 24-hydroxylase activity. This inhibits calcitriol production and, through 24-hydroxylase, converts 25-OHD to 24,25-dihydroxyvitamin D [24,25(OH)2D], which promotes antiresorptive effects on bone and positive calcium balance. This same sequence occurs less intensely with normal levels of PTH, PO4, and calcium. Calcitriol feeds back negatively on its own synthesis by suppressing 1-hydroxylase activity, stimulating 24-hydroxylase activity, decreasing PTH, increasing calcium, and increasing phosphate. Calcitriol is also degraded primarily through the enzyme 24-hydroxylase. 1-hydroxylase activity is classically thought of only in the kidney, but this enzyme is also present in bone (Fig. 13-2).

7. **What are the classical and nonclassical effects of vitamin D and what is the role of the vitamin D receptor?**
   Calcitriol acts classically on intestine, bone, kidney, and parathyroid gland to help regulate calcium and phosphate metabolism. When calcitriol activates the parathyroid vitamin D receptor (VDR), it decreases PTH mRNA synthesis by inhibiting the pre-pro-PTH gene at the vitamin D response element. This decreases PTH synthesis within the chief cell of the parathyroid gland

Figure 13-2. Vitamin D metabolism.

and ultimately lowers PTH levels. Additionally, calcitriol increases intestinal calcium and phosphate absorption, increases bone calcium and phosphate resorption, enhances bone turnover, and enhances renal calcium and phosphate reabsorption. The VDR is a nuclear hormone receptor that is also regulated by calcium and PTH. Many proteins are downregulated and upregulated by the activated VDR. Downregulated proteins include PTH, 1-hydroxylase, bone matrix protein, bone sialoprotein, type I collagen, interferons, interleukins, tumor necrosis factor (TNF), epidermal growth factor receptors, renin, and PPAR Gamma 2. Upregulated proteins include osteopontin, matrix Gla protein, type IV collagen, interleukins, VDR, calcium sensing receptor (CaR), and 24-hydroxylase. By activating the VDR, calcitriol has many (nonclassical) effects other than those related to calcium and phosphorus metabolism. VDR activation may ameliorate arterial calcification, retard neuronal degeneration, enhance host defenses against bacterial infection and tumor growth, enhance Sertoli cell function and spermatogenesis, enhance insulin synthesis and secretion from pancreatic beta cells, and assist with glycogen and transferrin synthesis in liver parenchymal cells. Additionally, calcitriol has antiproliferative and prodifferentiating effects on myeloid cell precursors, cardiac and smooth muscle cells, and a variety of skin cells, including keratinocytes, fibroblasts, hair follicles, and melanocytes.

8. **What is the CaR and what role does it play in calcium metabolism?**
   The CaR is a membrane-bound receptor located in many tissues in the body including low levels in pancreatic beta cells and thyroid C cells. The major function of the CaR is to keep calcium in the normal range and prevent hypercalcemia. The most important locations of the CaR are the parathyroid glands and the renal tubular cells. In the chief cells of the parathyroid, the CaR has a large extracellular domain of 700 amino acids (primary calcium binding site), a transmembranous portion of seven segments (primary calcimimetic binding site), and a cytoplasmic carboxyl-terminal component of about 200 amino acids (primary effector site for metabolic changes). The CaR belongs to a subfamily C of the G protein–coupled receptor family. The CaR senses the minutest change in ionized calcium and regulates PTH secretion in attempt to maintain steady-state calcium levels. These changes center around a set point for calcium-regulated PTH release. The set point is the calcium concentration at which PTH values are midway between the maximum and minimum achievable PTH levels. Cinacalcet, a calcimimetic, binds to the transmembranous portion of the CaR, making it markedly more responsive to any given level of ambient calcium. After it is activated by calcium, the CaR activates phospholipase C, inhibits adenylate cyclase, and opens nonselective cation channels. This results in increased

cytoplasmic calcium by mobilizing calcium from thapsigargin-sensitive intracellular stores and influx of Ca through voltage-insensitive cation channels. These CaR-induced changes in intracellular calcium act on the calcium response element of the pre-pro-PTH gene to decrease PTH mRNA synthesis. The net result of these CaR-mediated events in parathyroid chief cells is reduced PTH secretion, suppressed PTH mRNA levels, and decreased parathyroid gland hyperplasia. Secretion of PTH by the parathyroid glands includes Intact PTH (iPTH) and carboxy-terminal PTH fragments (CPTH). Intact PTH acts directly on bone PTH receptors. CPTH remains in the circulation much longer and at higher concentrations than iPTH and was previously thought to be inactive. Recent data suggest that CPTH fragments can exert direct effects on bone cells through a novel class of CPTH receptors. CPTH fragments accumulate in renal failure. PTH functions to keep calcium in the normal range and helps prevent hypocalcemia.

9. **What is the function of the CaR in the kidney?**
   In the kidney, as in the parathyroid gland, the CaR functions to prevent hypercalcemia. Activation of the CaR located on the basolateral membrane in the thick ascending limb of Henle's loop decreases tubular reabsorption of calcium and increases excretion. Activation of the renal CaR generates an arachidonic acid metabolite that inhibits the luminal potassium channel and the sodium-potassium ATPase pump on the basolateral membrane. This diminishes the lumen-positive electrical gradient needed for passive calcium and magnesium reabsorption. Thus there is less reabsorption and more excretion of calcium. Because PTH is decreased by the CaR activated in the parathyroid gland, there is less PTH-mediated distal tubular reabsorption of calcium, net calcium loss, and lower plasma calcium.

10. **What are the overall effects of PTH and vitamin D on calcium metabolism?**
    Plasma calcium must be maintained within a narrow concentration range because of the key role it plays in a diverse array of physiological processes, including intracellular signal transduction, muscle contraction, and neuronal transmission. Regulation of plasma calcium depends on normal amounts of PTH and calcitriol. Both hormones are also necessary for normal bone health. PTH and calcitriol provide the main control of serum calcium. Both PTH and calcitriol increase bone resorption by increasing osteoclast activity. At physiological levels, PTH and calcitriol also increase bone formation. Because osteoclasts have no known receptors for either hormone, PTH and calcitriol stimulate osteoclast activity indirectly. Both hormones promote normal bone formation by action on the osteoblast line of cells. PTH enhances the activity of osteoblasts, which secrete factors such as interleukin-6 (IL-6) that stimulate osteoclastic bone resorption. Calcitriol promotes osteoclast differentiation from promonocytes to monocytes to macrophages and finally to osteoclasts. This is accompanied by an increase in osteoclast number and activity and decreased collagen synthesis. In addition, calcitriol increases calcium transport from bone to blood and maintains a favorable calcium-phosphate product necessary for normal bone mineralization. These actions occur partly by stimulating osteoblast production of a membrane-bound protein called receptor activator of NF-B ligand (RANKL). RANKL acts on its receptor in osteoclasts and their precursor cells. Higher PTH and calcitriol levels increase bone resorption abnormally and may cause hypercalcemia. Bone resorption is the major mechanism of most hypercalcemia (see Table 13-4). PTH and calcitriol act on the kidney to increase Ca reabsorption. PTH increases renal phosphate excretion, and calcitriol increases its reabsorption. PTH has no direct effect on the intestine, but calcitriol increases both calcium and phosphate absorption. The higher calcium and calcitriol provide negative feedback on PTH secretion, whereas higher phosphate levels provide positive feedback. The net effect is normal bone function and plasma calcium at physiological levels of PTH and calcitriol and loss of bone mineral and hypercalcemia at high levels of the two hormones.

11. **How do calcium and phosphate interact with calcium-regulating hormones?**
    Table 13-1 summarizes the main factors controlling serum calcium. The arrows show direct actions of factors in the left column on factors in the top row, whereas the plus (+) and minus (−) signs show indirect actions. As a rule, the direct effects predominate as the net effect. Table 13-2 outlines the specific effects of each of these factors.

TABLE 13-1. INTERACTION OF FACTORS CONTROLLING SERUM CALCIUM

	PTH	1,25(OH)$_2$D	Calcitonin	Calcium	PO$_4$
PTH	—	↑+	+	↑+	↓↑+
1,25(OH)$_2$D	↓−	↓−	+	↑	↑
Calcitonin	+	+	—	↓	↓
Calcium	↓	↓	↑	—	↓
PO$_4$	↑+	↓	—	↓	—

PO$_4$, phosphate; PTH, parathyroid hormone.

TABLE 13-2. SUMMARY OF CALCIUM AND PHOSPHATE CONTROL

Variable	Direct Action
PTH	Increased bone resorption of calcium and phosphate
	Increased distal renal tubular calcium reabsorption
	Decreased renal tubular phosphate reabsorption
	Increased renal production of 1,25(OH$_2$)D
	Net effect: increased serum calcium and decreased phosphate
1,25(OH)$_2$D	Increased bone resorption of calcium and phosphate
	Increased renal reabsorption of calcium and phosphate
	Increased gut absorption of calcium and phosphate
	Decreased parathyroid production of PTH
	Decreased renal production of 1,25(OH)$_2$D
	Net effect: increased serum calcium and phosphate
Calcitonin	Decreased bone resorption of calcium and phosphate
	Decreased renal reabsorption of calcium and phosphate
	Decreased gut absorption of calcium and phosphate
	Net effect: decreased serum calcium and phosphate
Calcium	Decreases PTH synthesis and secretion
	Decreases 1,25(OH)$_2$D production in the kidney
	Increases calcitonin release from the thyroid C cells
	Decreases phosphate
Phosphate	Decreases 1,25(OH)$_2$D production in the kidney
	Decreases calcium Increases PTH synthesis in parathyroid chief cells

PTH, parathyroid hormone.

12. **List the main causes of hypercalcemia.**
The mnemonic VITAMINS TRAP (Pont, 1989) includes most causes of hypercalcemia:

V = Vitamins	T = Thiazide diuretics (drugs)
I = Immobilization	R = Rhabdomyolysis
T = Thyrotoxicosis	A = AIDS
A = Addison's disease	P = Paget's disease, parenteral nutrition, pheochromocytoma, parathyroid disease
M = Milk-alkali syndrome	
I = Inflammatory disorders	
N = Neoplastic-related disease	
S = Sarcoidosis	

13. **How do various causes of hypercalcemia increase the serum calcium?**
True hypercalcemia results from altered bone resorption, renal tubular reabsorption, and gut absorption of calcium. Although the bone (resorption and formation), kidney (reabsorption and excretion), and gut (absorption and secretion) have two major processes involved with mineral metabolism, only resorption, reabsorption, and absorption play a significant role in hypercalcemia. An exception to this rule occurs when decreased renal function from renal or prerenal disease impairs calcium filtration and excretion. In Fig. 13-3, solid arrows represent potential causes of increased calcium, and dashed arrows represent potential causes of decreased calcium.

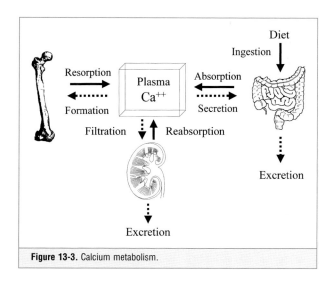

Figure 13-3. Calcium metabolism.

14. What are the mechanisms and causes of hypercalcemia?

From the preceding discussions, one appreciates that mechanisms of hypercalcemia are usually multifactorial. However, most hypercalcemic syndromes have a primary or predominant mechanism, as outlined in Table 13-3. Most resorptive hypercalcemia is humoral (PTH-related peptide [PTHrP], transforming growth factor-α [TGFα], TNF), or local osteolytic hypercalcemia

TABLE 13-3. MECHANISMS AND CAUSES OF HYPERCALCEMIA

Primary Mechanism	Cause of Hypercalcemia
Increased bone resorption	Hyperparathyroidism
	Local osteolytic hypercalcemia
	Humoral hypercalcemia of malignancy
	Thyrotoxicosis
	Pheochromocytoma
	Excessive vitamin A (usually >25,000 IU/day)
	Lithium carbonate
	Immobilization
	Addison's (possible sensitivity to thyroid hormone)
Increased renal reabsorption or decreased excretion	Milk-alkali syndrome
	Rhabdomyolysis
	Thiazide diuretics
	FHH
	Renal failure
	Lithium carbonate
Increased gut absorption	Excessive vitamin D (usually >10,000 IU/day)
	Berylliosis
	Candidiasis
	Coccidioidomycosis
	Eosinophilic granuloma
	Histoplasmosis
	Sarcoidosis
	Silicone implants
	Tuberculosis
	Inflammatory disorders
	AIDS
	Lymphomas

AIDS, acquired immunodeficiency syndrome; FHH, familial hypocalciuric hypercalcemia.

(PTHrP, interleukins, prostaglandins). Most increased calcium absorption occurs in response to excess 1,25(OH)2D produced by granulomas or tumors. Ninety percent of hypercalcemia results from hyperparathyroidism or cancer.

KEY POINTS: HYPERCALCEMIA

1. Therapy for hypercalcemia should be directed at the underling etiology, including excess bone resorption, renal tubular reabsorption, and gut absorption.

2. Although there are over 30 major causes of hypercalcemia, hyperparathyroidism and hypercalcemia of malignancy account for more than 90%.

3. Most patients with severe hypercalcemia require normal saline hydration and multiple drug therapy, but most therapies for hypercalcemia inhibit bone resorption.

4. Zoledronic acid is the most potent bisphosphonate approved for treatment of hypercalcemia and has the advantage over pamidronate of a shorter infusion time and a longer duration of action.

5. Cinacalcet is a calcimimetic approved for treatment of secondary hyperpara thyroidis (HPT) and parathyroid carcinoma. Cinacalcet can reduce parathyroid hormone (PTH) to normal and lowers calcium and phosphate in patients with secondary HPT of renal disease. Although not approved for such, cinacalcet also lowers PTH and calcium in primary HPT.

15. **What is the relative frequency of skeletal lesions in patients with advanced cancer?**
The relative frequency is as follows: myeloma 95% to 100%, breast and prostate 70%, thyroid 60%, bladder 40%, lung 35%, renal 25%, and melanoma 14% to 45%. Common sites of bone metastases are ribs, spine, pelvis, and proximal extremities.

16. **What is the incidence of hypercalcemia in patients with cancer?**
Hypercalcemia affects 10% to 20% of patients with cancer. It is most common in squamous cell carcinoma of the lung, head, and neck, renal cell carcinoma, breast cancer, multiple myeloma, and lymphoma.

17. **What are the multiple endocrine neoplasia syndromes?**
Multiple endocrine neoplasia (MEN) is associated with three familial syndromes, two of which present with hypercalcemia due to hyperparathyroidism. MEN 1, or Wermer syndrome, includes the three Ps: pituitary, parathyroid, and pancreatic tumors. Hypercalcemia due to hyperparathyroidism is usually the first feature of this syndrome to appear. MEN 2 has two variants. Patients with MEN 2a, or Sipple syndrome, have medullary carcinoma of the thyroid (MCT), pheochromocytoma, and hyperparathyroidism. Patients with MEN-IIb have MCT, pheochromocytoma, multiple mucosal neuromas, and marfanoid habitus; they usually do not have hyperparathyroidism. Relative to sporadic hyperparathyroidism, parathyroid tumors in the MEN syndromes are more often bilateral, hyperplastic, and malignant.

18. **How would you diagnose familial hypocalciuric hypercalcemia?**
Familial hypocalciuric hypercalcemia (FHH), also called benign familial hypercalcemia, is due to an autosomal dominant genetic mutation resulting in an inactivating mutation for the CaR on the membranes of parathyroid and renal tubular cells. The most important diagnostic features of FHH are the combination of no symptoms, a family history of benign hypercalcemia, mild hypercalcemia, normal-to-high serum levels of PTH, and decreased renal clearance of calcium

(fractional excretion of calcium [FECa] <1%). The clinical importance of FHH is to distinguish it from primary hyperparathyroidism to avoid needless and ineffective parathyroidectomy. Patients with primary hyperparathyroidism usually have a FECa greater than 2%.

19. **What is the likely cause of hypercalcemia in the following patient?**
    An 18-year-old man has presented with calcium values of 10.5 to 11.8 for 2 years, as well as a normal physical examination and a family history of hypercalcemia. Current laboratory values are as follows: calcium 11.5 mg/dL, intact PTH 70 pg/mL (normal NL<65), serum creatinine (Cr) 1.0 mg/dL, random urine calcium 5 mg/dL, and urine Cr 90 mg/dL. Because circulating proteins bind 40% of the calcium, the kidney filters only 60%. Plasma calcium available for filtration is 0.6 × 11.5 or 6.9 mg/dL:

    $$FECa = [UCa/PCa]/[UCr/PCr] = [UCa/PCa] \times [PCr/UCr]$$
    $$FECa = [5 \text{ mg/dL}/6.9 \text{ mg/dL}] \times [1 \text{ mg/dL}/90 \text{ mg/dL}] \times 100\% = 0.8\%,$$

    where UCa = urine calcium, UCr = urine creatinine, PCa = plasma calcium, and PCr = plasma creatinine. The history, physical, laboratory, and FECa of less than 1% support the diagnosis of FHH.

20. **What therapy is useful for hypercalcemia?**
    Most patients with severe hypercalcemia require treatment with multiple drugs. Give the lowest amount and least frequent dose that will achieve and maintain acceptable serum calcium. The usual order of therapy includes normal saline, calcitonin, zoledronic acid, and glucocorticoids, if indicated. Give furosemide after good hydration primarily to avoid volume overload and improve urinary volume. Plicamycin is no longer available for clinical use. Use gallium nitrate rarely for severe hypercalcemia of malignancy that is refractory to all other therapy. Consult with nephrology and consider dialysis for acute management of severe and refractory hypercalcemia and hypercalcemic crisis (Table 13-4).

TABLE 13-4. THERAPY FOR HYPERCALCEMIA

Therapy	Dose	Route	Monitor/Comment
Saline	250–1000 mL/h	IV	Cardiopulmonary function with examination, CVP/PCWP and CXR.
Furosemide	20–80 mg every 2–4 h or 40 mg/h CI	IV	Serum and urine electrolytes. Replace K, Mg, and PO_4 based on serum levels and urinary losses.
Salmon calcitonin	4–8 IU/kg every 6–12 h	IM, SC	Allergic reaction. Give a skin test of 1 IU intradermally before treatment.
Prednisone/ methylpred- nisolone	20 mg 2–3 times a day	PO/IV	Possible adjunct to calcitonin. Effective in $1,25(OH)_2D$ associated hypercalcemia.
Zoledronic acid	4 mg IV over 15 min every 2–4 weeks PRN	IV	Drug of choice for malignancy-associated hypercalcemia. Caution with CKD and myeloma.
Pamidronate	30–90 mg over 2–24 h every 1–3 weeks PRN	IV	Infuse over at least 4 hours in severe renal failure (GFR<30 mL/ minute).

(Continued)

TABLE 13-4. THERAPY FOR HYPERCALCEMIA (CONTINUED)

Therapy	Dose	Route	Monitor/Comment
Cinacalcet	30–90 mg b.i.d.–q.i.d.	PO	Take with meals. Monitor PTH, Ca, and PO_4 at least 12 h after dose.
Gallium nitrate	200 mg/m²/day CI over 4 h PRN for 5 days	IV	Avoid in renal failure. Monitor Cr, PO_4, and CBC.
Dialysis	Low or no calcium dialysate	HD/PD CVVHD	Hypercalcemic crisis or refractory hypercalcemia. Useful in renal failure. May require PO_4 addition to dialysate. Nephrologic consultation.

b.i.d., twice daily; BSA, body surface area; CBC, complete blood count; CI, continuous infusion; CKD, chronic kidney disease; Cr, creatinine; CVP, central venous pressure; CVVHD, continuous venovenous hemodialysis; CXR, chest radiograph; GFR, Glomerular Filtrating Rate; HD, hemodialysis; IM, intramuscularly; IV, intravenously; K, potassium; Mg, magnesium; Na, sodium; PCWP, pulmonary capillary wedge pressure; PD, peritoneal dialysis; PO, orally; PO_4, phosphate; PRN, as needed; PT, prothrombin time; PTT, partial thromboplastic time; q.i.d., four times daily; SC, subcutaneously.

21. **Describe the mechanisms of action of drug therapies for hypercalcemia.**
See Table 13-5.

TABLE 13-5. MECHANISM OF ACTION OF HYPERCALCEMIC THERAPY

Drug	Mechanism of Action
Saline	Dilutes serum calcium by volume expansion and increases urinary flow and calcium excretion
Furosemide	Impairs renal sodium and calcium reabsorption in Henle's loop, increasing urinary flow and calcium excretion
Calcitonin	Binds to receptors on osteoclasts, inhibiting osteoclast activity and decreasing bone resorption; also decreases renal reabsorption
Glucocorticoids	Antagonism of vitamin D causing decreased absorption and reabsorption; in tumoral states, may be tumor lytic and decrease production of OAFs and vitamin D
Bisphosphonates	Impair osteoclast differentiation, recruitment, motility, and attachment; incorporate into bone matrix, making the matrix resistant to hydrolysis; overall effect is decreased bone resorption
Cinacalcet	Calcimimetic that binds to the CaR, making it markedly more responsive to calcium activation

(Continued)

TABLE 13-5.	MECHANISM OF ACTION OF HYPERCALCEMIC THERAPY (CONTINUED)
Drug	**Mechanism of Action**
Gallium nitrate	Adsorbs to and decreases solubility of hydroxyapatite crystals, decreasing bone resorption
Dialysis	Direct removal of calcium from blood

OAFs, osteoclast-activating factors.
Note: For long-term hypocalcemic effects, drug therapy for hypercalcemia must antagonize one of the three main causes of hypercalcemia: bone resorption, renal reabsorption, or gut absorption. All hypercalcemia results from some abnormality in one of the three. Thus one of these etiologies should be considered when choosing drug therapy. As noted, most drug therapy for hypercalcemia impairs bone resorption.

22. How might calcimimetic drugs be useful in therapy of hypercalcemia?

On March 8, 2004, the U.S. Food and Drug Administration (FDA) approved the first-in-class oral calcimimetic for clinical use, cinacalcet. Calcimimetics are potentially the most useful drugs for treatment of hypercalcemia caused by hyperparathyroidism. Cinacalcet remains the only calcimimetic available for patient care. It acts by increasing the sensitivity of the CaR to calcium activation (see questions 8 and 9). This increased sensitivity shifts the PTH-calcium curve to the left, decreasing the responsiveness of parathyroid cells to the PTH stimulatory effects of low extracellular calcium and increasing the sensitivity of parathyroid cells to the PTH suppressive effects of high calcium. By increasing CaR calcium sensitivity in Henle's loop, cinacalcet increases renal calcium excretion. The net effect is a dose-dependent marked reduction in PTH secretion, a decrease in PTH-induced hypercalcemia, an increase in urinary calcium excretion, and a drop in serum calcium. Currently cinacalcet is FDA approved for treatment of secondary hyperparathyroidism from renal failure and PTH and calcium excess from parathyroid carcinoma. Although not approved for such, cinacalcet has successfully improved hypercalcemia caused by primary hyperparathyroidism, FHH, and lithium induced hypercalcemia (see question 23).

23. How does lithium cause hypercalcemia?

Lithium decreases urinary calcium by competitive inhibition of the CaR in the thick ascending limb of Henle's loop, causing increased calcium reabsorption, decreased calcium excretion, and hypercalcemia. Thus urinary calcium may be lower in lithium-treated patients such as those with FHH. Lithium also decreases the sensitivity of the parathyroid CaR to calcium and shifts the PTH-calcium curve in the parathyroid chief cells to the right. Thus for any given calcium level, there is less suppression of PTH secretion and synthesis and higher PTH levels. Unlike in hyperparathyroidism, serum phosphate tends to be normal and magnesium higher in lithium-treated patients. Because hypercalcemia and elevated PTH may persist after lithium is discontinued, therapy other than just discontinuing lithium may be indicated if the hypercalcemia is symptomatic. Cinacalcet has successfully corrected or ameliorated PTH and serum Ca levels in these patients. This is expected because cinacalcet sensitizes the CaR to calcium and shifts the PTH-calcium curve to the left.

WEBSITES

1. American Academy of Family Physicians. Available at http://www.aafp.org/afp/20030501/1959.html

2. National Cancer Institute. Available at http://www.meb.uni-bonn.de/cancer.gov/CDR0000062737.html

3. Zometa International: Zoledronic acid review. Available at http://www.zometa.com/monographs.html

BIBLIOGRAPHY

1. Bergua C, Torregrosa JV, Cofán F, et al: Cinacalcet for the treatment of hypercalcemia in renal transplanted patients with secondary hyperparathyroidism. Transplant Proc 39:2254–2255, 2007.

2. Bringhurst FR, Demay MB, Kronenberg HM: Hormones and disorders of mineral metabolism. In Kronenberg HM, Melmed S, Polonsky KS, et al, editors, Williams textbook of endocrinology, Philadelphia, 2008, Saunders Elsevier, pp. 1203–1268.

3. Brown EM: Familial hypocalciuric hypercalcemia and other disorders with resistance to extracellular calcium. Endocrinol Metab Clin North Am 29:503–522, 2000.

4. Body JJ: Current and future directions in medical therapy: hypercalcemia. Cancer 88(Suppl 12):3054–3058, 2000.

5. Casez JP, Pfammatter R, Nguyen QV: Relevance of parathyroid hormone and parathyroid hormone-related protein measurements. Eur J Intern Med 12:344–349, 2001.

6. Carroll MF, Schade, DS: A practical approach to hypercalcemia. Am Fam Physician 67:1959–1966, 2003.

7. Festen-Spanjer B, Haring CM, Koster JB, et al: Correction of hypercalcaemia by cinacalcet in familial hypocalciuric hypercalcaemia. Clin Endocrinol 68:324–325, 2008.

8. Jacobs TP, Bilezikian JP: Clinical review: rare causes of hypercalcemia. J Clin Endocrinol Metab 90:6316–6322, 2005.

9. Kaye TB: Hypercalcemia. How to pinpoint the cause and customize treatment. Postgrad Med 97:153–155, 159–160, 1995.

10. Major P: The use of zoledronic acid, a novel, highly potent bisphosphonate, for the treatment of hypercalcemia of malignancy. Oncologist 7:481–491, 2002.

11. Major PP, Coleman RE: Zoledronic acid in the treatment of hypercalcemia of malignancy: results of the international clinical development program. Semin Oncol 28:17–24, 2001.

12. Mihai R, Wass JAH, Sadler GP: Asymptomatic hyperparathyroidism—need for multicentre studies. Clin Endocrinol 68:155–164, 2008.

13. Nishi SPE, Barbagelata NA, Atar S, et al: Hypercalcemia-induced ST-segment elevation mimicking acute myocardial infarction. J Electrocardiol 39:298–300, 2006.

14. Pont A: Unusual causes of hypercalcemia. Endocrinol Metab Clin North Am 18:753–764, 1989.

15. Popovtzer MM: Disorders of calcium, phosphorus, vitamin D, and parathyroid hormone activity. In Schrier RW, editor, Renal and electrolytes disorders, Philadelphia, 2003, Lippincott Williams & Wilkins, pp. 216–277.

16. Rabbani SA: Molecular mechanism of action of parathyroid hormone related peptide in hypercalcemia of malignancy: therapeutic strategies [review]. Int J Oncol 16:197–206, 2000.

17. Shoback DM, Bilezikian JP, Turner SA, et al: The calcimimetic cinacalcet normalizes serum calcium in subjects with primary hyperparathyroidism. J Clin Endocrinol Metab 88:5644–5649, 2003.

18. Silverberg SH, Rubin MR, Faiman C, et al: Cinacalcet hydrochloride reduces the serum calcium concentration in inoperable parathyroid carcinoma. J Clin Endocrinol Metab 92:3803–3808, 2007.

19. Sloand JA, Shelly MA: Normalization of lithium-induced hypercalcemia and hyperparathyroidism with cinacalcet hydrochloride. Am J Kidney Dis 48:832–837, 2006.

20. Thakker RV: Multiple endocrine neoplasia type I. Endocrinol Metab Clin North Am 29:541–567, 2000.

CHAPTER 14

HYPERPARATHYROIDISM

Leonard R. Sanders

1. **What is hyperparathyroidism?**
   Hyperparathyroidism (HPT) is a clinical syndrome causing specific symptoms and signs that result from elevated parathyroid hormone (PTH), PTH-induced bone resorption, and hypercalcemia. The three types of HPT are primary, secondary, and tertiary.

2. **How common is primary HPT?**
   The prevalence of primary HPT in the United States is 28 in 100,000; the female-to-male ratio is 2:1 to 3:1. The incidence increases with age, and postmenopausal women have an incidence 5 times higher than the general population.

3. **What causes primary HPT?**
   Primary HPT is characterized by abnormal regulation of PTH secretion by calcium, resulting in excessive PTH secretion. Although the cause of HPT is not known, increased PTH secretion is due in part to an elevation of the set point and a change in the slope of the calcium-PTH curve, causing relative nonsuppressibility of PTH secretion. Expression of the calcium-sensing receptor (CaR) is reduced in parathyroid adenomas and hyperplasia and may be partly responsible for this relative PTH nonsuppressibility.

4. **What anatomic alterations occur in HPT?**
   Most hyperparathyroid patients (85%) have single parathyroid adenomas, 5% have multiple adenomas, 10% have four-gland hyperplasia, and fewer than 1% have parathyroid carcinomas. Normal parathyroid glands weigh less than 50 mg each. The average weight of parathyroid adenomas is 0.5 to 5 g; however, they may be more than 25 g. The largest reported tumor weighed 120 g, and the largest number of glands reported in one patient was eight.

5. **How do you diagnose HPT?**
   Persistent hypercalcemia with increased serum PTH levels makes the diagnosis of HPT. Associated low fasting serum phosphate makes the diagnosis of primary HPT more likely. Suspect HPT whenever the patient has documented hypercalcemia. Because symptoms of HPT are nonspecific or absent (see question 12), one must base the diagnosis primarily on laboratory studies. Furthermore, most patients with mild HPT have no specific symptoms or signs. Most cases are suspected after finding an elevated calcium value on routine laboratory screening.

6. **How does age complicate the diagnosis of HPT?**
   The laboratory normal range for intact PTH (10–65 pg/mL) and calcium (9–10.5 mg/dL) may not apply in the elderly. PTH levels normally decrease with age. A 50 year old should not have intact PTH levels exceeding 40 to 50 pg/mL. Thus normal PTH levels may exist in HPT in older patients. Furthermore, calcium levels decline with age, and high normal calcium levels (10 mg/dL) are probably abnormally high over the age 50.

7. **How might you make the diagnosis of primary HPT more certain before recommending parathyroidectomy?**

Obtain at least three fasting samples for calcium, ideally with no venous occlusion, and two PTH measurements at least several weeks apart. Ensure that the patient has normal renal function. Discontinue any thiazide diuretic for at least 1 week before measurement. Total calcium measurement is sufficient if albumin and total protein are normal. If not, measure ionized calcium or correct for the protein change (see Chapter 13). If calcium is elevated and PTH is high or high normal, primary HPT is usually present. If calcium is not elevated and PTH is high, measure 25-hydroxyvitamin D levels. To exclude vitamin D deficiency, levels should be greater than 30 ng/mL. Use the immunoradiometric (IRMA) or bio-intact immunochemiluminometric (ICMA) assays that are specific for intact PTH.

8. **When lab results are not specific for primary HPT, what other classic laboratory changes may help with diagnosis?**

Increased chloride (Cl) and decreased phosphate (PO4) with a Cl/PO4 ratio of greater than 33, elevated urinary pH (>6.0), and increased alkaline phosphatase concentrations support the diagnosis of primary HPT but are not specific. Assess PTH-related protein (PTHrP) in any patient with suspected malignancy and hypercalcemia. Ectopic PTH is rare and should be considered only if the patient has evidence of malignancy or a negative neck exploration for HPT.

9. **What differentiates familial hypocalciuric hypercalcemia from primary HPT?**

If measured PTH is borderline or normal but PTH is inappropriately increased for the level of calcium, consider familial (benign) hypocalciuric hypercalcemia (FHH). Calculate the fractional excretion of calcium (FECa) (see Chapter 13). The FECa in FHH is less than 1%. If the FECa is low, test family members to confirm the diagnosis. If positive, FHH is probably present. Avoid neck exploration, which will have no effect on reversing the hypercalcemia.

10. **How does chronic kidney disease (CKD) complicate the diagnosis of HPT?**

Renal failure increases serum phosphate and decreases 1,25-dihydroxyvitamin D (calcitriol) levels. Because phosphate directly stimulates and calcitriol directly inhibits PTH secretion, serum PTH levels increase in renal failure. In addition, increased phosphate and decreased calcitriol decrease serum calcium. The resulting absolute or relative hypocalcemia further increases PTH secretion. Symptoms and signs of renal insufficiency may be identical to those of HPT, including lethargy, depression, anorexia, nausea, constipation, and weakness. Thus unless overt, the diagnosis of primary HPT may be more difficult in renal failure. Before parathyroidectomy for presumed primary HPT, tissue localization with technetium-99m sestamibi scan may be appropriate.

11. **What changes occur in renal failure that may complicate the PTH assay?**

In renal failure, PTH increases above the normal range because of the stimulatory effects of high phosphate and low calcitriol. In addition, a molecular fragment of PTH (7–84) that has antagonistic actions to those of intact PTH accumulates in renal failure and cross-reacts with the intact molecule in the intact two-site assays. For this reason, patients with renal failure may have measured levels of intact PTH greater than 1.5 times that of normal subjects to maintain physiologic PTH (1–84) concentrations. Bio-intact or whole-PTH assays eliminate this cross-reactivity.

12. **What are the symptoms and signs of primary HPT?**

More than 85% of primary hyperparathyroid patients are asymptomatic. However, neurologic, gastrointestinal, musculoskeletal, and vascular changes all can occur in primary HPT. The classic phrase for many of these features is "stones, bones, abdominal groans, and psychic moans." Kidney stones occur in 15% to 20% of patients with primary hyperparathyroidism. Proximal muscle weakness is also characteristic. Other characteristic symptoms and signs and their probable cause are outlined in Table 14-1.

TABLE 14-1.   HYPERPARATHYROIDISM: SYMPTOMS AND SIGNS AND THEIR PROBABLE CAUSES

Symptoms and Signs	Probable Cause
Renal: hypercalciuria, nephrolithiasis, nephrocalcinosis, polyuria, polydipsia, renal insufficiency	Parathyroid hormone (PTH) stimulates bone resorption, hypercalcemia, bicarbonaturia, and phosphaturia, causing decreased tubular responsiveness to antidiuretic hormone (ADH), polyuria, calcium oxalate and phosphate crystallization, nephrocalcinosis, and renal insufficiency
Neuromuscular: weakness, myalgia	Prolonged excessive PTH arguably causes direct neuropathy with abnormal nerve conduction velocities (NCVs) and characteristic electromyographic changes and myopathic features on muscle biopsy
Neurologic and psychiatric: memory loss, depression, psychoses, neuroses, confusion, lethargy, fatigue, paresthesias	PTH and calcium cause peripheral neuropathy with abnormal NCVs and central nervous system damage with abnormal electroencephalographic changes
Skeletal: bone pain, osteitis fibrosa, osteoporosis, and subperiosteal skeletal resorption	PTH increases bone resorption and acidosis with subsequent bone buffering and bone loss of calcium and phosphate
Gastrointestinal: abdominal pain, nausea, peptic ulcer, constipation, and pancreatitis	Hypercalcemia stimulates gastrin secretion, decreases peristalsis, and increases the calcium-phosphate product with calcium-phosphate deposition and obstruction in pancreatic ducts
Hypertension	Hypercalcemia causes vasoconstriction, and parathyroid hypertensive factor (PHF) may increase blood pressure
Arthralgia, synovitis, arthritis	HPT is associated with increased crystal deposition from calcium phosphate (para-articular calcification), calcium pyrophosphate (pseudogout), and uric acid/urate (gout)
Band keratopathy	Calcium-phosphate precipitation in medial and limbic margins of cornea
Anemia	Unknown

13. **What is band keratopathy?**

Band keratopathy is a classic but unusual sign of HPT characterized by an irregular region of calcium phosphate deposition at the medial and lateral limbic margins of the outer edge of the cornea. The location is believed to be a result of diffusion of carbon dioxide from air-exposed areas of the cornea, leaving an alkaline environment that favors precipitation of calcium phosphate crystals. Band keratopathy occurs only with a high calcium-phosphate product. Diagnosis is made by ophthalmologic slit-lamp examination. It differs from arcus senilis, an age-related, linear, concentric gray crescent separated from the extreme periphery (limbus corneae) by a rim of clear cornea that with time completely encircles the cornea.

14. What are the classic radiographic findings in HPT?

Because most patients are diagnosed early, there are usually no radiographic findings related to HPT. If HPT is prolonged, osteopenia develops. However, the classic radiographic finding is subperiosteal bone resorption along the radial aspect of the middle and distal phalanges and distal clavicles. Salt-and-pepper skull is another classic finding. Because cortical bone loss is higher in HPT, bone densitometry of the distal radius is a good way to follow patients for osteopenia who do not have parathyroidectomy.

15. What is the differential diagnosis of primary HPT?

Because the main abnormality in primary HPT is hypercalcemia, the differential diagnosis initially is that of hypercalcemia (see Chapter 13). A history and physical examination focused on symptoms and signs (see question 12) may suggest one of the causes of hypercalcemia. If hypercalcemia is mild and history and physical examination are nonspecific, primary HPT is likely. The two most common causes of hypercalcemia are primary HPT and malignancy. In humoral hypercalcemia of malignancy (HHM), the tumor usually produces a PTH-like hormone called PTHrP.

16. What lab tests help to distinguish the three types of HPT?

See Table 14-2.

TABLE 14-2. PARATHYROID HORMONE AND CALCIUM IN HYPERPARATHYROIDISM		
	PTH	**Calcium**
Primary	Normal ↑	↑
Secondary	↑	↓ Normal
Tertiary	↑↑	↑

17. What pathophysiologic changes occur in primary HPT?

Primary HPT is idiopathic and results from excessive secretion of PTH from parathyroid adenomas, hyperplasia, or rarely carcinoma. The increased PTH causes hypercalcemia. PTH is inappropriately normal or high.

18. What pathophysiologic changes occur in secondary HPT?

Secondary HPT is excessive PTH secretion as a secondary response to hypocalcemia. Hyperphosphatemia and low levels of calcitriol also stimulate PTH secretion. Renal failure is the most common cause of secondary HPT. Other causes of hypocalcemia are renal calcium leak, dietary calcium malabsorption, and vitamin D deficiency. Hypocalcemia causes parathyroid hyperplasia. Attempting to return the calcium to normal, the enlarged glands secrete excessive PTH. In renal failure, phosphorus increases because of decreased renal function. The increased phosphorous stimulates PTH secretion and decreases 1,25(OH)2D and calcium. The lower calcium and vitamin D also increase PTH synthesis and secretion. Thus controlling phosphorus levels with diet and phosphate binders and appropriate calcitriol supplementation may delay onset of secondary hyperparathyroidism of renal failure.

19. What pathophysiologic changes occur in tertiary HPT?

Tertiary HPT results from progression of secondary HPT. In tertiary HPT, prolonged hypocalcemia causes development of autonomous parathyroid function and hypercalcemia. Spontaneous change from low or normal calcium levels to hypercalcemia marks the transition from secondary to tertiary HPT. In tertiary HPT, PTH levels are usually approximately 10 to 20 times normal. This most commonly occurs in chronic renal failure. PTH remains elevated despite vitamin D therapy and correction of hyperphosphatemia. Hypercalcemia remains despite discontinuation of vitamin D and calcium supplements. Tertiary HPT usually requires resection of at least three and a half parathyroid glands to correct the hypercalcemia. However, discontinue vitamin D and give a trial of cinacalcet therapy before surgical referral.

20. **How is HHM distinguished from primary HPT?**
   The main distinguishing features are the levels of intact PTH, PTHrP, and 1,25(OH)$_2$D. The classic and most common patterns of these hormones are shown in Table 14-3. Primary HPT usually has elevated levels of intact PTH. PTHrP levels, when measured, are low. Malignancy-associated hypercalcemia, in contrast, has low levels of intact PTH, but 80% of cases have increased levels of PTHrP and 20% have both low intact PTH and PTHrP. Thus measuring the two hormones distinguishes all three disorders (see question 21).

TABLE 14-3. HYPERCALCEMIA, PRIMARY HPT, AND MALIGNANCY				
	Intact PTH	PTHrP	1,25(OH)$_2$D	Calcium
Primary HPT	↑	↓	↑	↑
PTHrP malignancy	↓	↑	↓	↑
Non-PTHrP malignancy	↓	↓	↓	↑

HPT, hyperparathyroidism; PTHrP, parathyroid hormone–related protein.

21. **How do PTHrP and PTH differ?**
   PTHrP consists of three protein forms with 139, 141, and 173 amino acids. The first 139 amino acids are the same among the three forms. Eight of the first 13 N-terminal amino acids are identical to intact PTH (1–84), allowing PTHrP to stimulate the same receptors as PTH and to have similar biological effects. The two hormones have different effects on levels of 1,25(OH)$_2$D, partly because of their different secretion patterns. Both PTH (in primary HPT) and PTHrP (in HHM) stimulate receptors that activate renal 1α-hydroxylase. However, continuous secretion of PTHrP by malignant tumors probably downregulates these receptors, inhibiting 1α-hydroxylase activity and decreasing 1,25(OH)$_2$D production. Continuous infusion of PTH causes similar decreases in 1,25(OH)$_2$D. Nevertheless, other mechanisms may decrease 1,25(OH)$_2$D in PTHrP associated HHM. HHM may have an associated 5-10X increase in the phosphaturic factor, fibroblast growth factor 23 (FGF-23). FGF-23 inhibits 1α-hydroxylase activity and decreases 1,25(OH)$_2$D levels. Higher levels of calcium in HHM may also decrease 1α-hydroxylase activity and 1,25(OH)$_2$D levels.

22. **What hormonal and laboratory changes occur in HPT?**
   Secretion of PTH in HPT is intermittent; intermittent secretion avoids downregulation and results in increased 1,25(OH)$_2$D. In addition, serum calcium levels are higher in HHM than in HPT. The higher calcium levels further decrease production of 1,25(OH)$_2$D. Thus 1,25(OH)$_2$D levels tend to be high in HPT and low in HHM. Traditional associations of primary HPT include mild renal tubular acidosis, hypophosphatemia, hyperchloremia, and an increased ratio of chloride to phosphate. Unfortunately such associations are nonspecific and too insensitive to be of diagnostic use. However, the triad of elevated PTH, hypercalcemia, and hypophosphatemia make the diagnosis of primary HPT likely.

23. **What PTH assay is most useful in the workup of hypercalcemia?**
   Intact PTH has 84 amino acids, is 70% metabolized by the liver, is 20% metabolized by the kidneys, has a half-life of 2 minutes; and less than 1% of the secreted hormone remains to interact physiologically with PTH receptors. Although the first 34 amino acids of the N-terminus contain the full biologic activity of the hormone, intact PTH (1–84) is the active hormone in vivo. The preferred assays for measurement are the ICMA and IRMA for intact PTH; both are highly sensitive and specific. Because of availability, the IRMA is more commonly used. At times, a midmolecule assay for PTH will support the clinical diagnosis of HPT when the ICMA and IRMA assays are both negative. The IRMA also measures a 7–84 amino acid fragment of intact PTH (1–84). The newer scantibodies (whole PTH) and bio-intact PTH assays measure the true intact PTH molecule. These assays were felt to be potentially more useful in patients with renal failure; however, they have not been more clinically useful than the usual IRMA. A rapid PTH is often measured preoperatively and intraoperatively 10 minutes post-parathyroidectomy. At least a 50% reduction in PTH indicates a successful operation.

24. **What methods best localize the parathyroid tumor in HPT?**
   Technetium-99m sestamibi single proton emission computed tomography (SPECT) scintigraphy may be greater than 85% to 90% sensitive, specific, and accurate and therefore is the procedure of choice. Sestamibi scanning is most accurate for localizing parathyroid adenomas and is much less useful for parathyroid hyperplasia. Ultrasonography is usually a complementary test for localization and, combined with sestamibi scanning, increases sensitivity to 95%. Less commonly used localization studies that may be useful include intraoperative guidance with a γ-probe, cervical computed tomography (CT), magnetic resonance imaging, positron emission tomography (PET), intravenous digital subtraction angiography (IVDSA), arteriography, and selective venous sampling.

KEY POINTS: HYPERPARATHYROIDISM

1. Primary hyperparathyroidism (HPT) is associated with hypercalcemia, osteoporosis, nephrolithiasis, and symptoms associated with these conditions.

2. The new recommendations for surgery in patients with asymptomatic HPT are as follows: serum calcium >1 mg/dL above the upper normal limit, hypercalciuria >400 mg/24 h, decreased creatinine clearance <70% of age-matched normal persons, reduced bone density with T-score less than −2.5, age <50 years, and calcium nephrolithiasis.

3. It is never wrong to recommend surgery for treatment of asymptomatic HPT if the patient has no contraindications to surgery and has access to a skilled parathyroid surgeon.

4. Advantages of parathyroid surgery include cure of HPT and hypercalcemia in most cases with a single operation, no need for regular prolonged follow-up, decreased fracture rate, and increased bone mass in most patients.

5. Most surgeons prefer preoperative localization studies before minimally invasive parathyroidectomy, before reoperative parathyroid surgery, and for suspected bilateral disease.

25. **When should you use preoperative localization of a parathyroid adenoma?**
   For bilateral neck exploration, the statement suggested by John Doppman at the 1990 NIH Consensus Development Conference generally holds true today that the greatest challenge in preoperative localization of the parathyroid adenoma is locating an experienced parathyroid

surgeon (Bilezikian 2002). More than 90% to 95% of the time, a skilled parathyroid surgeon can localize and remove a parathyroid adenoma without preoperative localization. For this reason, preoperative localization before standard bilateral neck exploration is not usually necessary. However, minimally invasive parathyroidectomy (MIP) using a small incision localized to one side of the neck is becoming the state-of-the-art surgical approach to treat primary HPT. Most surgeons require preoperative localization studies before MIP, reoperative parathyroid surgery, and surgery for suspected bilateral disease.

26. **Do all asymptomatic patients with HPT require surgical treatment?**
No. Many asymptomatic patients with mild primary HPT do not require surgery (see question 27). However, the only definitive therapy for HPT is parathyroidectomy, and it is usually appropriate to recommend parathyroidectomy for patients with asymptomatic primary HPT if they have access to an experienced parathyroid surgeon. Advantages of parathyroid surgery are cure of HPT and hypercalcemia in most cases with a single operation, no need for regular prolonged follow-up, decreased fracture rate, increased bone mass in most patients, and decreased cardiovascular disease.

27. **What are the indications for parathyroidectomy as recommended by the April 2002 National Institutes of Health–sponsored workshop on asymptomatic HPT?**
    1. Hypercalcemia >1.0 mg/dL above the upper normal limit
    2. Hypercalciuria >400 mg/24 h
    3. Decreased creatinine clearance 30% from baseline or <70% of age-matched normal persons
    4. Reduced bone density by dual-energy x-ray absorptiometry (DEXA) (T-score < −2.5)
    5. Age <50 years with mild hypercalcemia
    6. Calcium nephrolithiasis
    7. When good follow-up is not possible or inadvisable because of medical illness

28. **How should you monitor patients with asymptomatic HPT who have not had parathyroidectomy?**
Initially measure serum calcium, creatinine, PTH, 24-hour urine calcium, creatinine clearance, FECa, abdominal radiograph (KUB), and DEXA bone densitometry. Measure serum calcium biannually. Obtain three-site bone densitometry (lumbar spine, femur, and forearm) serum creatinine, and estimated creatinine clearance or glomerular filtration rate (GFR) annually. Schedule office visits every 6 months and as needed. Evaluate for symptoms of HPT. Make sure patients maintain adequate hydration, exercise, and a normal calcium diet. Avoid thiazide diuretics, lithium, and excessive calcium input. Alert the primary physician to watch for medical illness predisposing to dehydration.

29. **How would you estimate the creatinine clearance or GFR without doing a 24-hour urine collection?**
Use either the Cockroft-Gault formula or the MDRD equation, noting that the MDRD equation is the best equation for estimating GFR but is difficult to calculate. However, the MDRD calculation of GFR is easy if one has Internet access (see http://nkdep.nih.gov/professionals/gfr_calculators/orig_con.htm).
Cockroft-Gault Formula:

$$CCr = (140 - age) \times \text{ideal body weight(kg)} / [72 \times \text{serum } Cr(mg/dL)] \times (0.85 \text{ if female})$$

MDRD equation:

$$GFR(mL/min/1.73 \text{ m}^2) = 186 \times (Pcr)^{-1.154} \times (age)^{-0.203}$$
$$\times (0.742 \text{ if female}) \times (1.210 \text{ if African American})$$

30. **How would you estimate the GFR for a 60-year-old Caucasian woman with serum creatinine of 0.8 mg/dL and a weight of 60 kg?**

Crockroft-Gault Forumula:

$$CCr = (140 - 60) \times 60 \text{ kg} \times 0.85/(72 \times 0.8 \text{ mg/dL}) = 83 \text{ mL/min}$$

MDRD Equation:

$$GFR = 60 \text{ mL/min}/1.73 \text{ m}^2$$

31. **How would you estimate the 24-hour urine calcium excretion without doing a 24-hour urine collection?**

A good estimate of the 24-hour urine calcium excretion is 1.1 times the calcium-to-creatinine ratio on a random urine specimen. An example in the same patient as in question 30 follows:

$$UCa = 20 \text{ mg/dL and } UCr = 70 \text{ mg/dL Calcium/creatinine} = 20/70 = 0.286 \text{ g}$$

Estimated 24-hour urinary calcium excretion is 1.1×286 mg/day $= 315$ mg/day. Because normal 24-hour urinary calcium is up to 4 mg/kg/day or about 240 mg/day in a 60-kg woman, the urinary calcium is elevated, as would be expected in HPT. However, it is not elevated to a degree that requires surgical recommendation in an asymptomatic patient with normal renal function for age.

32. **What therapeutic options are available for patients unable to undergo surgery for HPT?**

Calcimimetics bind to the extracellular calcium-sensing receptor on parathyroid cells and alter their sensitivity to extracellular calcium. This shifts the calcium-PTH curve to the left, increasing parathyroid sensitivity to the suppressive effects of calcium at all concentrations. Cinacalcet, a calcimimetic, is available for treatment of secondary HPT in end-stage renal disease and parathyroid carcinoma. Although not yet approved for treatment of primary HPT, cinacalcet effectively reduces PTH and calcium in primary HPT. Cinacalcet also decreases calcium reabsorption from the renal tubule and increases calcium excretion. Bisphosphonates inhibit osteoclast-mediated bone resorption and can increase bone mass in osteopenic patients with HPT. Raloxifene may also preserve bone mass if bisphosphonates are not tolerated. Estrogens preserve bone mass but should not be used routinely for osteopenia in HPT because of an associated potential risk of breast cancer and cardiovascular disease. Angiographic ablation or percutaneous alcohol injection of parathyroid tissue can also be tried.

33. **How would you evaluate and treat a patient with normocalcemic HPT?**

Normocalcemic HPT (NCHPT) manifests with an elevated PTH and a normal corrected calcium level. Recent studies suggest that NCHPT is more common than previously thought and may present with complications similar to hypercalcemic HPT. Evaluate and treat for secondary causes of HPT such as vitamin D deficiency, CKD, and renal hypercalciuria. Perform ionized calcium to confirm the normocalcemia. After secondary HPT has been ruled out, follow and treat these patients similar to those with hypercalcemic HPT. However, referral for parathyroid surgery should not be routine but based on symptoms and signs (see questions 27 and 28).

WEBSITES

1. AACE/AAES Position Statement on the diagnosis and management of Primary Hyperparathyroidism. Available at http://www.aace.com/pub/pdf/guidelines/ hyperparathyroidPS.pdf (available to AACE members only at AACE website)

2. EMedicine: Primary Hyperparathyroidism review. Available at http://www.emedicine.com/ RADIO/topic355.htm

3. Good review of all aspects of parathyroid disease. Available at http://www.parathyroid.com

4. Algorithm for preoperative localization in primary hyperparathyroidism. Available at http://www.viamedica.pl//gazety/gazetax2ang/darmowy_pdf.phtml? indeks=18&indeks_art=284&VSID=90da16d

5. Surgical rounds: Normocalcemic primary hyperparathyroidism: How new technology affects an old diagnosis. Available at http://www.surgicalroundsonline.com/issues/articles/2007-06_03.asp

BIBLIOGRAPHY

1. Ambrogini E, Cetani F, Cianferotti L, et al: Surgery or surveillance for mild asymptomatic primary hyperparathyroidism: a prospective, randomized clinical trial. J Clin Endocrinol Metab 92:3114–3121, 2007.

2. Bilezikian JP, Potts JT, Fuleihan H, et al: Summary statement from a workshop on asymptomatic primary hyperparathyroidism: a perspective for the 21st century. J Clin Endocrinol Metab 87:5353–5361, 2002.

3. Bilezikian JP, Silverberg SJ: Asymptomatic primary hyperparathyroidism. N Engl J Med 350:1746–1751, 2004.

4. Bringhurst FR, Demay MB, Kronenberg HM: Hormones and disorders of mineral metabolism. In Kronenberg HM, Melmed S, Polonsky KS, et al, editors, *Williams textbook of endocrinology*, Philadelphia, 2008, Saunders Elsevier, pp. 1203–1268.

5. Farford R, Presutti J, Moraghan TJ: Nonsurgical management of primary hyperparathyroidism. Mayo Clin Proc 82:351–355, 2007.

6. Helene Siilin, Jonas Rastad, Östen Ljunggren, Ewa Lundgren: Disturbances of calcium homeostasis consistent with mild primary hyperparathyroidism in premenopausal women and associated morbidity. J. Clin Endocrinol Metab 93:47–53, 2008.

7. Kukora JS, Zeiger MA, Clark OH, et al: AACE/AAES Position statement on diagnosis and management of primary hyperparathyroidism. Endocr Pract 11:49–54, 2005.

8. Lowe H, McMahon DJ, Rubin MR, et al: Normocalcemic primary hyperparathyroidism: further characterization of a new clinical phenotype. J Clin Endocrinol Metab 92:3001–3005, 2007.

9. Maruani G, Hertiga A, Paillard M, et al: Normocalcemic primary hyperparathyroidism: evidence for a generalized target-tissue resistance to parathyroid hormone. J Clin Endocrinol Metab 88:4641–4648, 2003.

10. Peacock M, Bilezikian JP, Klassen PS, et al: Cinacalcet hydrochloride maintains long-term normocalcemia in patients with primary hyperparathyroidism. J Clin Endocrinol Metab 90:135–141, 2005.

11. Quiros RM, Alioto J, Wilhelm SM, et al: An algorithm to maximize use of minimally invasive parathyroidectomy. Arch Surg 139:501–507, 2004.

12. Rubello D, AL-Nahhas A, Khan S: Is there an ideal algorithm in preoperative localization of primary hyperparathyroidism? Nucl Med Rev 9:105–107, 2006.

CHAPTER 15

HYPERCALCEMIA OF MALIGNANCY

Michael T. McDermott

1. **What are the two major categories of hypercalcemia of malignancy?**
   - Humoral hypercalcemia of malignancy (HHM)
   - Local osteolytic hypercalcemia (LOH)

2. **What types of cancer are associated with HHM?**
   Carcinoma of the lung, particularly squamous cell carcinoma, is the most common. Other tumors associated with this disorder include squamous cell carcinomas of the head, neck, and esophagus and adenocarcinomas of the breast, kidney, bladder, pancreas, and ovary.

3. **What is the cause of HHM?**
   HHM results when solid malignancies, both solitary and metastatic, secrete into the circulation one or more substances that cause hypercalcemia. The humoral mediator identified in more than 90% of cases is parathyroid hormone–related peptide (PTHrp). Other humoral substances that are occasionally secreted and contribute to the development of hypercalcemia include transforming growth factor-alpha (TGFα), tumor necrosis factor (TNF), and various interleukins and cytokines.

4. **What is PTHrp?**
   PTHrp is a protein that has sequence homology with the first 13 amino acids of parathyroid hormone (PTH). Both PTH and PTHrp bind to a common receptor (PTH/PTHrp receptor), resulting in stimulation of bone resorption and inhibition of renal calcium excretion. PTHrp is found in high concentrations in breast milk and amniotic fluid, but it can be detected in almost every tissue in the body; it is increased in the circulation during pregnancy. Its physiologic endocrine function may be to govern the transfer of calcium from the maternal skeleton and bloodstream into the developing fetus and into breast milk. As a generalized paracrine factor, it also regulates growth and development of many tissues, most prominently the skeleton and breast.

5. **How does PTHrp cause hypercalcemia in patients with cancer?**
   Elevated circulating levels of PTHrp stimulate generalized bone resorption, flooding the bloodstream with excessive calcium; PTHrp also acts on the kidneys, preventing excretion of the increased calcium load. This combination produces an increase in the serum calcium concentration. Hypercalcemia induces polyuria, which leads to dehydration with impaired renal function, further reducing calcium excretion and leading to a cycle of progressive and eventually life-threatening hypercalcemia.

6. **How do you make a diagnosis of HHM?**
   Hypercalcemia in any patient with a known malignancy should make one suspect this diagnosis. Occasionally, however, a raised serum calcium is the first clue to an underlying cancer. The key to the diagnosis is a suppressed serum intact PTH level; this finding reliably excludes hyperparathyroidism, the other leading cause of hypercalcemia. Serum PTHrp levels are nearly always high, but this expensive test is not necessary for diagnosis in most instances. If a patient

meeting these diagnostic criteria does not have a known tumor, a careful search for an occult malignancy should be undertaken.

7. **What types of cancer are associated with LOH?**
Breast cancer with skeletal metastases, multiple myeloma, and lymphoma are the major cancers associated with LOH.

KEY POINTS: HYPERCALCEMIA OF MALIGNANCY

1. Hypercalcemia of malignancy is most often due to tumor production of parathyroid hormone–related peptide (PTHrp), which binds to parathyroid hormone (PTH) and PTH/PTHrp receptors to stimulate bone resorption.

2. The key diagnostic test in hypercalcemic patients is measurement of serum PTH, which is elevated or high normal in primary hyperparathyroidism but low or undetectable in hypercalcemia of malignancy and most other hypercalcemic disorders.

3. The development of hypercalcemia of malignancy portends a poor prognosis in most cancer patients, because it tends to occur with advanced tumor stages.

4. Serum calcium levels can be lowered effectively in patients with hypercalcemia of malignancy by the intravenous administration of saline and bisphosphonates.

8. **What is the cause of LOH?**
LOH generally occurs when cancer cells are present in multiple sites throughout the skeleton. The pathogenesis involves the elaboration by malignant cells of osteoclast-stimulating factors directly onto the surface of bone. Such factors include PTHrp, lymphotoxin, interleukins, transforming growth factors, prostaglandins, and procathepsin D.

9. **How do you make a diagnosis of LOH?**
The diagnosis is fairly straightforward when a patient with one of the previously noted malignancies develops hypercalcemia. Again, the key is demonstration of a suppressed serum intact PTH, indicating that hyperparathyroidism is not the culprit. Patients without a known malignancy should have a complete blood count, serum and urine protein electrophoresis, and bone scan; if these studies are not informative, a bone marrow biopsy should be performed.

10. **Can lymphomas cause hypercalcemia by other mechanisms?**
Some lymphomas express 1α hydroxylase activity. This enzyme converts 25-hydroxyvitamin D to 1,25-dihydroxyvitamin D, which then stimulates increased intestinal calcium absorption and bone resorption. This may eventually lead to hypercalcemia, particularly in patients who have reduced renal calcium excretion due to dehydration or intrinsic renal disease.

11. **What is the prognosis for patients with hypercalcemia of malignancy?**
Because hypercalcemia generally correlates with far-advanced disease, the overall prognosis is quite poor. In one study, the median survival of patients who developed hypercalcemia was only 30 days. Effective treatments are available to reduce the serum calcium levels, however.

12. **How do you treat hypercalcemia of malignancy?**
Treatment of the underlying malignancy is the most effective measure. For symptomatic patients, rapid reduction of serum calcium is also indicated. An intravenous saline infusion (200–500 ml/h, if tolerated) to enhance renal calcium excretion should be the initial measure in most patients. Furosemide 20 to 40 mg intravenous (IV) can be added after adequate hydration

is achieved. Anti-resorptive medications should be given concomitantly. The most effective of these are the intravenous bisphosphonates. Suggested treatment regimens are as follows:

Medications	Dosage
Zoledronic acid (Zometa)	4 mg in 50 mL NS IV over 15 min
Pamidronate (Aredia)	60–90 mg in 250–500 mL NS IV over 2–4 h
Plicamycin	25 mg/kg IV over 4–6 h
Calcitonin	4–8 IU/kg SQ or intramuscular twice daily
Gallium Nitrate	100–200 mg/m^2/24 h for 5 days
Prednisone	60 mg daily for 10 days

IV, intravenous; NS, normal saline; SQ, subcutaneous.

BIBLIOGRAPHY

1. Bilezikian JP: Management of acute hypercalcemia. N Engl J Med 326:1196–1203, 1992.

2. Grill V, Ho P, Body JJ, et al: Parathyroid hormone related protein: elevated levels in both humoral hypercalcemia of malignancy and hypercalcemia complicating metastatic breast cancer. J Clin Endocrinol Metab 73:1309–1315, 1991.

3. Hortobagyi GN, Theriault RL, et al: Efficacy of pamidronate in reducing skeletal complications in patients with breast cancer and lytic bone metastases. N Engl J Med 335:1785–1791, 1996.

4. Major P, Lortholary A, Hon J, et al: Zoledronic acid is superior to pamidronate in the treatment of hypercalcemia of malignancy: a pooled analysis of two randomized controlled clinical trials. J Clin Oncol 19:338–367, 2001.

5. Mundy GR, Guise TA: Hypercalcemia of malignancy. Am J Med 103:134–145, 1997.

6. Nussbaum SR, Younger J, et al: Single dose intravenous therapy with pamidronate for the treatment of hypercalcemia of malignancy. Comparison of 30, 60 and 90 mg doses. Am J Med 95: 297–304, 1993.

7. Ralston SH, Gallacher SJ, Patel U, et al: Cancer associated hypercalcemia: morbidity and mortality. Clinical experience in 126 treated patients. Ann Intern Med 112:499–504, 1990.

8. Roodman GD. Mechanisms of bone metastasis. N Engl J Med 350:1655–1664, 2004.

9. Stewart AF: Hypercalcemia associated with cancer. N Engl J Med 352:373–379, 2005.

10. Stewart AF, Broadus AE: Parathyroid hormone related proteins: coming of age in the 1990s. J Clin Endocrinol Metab 71:1410–1414, 1990.

CHAPTER 16

HYPOCALCEMIA

Reed S. Christensen and Jenny L. Ryan

1. **Define hypocalcemia.**
   Hypocalcemia is the state in which the serum ionized calcium level drops below the normal range of 1.0 to 1.3 mmol/L. This corresponds, under normal conditions, to a total serum calcium level of 2.1 to 2.5 mmol/L (8.5–10.5 mg/dL).

2. **How are serum calcium and serum albumin levels related?**
   Approximately 50% of serum calcium is bound to albumin, other plasma proteins, and related anions, such as citrate, lactate, and sulfate. Of this, 40% is bound to protein, predominantly albumin, and 10% to 13% is attached to anions. The remaining 50% is unbound or ionized calcium. The total serum calcium level reflects both the bound and the unbound portions with a normal range of 2.1 to 2.5 mmol/L (8.5–10.5 mg/dL).

3. **How is the total serum calcium corrected for a low serum albumin level?**
   Total serum calcium levels are corrected for hypoalbuminemia by adding 0.8 mg/dL to the serum calcium level for every 1.0 gm/dL that the albumin level is below 4.0 gm/dL. The adjusted level of total serum calcium correlates with the level of ionized calcium, which is the physiologically active form of serum calcium.

   $$\text{Corrected Ca (mg/dL)} = \text{serum Ca (mg/dL)} + 0.8(4.0 - \text{measured albumin g/dL})$$

4. **What is the most common cause of low total serum calcium?**
   Hypoalbuminemia. The ionized calcium concentration is normal. Low serum albumin is common in chronic illness and malnutrition.

5. **What factors other than albumin influence the levels of serum ionized calcium?**
   Serum pH influences the level of ionized calcium by causing decreased binding of calcium to albumin in acidosis and increased binding in alkalosis. As an example, respiratory alkalosis, seen in hyperventilation, causes a drop in the serum ionized calcium level. A shift of 0.1 pH unit is associated with an ionized calcium change of 0.04 to 0.05 mmol/L. Increased levels of chelators, such as citrate, that may occur during large volume transfusions of citrate-containing blood products, also may lower the levels of ionized calcium. Heparin may act similarly.

6. **How is serum calcium regulated?**
   Three hormones maintain calcium homeostasis: parathyroid hormone (PTH), vitamin D, and calcitonin. PTH acts in three ways to raise serum calcium levels: (1) stimulates osteoclastic bone resorption; (2) increases conversion of 25-hydroxyvitamin D to 1,25-dihydroxyvitamin D, increasing intestinal calcium absorption; and (3) increases renal reabsorption of calcium. Calcitonin decreases the level of serum calcium by suppressing osteoclast activity in bone. The interplay of these hormones maintains calcium levels within a narrow range in a normal individual. Calcium levels are also influenced by the presence or absence of hyperphosphatemia.

7. **What steps in vitamin D metabolism may influence serum calcium levels?**
Vitamin D is obtained through the diet or is formed in the skin in the presence of ultraviolet light. Vitamin D is converted to 25-hydroxyvitamin D in the liver and finally to 1,25-dihydroxyvitamin D, the most active form of vitamin D, in the kidney. 1,25 dihydroxyvitamin D acts directly on intestinal cells to increase calcium absorption. Deficiency in any of these steps may cause hypocalcemia.

8. **What are the major causes of hypocalcemia?**
The multiple organ and hormonal regulatory systems involved in calcium homeostasis create the potential for multiple causes of hypocalcemia. The etiology of hypocalcemia must be considered in relation to the level of serum albumin, the secretion of PTH, and the presence or absence of hyperphosphatemia. Initially, hypocalcemia may be approached by looking for failure in one or more of these systems. The systems primarily involved are the parathyroid glands, bone, kidney, and liver; the following shows the clinical entity followed by its mechanism(s):
   - **Hypoparathyroidism:** Decreased PTH production
   - **Hypomagnesemia:** Decreased PTH release, responsiveness, and action
   - **Citrate toxicity from massive blood transfusion:** Complexing of calcium with citrate
   - **Pseudohypoparathyroidism:** PTH ineffective at target organ
   - **Liver disease:** Decreased albumin production, decreased 25-hydroxyvitamin D production, drugs that stimulate 25-hydroxyvitamin D metabolism
   - **Renal disease:** Renal calcium leak, decreased 1,25-dihydroxyvitamin D production, elevated serum phosphate (PO_4) from decreased PO_4 clearance; drugs that increase renal clearance of calcium
   - **Bone disease:** Drugs suppressing bone resorption; "hungry bone syndrome"—recovery from hyperparathyroidism or hyperthyroidism
   - **Phosphate load:** Endogenous—tumor lysis syndrome, hemolysis, and rhabdomyolysis; exogenous: phosphate-containing enemas, laxatives, and phosphorus burns
   - **Pancreatitis:** Sequestration of calcium in the pancreas; other
   - **Toxic shock syndrome, other cortical illness:** Decreased PTH production or PTH resistance

9. **What physical signs suggest hypocalcemia?**
Chvostek's and Trousseau's signs are useful in detecting hypocalcemia. Chvostek's sign is a facial twitch elicited by tapping over the zygomatic arch. Trousseau's sign is a forearm spasm induced by inflation of an upper arm blood pressure cuff for up to 3 minutes. It is important to note that 4% to 25% of normal individuals have a positive response.

10. **What laboratory tests are clinically useful in distinguishing among the causes of hypocalcemia?**
Table 16-1 summarizes the laboratory findings in the conditions listed.

TABLE 16-1. DIFFERENTIAL DIAGNOSIS OF LABORATORY EVALUATION OF HYPOCALCEMIA

	Calcium	Phosphate	PTH	25-OH Vitamin D	1,25 (OH)$_2$ Vitamin D
Hypoparathyroidism	↓	↑	↓	Normal	↓
Pseudohypoparathyroidism	↓	↑	↑	Normal	↓ or Normal
Liver disease	↓	↓	↑	↓	↓ or Normal
Renal disease (secondary hyperparathyroidism)	↓	↑	≠↑	Normal	↓ or Normal

PTH, parathyroid hormone.

11. **Describe the symptoms of hypocalcemia.**
    - Early symptoms: numbness and tingling involving fingers, toes and circumoral region
    - Neuromuscular symptoms: cramps, fasciculations, laryngospasm, and tetany
    - Cardiovascular symptoms: arrhythmias, bradycardia, and hypotension
    - CNS symptoms: irritability, paranoia, depression, psychosis, organic brain syndrome, and seizures; "cerebral tetany," not a true seizure (see question 13), may also be seen in hypocalcemia; subnormal intelligence has also been reported
    - Chronic symptoms: papilledema, basal ganglia calcifications, cataracts, dry skin, coarse hair, and brittle nails

    Symptoms reflect the absolute calcium concentrations and the rate of fall in calcium concentration. Individuals may be unaware of symptoms because of gradual onset and may realize an abnormality only when their sense of well-being improves with treatment.

12. **What radiographic findings may be present with hypocalcemia?**
    Calcifications of basal ganglia may occur in the small blood vessels of that region. These occasionally may cause extrapyramidal signs but usually are asymptomatic. Of note, 0.7% of routine computed tomographic (CT) scans of the brain show calcification of the basal ganglia.

13. **What is cerebral tetany, and how does it differ from a true seizure?**
    Cerebral tetany is manifested by generalized tetany without loss of consciousness, tongue biting, incontinence, or postictal confusion. Anticonvulsants may relieve the symptoms but, because they enhance 25-hydroxyvitamin D catabolism, they also may worsen the hypocalcemia.

KEY POINTS: HYPOCALCEMIA

1. Serum calcium levels must be corrected for serum albumin levels in hypocalcemia.
2. Multiple organ systems, minerals, anions, and drugs affect calcium levels and must be considered when evaluating hypocalcemia.
3. Hypocalcemia is a frequent problem in trauma and intensive care settings and is often a result of intravenous agents.
4. 1,25-dihydroxyvitamin D is the treatment for hypocalcemia in hypoparathyroidism and renal failure.
5. PTH is not currently a treatment for hypocalcemia.

14. **How does hypocalcemia affect cardiac function?**
    Calcium is involved in cardiac automaticity and is required for muscle contraction. Hypocalcemia can therefore result in arrhythmias and reduced myocardial contractility. This decrease in the force of contraction may be refractory to pressor agents, especially those that involve calcium in their mechanism of action. Through this process, beta-blockers and calcium channel blockers can exacerbate cardiac failure. With low serum calcium, the Q-T interval is prolonged, and ST changes may mimic myocardial infarction. Although the relationship is variable, the calcium level correlates moderately well with the interval from the Q-wave onset to the peak of the T-wave.

15. **What are the potential ophthalmologic findings in hypocalcemia?**
    Papilledema may occur with subacute and chronic hypocalcemia. Patients are most often asymptomatic, and the papilledema usually resolves with normalization of the serum calcium level. If symptoms develop or if papilledema does not resolve when the patient is

normocalcemic, a cerebral tumor and benign intracranial hypertension must be excluded. Optic neuritis with unilateral loss of vision occasionally develops in hypocalcemic patients. Lenticular cataracts also may occur with long-standing hypocalcemia but usually do not increase in size after hypocalcemia is corrected.

16. **With which autoimmune disorders is hypocalcemia sometimes associated?**
Hypoparathyroidism may result from autoimmune destruction of the parathyroid glands. This disorder has been associated with adrenal, gonadal, and thyroid failure, as well as with alopecia areata, vitiligo, and chronic mucocutaneous candidiasis. This combination of conditions, each associated with organ-specific autoantibodies, has been termed the autoimmune polyglandular syndrome, type 1.

17. **Hypocalcemia is frequently encountered in intensive care settings. What are the potential causes?**
Low total serum calcium levels are found in 70% to 90% of intensive care patients and result from multiple causes including:
- Hypoalbuminemia
- Administration of anionic loads causing chelation (i.e., citrate, lactate, oxalate, bicarbonate, phosphate, ethylenediaminetetraacetic acid, and radiographic contrast)
- Rapid blood transfusion with citrate ion as a preservative and anticoagulant therapy
- Parathyroid failure and decreased vitamin D synthesis in severe illness
- Sepsis inducing some degree of resistance to the biologic effects of PTH

Because of all the above factors, it is recommended that ionized serum calcium rather than total serum calcium be measured in patients with severe illness.

18. **Hypercalcemia is not unusual in patients with cancer. What conditions may lead to hypocalcemia in this patient group?**
- Tumor lysis syndrome from hyperphosphatemia and associated formation of intravascular and tissue calcium-phosphate complexes
- Multiple chemotherapeutic agents and antibiotics (amphotericin B and aminoglycosides) induce hypomagnesemia; hypomagnesemia impairs secretion of PTH and causes resistance to PTH in skeletal tissue
- Thyroid surgery and neck irradiation with transient or permanent hypoparathyroidism
- Medullary carcinoma of the thyroid and pheochromocytoma; may secrete calcitonin and on rare occasions cause hypocalcemia

19. **What drugs may cause hypocalcemia?**
Phenobarbital, phenytoin, primidone, rifampin, and glutethimide increase hepatic metabolism of 25-hydroxyvitamin D and may thereby cause hypocalcemia. Aminoglycosides, diuretics (furosemide), and chemotherapeutic agents that induce renal magnesium wasting, and laxatives or enemas that create a large phosphate load, also may be associated with hypocalcemia. Ketoconazole, isoniazid, heparin, fluoride, bisphosphonates, foscarnet, and glucagon may also induce hypocalcemia by a variety of mechanisms.

20. **Which vitamin D metabolite is best for assessing total body vitamin D stores, 25-hydroxyvitamin D or 1,25-dihydroxyvitamin D?**
The serum level of 25-hydroxyvitamin D best reflects the total body stores of vitamin D. The conversion of 25-hydroxyvitamin D to 1,25-dihydroxyvitamin D is tightly controlled and the level of serum 1,25-dihydroxyvitamin D is maintained despite significant vitamin D depletion. Increases in PTH (secondary hyperparathyroidism) stimulate increased conversion of 25-hydroxyvitamin D to 1,25-dihydroxyvitamin D in this situation.

21. **How is hypocalcemia treated?**

Asymptomatic hypocalcemia requires supplementation with oral calcium and vitamin D derivatives to maintain the serum calcium level at least in the range of 7.5 to 8.5 mg/dL. When the serum calcium falls acutely to a level where the patient is symptomatic, intravenous administration is recommended. The dosage of calcium depends on the amount of elemental calcium present in a given preparation (Table 16-2). For a hypocalcemic emergency, 90 mg of elemental calcium may be given as a intravenous bolus, or alternatively 100 to 300 mg of elemental calcium may be given intravenously over 10 minutes, followed by and infusion of 0.5 to 2.0 mg/kg/h.

TABLE 16-2. ELEMENTAL CALCIUM CONTENT OF COMMONLY USED PREPARATIONS		
Preparation	**Oral Dose**	**Elemental Calcium (mg)**
Calcium citrate		
Citracal	950 mg	200
Calcium acetate		
PhosLo	667 mg	169
Calcium carbonate		
Tums	500 mg	200
Tums Ex	750 mg	300
Oscal	625 mg	250
Oscal 500	1250 mg	500
Calcium 600	1500 mg	600
Titralac (suspension)	1000 mg/5 mL	400
Intravenous Agent	**Volume**	**Elemental Calcium (mg)**
Calcium chloride	2.5 mL of 10% solution	90
Calcium gluconate	10 mL of 10% solution	90
Calcium gluceptate	5 mL of 22% solution	90

22. **When is treatment with 1,25 dihydroxyvitamin D (calcitriol) indicated?**

Under normal conditions, 25-hydroxyvitamin D is converted to 1,25-dihydroxyvitamin D (calcitriol) in the kidney under the stimulatory influence of PTH. Two conditions can therefore make the body unable to produce adequate amounts of calcitriol: hypoparathyroidism and renal failure. Because calcitriol is essential for normal intestinal calcium absorption, oral calcitriol (Rocaltrol) supplementation is indicated in patients who have either hypoparathyroidism or chronic renal failure. Of note, because vitamin D has weak biological activity, these patients may be given large dosages of vitamin D (50,000–100,000 U/day) if calcitriol is unavailable.

23. **Can recombinant human PTH (rhPTH) be used in the treatment of hypocalcemia?**

Subcutaneous injections of rhPTH have been shown to be effective in normalizing serum calcium levels in hypoparathyroidism. The therapy is not approved, however, and is considered experimental.

BIBLIOGRAPHY

1. Bringhurst FR, Demay MB, Kronenberg HM: Hypocalcemic disorders. In Larsen PR, editor, *Williams textbook of endocrinology*, ed 10, Philadelphia, 2003, W.B. Saunders, pp. 1340–1348.

2. Kastrup EK, editor: *Drug facts and comparisons*, St. Louis, 2003, Wolters Kluwer Health, pp. 27–29, 112–113.

3. Lebowitz MR, Moses AM: Hypocalcemia. Semin Nephrol 12:146–158, 1992.

4. Lind L: Hypocalcemia and parathyroid hormone secretion in critically ill patients. Crit Care Med 28:93–98, 2000.

5. McEvoy GK, editor: Calcium salts. In *AHFS drug information*, Bethesda, MD, 2007, American Society of Health-System Pharmacists, pp. 2655–2661.

6. Olinger ML: Disorders of calcium and magnesium metabolism. Emerg Med Clin North Am 7:795–822, 1989.

7. Potts JT: Hypocalcemia. In Kasper DL, editor, *Principles of internal medicine*, ed 16, New York, 2005, McGraw-Hill, pp. 2263–2268.

8. Shane E: Hypocalcemia: pathogenesis, differential diagnosis and management. In Favus MJ, editor, *Primer on the metabolic bone diseases and disorders of mineral metabolism*, ed 4, Philadelphia, 1999, Lippincott Williams & Wilkins, pp. 223–226.

9. Winer KK, Yanovski JA, Sarani B, Cutler GB: A randomized, cross-over trial of once-daily versus twice-daily parathyroid hormone 1–34 in treatment of hypoparathyroidism. J Clin Endocrinol Metab 83:3480–3486, 1998.

10. Zaloga GP: Hypocalcemia in critically ill patients. Crit Care Med 20:251–262, 1992.

11. Dickerson RN: Treatment of hypocalcemia in critical illness. Nutrition 23:358–361, 436–437, 2007.

CHAPTER 17

NEPHROLITHIASIS

Leonard R. Sanders

1. **Define hypercalciuria, kidney stones, renal calculi, nephrolithiasis, urolithiasis, renal lithiasis, and nephrocalcinosis.**
   Hypercalciuria is urinary excretion greater than 300 mg/day of calcium in men and greater than 250 mg/day in women. A more accurate definition is urinary calcium excretion greater than 4 mg/kg ideal body weight/day in either sex. Kidney stones, renal calculi, nephrolithiasis, urolithiasis, and renal lithiasis are synonymous terms that define the clinical syndrome of formation and movement of stones in the urinary collecting system. Renal calculi are abnormally hard, insoluble substances that form in the renal collecting system. Nephrocalcinosis is deposition of calcium salts in the renal parenchyma.

2. **Who is at risk of developing kidney stones?**
   The average prevalence of kidney stones in the United States is approximately 5%, with the lifetime risk of developing a stone being 13% in men and 7% in women. The yearly cost of kidney stone disease to the nation is more the $2.5 billion. Fifty percent of stone patients have a recurrence within 5 years. Stones occur most commonly between ages 18 and 45, in men 2 times more often than women, and in Caucasians more than other races. Women have had more stones in recent years possibly because of increased calcium and protein intake and increased exercise (dehydration). Risk factors include a family history of stones, obesity, diabetes mellitus, hypertension, autosomal dominant polycystic kidney disease, medullary sponge kidney, renal tubular acidosis, urine volume less than 2 L/day, dietary sodium greater than 2 g/day, low water intake, and high protein intake (see question 4).

3. **What are the composition and approximate frequency of most kidney stones?**
   There are six major types of stones as outlined in Figure 17-1. The figure also shows the approximate frequency of occurrence of each type of stone.

4. **What are the main causes of nephrolithiasis?**
   The most common causes of nephrolithiasis are the various types of idiopathic hypercalciuria (IH): absorptive hypercalciuria (AH) types AH-I to AH-III (renal phosphate leak) and renal hypercalciuria (RH). Other causes include primary hyperparathyroidism, hyperoxaluria, hyperuricosuria, hypocitraturia, hypomagnesuria, infection stones, gouty diathesis, renal tubular acidosis, cystinuria, and possibly nanobacteria. Rarely, kidney stones may form from xanthine, triamterene, monosodium urate, ephedrine, guaifenesin, and indinavir (protease inhibitor). Patients with idiopathic nephrolithiasis make up 10% to 20% of stone formers and have no identifiable cause after routine workup.

5. **Describe the conditions associated with both renal stone disease and hypercalciuria.**
   Calcium stones account for 80% of all kidney stones. Approximately 40% to 50% of calcium stone formers have hypercalciuria. Of those with hypercalciuria, 40% have IH, 5% have primary hyperparathyroidism, and 3% have renal tubular acidosis. Other causes of hypercalciuria include

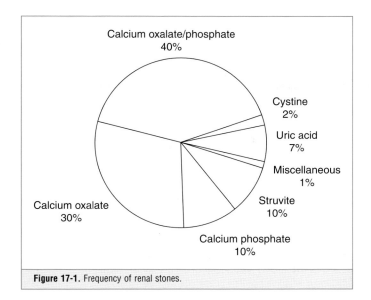

Figure 17-1. Frequency of renal stones.

excessive dietary vitamin D, excessive calcium and alkali intake, sarcoidosis, Cushing's syndrome, hyperthyroidism, Paget's disease of bone, and immobilization.

6. **What are the most important causes of normocalciuric calcium nephrolithiasis?**
   The most important and most common causes of normocalciuric calcium nephrolithiasis are hypocitraturia (50%), hyperuricosuria (25%), hyperoxaluria (10%), and urinary stasis (5%).

7. **Describe the process of renal stone formation.**
   Initially, urinary crystallization or precipitation of sparingly soluble salts and acids occurs. Nucleation follows as the initial crystals and urinary matrix ions form a stable framework for crystal enlargement through growth and aggregation. After they are sufficiently large, crystals become trapped in a narrow portion of the urinary collecting system, forming a nidus for further stone growth. Usually stones originate in the renal papilla and may detach, move distally, and cause obstruction. Common sites for obstruction are the ureteropelvic junction, midureter, and ureterovesical junction.

8. **Discuss the pathophysiologic factors that influence formation of renal stones.**
   Renal stones result from hereditary or acquired disorders causing supersaturation of stone precursors, deficiency of stone inhibitors, and possibly excess promoters. Supersaturation causes crystallization with mineral precursors, such as calcium oxalate. Calcium oxalate crystals bind to anionic, sialic-acid-containing glycoproteins on the apical surface of renal tubular epithelial cells, allowing further growth. Other factors that increase stone formation include urinary stasis (medullary sponge kidney), decreased flow (obstruction), increased urine ammonium (infection), dehydration (concentrated urine), and increased level of urinary alkalinity (renal tubular acidosis [RTA]). Type I RTA promotes stone formation through the increased release of calcium and phosphorus from bone to buffer the acidemia, with resulting hypercalciuria and hyperphosphaturia. The acidemia enhances proximal tubule reabsorption of citrate with resulting hypocitraturia. The alkaline urine of RTA promotes precipitation of calcium phosphate stones. Acidemia with a positive urine anion gap (UNa + UK − UCl) is a clue to the presence of RTA.

9. **What are the main chemical precursors of renal stones?**

   Relatively high concentrations of salt and acid solutes are the main determinants of crystalluria and stone formation. Calcium oxalate is most common and is supersaturated to 4 to 5 times its solubility in normal urine. Other precursors are calcium phosphate (hydroxyapatite) and calcium phosphate monohydrate (brushite). Uric acid, cystine, struvite (magnesium ammonium phosphate), and mucoprotein are undersaturated stone precursors. Drugs such as ascorbic acid (conversion to oxalate) and triamterene (nidus for stone formation) also may promote renal stone formation.

10. **What are the main inhibitors of renal stone formation? How do they work?**

    Inhibitors include urinary citrate, pyrophosphate, magnesium, nephrocalcin, uropontin, glycosaminoglycans, and Tamm-Horsfall protein. Most of these bind crystal precursors; for example, citrate binds calcium, making it less available to bind to oxalate. Inhibitors improve solubility and impair precipitation, nucleation, crystal growth, or aggregation. They also compete with stone precursor minerals, such as calcium oxalate, for binding to the apical surface of epithelial cells and inhibit epithelial cell adhesion and internalization of calcium oxalate crystals. Finally, inhibitors impair stone precursor transformation to a focus for crystallization and stone growth.

11. **What is nephrocalcin? What role does it play in formation of renal stones?**

    Nephrocalcin is an anionic protein produced by the proximal renal tubule and the loop of Henle. It normally inhibits the nucleation, crystal growth, and aggregation phases of stone formation. However, nephrocalcin isolated from some stone formers has defective structure and function and is found in the matrix of many calcium stones. Thus nephrocalcin may have a dual role in stone formation. When normal, it acts as an inhibitor of stone formation. When abnormal, it may act as a promoter by binding calcium and forming a nidus for crystallization.

12. **What are promoters of renal stone formation?**

    Promoters of renal stone formation are poorly characterized but are believed to be primarily urinary mucoproteins and glycosaminoglycans. Under certain conditions, promoters enhance the formation of renal stones.

13. **What are the basic determinants of serum calcium?**

    In the serum, calcium is 40% protein bound, 10% complexed, and 50% ionized. The three sources of serum calcium are intestinal absorption, bone resorption, and renal reabsorption. Intestinal calcium absorption is a variable proportion of the intake (30%–70%). Ninety percent of calcium absorption occurs in the small intestines and 10% in the cecum and ascending colon. Renal calcium reabsorption is a variable portion of the filtered load (95%–99.5%). The net flux of calcium from bone varies, depending on changes in the intestines and kidney. Under normal physiologic conditions, flux of calcium into and out of bone is the same. Parathyroid hormone (PTH) and vitamin D control normal bone, gastrointestinal, and renal handling of calcium.

14. **How does the kidney handle calcium?**

    Approximately 60% of the serum calcium is ionized or complexed and freely filtered by the glomerulus. The kidney reabsorbs 98% of the filtered calcium passively throughout the nephron. Sixty percent reabsorption occurs in the proximal convoluted tubule, 30% in the loop of Henle, and 10% in the distal tubule. Furosemide impairs calcium reabsorption in the loop of Henle and increases urinary calcium excretion. Thiazide diuretics impair distal tubule reabsorption of sodium, which increases intracellular negativity and calcium reabsorption. PTH increases distal tubular calcium reabsorption by enhancing calcium channel activity.

15. **Calculate the normal filtered and excreted load of calcium per day.**
The serum calcium is normally 10 mg/dL. The kidney filters complexed and free calcium, which makes up 60% of the total or 6 mg/dL. The normal glomerular filtration rate (GFR) = 120 mL/min. Thus the filtered load of calcium is 6 mg/100 mL × 120 mL/min × 1440 min/day = 10,368 mg/day. Because the kidney reabsorbs 98% of the filtered calcium, only 2% is excreted. Thus normally the kidney excretes about 200 mg of calcium/day (10,368 mg/day × 0.02 = 207 mg/day). If the excreted calcium increases to 5%, the urinary calcium increases to 500 mg/day.

KEY POINTS: INCIDENCE AND ETIOLOGY OF NEPHROLITHIASIS

1. Kidney stones are increasingly more common, possibly because of excessive dietary protein and calcium and exercise without adequate hydration.

2. Approximately 10% of the U.S. population has a lifetime risk for at least one kidney stone.

3. Stones form because of supersaturation of urinary stone precursors (such as calcium and oxalate), insufficient stone inhibitors (such as citrate), abnormal urine pH, or insufficient urine volume.

4. Stones are most commonly calcium based and result from hypercalciuria caused by excess absorption of dietary calcium, resorption of bone calcium, and unusually decreased renal calcium reabsorption.

5. Restricting dietary calcium without restricting dietary oxalate increases oxalate absorption and calcium oxalate stones.

16. **How do serum calcium and dietary sodium affect hypercalciuria?**
To help prevent hypercalcemia, nonrenal elevation in serum calcium causes increased filtered calcium and increased urinary calcium. Increased sodium delivery to the loop of Henle and the distal tubule also increases urinary calcium. In non–stone formers, urinary calcium excretion increases about 40 mg for each 100 mEq sodium excretion. In hypercalciuric stone formers, calcium excretion increases up to 80 mg per each 100 mEq of sodium. Because urinary sodium excretion equals dietary sodium input, restricting dietary sodium decreases urinary calcium excretion. In stone patients, recommended daily dietary sodium is no more than 100 mEq (2300 mg).

17. **What are the etiology and pathophysiology of IH?**
IH affects 10% of the general population and 40% of stone formers. The four types of IH are AH-I to AH-III and RH. AH-I and AH-II result from increased intestinal sensitivity to calcitriol with intestinal calcium hyperabsorption and increased numbers of vitamin D receptors in osteoblasts causing increased bone resorption and resorptive hypercalciuria. The latter accounts for decreased bone mass seen in many AH-I and some AH-II patients. AH-III, an unusual disorder, is due to a renal phosphate leak with urinary loss of phosphate, decreased serum phosphate, increased renal calcitriol production, and increased intestinal calcium absorption. The phosphaturic factor, fibroblast growth factor 23, is increased in some patients with calcium nephrolithiasis, hypophosphatemia, and renal phosphate leak. RH is characterized by impaired tubular reabsorption of calcium, causing decreased serum calcium, increased PTH and calcitriol, increased bone resorption, and increased intestinal calcium absorption.

18. **Distinguish among the various forms of IH.**
    See Table 17-1.

TABLE 17-1. FORMS OF IH				
Lab Value	AH-I	AH-II	AH-III	RH
Serum calcium	Normal	Normal	Normal	Normal
Serum phosphorus	Normal	Normal	↓	Normal
Serum intact PTH	Normal	Normal	Normal	↑
24-hour urinary calcium (1-gm calcium diet)	↑	↑	↑	↑
Urine Ca/Cr ratio (1-gm calcium load)	↑	↑	↑	↑
24-hour urinary calcium (400-mg calcium diet)	↑	Normal	↑	↑
Fasting urinary calcium (mg/dL GFR)	Normal	Normal	↑	↑

AH, absorptive hypercalciuria; Ca/Cr, calcium/creatinine; GFR, glomerular filtration rate; IH, idiopathic hypercalciuria; PTH, parathyroid hormone; RH, renal hypercalciuria.

19. **When is it necessary to distinguish among the various forms of IH?**
    Only complicated nephrolithiasis unresponsive to usual therapy requires differentiation (see Internet reference on hypercalciuria review at the end of the chapter).

20. **Explain the differences in serum levels of phosphorus and PTH in AH-III and RH.**
    Serum phosphorus is low in AH-III because of a primary renal phosphate leak. Intact PTH is high in RH because the primary defect is decreased renal tubular calcium reabsorption, causing relative hypocalcemia that stimulates PTH.

21. **Explain the differences in 24-hour calcium urine levels on a restricted calcium diet.**
    In AH-II, the 24-hour urine calcium normalizes on a restricted calcium diet (400 mg/day) because the absorptive excess is not as severe. However, the 24-hour urine calcium during calcium restriction remains high in AH-I, AH-III, and RH: AH-I because of marked calcium hyperabsorption, AH-III because hypophosphatemia decreases renal tubular reabsorption of calcium, and RH because decreased renal tubular reabsorption is the primary defect.
    High 24-hour urinary calcium is greater than 4 mg/kg ideal body weight. Normal 24-hour urinary calcium on a 400-mg/day calcium restriction is less than 200 mg/day. Normal fasting urine calcium is less than 0.11 mg/100 mL GFR. Normal urine Ca/Cr is less than 0.20 after a 1-g oral load of calcium.

22. **Define low serum phosphorus level on an 800-mg/day phosphorus-restricted diet.**
    Low serum phosphorus is less than 2.5 mg/dL on an 800-mg/day phosphorus diet.

23. **What causes hyperoxaluria?**
    Approximately 14% of urinary oxalate comes from dietary absorption and the remainder from metabolism of glyoxylate and ascorbic acid. Increased oxidation of glyoxylate to oxalate occurs in the rare autosomal recessive hereditary hyperoxaluria. The clinically more important enteric hyperoxaluria occurs with small bowel resection, bypass, or inflammation. Small bowel disease

may cause bile salt and fat malabsorption resulting in increased delivery of bile salts and fats to the colon. Bile salts damage colonic mucosa, increasing colonic permeability and oxalate absorption. Intestinal fatty acids are negatively charged and bind calcium and magnesium, decreasing calcium and magnesium available for binding intestinal oxalate and leaving more oxalate free for intestinal absorption. Low calcium diets do the same. Because oxalate is primarily absorbed in the colon, patients with small bowel disease and an ileostomy do not hyperabsorb oxalate. Excessive dietary oxalate or ascorbic acid (>2 g/day) also leads to hyperoxaluria.

24. **Why is hyperoxaluria important in nephrolithiasis?**
Oxalate is a major component of the most commonly formed stones (calcium oxalate) and contributes to supersaturation. Previously it was felt to be a much stronger stimulus to calcium oxalate stone formation than calcium. Newer data suggest that calcium may be just as potent, however, and high urinary concentrations of either calcium or oxalate are powerful stimuli for calcium oxalate stone formation.

25. **How does hyperuricosuria contribute to renal stones?**
Approximately 25% of patients with symptomatic tophaceous gout develop uric acid stones. Excessive urinary uric acid (>600 mg/day) supersaturates the urine, crystallizes, and forms uric acid stones. However, most uric acid stone formers do not have gout, hyperuricemia, or hyperuricosuria. All do have a urinary pH less than 5.5, which promotes uric acid stone formation. Approximately 25% of calcium stone formers have hyperuricosuria. Monosodium urate may form a nidus for calcium phosphate and calcium oxalate deposition, or it may interfere with inhibitors, resulting in increased calcium stone formation. This disorder, called hyperuricosuric calcium nephrolithiasis, is characterized by normal serum calcium, urinary uric acid greater than 600 mg/day, urine pH greater than 5.5, and recurrent calcium stones.

26. **How does urinary pH relate to renal stones?**
Because uric acid has a pKa of 5.5, acid urine shifts the equilibrium so that the concentration of uric acid is greater than the concentration of sodium urate. At urine pH 6.5, only 10% will be in the form of uric acid and approximately 90% in the form of sodium urate. Because uric acid is 100 times less soluble than urate, uric acid stones are more likely to form in acid urine. This equilibrium is so important that uric acid stones virtually never develop unless the urinary pH is less than 5.5. Because of low urinary pH, uric acid stones occur more frequently in obesity and diabetes. Obesity and diabetes are associated with insulin resistance. This results in decreased insulin-dependent renal ammonia production, decreased urinary ammonium, a lower urinary pH, and a propensity for uric acid stones. Cystine stones are also more likely in acid urine, whereas calcium phosphate (brushite) stones usually form only in alkaline urine. Calcium oxalate stones may develop in either acid or alkaline urine.

27. **What conditions cause low levels of urinary citrate?**
Patients with hypocitraturia excrete less than 320 mg/day. IH occurs in less than 5% of patients with calcium stones, and secondary hypocitraturia may occur in 30%. Citrate is freely filtered by the glomerulus, 75% is reabsorbed by the proximal renal tubule, and little citrate is secreted. Most secondary causes of hypocitraturia decrease urinary citrate by increasing proximal renal tubular reabsorption. Secondary causes of low citrate include dehydration, metabolic acidosis, hypokalemia, thiazide diuretics, carbonic anhydrase inhibitors, magnesium depletion, renal tubular acidosis, and diarrhea. Diarrhea also causes direct gastrointestinal loss of citrate and magnesium.

28. **What is the role of diet in the formation of kidney stones?**
The high animal protein (beef, poultry, pork, and fish) intake of many Americans (>1.5–2 g/kg/day) acidifies the urine with phosphoric, sulfuric, and uric acids; decreases urinary citrate; increases urinary calcium; and increases risk for nephrolithiasis. Higher protein diets, such as

the Atkins Diet, worsen these effects. Increased sulfates and uric acid may act as cofactors in the formation of calcium oxalate and uric acid stones. High sodium intake increases urinary calcium (see question 16). High calcium intakes ($>$1200 mg) contribute to hypercalciuria. However, low calcium intakes ($<$600 mg) without low oxalate intake decrease oxalate binding in the gut, increase oxalate absorption, and increase urinary oxalate. High dietary oxalate (see Table 17-2) increases calcium oxalate crystalluria. Orange juice may help prevent kidney stones by increasing urinary potassium and citrate. Potassium citrate as Urocit-K is commonly prescribed to increase urinary citrate. From Micromedex, Urocit-K at 60 mEq/day raises urinary citrate by approximately 400mg/day and increases urinary pH by approximately 0.7 units. An 8-oz glass of orange juice supplies 12 mEq potassium and 38 mEq citrate (more than a 10 mEq/ 1080-mg tablet of Urocit-K). Cranberry juice has mixed reviews, but recent data suggest it should not be used in excess in stone disease because it may increase urinary oxalate. Citric acid juices (lemon and lime) supply little potassium and only one third as much citrate as orange juice. Although potassium citrate juices are more powerful at stone inhibition, nearly all citrate drinks are useful. An exception is grapefruit juice, which may increase stone formation by 30% to 50%. Be flexible with your patients' choice of fluid, because the importance of the fluid intake may outweigh some of the theoretical negatives of the particular drink.

TABLE 17-2. SELECTED HIGH-OXALATE FOODS

Fruits	Vegetables	Others
Rhubarb	Leafy dark greens	Roasted coffee
Raspberries	Spinach	Ovaltine
Blueberries	Mustard greens	Tea
Blackberries	Collard greens	Cocoa
Gooseberries	Cucumbers	Chocolate
Strawberries	Green beans	Nuts
Fruit cocktail	Beets	Peanuts
Tangerines	Sweet potatoes	Wheat germ
Purple grapes	Summer squash	Baked beans
Citrus peel	Celery	Tofu

(Adapted from Renal diseases and disorders. In Nelson JK, Moxness KE, Jensen MD, Gastineau CF, editors, *Mayo Clinic Diet Manual,* ed 7, St. Louis, 1994, Mosby, pp. 315-362.)

29. **Summarize the presenting symptoms and signs of renal stones.**
    Approximately 30% of renal stones are asymptomatic and are found incidentally on radiographic studies. Seventy percent of renal stones are symptomatic. Patients may present with a dull ache in the posterior flank. However, the classic symptom of renal stones is excruciating pain that waxes and wanes. The pain starts in the posterior lumbar area and then radiates anteroinferiorly into the abdomen, groin, genital region, and medial thigh. Intense pain may last several hours and be followed by dull flank pain. Nausea, vomiting, sweating, fever, chills, and hematuria may occur. Patients with renal colic appear acutely ill and restless and move from side to side, attempting to relieve the pain. Physical examination shows tenderness and guarding of the respective lumbar area. Deep palpation worsens discomfort, but rebound tenderness is absent. Urinary tract infection may be present. Obstruction, if present, is usually unilateral. Clinical evidence of renal failure is usually absent.

30. **What elements of the history and physical examination are important in patients with kidney stones?**
Obtain present, past, and family histories and ask about previous stone disease. Because all of the following may be associated with stones, ask about use of guaifenesin, ephedrine, indinavir, triamterene, sulfonamides, and vitamins A, C, and D. Determine fluid intake and sources of excess calcium, salt, oxalate, uric acid, and protein. Physical examination is generally not helpful except during acute disease (see question 29).

31. **What lab tests are appropriate in the diagnosis of kidney stones?**
Evaluate urine for pH, hematuria, pyuria, bacteriuria, and crystalluria. If pH is high or bacteriuria is seen, perform urine culture. Perform appropriate radiographic studies (see question 35). Have the patient strain all urine and save the stone, if passed, for stone analysis. If this is the patient's first stone, the pain subsides, and the stone is less than 5 mm, follow-up for several months is acceptable. More than 50% of stones in the proximal ureter and 75% of stones in the distal ureter less than 5 mm pass spontaneously. Order a chemistry panel that includes serum sodium, potassium, chloride, carbon dioxide, creatinine, calcium, albumin, phosphorus, magnesium, and uric acid. Consider serum PTH and random urine for determination of the Ca/Cr ratio. If the patient has continued symptoms, if the stone is larger than 5 mm, or if obvious obstruction is present, consult a urologist and plan for a more extensive evaluation. Include a 24-hour urine test for creatinine, sodium, calcium, phosphorus, magnesium, oxalate, citrate, and uric acid.

32. **Summarize the therapeutic approach to patients with kidney stones.**
Unless contraindicated, all patients should increase fluid intake to at least 2 L/day or enough to increase urine output to more than 2 L/day; restrict dietary sodium to 2 g/day; restrict protein to less than 1 g/kg ideal body weight per day; decrease animal protein intake; avoid grapefruit juice; consume 1000 to 1200 mg/day of dietary calcium; and avoid excessive calcium, calcium supplements, oxalate, and vitamin C.

KEY POINTS: TREATMENT OF NEPHROLITHIASIS

1. Therapy of kidney stones includes daily intake of 10 to 12 eight-ounce glasses of fluid, increased intake of citrate-containing drinks, 1000 to 1200 mg of dietary calcium, and no more than 2300 mg of sodium and 1 g/kg of protein.

2. Avoid grapefruit juice and excessive calcium, oxalate, and vitamin C.

3. Although potassium citrate is preferred for urinary alkalization and citrate replacement, orange and cranberry juice contain potassium citrate and may supplement or substitute for potassium citrate medication if cost or intolerance is an issue.

4. Citrus beverages such as lemon and lime may also be beneficial.

33. **Describe the clinical significance of urinalysis in patients with renal stones.**
Most stone formers have macroscopic or microscopic hematuria. The remainder of the urinalysis is usually normal. Crystals are normally absent in warm, freshly voided urine and, if present, suggest a diagnosis. However, most urine specimens cool before examination, and crystals may form in normal urine with time and cooling. Thus by the time urine is usually examined most crystalluria has little clinical significance. An exception is the presence of cystine crystals, which are diagnostic of cystinuria. Persistently acidic urine (pH <5.5) suggests uric acid or cystine stones. Persistently alkaline urine (pH >7.0–7.5) and recurrent urinary tract infection strongly suggest struvite stones. Struvite stones never form unless the urine pH is alkaline.

34. **What are the characteristics of urinary crystals in patients with renal stones?**
Calcium oxalate monohydrate crystals may be dumbbell-shaped, needle-shaped, or oval, with the latter resembling red blood cells. Calcium oxalate dihydrate crystals are pyramid-shaped and have an envelope appearance. Calcium phosphate and uric acid crystals are too small for standard light microscopic resolution and look like amorphous debris. Uric acid crystals are characteristically yellow-brown. Less commonly, uric acid dihydrate crystals may be rhomboid-shaped or resemble the six-sided diamonds on a deck of cards. Because all of these crystals may be found in normal urine, they are not necessarily diagnostic of disease. However, cystine crystals always mean cystinuria and are flat, hexagonal plates, resembling benzene rings. Struvite (magnesium ammonium phosphate) crystals are rectangular prisms that resemble coffin lids.

35. **How do radiographic tests help to evaluate patients with renal stones?**
A plain radiograph of the abdomen (KUB) should be obtained in all stone formers and shows stones with the following features: calcium (small, dense, and circumscribed); cystine (faint, soft, and waxy); struvite (irregular and dense). Uric acid stones are radiolucent and not seen. Intravenous pyelography (IVP) localizes stones in the urinary tract and shows degree of obstruction. Radiolucent obstruction on IVP suggests a uric acid stone. Ultrasonography reveals size and location of larger stones, is sensitive for diagnosing obstruction, and may be best when radiation should be avoided as in pregnancy. Non-contrast-enhanced helical CT scanning is the most sensitive, specific, and accurate procedure for localizing kidney stones. Order the CT scan as a CT urogram with 5-mm cuts and without contrast to alert the radiologist to look at the kidneys, ureters, and bladder. Indinavir stones are not seen by KUB or CT scan and are diagnosed by suspicion from history, physical examination, and signs of obstruction.

36. **Which medications are useful for treating the various stone-forming conditions?**
See Table 17-3.

TABLE 17-3. ORAL DRUG THERAPY FOR RENAL STONES

Disorder	Drug	Dosage
Absorptive type I	Hydrochlorothiazide	25–50 mg b.i.d.
	Potassium citrate	10–30 mEq t.i.d.
	Cellulose sodium phosphate	5 gm 1–3 times/day with meals
	Magnesium gluconate	1–1.5 g b.i.d. and as needed
Absorptive type II	Hydrochlorothiazide	25–50 mg/day as needed
Renal phosphate leak	Neutral sodium phosphate	500 mg t.i.d.
RH	Hydrochlorothiazide	25–50 mg b.i.d.
Hypocitraturia	Potassium citrate	10–30 mEq t.i.d.
Hyperuricosuria	Potassium citrate	10–30 mEq t.i.d.
	Allopurinol	200–600 mg/day
Enteric hyperoxaluria	Potassium citrate	10–30 mEq t.i.d.
	Magnesium gluconate	1–1.5 g b.i.d.
	Calcium citrate	950 mg q.i.d.
	Calcium carbonate	250–500 mg q.i.d.
	Cholestyramine	4 g t.i.d.
	Pyroxidine	100 mg/day

(Continued)

TABLE 17-3. ORAL DRUG THERAPY FOR RENAL STONES (CONTINUED)		
Disorder	**Drug**	**Dosage**
Cystinuria	Potassium citrate	10–30 mEq t.i.d.
	α-Mercaptopropionylglycine	250–500 mg q.i.d.
	D-Penicillamine	250–500 mg q.i.d.
	Pyridoxine	50 mg/day
Struvite stones	Acetohydroxamic acid	250 mg 2–4 times/day

b.i.d., twice daily; q.i.d., four times daily; t.i.d., three times daily.
Note: Dosages are estimated ranges and not absolute recommendations. Each drug must be adjusted according to the patient's tolerance. Use the lowest dosage necessary to attain the desired effect and avoid side effects. Always use drug therapy in addition to appropriate dietary changes and fluid input. Potassium citrate is better tolerated in lower dosages taken three times a day. However, twice-daily dosing may improve compliance. Potassium citrate is often required to correct thiazide-induced hypokalemia and hypocitraturia (see question 37).

37. **What are special considerations in the drug therapy of nephrolithiasis?**
    Potassium citrate and not sodium citrate for alkalinization of urine to a pH greater than 7.0 is recommended for uric acid and cystine stones. Cystine stone formers require higher fluid intake to reduce urinary cystine below its solubility limit of 200 to 250 mg/L. Sodium citrate increases urinary sodium and calcium, and in alkaline urine, sodium urate may increase calcium stone formation. Fluid and potassium citrate often is the only therapy necessary for uric acid stones if uricosuria is less than 800 mg/day. Use allopurinol with potassium citrate if uric acid stones continue or hyperuricemia is more severe. Use cellulose sodium phosphate (CSP) only for refractory stone disease in AH-I. CSP binds calcium and magnesium in the gut, decreases absorption of both, and may worsen osteopenia and increase urinary oxalate. Replace magnesium as required. Monitor bone mass and treat osteopenia as necessary.

38. **Why are thiazide diuretics the first-line therapy for hypercalciuria-induced nephrolithiasis?**
    Thiazides are first-line therapy because they increase proximal (indirectly) and distal (directly) tubular reabsorption of calcium. However, thiazides can cause depletion of potassium and citrate, which should be replaced with potassium citrate. Avoid triamterene, which can cause kidney stones. If potassium supplementation is added, use amiloride with caution to avoid hyperkalemia. The thiazide-like diuretics, chlorthalidone (12.5–50.0 mg daily) or indapamide (2.5–5.0 mg daily), may be preferred to hydrochlorothiazide for the convenience of once-daily dosing. Additionally, indapamide is less likely to cause lipid disturbances associated with the higher thiazide dosages needed to reduce urinary calcium.

39. **How should you treat a symptomatic patient with a renal stone 1 to 2 cm in size?**
    Apply the therapeutic options in question 32. Many urologists treat symptomatic patients with calcium stones 1 to 2 cm in size in the renal pelvis or a significant proximally obstructing stone (0.5–2.0 cm) with extracorporeal shock wave lithotripsy (ESWL). If the stone is too large or too hard, as estimated by CT scan, or is not in a good location for ESWL, percutaneous stone removal or a ureteroscopic approach may be indicated (see question 40). Additionally, because of higher stone free rates, many urologists choose percutaneous nephrolithotomy (PCNL) for 1- to 2-cm stones. Distal ureteral stones are best managed with ureteroscopic stone extraction or in situ ESWL.

40. **How should you treat an asymptomatic patient with a renal stone of the same size?**
    The asymptomatic patient is a toss-up. Each expert has an opinion based on the experience of the local medical community. Many asymptomatic stones can be followed without intervention other than that noted in question 32. Specifics of stone location, duration, and overall patient health are important in the decision. Recurrent, enlarging, or multiple asymptomatic stones probably should be treated. Nephrology and urology consultations are appropriate. Other forms of lithotripsy include percutaneous ultrasonic lithotripsy and endoscopic ultrasonic lithotripsy. Intracorporeal lithotripsy uses the holmium:yttrium aluminum garnet laser and electrohydraulic lithotripsy.

41. **What treatment should be used if the stone is larger than 3 cm?**
    If the stone is larger than 3 cm, lithotripsy usually fails. The initial approach to patients with stones of this size is PCNL. However, many urologists choose this therapy for stones larger than 1.5 cm. Open lithotomy is now unusual. Therapy for stones larger than 2 cm depends on the patient's overall status, wishes, and experiences and the experiences of the patient's physician and urologist.

WEBSITES

1. EMedicine: Nephrolithiasis. Available at: http://www.emedicine.com/med/TOPIC1600.HTM

2. EMedicine: Hypercalciuria review. Available at: http://www.emedicine.com/med/topic1069.htm

3. EMedicine: Hyperuricemia and gout review. Available at: http://www.emedicine.com/med/topic3028.htm

4. EMedicine: Hypocitraturia review. Available at: http://www.emedicine.com/med/topic3030.htm

5. EMedicine: Intracorporeal lithotripsy. Available at: http://www.emedicine.com/med/topic3034.htm

6. Food and health communications: Diet and Kidney Stones. Available at: http://www.foodandhealth.com/cpecourses/kidney.php?print=yes

7. National Institute of Diabetes & Digestive & Kidney Diseases (NIDDK), National Institutes of Health. Available at: http://kidney.niddk.nih.gov/kudiseases/topics/stones.asp

8. Nephrolithiasis review questions. Available at: http://www.turner-white.com/memberfile.php?PubCode=hp_oct06_rqnephro.pdf

BIBLIOGRAPHY

1. Alan G, Wasserstein AG: Nephrolithiasis. Am J Kidney Dis 45:422–428, 2005.

2. Bhandari A, Menon M: Nephrolithiasis: reducing the risk of recurrence. Contemp Urol 15:36–52, 2003.

3. Cameron MA, Khashayar Sakhaee K: Uric acid nephrolithiasis. Urol Clin North AM 34:335–346, 2007.

4. Frick KK, Bushinsky DA: Molecular mechanisms of primary hypercalciuria. J Am Soc Nephrol 14:1082–1095, 2003.

5. Gettman MT: Effect of cranberry juice consumption on urinary stone risk factors. J Urol 174:590–594, 2005.

6. Lieske JC, Peña de la Vega LS, Gettman MT, et al: Diabetes mellitus and the risk of urinary tract stones: a population-based case-control study. Am J Kidney Dis 48:897–904, 2006.

7. Monk RD, Bushinsky DA: Kidney Stones. In Kronenberg HM, Melmed S, Polonsky KS, et al, editors, *Williams textbook of endocrinology*, Philadelphia, 2008, Saunders Elsevier, pp. 1311–1326.

8. Park S, Pearle MS: Pathophysiology and management of calcium stones. Urol Clin North Am 34:323–334, 2007.

9. Reddy ST, Wang CY, Sakhaee K: Effect of low-carbohydrate high-protein diets on acid–base balance, stone-forming propensity, and calcium metabolism. Am J Kidney Dis 40:265–274, 2002.

10. Rendina D, Mossetti G, De Filippo G, et al: Fibroblast growth factor 23 is increased in calcium nephrolithiasis with hypophosphatemia and renal phosphate leak. J Clin Endocrinol Metab 91:959–963, 2006.

11. Rivers K, Shetty S, Menon M: When and how to evaluate a patient with nephrolithiasis. Urol Clin North Am 27:203–213, 2000.

12. Wimpissinger F,Türk C, Kheyfets O, et al: The silence of the stones: asymptomatic ureteral calculi. J Urol 178:1341–1344, 2007.

13. Zheng W, Denstedt JD: Intracorporeal lithotripsy. Update on technology. Urol Clin North Am 27:301–313, 2000.

14. Lotan Y, Pearls MS: Economics of stone management. Urol clin North Am 34:443–453, 2007.

15. Sur RL, Preminger GM: Medical treatment: worthwhile and when? EAU Update Series 3(1):10–16, 2005.

PITUITARY INSUFFICIENCY

William J. Georgitis

CHAPTER 18

1. **What causes pituitary insufficiency?**

   Pituitary insufficiency (hypopituitarism) results from pituitary, hypothalamic, or parasellar diseases that disrupt normal pituitary function by displacing, infiltrating, or destroying the hypothalamic-pituitary unit. Pituitary insufficiency is present when inadequate amounts of one or more of the following anterior or posterior pituitary hormones is secreted (Fig. 18-1).

Adenohypophysis	Neurohypophysis
Growth hormone (GH)	Antidiuretic hormone (ADH)
Prolactin (PRL)	Oxytocin (OXT)
Adrenocorticotropic hormone (ACTH)	
Thyroid-stimulating hormone (TSH)	
Luteinizing hormone (LH)	
Follicle-stimulating hormone (FSH)	

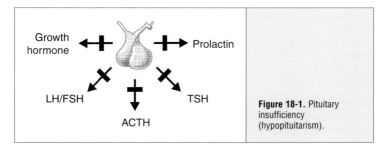

Figure 18-1. Pituitary insufficiency (hypopituitarism).

2. **When the pituitary stalk is severed, what happens to anterior pituitary hormone levels?**

   Serum levels of anterior pituitary hormones secreted in response to hypothalamic releasing hormones decline; this is true for TSH, LH, FSH, GH, and ACTH. In contrast, PRL levels rise. This unique response among pituitary hormones results from a decline in hypothalamic dopamine, the inhibitor of lactotrope PRL secretion.

3. **Which parasellar disorders cause pituitary dysfunction?**

   Processes adjacent to the sella that cause hypopituitarism include meningiomas, chordomas, craniopharyngiomas, optic nerve gliomas, carotid aneurysms, sphenoid sinus mucoceles, nasopharyngeal carcinomas, and pineal dysgerminomas.

4. **What is a craniopharyngioma?**

Craniopharyngioma is a squamous cell tumor that arises from Rathke's pouch remnants. It is the most common tumor in the region of the hypothalamus and pituitary in children but is relatively uncommon in adults. Two thirds of craniopharyngiomas are located in a suprasellar position. One third extend into or are confined within the sella. Most are cystic, but some contain both cystic and nodular components. The cystic portions characteristically contain a viscous yellow-brown fluid resembling motor oil. Sometimes the outer border of the tumor becomes calcified resembling an eggshell on radiographs. Best demonstrated with computed tomography (CT), calcifications are present in 75% of children but in only 35% of adults. Surgery is indicated for both treatment and pathologic confirmation.

5. **How does a pineal dysgerminoma present?**

Most often this tumor, comprising large undifferentiated germ cells and reactive lymphocytes, occurs in young males. Dysgerminomas associated with pituitary insufficiency can arise in the suprasellar region and also originate from the pineal region spreading to involve the hypothalamus. Simultaneous disruption of both posterior and anterior pituitary functions, hydrocephalus, and paralysis of upward gaze (Parinaud's palsy) may be presenting features. Patients often present with a combination of secondary hypogonadism and polyuria with polydipsia from neurogenic diabetes insipidus in addition to the neurologic signs associated with the mass or associated hydrocephalus.

6. **What is pituitary apoplexy?**

Apoplexy means loss of consciousness followed by paralysis. Classic pituitary apoplexy is an acute life-threatening event characterized by severe headache and collapse, with evidence of pituitary hemorrhage. An expanding hemorrhagic mass arising most often from an infarcted pituitary adenoma may compress parasellar structures, including cranial nerves coursing through the adjacent cavernous sinuses. Ocular paralysis and ptosis from involvement of the third, fourth, and sixth cranial nerves, as well as facial nerve involvement, contribute the component of paralysis necessary to fulfill the definition of apoplexy. Following an episode of pituitary apoplexy, anterior pituitary insufficiency is common. Posterior pituitary functions are almost always preserved. Most patients recover spontaneously and often do not require emergent surgical intervention.

Subacute forms of pituitary necrosis occur in patients with diabetes mellitus and sickle cell disease. Radiologic evidence of pituitary infarction even when unaccompanied by catastrophic symptoms and signs always deserves a comprehensive functional evaluation of the pituitary.

7. **Define empty sella.**

Empty sella refers to the absence or relative absence of the pituitary gland on radiologic imaging of the sella turcica. The term *sella turcica* (Latin sella = saddle and turcica = Turkish) stems from the resemblance of the cuplike prominence of the sphenoid bone that contains the pituitary to saddles used by Turks. These saddles with front and back supports differed from the Roman equestrian style of riding on a cloth tied to a horse's back.

8. **What is the distinction between primary and secondary empty sella?**

Primary empty sella is probably a normal anatomic variant or perhaps arises secondary to a congenital defect in the diaphragm sella. The sella is not actually empty but contains cerebrospinal fluid. The pituitary gland is flattened against the walls of the sella. Hypopituitarism with signs of symptomatic dysfunction occurs in less than 10% of the patients with primary empty sella.

Secondary empty sella is the end result of infarction, surgical removal, or irradiation of a tumor.

9. **What is Sheehan's syndrome? How common is it?**

Sheehan's syndrome is an acquired form of empty sella syndrome due to ischemic pituitary necrosis generally following child birth complicated by severe blood loss and hypotension.

Thirty percent of women suffering postpartum hemorrhage with blood loss of sufficient severity to cause vascular collapse eventually may demonstrate a spectrum of anterior pituitary insufficiency from mild to severe. Difficulties with lactation followed by persistent amenorrhea postpartum are features of this syndrome. If secondary adrenal insufficiency accompanies secondary hypogonadism, loss of axillary and pubic hair may also be a feature of the syndrome. Axillary and pubic hair are dependent on androgens and will only be lost if both adrenal and gonadal androgens are severely deficient.

10. **Do the clinical presentations of pituitary insufficiency differ between children and adults?**
In children, a signal of hypopituitarism is growth failure. In adolescents, abnormalities in sexual maturation such as failure to achieve puberty or arrest in sexual maturation may signal pituitary malfunction. Puberty occurs over a time span of several years when patients often change providers from pediatricians to family practitioners and internists. Signs of pituitary insufficiency can easily be overlooked.

In adults, symptoms and signs of hypogonadism dominate the clinical picture. Older patients often fail to complain about declining sexual function or libido, and the hypogonadal complaints lack specificity for hypopituitarism because they are so prevalent in the elderly. Features of hypothyroidism and adrenal insufficiency may be similarly insidious.

11. **Is there an easy way to tell whether the sella turcica is enlarged?**
An old axiom instructs that if a dime (diameter = 16 mm) fits within the sella on lateral skull films, enlargement of the sella turcica is probably present. Exceeding this dimension by any modern imaging modality should raise concern about pituitary enlargement.
The most common cause a pituitary enlargement is pituitary adenoma. Pituitary tumors comprise 10% to 15% of intracranial neoplasms and are present in 6% to 23% of pituitary glands carefully inspected at autopsy. Carcinoma of the pituitary is extremely rare and reported in the medical literature by case reports rather than large patient series. Metastases to this anatomical region from primary tumors elsewhere in the body are also rare and more often involve the highly vascular hypothalamus. Often metastatic spread of breast cancer or other aggressive neoplasms will result in both secondary hypopituitarism and diabetes insipidus.

12. **What tests should be considered for hypopituitary patients?**
The evaluation should include assessment of anterior pituitary hormones, radiographic imaging by CT or magnetic resonance imaging to assess anatomy, and formal visual fields testing. The tests for anterior pituitary function usually include serum levels of testosterone (men), estradiol (women), LH, FSH, thyroxine (T4), TSH, PRL, GH (children), and cortisol (before and after intravenous ACTH administration). Nocturia, polyuria, or polydipsia suggest the need to test for adequacy of vasopressin secretion by performing a water deprivation test.

13. **What is the Houssay phenomenon?**
Houssay, an Argentinian Nobel laureate, showed improvement in the diabetes of dogs rendered diabetic by pancreatectomy following hypophysectomy. He and other investigators subsequently demonstrated the diabetogenic actions of pituitary extracts. The clinical expression of the Houssay phenomenon sometimes appears in diabetic patients who demonstrate diminishing insulin requirements in the presence of hypopituitarism. The diabetic patient with recurrent and serious hypoglycemic episodes leading to major reductions in antihyperglycemic medications may have acquired hypopituitarism. The change is insulin sensitivity results from the acquired deficiencies of the insulin counterregulatory factors GH and cortisol. To grasp the significance of hormones counterregulatory to insulin in carbohydrate metabolism, consider that the diabetes seen with acromegaly also may improve or resolve after pituitary surgery, pituitary apoplexy, or octreotide therapy.

14. **What characteristics of adrenal insufficiency are present in ACTH-deficient patients?**
    Nonspecific symptoms, such as fatigue and weight loss, appear with ACTH deficiency. Serum sodium levels tend to be low, but potassium remains normal. Features of glucocorticoid deficiency are usually not as severe as those seen with primary adrenal failure. In women, axillary and pubic hair may diminish or disappear.

15. **Define secondary hypothyroidism.**
    Hypothyroidism is primary when the thyroid gland itself fails. Elevation of the serum TSH level is the most sensitive and specific test for the diagnosis of primary hypothyroidism because TSH levels increase as the thyroid's secretion of T4 declines. In secondary (or central) hypothyroidism, thyroid hormone deficiency is secondary to loss of TSH secretion by the pituitary gland or thyrotropin-releasing hormone (TRH) production by the hypothalamus. Symptoms and signs are similar to those seen in primary hypothyroidism but are generally milder. Even patients with massive pituitary tumors may not have obvious features of hypothyroidism. Laboratory tests abnormalities, like the symptoms and signs, are more subtle than those in primary hypothyroidism. TSH levels are often in the normal range but may be low, whereas serum T4 levels are decreased.

16. **Why are thyroid hormone levels low in secondary hypothyroidism?**
    Several defects explain the decline in thyroid hormone secretion in secondary hypothyroidism. TSH pulsatility in patients with pituitary macroadenomas is often abnormal, as depicted in Fig. 18-2. Both TSH pulse frequency and amplitude are decreased, resulting in loss or diminution of the normal nocturnal surge in TSH secretion. Circulating TSH molecules are also abnormal, having higher molecular weights than TSH molecules produced in normal individuals. Failure to remove sugar moieties during posttranslational processing by the Golgi apparatus appears to be the responsible mechanism. These higher molecular weight forms of TSH show decreased ability to stimulate thyroid hormone secretion by thyroid cells in bioassays.

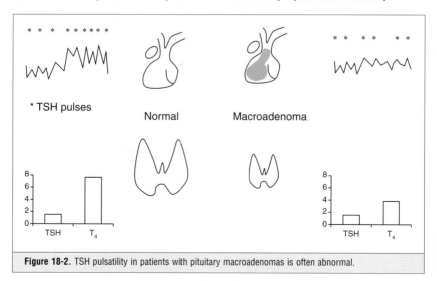

Figure 18-2. TSH pulsatility in patients with pituitary macroadenomas is often abnormal.

17. **What cortisol level is consistent with adrenal insufficiency?**
    Morning serum cortisols less than 10 ug/dL or ACTH-stimulated cortisol levels below 20 ug/dL are consistent with adrenal insufficiency. Plasma ACTH levels, when assayed properly, are elevated in primary adrenal insufficiency but are normal or low in secondary (central) adrenal insufficiency.

18. **Is secondary adrenal insufficiency as common as gonadotropin deficiency in patients with pituitary tumor?**
    No. The frequency of deficiency among the anterior pituitary hormones at the time of diagnosis of a pituitary tumor presents a spectrum of prevalence with GH > LH/FSH > TSH > ACTH. PRL deficiency rarely is recognized clinically. Posterior pituitary dysfunction with diabetes insipidus is so infrequent that its presence should suggest diseases primarily of hypothalamic or pineal origin, and deficiency of oxytocin is not usually considered at all. Most patients with pituitary adenomas have surprisingly intact anterior pituitary function before treatment and usually develop hypopituitarism only after surgical or radiation treatment. This is even true for most macroadenomas. The search for medical therapies as alternatives to pituitary tumor ablation by surgery and radiation continues to focus on preservation or restoration of normal pituitary function.

19. **Is life expectancy altered by hypopituitarism?**
    Yes. Life expectancy is shorter. All-cause mortality in patients with hypopituitarism is significantly increased approximately 1.7-fold. Women tend to fare worse than men, with observed/expected death ratios of 2.3 compared with 1.5, respectively. The increase is suspected to be due to vascular disease events but is probably multifactorial. Age and gonadal status appear to be independent risk factors, with hypogonadal patients having a better prognosis than eugonadal hypopituitary patients.

20. **Are health-related costs greater for patients with hypopituitarism?**
    A Swedish endocrine unit reported that hypopituitary patients have almost 2-fold higher direct health-related costs per annum. They also claim disability pensions and take a 1.6-fold greater number of sick days than the general population. None of the studied populations were on growth hormone replacement.

KEY POINTS: PITUITARY INSUFFICIENCY

1. The rise in prolactin from the loss of hypothalamic dopamine inhibitory tone sets it apart from other pituitary hormones that all decline after the loss of hypothalamic-releasing hormones.

2. The most important hormone deficiency to identify and treat in patients with anterior pituitary disease is cortisol deficiency. Acute adrenal insufficiency may be life threatening.

3. Replacement with thyroid hormone alone without concomitant adrenal hormone replacement in a patient with both thyroid and adrenal deficiency increases the risk for acute adrenal crisis.

4. Serum TSH can be low, normal, or mildly elevated in secondary hypothyroidism.

5. Aldosterone deficiency generally does not occur in hypopituitarism because the principal physiologic regulator of aldosterone secretion is the renin-angiotensin system not adrenocorticotropic hormone.

21. **What is the most important hormone deficiency to identify and treat in patients with anterior pituitary disease?**
    Inadequate cortisol secretion is the most important to identify and treat. Acute adrenal insufficiency may be life threatening.

22. **Why is aldosterone deficiency generally absent in hypopituitarism?**
    Secretion of aldosterone is regulated primarily by the renin-angiotensin axis, and therefore aldosterone secretion is normal in patients with hypopituitarism. However, hyponatremia

may still be a clue to hypopituitarism because it may result from either thyroid hormone or glucocorticoid deficiency and will be corrected with appropriate thyroid hormone or glucocorticoid replacement therapy (or both).

23. **Is anterior pituitary hormone deficiency always a commitment to lifelong replacement?**

Yes, in most cases, but there are important exceptions. Primary hypothyroidism sometimes causes significant pituitary hyperplasia with hyperprolactinemia and may present as amenorrhea-galactorrhea in women or as impotence and impaired libido in men. Dramatic reduction of pituitary size, normalization of serum PRL levels, and resolution of the hypogonadism usually occur with thyroid replacement. Hypopituitarism from hemochromatosis, an inherited disorder of iron storage, in rare cases, has also improved with therapy directed at the underlying disorder. Another example is seen in certain patients with pituitary macroadenomas. Mild elevations in serum PRL and deficiencies of other anterior pituitary hormones, especially ACTH, sometimes resolve immediately after surgical excision of the tumor.

24. **When one hormone deficiency in hypopituitarism is diagnosed, why is it important to define whether other hormone deficiencies are present?**

Replacement with thyroid hormone alone in a patient with coexistent adrenal deficiency may precipitate an acute adrenal crisis. Furthermore, vasopressin deficiency may be masked by adrenal insufficiency. After glucocorticoid replacement, central diabetes insipidus may appear and require specific treatment with a vasopressin analogue.

25. **What is the treatment of pituitary insufficiency?**

The treatment of pituitary insufficiency consists of replacing the hormones normally made by the pituitary gland or by the endocrine glands regulated by the anterior pituitary hormones. Thus patients with hypopituitarism are usually treated with replacement doses of thyroid hormone, glucocorticoids, and sex steroids. Patients with diabetes insipidus are treated with a vasopressin preparation.

26. **Who should receive GH treatment?**

Treatment is indicated for children with short stature, open epiphyses, and documented congenital or acquired GH deficiency. Evidence is also accumulating that adults with GH deficiency may benefit from GH replacement, although the cost-effectiveness of this intervention is an unsettled issue.

TOP SECRETS

1. Diabetes insipidus may be masked by concomitant secondary pituitary deficiency and appear after replacement with thyroid hormone and cortisol.

2. Most patients with macroadenomas of the pituitary do not manifest signs and symptoms of hypopituitaranism until after treatment with surgery or radiation.

3. Diabetes mellitus in acromegaly may improve or resolve after treatment for the growth hormone excess.

WEBSITE

Pituitary Foundation. Available at: www.pituitary.org.uk

BIBLIOGRAPHY

1. Arafah B: Reversible hypopituitarism in patients with large nonfunctioning pituitary adenomas. J Clin Endocrinol Metab 62:1173–1179, 1986.

2. Bates AS, Van't Hoff W, Jones PJ, Clayton RN: The effect of hypopituitarism on life expectancy. J Clin Endocrinol Metab 81:1169–1172, 1996.

3. Cummings DE, Merriam GR: Age-related changes in growth hormone secretion: should the somatopause be treated? Semin Reprod Endocrinol 17:311–325, 1999.

4. Ehrnborg C, Hakkaart-Van Roijen L, Jonsson B, et al: Cost of illness in adult patients with hypopituitarism. Pharmacoeconomics 17:621–628, 2000.

5. Gama R, Smith MJ, Wright J, Marks V: Hypopituitarism in primary haemochromatosis: recovery after iron depletion. Postgrad Med J 71:297–298, 1995.

6. Hazouard E, Piquemal R, Dequin PF, et al: Severe non-infectious circulatory shock related to hypopituitarism. Intensive Care Med 25:865–868, 1999.

7. Lurie SN, Doraiswamy PM, Husain MM, et al: In vivo assessment of pituitary gland volume with magnetic resonance imaging: the effect of age. J Clin Endocrinol Metab 71:505–508, 1990.

8. Schmidt DN, Wallace K: How to diagnose hypopituitarism. Learning the features of secondary hormonal deficiencies. Postgrad Med 104:77–87, 1998.

9. Vance ML: Hypopituitarism. N Engl J Med 330:1651–1662, 1994.

10. Webb SM, Rigla M, Wagner A, et al: Recovery of hypopituitarism after neurosurgical treatment of pituitary adenomas. J Clin Endocrinol Metab 84:3696–3700, 1999.

CHAPTER 19

NONFUNCTIONING PITUITARY TUMORS

Michael T. McDermott

1. **Name the functioning pituitary tumors.**
   Prolactin-secreting tumors, growth hormone-secreting tumors, corticotropin (adrenocorticotropic hormone [ACTH])-secreting tumors, thyrotropin (thyroid-stimulating hormone [TSH])-secreting tumors, and gonadotropin (follicle-stimulating hormone [FSH]/ luteinizing hormone [LH])-secreting tumors are the major functioning pituitary neoplasms. Some tumors secrete a mixture of hormones.

2. **What is a nonfunctioning pituitary tumor?**
   A nonfunctioning pituitary tumor arises from cells of the pituitary gland but does not secrete clinically detectable amounts of a pituitary hormone. These tumors are usually benign adenomas.

3. **What is the alpha subunit?**
   The alpha subunit is a component of three pituitary hormones: TSH, LH, and FSH. Each of these hormones consists of the common alpha subunit and a specific beta subunit (TSH beta, LH beta, and FSH beta). The alpha and beta subunits normally combine before the intact hormone is secreted into the circulation. Some nonfunctioning pituitary tumors actually synthesize and secrete measurable amounts of the free alpha subunit, which may therefore serve as a tumor marker.

4. **What other lesions can resemble nonfunctioning pituitary tumors?**
   Tumors that are not of pituitary origin may be found within the sella turcica; examples include metastatic carcinomas, craniopharyngiomas, meningiomas, and neural tumors. Nonneoplastic Rathke's pouch cysts, arterial aneurysms, and infiltrative pituitary diseases, such as sarcoidosis, histiocytosis, tuberculosis, lymphocytic hypophysitis, and hemochromatosis, may also be seen in this location.

5. **Differentiate between a microadenoma and a macroadenoma.**
   A pituitary microadenoma is less than 10 mm in its largest dimension, whereas a macroadenoma is 10 mm or larger. A macroadenoma may be contained entirely within the sella turcica or may have extrasellar extension.

6. **Which structures may be damaged by growth of a pituitary tumor outside the sella turcica?**
   Pituitary tumors that grow superiorly may compress the optic chiasm and pituitary stalk. Those that grow laterally can invade the cavernous sinuses and compress cranial nerves III, IV, and VI or the internal carotid artery. Inferior growth may erode into the sphenoid sinus. Anterior and posterior growth often erodes the bones of the tuberculum sellae and dorsum sellae, respectively (Fig. 19-1).

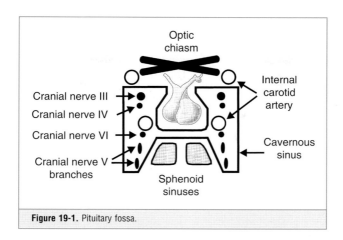

Figure 19-1. Pituitary fossa.

7. **What are the clinical features of nonfunctioning pituitary tumors?**
Many nonfunctioning pituitary tumors are asymptomatic and are discovered incidentally during cranial imaging procedures performed for other reasons. This is true of both microadenomas (<10 mm) and macroadenomas (≥10 mm). Nonfunctioning pituitary tumors that cause symptoms are usually large, space-occupying macroadenomas that compress nearby neurologic or vascular structures. Common clinical manifestations include headaches, visual field defects, visual loss, and extraocular nerve palsies. Pituitary insufficiency also may result from destruction of the remaining normal pituitary tissue.

8. **What anatomic evaluation is necessary for a pituitary tumor?**
Magnetic resonance imaging (MRI) or computed tomography (CT) of the pituitary gland and parasellar regions often allows a precise diagnosis and determines the presence and extent of extrasellar invasion. Visual field testing helps to assess function of the optic chiasm and tracts. Angiography may be necessary in some cases to rule out the presence of an aneurysm.

9. **What evaluation is necessary to determine that a pituitary tumor is nonfunctioning?**
A thorough history and physical examination must be performed to detect any signs or symptoms of overproduction of pituitary hormones. Hormone testing should include measurement of serum prolactin, insulin-like growth factor 1 (IGF-1), TSH, free thyroxine (free T_4), LH, FSH, testosterone (men), estradiol (women), and 24-hour urinary free cortisol excretion. Serum alpha subunit, when available, is also helpful.

10. **Does an elevated level of serum prolactin mean that a tumor is functioning?**
No. Secretion of prolactin is negatively regulated by hypothalamic inhibitory factors, such as dopamine, which reach the anterior pituitary gland through the pituitary stalk. Stalk compression from a nonfunctioning tumor can impair dopamine delivery and thus increase the release of prolactin from the normal pituitary gland. The serum prolactin rarely exceeds 100 ng/mL in such cases, whereas it is usually much higher with prolactin-secreting tumors.

11. **What is the primary treatment for a nonfunctioning pituitary tumor?**
Asymptomatic microadenomas can be managed with observation by serial imaging studies. Asymptomatic macroadenomas ($\geq$1 cm) should be considered for surgical removal although serial observation is an option if the tumor does not grow and does not cause significant patient anxiety.
The treatment of choice for symptomatic tumors is transsphenoidal surgery, in which access to the pituitary gland is gained through the sphenoid sinus. Radiation therapy may be used if surgery is contraindicated or not desired. Medications, such as bromocriptine, are rarely helpful.

KEY POINTS: NONFUNCTIONING PITUITARY TUMORS

1. Nonfunctioning pituitary tumors cause symptoms primarily by mass effects, resulting in compression of the pituitary stalk and optic chiasm, invasion of the cavernous sinuses, and erosion into the bony sella turcica.

2. Nonfunctioning pituitary tumors do not produce detectable levels of pituitary hormones but may raise serum prolactin levels modestly by pituitary stalk compression, interfering with the flow of dopamine from the hypothalamus.

3. Lesions that can resemble pituitary tumors include metastatic carcinomas, craniopharyngiomas, meningiomas, neural tumors, Rathke's pouch cysts, aneurysms, and infiltrative pituitary diseases.

4. Treatment for nonfunctioning pituitary tumors $\geq$1.0 cm in size is transsphenoidal surgery with subsequent radiation therapy or close monitoring for incompletely resected tumors.

5. Diabetes insipidus or secretion of inappropriate antidiuretic hormone (ADH) (SIADH) may occur in the immediate postoperative period and must be managed appropriately.

6. Anterior pituitary hormone deficiencies (hypopituitarism) can occur months to years after pituitary tumor removal, particularly if radiation therapy was used.

12. **Is postoperative radiation therapy recommended for incompletely resected tumors?**
Older literature, primarily from uncontrolled studies, suggests that postoperative radiation therapy is beneficial. Currently, however, most experts advise radiation only for large tumor remnants that compress vascular or neural structures. Many centers are now using stereotactic rather than conventional radiation therapy in these situations to deliver a greater focused radiation dose to neoplastic tissue with less radiation exposure to surrounding structures. Residual disease of lesser severity may be monitored with imaging studies and not treated unless growth occurs.

13. **What endocrine complications occur in the immediate postoperative period?**
Transient diabetes insipidus (vasopressin deficiency) manifested by high-volume urine output is common in the first few days. It may be followed by a short period (1–2 days) of water intoxication (vasopressin excess) causing hyponatremia. Both conditions result from reversible trauma or edema of the neurohypophysis, where vasopressin is stored. Fluid balance and serum electrolytes must therefore be closely monitored. Secondary adrenal insufficiency is of little immediate concern because high-dose dexamethasone is often given to prevent cerebral edema, but it may sometimes become apparent after dexamethasone is stopped. Deficiencies of other pituitary hormones do not tend to be an early postoperative problem if they were normal preoperatively.

14. **What is the management of postoperative diabetes insipidus and water intoxication?**
   Mild postoperative diabetes insipidus can be managed with isovolumetric, isotonic fluid replacement. More severe cases should be treated with desmopressin (DDAVP), 0.25 to 0.5 mL (1–2 μg) two times a day intravenously or subcutaneously or with aqueous vasopressin, 5 units subcutaneously every 4 to 6 hours, until urine volumes become normal. If hyponatremia develops, vasopressin must be reduced or stopped and free water intake restricted. If diabetes insipidus persists beyond 1 week, patients may be switched to intranasal DDAVP, 0.1 to 0.2 mL once or twice daily, or oral DDAVP tablets, 0.1 to 0.4 mg daily.

15. **What endocrine problems may occur during long-term follow-up?**
   Deficiency of one or more pituitary hormones may develop weeks, months, or years after treatment, especially if radiation was given. The only major concern in the first month is adrenal insufficiency. During this time one should question the patient about symptoms suggesting this disorder and, if they are present, obtain a morning cortisol level. If the cortisol level is low, hydrocortisone replacement should be initiated and the patient retested in 3 to 6 months with a cosyntropin stimulation test. At that time serum free T_4, TSH, IGF-1, LH, FSH, testosterone (men), and estradiol (women) should also be checked and replacement therapy considered for any identified deficiencies. It is recommended that these tests then be monitored at 6 months, 1 year, and annually thereafter.

16. **Summarize the long-term management of pituitary insufficiency.**
   See Table 19-1.

TABLE 19-1. LONG-TERM MANAGEMENT OF PITUITARY INSUFFICIENCY	
Deficiency	**Replacement Regimen**
Adrenal insufficiency	Hydrocortisone, 10–15 mg a.m., 5–10 mg p.m.
Hypothyroidism	Levothyroxine, 1.6 μg/kg/day
Hypogonadism (men)	Androgel, 5–10 g q.d. Testim gel, 5–10 g q.d.
Hypogonadism (women)	Oral or transdermal contraceptives Oral or transdermal postmenopausal hormone replacement
Growth hormone (GH)	GH 0.3 mg q.d. subcutaneously
Diabetes insipidus	DDAVP nasal spray, 0.1–0.2 mL q.d–b.i.d. DDAVP tablets, 0.1–0.4 mg q.d.–b.i.d.

b.i.d., twice daily; DDAVP, desmopressin; q.d., daily.

17. **Describe the clinical features of pituitary carcinomas.**
   Pituitary carcinomas, which are extremely rare, expand rapidly and cause mass effects. Some secrete hormones causing endocrine syndromes similar to those seen with adenomas. Metastatic disease to the central nervous system, cervical lymph nodes, liver, and bone are commonly associated.

18. **What is the treatment for pituitary carcinoma?**
   Transsphenoidal surgery is the primary therapy, followed by postoperative radiation. No significant use of chemotherapy has been reported for pituitary carcinoma.

19. **What is the prognosis for pituitary carcinoma?**
The mean survival is approximately 4 years.

20. **Which cancers metastasize to the pituitary gland?**
Metastatic disease to the pituitary gland occurs in approximately 3% to 5% of patients with widely disseminated carcinoma. The most commonly reported primary tumors are breast, lung, kidney, prostate, liver, pancreas, nasopharynx, plasmacytoma, sarcoma, and adenocarcinoma of unknown primary site.

BIBLIOGRAPHY

1. Arafah BM, Kailani SH, Nekl KE, et al: Immediate recovery of pituitary function after transsphenoidal resection of pituitary macroadenomas. J Clin Endocrinol Metab 79:348–354, 1994.

2. Arafah BM, Prunty D, Ybarra J, et al: The dominant role of increased intrasellar pressure in the pathogenesis of hypopituitarism, hyperprolactinemia, and headaches in patients with pituitary adenomas. J Clin Endocrinol Metab 85:1789–1793, 2000.

3. Barker FG, Klibanski A, Swearingen B: Transsphenoidal surgery for pituitary tumors in the United States 1996–2000: mortality, morbidity, and effects of hospital and surgeon volume. J Clin Endocrinol Metab 88:4709–4719, 2003.

4. Branch CL Jr, Laws ER Jr: Metastatic tumors of the sella turcica masquerading as primary pituitary tumors. J Clin Endocrinol Metab 65:469–474, 1987.

5. Gittoes NJL: Review: current perspectives on the pathogenesis of clinically non-functioning pituitary tumours. J Endocrinol 157:177–186, 1998.

6. Kaltsas GA, Mukherjee JJ, Plowman PN, et al: The role of cytotoxic chemotherapy in the management of aggressive and malignant pituitary tumors. J Clin Endocrinol Metab 83:4233–4238, 1998.

7. Katznelson L, Alexander JM, Klibanski A: Clinically nonfunctioning pituitary adenomas. J Clin Endocrinol Metab 76:1089–1094, 1993.

8. Klibanski A, Zervas NT: Diagnosis and management of hormone-secreting pituitary adenomas. N Engl J Med 324:822–831, 1991.

9. Mountcastle RB, Roof BS, Mayfield RK, et al: Case report: pituitary adenocarcinoma in an acromegalic patient: response to bromocriptine and pituitary testing: a review of the literature on 36 cases of pituitary carcinoma. Am J Med Sci 298:109–118, 1989.

10. Mukherjee JJ, Islam N, Kaltsas G, et al: Clinical, radiological and pathological features of patients with Rathke's cleft cysts: tumors that may recur. J Clin Endocrinol Metab 82:2357–2362, 1997.

11. Pernicone PJ, Scheithauer BW, Sebo TJ, et al: Pituitary carcinoma: a clinicopathological study of 15 cases. Cancer 79:804–812, 1997.

12. Shimon I, Melmed S: Management of pituitary tumors. Ann Intern Med 129:472–483, 1998.

13. Shin JL, Asa SL, Woodhouse LJ, et al: Cystic lesions of the pituitary: clinicopathological features distinguishing craniopharyngioma, Rathke's cleft cyst, and arachnoid cyst. J Clin Endocrinol Metab 84:3972–3982, 1999.

14. Swords FM, Allan CA, Plowman PN: Stereotactic radiosurgery XVI: a treatment for previously irradiated pituitary adenomas. J Clin Endocrinol Metab 88:5334–5340, 2003.

15. Wilson CB: Extensive personal experience: surgical management of pituitary tumors. J Clin Endocrinol Metab 82:2381–2385, 1997.

CHAPTER 20

PROLACTIN-SECRETING PITUITARY TUMORS

Virginia Sarapura

1. **Describe the normal control of prolactin secretion. How is it altered in prolactin-secreting tumors?**

   Multiple factors affect prolactin secretion (Fig. 20-1). However, the principal influence on prolactin secretion is tonic inhibition by dopamine input from the hypothalamus. Dopamine interaction with receptors of the D2 subtype on pituitary lactotroph membranes activates the inhibitory G-protein, leading to decreased adenylate cyclase activity and decreased levels of cyclic adenosine monophosphate (cAMP). In prolactin-secreting pituitary adenomas, a

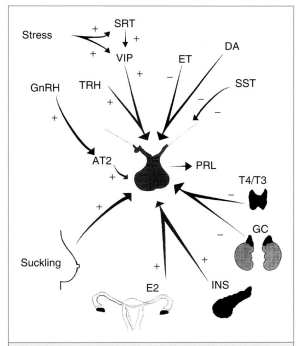

Figure 20-1. The multiple pathways controlling prolactin secretion. Plus (+), stimulatory effect; minus (−), inhibitory effect. Input from above the pituitary gland (depicted) arises in the hypothalamus; input from below arises in the breast nipple, ovary, pancreas, adrenal gland, and thyroid gland, as depicted. AT2, angiotensin 2; DA, dopamine; E2, estradiol; ET, endothelin; GC, glucocorticoids; GnRH, gonadotropin-releasing hormone; INS, insulin; PRL, prolactin; SRT, serotonin; SST, somatostatin; T4/T3, thyroxine/triiodothyronine; TRH, thyrotropin-releasing hormone; VIP, vasoactive intestinal peptide.

monoclonal population of cells autonomously produces prolactin, escaping the normal physiologic input of dopamine from the hypothalamus. In almost all cases, responsiveness to a pharmacological dose of dopamine is maintained.

2. **What are the normal levels of serum prolactin? Are they different in men and women? What levels are seen in patients with prolactin-secreting tumors?**
The normal serum prolactin level is less than 15 or 30 ng/mL, depending on the laboratory. Women tend to have slightly higher levels than men, probably because of estrogen stimulation of prolactin secretion. In patients with prolactin-secreting tumors, the levels are usually greater than 100 ng/mL but may be as low as 30 to 50 ng/mL if the tumor is small. A level greater than 200 ng/mL is almost always indicative of a prolactin-secreting tumor. Very high prolactin levels may be found to be falsely normal because of the high-dose hook effect of the assay; if clinically indicated, the sample should be assayed again after dilution.

3. **What are the physiologic causes of an elevated prolactin level that must be considered in the differential diagnosis of prolactin-secreting tumors? What levels can be reached under these circumstances?**
The most important physiologic states in which prolactin is found to be elevated are pregnancy and lactation. During the third trimester of pregnancy, the prolactin level may reach 200 to 300 ng/mL. It then gradually decreases during the first months postpartum, despite continued lactation. Prolactin levels are also elevated during sleep, strenuous exercise, stress, and nipple stimulation. In these cases, the elevation is mild, below 50 ng/mL.

4. **List the abnormal causes of an elevated serum prolactin level other than a prolactin-secreting tumor, and state the mechanism underlying the abnormal prolactin production.**
See Table 20-1.

TABLE 20-1.   ABNORMAL CAUSES OF ELEVATED SERUM PROLACTIN LEVEL OTHER THAN PROLACTIN-SECRETING TUMOR AND UNDERLYING MECHANISM OF ABNORMAL PROLACTIN PRODUCTION

Causes	Mechanism
1. Pituitary stalk interruption Trauma Surgery Pituitary, hypothalamic, or parasellar tumors Infiltrative disorders of the hypothalamus	Interference with the hypothalamic-pituitary pathways: prolactin production increases because the tonic inhibition of prolactin secretion is interrupted; often accompanied by hypopituitarism
2. Pharmacologic agents Phenothiazines Tricyclic antidepressants Alpha-methyldopa Metoclopramide Cimetidine Estrogens	Specific interference with dopaminergic input to the pituitary gland

(Continued)

TABLE 20-1. ABNORMAL CAUSES OF ELEVATED SERUM PROLACTIN LEVEL OTHER THAN PROLACTIN-SECRETING TUMOR AND UNDERLYING MECHANISM OF ABNORMAL PROLACTIN PRODUCTION (CONTINUED)	
Causes	Mechanism
3. Hypothyroidism	Increased TRH that stimulates prolactin release
4. Renal failure and liver cirrhosis	Decreased metabolic clearance of prolactin; also increased production in chronic renal failure
5. Intercostal nerve stimulation	Mimicking of the stimulation caused by suckling
Chest wall lesions	
Herpes zoster	

TRH, thyrotropin-releasing hormone.

5. **What are the typical levels of serum prolactin associated with these causes?**
In all these cases, the prolactin level is usually mildly elevated, 30 to 50 ng/mL and rarely above 100 ng/mL.

6. **How does prolactin elevation result in gonadal dysfunction? What are the symptoms associated with gonadal dysfunction?**
Elevated prolactin levels suppress the hypothalamic-pituitary-gonadal axis by interference with the secretion of gonadotropin releasing hormone (GnRH) in the hypothalamus, resulting in a decrease in circulating levels of estrogen or testosterone. Symptoms include infertility, loss of libido, menstrual irregularity and amenorrhea in women, and loss of libido and impotence in men.

7. **What is galactorrhea? Do most patients with prolactin-secreting tumors present with this symptom?**
Galactorrhea is the discharge of milk from the breast not associated with pregnancy or lactation. Although a typical symptom of prolactin-secreting tumors, it may be absent in up to 50% of women, particularly when estrogen levels are very low. Galactorrhea is uncommon in men, and may be seen in conjunction with gynecomastia when decreased gonadal function results in a low ratio of testosterone to estrogen.

8. **Why do men with prolactin-secreting tumors often present with more advanced disease than do women?**
The major symptoms of elevated prolactin levels in men are decreased libido and impotence. These symptoms may be ignored or attributed to psychological causes. Many years may go by before an evaluation is sought, often when the patient develops headaches and visual field defects related to the mass effect of the tumor. Women are more likely to seek evaluation early in the disease process, when infertility or menstrual irregularities prompt an evaluation of their hormonal status. In addition, studies have suggested that large ($\geq$10 mm) and small (<10 mm) tumors may be biologically different from their onset. Also, it was found that there was no difference in the prevalence of large tumors between men and women; however, there was a much higher prevalence of small tumors in women. This suggests that factors in women, possibly estrogen, may promote the appearance of prolactin-secreting tumors, but when these appear, they may be smaller and less aggressive.

9. **What is the imaging technique of choice when a prolactin-secreting tumor is suspected? Why?**
   Magnetic resonance imaging (MRI) of the pituitary with a contrast agent, such as gadolinium, is the imaging technique of choice in the evaluation of pituitary tumors. In particular, discrimination of small tumors is improved. Computed tomographic scanning allows better visualization of bone structures, such as the floor of the sella, in cases of large tumors. However, the relationship of the tumor to other soft tissue structures, such as the cavernous sinuses and carotid arteries, is better visualized with MRI. Skull radiographs and tomograms are not helpful.

10. **Bone metabolism is altered when prolactin levels are elevated. What is the mechanism for this effect? Is it reversible?**
    The resulting decrease in circulating levels of estrogen or testosterone causes a corresponding decrease in osteoblastic bone formation and an increase in osteoclastic bone resorption. The consequence is a decrease in bone mineral density and progression to osteoporosis. Studies suggest that normalization of the prolactin level restores bone density in most but not all patients, particularly those affected at an early age before reaching the peak bone mass in the third decade of life.

KEY POINTS: PROLACTIN-SECRETING PITUITARY TUMORS

1. When a mild prolactin elevation is found (30–50 ng/mL), physiologic, pathologic, and iatrogenic causes must be excluded before making the diagnosis of a small prolactin-secreting tumor.

2. A prolactin level greater than 200 ng/mL is almost always indicative of a prolactin-secreting tumor, except during late pregnancy.

3. Elevated prolactin levels cause galactorrhea and suppress the hypothalamic-pituitary-gonadal axis, which results in hypogonadism and a progressive decrease in the bone mineral density.

4. Untreated prolactin-secreting tumors grow very slowly: less than 5% of small tumors are noticeably larger after 2 to 5 years.

5. Treatment with dopamine agonists is well tolerated and quickly effective in normalizing the prolactin level and shrinking the tumor mass of even very large prolactin-secreting tumors.

11. **If a prolactinoma is left untreated, what is the risk of tumor enlargement?**
    Many longitudinal studies agree that progression of the disease is rare and occurs at a slow pace. This is particularly true of small prolactin-secreting tumors (<10 mm), less than 5% of which will enlarge significantly over a 2- to 5-year period of observation. There is no reliable way to predict which patients will show progression. Spontaneous resolution, attributed to necrosis, has also been described in some patients, particularly after pregnancy.

12. **Is medical treatment available for prolactin-secreting tumors? What is the mode of action?**
    Medical treatment with dopamine agonists has been available since the early 1980s.
    The most commonly used drugs are bromocriptine and cabergoline; pergolide and Hydergine are also commercially available but are not approved specifically for treatment of prolactin-secreting tumors. These medications are highly effective in reducing both the prolactin level and tumor size.

13. Describe the mode of action of commonly used drugs.

Dopamine agonists bind to the pituitary-specific D2 dopamine receptors on the cell membrane of prolactin-secreting cells, decreasing intracellular levels of cAMP and Ca^{2+}. This results in inhibition of the release and synthesis of prolactin. An increase in cellular lysosomal activity causes involution of the rough endoplasmic reticulum and Golgi apparatus. The action of dopamine agonists on D1 dopamine receptors in the brain causes side effects of nausea and dizziness; dopamine agonists with more D2 specificity, such as cabergoline, are less likely to cause these side effects.

14. If a woman with a prolactin-secreting tumor becomes pregnant while on medical treatment, should the treatment be continued? Should she be allowed to breast-feed her infant?

Even though many studies have found that maternal treatment with dopamine agonists is safe to the fetus, it is recommended that the drug be stopped as soon as pregnancy is diagnosed. The risk of tumor reexpansion is low: less than 5% for small prolactin-secreting tumors and 15% to 35% for large tumors. Assessment of symptoms, particularly headaches, and visual field tests should be performed monthly; any evidence of tumor reexpansion should prompt the reinstitution of treatment. Breast-feeding does not appear to add any significant risk for these patients, but close follow-up should be continued.

15. How long does it take for medical treatment to reduce the serum prolactin level? To reduce the size of the tumor?

The onset of action of dopamine agonists is rapid, and because prolactin has a serum half-life of 50 minutes, a decrease in the prolactin level may be noted within 2 hours. However, normalization of the prolactin level may take weeks or months, with the maximal decrease usually seen by 3 months. A reduction in tumor size may be apparent within the first 48 hours and may be demonstrated by improvement in the visual fields, when these are affected by the tumor. Tumor shrinkage of at least 50% is usually evident by 3 months. Maximal tumor shrinkage, however, is not usually observed until after at least 6 to 12 months of treatment.

16. How long is medical treatment of prolactin-secreting tumors required? Why?

In general, lifelong treatment is required, because prolactin levels rise and tumors reexpand when treatment is interrupted, suggesting that the effect is mostly cytostatic. Recent reports, however, suggest that about 20% of cases may be cured after 2 to 5 years of treatment, and some evidence suggests that dopamine agonists may have a cytolytic effect.

17. When is surgical removal of a prolactin-secreting tumor indicated?

With the availability of dopamine agonists, surgery has become a secondary choice in the treatment of prolactin-secreting tumors, particularly because the long-term surgical cure rate for large tumors is only 25% to 50%. The principal indications for surgical treatment of a prolactin-secreting tumor are intolerance or resistance to dopamine agonists and acute hemorrhage into the tumor. A cerebrospinal fluid leak due to erosion of the floor of the sella turcica is another indication for surgical debulking and repair.

18. When is radiotherapy indicated to treat a prolactin-secreting tumor?

Radiotherapy has rarely been used because hypopituitarism is a common side effect. This complication is of critical concern, particularly in patients under treatment for infertility. However, radiotherapy may be a useful adjunct in patients who require additional treatment after surgery and who do not tolerate dopamine agonists. Some experts advocate the use of radiotherapy 3 months before attempting pregnancy in women with large tumors to avoid tumor reexpansion during pregnancy. The development of new stereotactic radiosurgical techniques, such as the gamma knife, may improve outcomes and minimize radiation side effects.

WEBSITES

1. National Institute for Diabetes, Digestive and Kidney Disorders. Available at: http://www.endocrine.niddk.nih.gov/pubs/prolact/prolact.htm

2. UpToDate—Patient Information. Available at: http://patients.uptodate.com/topic.asp?file=endocrin/8753

3. Pituitary Society—Information for Patients. Available at: http://www.pituitarysociety.org/public/specific/prolactinoma

BIBLIOGRAPHY

1. Bronstein MD: Prolactinomas and pregnancy. Pituitary 8:31–38, 2005.

2. Casanueva FF, Molitch ME, Schlechte JA, et al: Guidelines of the Pituitary Society for the diagnosis and management of prolactinomas. Clin Endocrinol (Oxf) 65:265–273, 2006.

3. Colao A, Abs R, Bárcena DG, et al: Pregnancy outcomes following cabergoline treatment: extended results from a 12-year observational study. Clin Endocrinol (Oxf) 68:66–71, 2008

4. Gillam MP, Molitch ME, Lombardi G, Colao A: Advances in the treatment of prolactinomas. Endocr Rev 27:485–534, 2006.

5. Molitch ME: Pharmacologic resistance in prolactinoma patients. Pituitary 8:43–52, 2005.

6. Schlechte JA: Long-term management of prolactinomas. J Clin Endocrinol Metab 92:2861–2865, 2007.

GROWTH HORMONE-SECRETING PITUITARY TUMORS

Mary H. Samuels

CHAPTER 21

1. What is the normal function of growth hormone in children and adults?

In children, growth hormone (GH) is responsible for linear growth. In children and adults, GH has many effects on intermediary metabolism, including protein synthesis and nitrogen balance, carbohydrate metabolism, lipolysis, and calcium homeostasis.

2. How are levels of GH normally regulated?

Pituitary secretion of GH is regulated by two hypothalamic hormones: stimulatory GH-releasing hormone (GH-RH) and inhibitory somatostatin. Secretion of GH is also affected by adrenergic and dopaminergic hormones, as well as by other central nervous system factors.

3. Does GH directly affect peripheral tissues?

No. Many (although not all) effects of GH are mediated by another hormone called somatomedin-C or insulin-like growth factor type 1 (IGF-1). IGF-1 is made by the liver and other organs in response to stimulation by GH. IGF-1 feeds back to the pituitary gland and suppresses GH secretion. Unlike GH, IGF-1 has a long half-life in plasma; thus plasma levels of IGF-1 are helpful in the diagnosis of GH abnormalities.

4. What are the clinical features of excessive production of GH in children?

In children who have not yet undergone puberty and whose long bones still respond to GH, excessive GH causes accelerated linear growth. The result is gigantism.

5. Describe the clinical features of excessive production of GH in adults.

In adults, excessive GH causes acromegaly. The pathologic and metabolic effects of acromegaly are summarized in Table 21-1.

6. What is the single best clue in examining a patient suspected of having acromegaly?

An old driver's license picture or other old photographs provide the best clues. Patients with acromegaly are often unaware of the gradual disfigurement due to the disease or attribute it to aging. Comparing serial photographs can help to establish the diagnosis, as well as date its onset.

7. From what do patients with acromegaly die?

Acromegaly increases cardiovascular and metabolic resk factors, including hypertension, glucose intolerance, cardiomyopathy, and sleep apena. The mortality from untreated or inadequately treated acromegaly is about double the expected rate in healthy subjects matched for age. Major causes of death include hypertension, cardiovascular disease, diabetes, pulmonary infections, and cancer.

8. In patients with acromegaly, are skin tags all over the neck and chest a relevant finding?

There appears to be an association between multiple skin tags and colonic polyps in acromegaly. Therefore the patient should undergo careful colonoscopic screening for polyps and colon cancer. However, even patients without active disease or skin tags may be at risk for colonic neoplasia and probably should be screened regularly, according to conventional guidelines.

TABLE 21-1. CLINICAL EFFECTS OF ACROMEGALY	
Clinical Effect	Cause
Coarse features	Periosteal formation of new bone
Enlarged hands and feet	Soft tissue hypertrophy
Excess sweating	Hypertrophy of sweat glands
Deepened voice	Hypertrophy of larynx
Skin tags	Hypertrophy of skin
Upper airway obstruction and sleep apnea	Hypertrophy of tongue and upper airway
Osteoarthritis	Hypertrophy of joint cartilage and osseous overgrowth
Carpal tunnel syndrome	Hypertrophy of joint cartilage and osseous overgrowth
Hypertension, congestive heart failure	Cardiac hypertrophy
Hypogonadism	Multifactorial
Diabetes mellitus, glucose intolerance	Insulin antagonism, other factors
Colonic polypss	Colonic hypertrophy

9. **The husband of the patient with acromegaly complains that he cannot sleep because his wife snores so loudly. Is this complaint relevant?**
Sleep apnea occurs in up to 80% of patients with acromegaly. It can be due to soft tissue overgrowth of the upper airway or to altered central respiratory control. Sleep apnea may contribute to morbidity and mortality in acromegaly by producing hypoxia and pulmonary hypertension.

10. **If I suspect that a patient may have acromegaly, what test should I order?**
The single best screening test for acromegaly is the plasma level of IGF-1. Because plasma levels of IGF-1 are independent of food intake, samples can be drawn any time of day. In adults, acromegaly is essentially the only condition that causes elevated IGF-1 levels. In children, IGF-1 levels are more difficult to interpret because growing children normally have higher levels than adults.

11. **The patient's IGF-1 level is not elevated, but I still think that she may have acromegaly. What other test should I do?**
The gold standard test to rule out acromegaly is the measurement of serum GH levels in the fasting state and after glucose suppression. Some patients with acromegaly have extremely elevated fasting levels of GH, and further testing is not necessary. Most patients, however, have GH levels that are only mildly elevated or overlap with levels in healthy subjects. Therefore, the diagnosis is usually made by measuring GH levels after a glucose tolerance test. Healthy subjects suppress GH levels after glucose, whereas patients with acromegaly show no suppression or an increase in GH levels. This test is unreliable in patients with diabetes mellitus.

12. **After the biochemical diagnosis of acromegaly or gigantism is made, what is the next step?**
Excessive secretion of GH is almost always due to a benign pituitary tumor. Therefore the next step is to obtain a radiologic study of the pituitary gland. The optimal study is magnetic resonance imaging (MRI) with special cuts through the pituitary gland. If MRI is not available, the best alternative study is a computed tomography (CT) scan with special cuts through the pituitary gland.

13. **What causes GH-secreting pituitary tumors?**

GH-secreting pituitary tumors have been shown to be monoclonal, suggesting that a spontaneous somatic mutation is a key event in neoplastic transformation of somatotrophs. Further studies have clarified the nature of the mutation in some GH tumors that appear to have an altered stimulatory subunit (G_S) of the G-proteins that regulate adenylate cyclase activity. In a mutated cell, alterations in the G_S subunit cause autonomous adenylate cyclase activity and elevated secretion of GH. However, the mutant G_S is found only in a subset of patients with acromegaly. The mechanism of GH regulation and tumor growth may differ in other patients with acromegaly.

14. **Are other endocrine syndromes possible in patients with acromegaly or gigantism?**

Yes. Otherwise acromegaly and gigantism would not be endocrine disorders. Three endocrine syndromes include acromegaly (Table 21-2).

TABLE 21-2. ENDOCRINE SYNDROMES ASSOCIATED WITH ACROMEGALY

Syndrome	Major Involved Organs	Clinical Findings	Other Clues
Multiple endocrine neoplasia type 1	Pituitary tumors		Autosomal dominant
(MEN 1)	Parathyroid hyperplasia	Hypercalcemia (most)	Check calcium levels in patients with acromegaly
	Islet-cell tumors	Peptic ulcer disease (if gastrinoma) Hypoglycemia (if insulinoma)	
McCune-Albright syndrome	Bones	Polyostotic fibrous dysplasia	Mostly in girls
	Skin	Café-au-lait spots	
	Gonads	Sexual precocity	
	Others		
Carney's complex	Heart	Cardiac myomas	Autosomal dominant
	Skin	Pigmented skin lesions	
	Adrenals	Pigmented nodular adrenal hyperplasia	
	Others	Many other tumors	

15. **Do other tumors besides pituitary tumors make GH and cause acromegaly or gigantism?**

Yes. Rare tumors of the pancreas, lung, ovary, and breast may produce GH. However, only one patient has been reported to develop clinical acromegaly from ectopic GH production (from a pancreatic tumor).

16. **Do tumors ever cause acromegaly or gigantism by making excessive GH-RH?**

Yes. More than 50 cases of GH-RH production by various tumors have been described. These tumors occur in the lung, gastrointestinal tract, or adrenal glands and cause acromegaly by stimulating pituitary secretion of GH. The clinical and biochemical features of acromegaly in such patients are indistinguishable from those of acromegaly due to a pituitary adenoma. Pituitary enlargement also occurs as a result of hyperplasia of somatotrophs. Some patients have had inadvertent transsphenoidal surgery before the correct diagnosis was made. Therefore the plasma level of GH-RH should be measured in any acromegalic patient with an extrapituitary abnormality or with hyperplasia on pituitary pathology.

17. **If MRI of the pituitary confirms a tumor in the acromegalic patient, what issues other than the metabolic effects of excessive GH should be considered?**
    1. Is the tumor making any other pituitary hormones besides GH? For example, many GH-secreting tumors also produce prolactin; rare tumors also make thyroid-stimulating hormone or other pituitary hormones. In patients with acromegaly, prolactin levels should be measured, as well as other hormones when clinically indicated.
    2. Is the tumor interfering with the normal function of the pituitary gland? Specifically, what are the patient's thyroid, adrenal, and gonadal function? Does the patient have diabetes insipidus? It is important to diagnose and treat pituitary insufficiency before therapy for the excessive secretion of GH, especially if the patient is scheduled for surgery.
    3. Is the tumor causing effects owing to its size and location? Possible effects include headache, visual field disturbances, and extraocular movement abnormalities. Formal visual fields examination should be carried out in patients with large pituitary tumors.

18. **How big are GH-secreting pituitary tumors?**
    GH-secreting tumors vary considerably in size, but most are larger than 1 cm in diameter when diagnosed (i.e., macroadenomas), and some can be very large. Tumor size is an important issue because it determines success rates of treatment.

KEY POINTS: ACROMEGALY

1. Acromegaly leads to gradual soft tissue enlargement and disfigurement over many years, and the patient may be unaware of the changes.

2. Acromegaly causes damage to bones, joints, the heart, and other organs and is associated with considerable morbidity and excess mortality.

3. The best screening test for acromegaly is an insulin-like growth factor type 1 level.

4. The best initial treatment for acromegaly is usually surgery, performed by an experienced pituitary surgeon.

5. There are new medical treatments for acromegaly that are effective in controlling the metabolic effects of excess growth hormone secretion.

19. **How should acromegaly or gigantism be treated?**
    The treatment of choice for GH-secreting tumors is transsphenoidal surgery by an experienced neurosurgeon. Most patients with microadenomas are cured, and larger tumors are debulked. Significant reduction in GH levels and improvement in symptoms typically follow surgery, even when further treatment is required. Certain patients may benefit from medical therapy with a somatostating analog before surgery to reduce surgical risks, including patients with congestive heart failure, severe sleep apnea, intubation problems, or other comorbidites of acromegaly. There are no conclusive data that presurgical treatment improves cure rates, however. Primary medical therapy with a somatostatin analog can be considered for carefully selected patients, such as those who are poor surgical candidates or who decline surgery.

20. **What if surgery does not cure the patient? Should I recommend radiation therapy?**
    Conventional radiation therapy of GH-secreting tumors causes a gradual decline in GH levels over many years and is not recommended as sole therapy. Stereotactic "radiosurgery" has been applied to pituitary tumors, including acromegaly. Stereotactic radiosurgery consists of applying a highly concentrated high-energy radiation therapy beam to the tumor, and it appears to be

more effective and to work more quickly than conventional radiation therapy for pituitary tumors. However, stereotactic radiosurgery still takes months to years to work. Therefore although it is not a good initial choice, radiation therapy is sometimes used after surgery for additional control of the residual tumor mass, or if medical therapy fails to control the metabolic effects of growth hormone excess. Many patients eventually develop hypopituitarism from radiation therapy.

21. **Are there any options for medical therapy of acromegaly?**
Two agents are effective: octreotide and pegvisomant.

22. **Discuss the mechanisms of action of octreotide.**
Most GH-secreting tumors have somatostatin receptors and respond to exogenous somatostatin with decreases in GH levels. The development of octreotide, a long-acting analog of somatostatin, was a major advance in the treatment of acromegaly.

23. **How effective is octreotide?**
Given as injections two or three times a day, octreotide leads to markedly decreased levels of GH in most acromegalic patients, with amelioration of many of the symptoms and side effects of acromegay. It also causes tumor shrinkage in some patients. However, it does not cure acromegaly; stopping the drug usually leads to increases in GH levels and tumor regrowth. Therefore octreotide must be given indefinitely or while waiting for radiation to take effect. Recently, long-acting depo forms of octreotide have been developed. Now most patients can be treated with an injection once a month rather than two to three times a day.

24. **Describe the mechanism of action of pegvisomant. When is it used?**
Pegvisomant, the newest therapeutic option for acromegaly, blocks GH action at peripheral receptors, improving IGF-1 levels, reducing clinical effects, and correcting metabolic defects. It does not appear to affect tumor size in the great majority of patients, but tumor size should be monitored, given the drug's mechanism of action. It is currently used for patients who are resistant to or do not tolerate octreotide.

25. **What are the side effects of octreotide and pegvisomant?**
Gastrointestinal side effects are common with octreotide, including abdominal bloating, mild diarrhea, nausea, and flatulence. The incidence of gallstones may be increased with octreotide, and therefore patients should be monitored with serial ultrasonography of the gallbladder. Pegvisomant appears to have few adverse effects, aside from rare elevations in liver function tests.

26. **How can one tell whether a patient has been cured of acromegaly?**
The criteria for cure of acromegaly are somewhat controversial. Older studies defined cure as a random GH level below 5 ng/mL. More recent studies have shown that this criterion is inadequate because patients with low levels of GH may still have acromegaly. Therefore more rigorous criteria have been developed depending on specific GH assays. For complete control of growth hormone secretion, it has recently been recommended that patients should have a normal IGF-1 level and GH levels less than 0.4 ng/mL following oral glucose.

27. **The patient has undergone transsphenoidal surgery for acromegaly and now has normal postoperative fasting levels of GH, suppressed levels of GH following oral glucose, and a normal level of IGF-1. How should the patient be followed?**
It appears that the patient is cured, but GH tumors can slowly regrow over years. At the least, measurements of GH, IGF-1, or both should be repeated every 6 to 12 months. Some physicians

also repeat a pituitary MRI at yearly intervals. The patient also requires monitoring for colonic neoplasia at regular intervals. In addition, one must assess whether the surgery damaged normal pituitary function by determining the patient's thyroid, adrenal, gonadal, and posterior pituitary function. Finally, the effects of surgery on visual fields should be assessed, especially if the patient had preoperative defects.

28. **The patient asks which symptoms and physical abnormalities will improve after cure is confirmed. What is the appropriate answer?**
Most soft tissue changes improve, including coarsening of facial features, increased size of hands and feet, upper airway hypertrophy, carpal tunnel syndrome, osteoarthritis, and excessive sweating. Hypertension, cardiovascular disease, and diabetes also improve. Unfortunately, bony overgrowth of the facial bones does not regress after treatment.

29. **For bonus points, name an actor with acromegaly and the movie in which he starred.**
Andre the Giant starred in *The Princess Bride*.

BIBLIOGRAPHY

1. Ben-Shlomo A, Melmed S: Acromegaly. Endocrinol Metab Clin North Am 30:565–583, 2001.
2. Colao A, Ferone D, Marzullo P, Lombardi G. Systemic complications of acromegaly: epidemiology, pathogenesis, and management. Endocr Rev 25:102–152, 2004.
3. Consensus statement: biochemical assessment and long-term monitoring in patients with acromegaly. Statement from a join consenses conference of the Growth Hormone Research Society and the Pituitary Society. J Clin Endocrinol Metab 89:3099–3102, 2004.
4. Freda PU: Somatostatin analogs in acromegaly. J Clin Endocrinol Metab 87:3013–3018, 2002.
5. Melmed, S, Casanueva F, Cavagnini F, et al: Consensus statement: medical management of acromegaly. Eur J Endocrinol 153:737–740, 2005.
6. Muller AF, Kopchick JJ, Flyvbjerg A, van der Lely AJ: Growth hormone receptor antagonists. J Clin Endocrinol Metab 89:1503–1511, 2004.

CHAPTER 22

GLYCOPROTEIN-SECRETING PITUITARY TUMORS

Robert C. Smallridge

1. **What are glycoprotein hormones?**

   The glycoprotein hormones are luteinizing hormone (LH), thyrotropin (TSH), follicle-stimulating hormone (FSH), and chorionic gonadotropin (CG). Glycoprotein hormones are composed of two noncovalently bound subunits. The alpha subunit (α-SU) is similar among all four hormones. In contrast, the beta subunit (β-SU) is unique both immunologically and biologically for each hormone; these subunits are identified as LHβ, FSHβ, TSHβ, and βCG.

2. **Name two types of glycoprotein-secreting pituitary tumors.**

Type	Secretory Products
Gonadotropinomas	LH, FSH, LHβ, FSHβ, α-SU
Thyrotropinomas (TSHomas)	TSH, α-SU

3. **Do pituitary tumors secrete only a single hormone?**

   No. Many tumors make two or more hormones or subunits. In some circumstances, sufficient quantities of multiple hormones are secreted to produce clinical symptoms characteristic of several syndromes within the same patient.

4. **Under what circumstances should a TSH-secreting tumor be considered?**
   - Suspected hyperthyroidism
   - Increased serum free thyroxine (T_4) or FT_4 index
   - Detectable serum TSH

5. **Describe the differential diagnosis for patients with a transient increase in serum total T_4 and a detectable or elevated level of serum TSH.**

   Exogenous
   - L-Thyroxine (L-T_4) therapy (noncompliant patient who took L-T_4 the day blood was drawn)
   - Other drugs (amiodarone, ipodate, amphetamines)

   Endogenous (subgroup of nonthyroidal illness)
   - Acute psychiatric illness
   - Acute liver disease

6. **Describe the differential diagnosis for patients with a permanent increase in serum total T_4 and detectable or elevated level of serum TSH.**

   Binding protein disorders
   - Excessive thyroxine-binding globulin (TBG)
   - Abnormal thyroxine-binding prealbumin (TBPA) (transthyretin)
   - Familial dysalbuminemic hyperthyroxinemia (FDH)
   - T_4 autoantibody
   - TSH heterophile antibody (requires separate cause for T_4 elevation)

Inappropriate TSH secretion
- Resistance to thyroid hormone (generalized, central)
- Pituitary tumor

7. **What tests are useful in the differential diagnosis of the patient with an elevated serum total T_4 and a detectable or elevated serum TSH?**
The history and physical examination usually rule out medications and nonthyroidal illnesses. The most important laboratory test is the free T_4. A normal free T_4 strongly suggests one of the binding protein disorders. An elevated free T_4, in contrast, generally narrows the differential to two disorders: a thyroid hormone resistance syndrome or a TSH-secreting pituitary tumor. Clinical thyrotoxicosis is commonly present in patients with either condition. One should confirm the abnormal test results in a second laboratory before initiating a workup for these uncommon disorders.

8. **How can one distinguish between the hyperthyroid patient with thyroid hormone resistance and the patient with a pituitary tumor?**
TSH tumors may secrete α-SU in excess of the whole TSH molecule. The molar ratio of serum α-SU to TSH is increased in many patients with TSH tumors but normal in thyroid hormone resistance. A thyrotropin-releasing hormone (TRH; protirelin) test is also helpful. Fewer than 20% of patients with a tumor have a twofold increase in serum TSH after TRH, whereas those with resistance respond briskly. If tumor is suspected after both tests, a magnetic resonance imaging (MRI) scan of the pituitary should be obtained. Most TSH tumors (approximately 90%) are macroadenomas (i.e., $\geq$10 mm). Most microadenomas (<10 mm) are also visualized, but rarely sampling of inferior petrosal sinus blood has helped localize the tumor. Dynamic MRI scan or somatostatin receptor scintigraphy (OctreoScan) is also useful. Chronic (2-month) administration of a long-acting somatostatin analog decreases serum free T_4/T_3 and TSH in patients with TSH tumors.

9. **Describe how to calculate an α/TSH molar ratio.**
TSH values are expressed as μU/mL (or mU/L). One must know the bioactivity and convert these units to ng/mL, the units of α-SU. Furthermore, the molecular weight of the subunit is only half the molecular weight of the whole TSH molecule; this fact also must be considered in calculating the molar ratio. From a practical standpoint, the following formula can be used:

$$\text{molar ratio} = [\alpha\text{-SU(ng/mL)}/\text{TSH}(\mu\text{U/mL})] \times 10$$

10. **Name the treatment of choice for TSH-secreting tumors and its likelihood of success.**
Pituitary surgery is the treatment of choice, but it is curative in only one third of patients. Results are somewhat better if surgery is followed by radiation therapy. Because more microadenomas are being identified, results are improving.

11. **How effective is radiation as the sole therapy?**
Because so few cases have been reported, results are uncertain.

12. **List the medical therapies used for TSH-secreting tumors.**
Octreotide (somatostatin analog) decreases TSH in more than 90% of cases and normalizes free T_4 in 75% of cases. Tumor size decreases, and vision improves. Long-acting (monthly) analogs are effective.
Bromocriptine has limited success.
Dexamethasone reduces TSH, but its side effects exclude long-term use.
Iopanoic acid is effective preoperatively.

13. **Summarize the role of thyroid gland ablation in the treatment of TSH-secreting tumors.**

Thyroidectomy and [131]iodine have been contraindicated. Thyroid ablation does not control TSH secretion and may enhance pituitary activity and growth, although recently two patients were followed 8 and 12 years without tumor growth.

14. **Do all patients with an enlarged pituitary gland and an elevated level of serum TSH have thyrotropinomas?**

No. Patients with long-standing hypothyroidism may develop pituitary hyperplasia, producing a pseudotumor (Fig. 22-1). The pituitary mass can extend into the suprasellar region and cause visual field defects. Serum T_4 is always low, and shrinkage of the enlarged gland usually occurs with L-T_4 replacement therapy. Hyperplasia of lactotrophs, in addition to thyrotrophs, may result in elevated prolactin levels. No patient should undergo pituitary gland surgery without a preoperative measurement of serum T_4 and TSH.

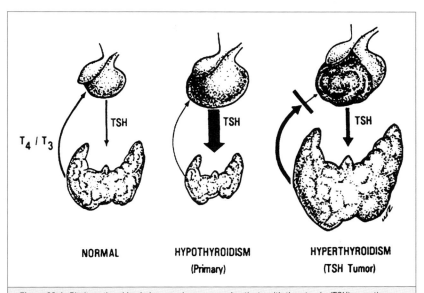

NORMAL

HYPOTHYROIDISM
(Primary)

HYPERTHYROIDISM
(TSH Tumor)

Figure 22-1. Pituitary-thyroid axis in normal persons and patients with thyrotropin (TSH)-secreting pituitary tumors. On the left is the appropriate feedback loop in euthyroid persons, with the width of the arrows representing the normal serum concentration of TSH and thyroxine (T_4). The middle figure depicts a small thyroid gland due to primary hypothyroidism. The low T_4 levels result in markedly increased secretion of TSH and, in some patients, a generalized hyperplasia of the anterior pituitary gland. On the right is an autonomous pituitary tumor secreting TSH. Serum TSH levels may vary greatly but in all cases are sufficiently biologically active to increase levels of T_4 above normal. The elevated T_4 level has little, if any, ability to suppress tumor function.

15. **What clinical features raise suspicion of a TSH-secreting pseudotumor?**

Almost all patients have symptoms of hypothyroidism, and the serum T_4 concentration is always low. The underlying abnormality is usually autoimmune thyroiditis, predominantly a disease of women. Approximately 80% of reported cases of pituitary enlargement with hypothyroidism were in women, whereas only 55% of true TSH tumors have occurred in women. In children, precocious puberty may occur. Thyroid antibodies are present in more than 75% of cases with pseudotumor, compared with about 10% of patients with TSH tumors that produce hyperthyroidism.

16. **Does the presence of abnormal visual fields help to distinguish between patients with pituitary hyperplasia due to primary hypothyroidism and patients with TSH-secreting tumors?**

No. Abnormal visual fields have been reported in 28% of patients with pituitary hyperplasia compared with 42% of patients with tumors. In contrast, patients with thyroid hormone resistance have normal vision.

17. **Does family history provide any clues in distinguishing these disorders?**

In pseudotumor from thyrotroph hyperplasia, the family history may be positive for the presence of autoimmune diseases (e.g., thyroiditis, Graves' disease, type 1 diabetes mellitus, rheumatoid arthritis, lupus erythematosus, Sjögren's syndrome, vitiligo, Addison's disease, pernicious anemia). In TSH tumors, family history is of no use. Most cases of generalized thyroid hormone resistance are familial with autosomal dominant inheritance (i.e., 50% of the family have the biochemical abnormalities).

18. **Which hormones are elevated in the serum of patients with gonadotroph adenomas?**

Serum FSH is increased much more often than LH. An increase in α-SU is not specific for gonadotrophs because it may also derive from thyrotrophs. Furthermore, an α/LH (or FSH) molar ratio has not been clinically useful.

KEY POINTS: GLYCOPROTEIN-SECRETING PITUITARY TUMORS

1. Glycoprotein-secreting pituitary tumors include gonadotropinomas (luteinizing hormone or follicle-stimulating hormone secreting) and thyrotropin (TSH)-omas.
2. Hyperthyroid patients with detectable serum TSH should always be evaluated for inappropriate TSH secretion (either a TSH tumor or thyroid hormone resistance).
3. TSH tumors are best managed by transsphenoidal surgery and possibly long-term use of octreotide analog.
4. Gonadotropinomas often present with neurologic symptoms due to mass effect and require pituitary surgery.
5. Hypothyroidism can produce thyrotroph hyperplasia and pituitary pseudotumors.

19. **List the presenting symptoms of patients with gonadotropinomas.**

Mass effect (common)
- Large tumors with extrasellar growth
- Visual impairment/diplopia
- Headaches
- Apoplexy
- Hypopituitarism

Endocrine excesses (uncommon)
- Ovarian hyperstimulation
- Testicular enlargement
- Precocious puberty

20. **When gonadotropin levels are elevated, how can one distinguish clinically between a gonadotroph adenoma and primary hypogonadism?**
This distinction can be difficult, especially in women, because their levels of LH and FSH increase after menopause. This is probably why most gonadotroph adenomas have been recognized in men. Historically, men with such tumors experienced a normal puberty and may have fathered children.
On examination, testicular size may be normal. In contrast, men with hypogonadism may have had abnormal pubertal development or a history of testicular injury; the testes are small.

21. **What laboratory tests are helpful?**
In primary hypogonadism, both FSH and LH are increased, whereas FSH is elevated, but LH is usually normal in patients with gonadotropinomas. When LH is high in men with gonadotropinomas, testosterone also is high rather than low, as in hypogonadism. For unexplained reasons, approximately one third of patients with a tumor have an anomalous rise in serum FSH or LHβ when given a TRH injection. An MRI scan of the pituitary reveals a large tumor. Occasionally, a patient with long-standing hypogonadism may have some degree of pituitary enlargement.

22. **How are gonadotropinomas treated?**
Pituitary surgery is the treatment of choice. Although complete cure is often impossible, substantial reduction in tumor size and hormone secretion is common. Reduced hormone secretion provides a convenient marker for monitoring recurrence of tumor; an abrupt increase in FSH or α-SU should prompt a repeat imaging study. Radiation therapy is often given after surgery in the hope of delaying tumor recurrence.

23. **Is medical therapy effective?**
Agonist analogs of gonadotropin-releasing hormone (GnRH) reduce secretion from normal gonadotrophs. Unfortunately, they usually have the opposite effect on gonadotropinomas. An antagonist analog (Nal-Glu-GnRH) has effectively reduced serum FSH in a small group of men with gonadotropinomas but did not reduce tumor size. Bromocriptine has reduced hormone levels in an occasional patient, whereas octreotide has reduced α-SU and improved visual fields in certain patients. Cabergoline can reduce estradiol levels and ovarian size in women with ovarian hyperstimulation.

24. **Are pituitary tumors malignant?**
Carcinomas are rare but occasionally have been reported for
   ■ ACTH
   ■ PRL
   ■ GH
   ■ TSH ($n = 2$)

25. **What causes pituitary tumors?**
   ■ Oncogene overexpression (e.g., pituitary tumor transforming gene, others)
   ■ Silencing of tumor suppressor genes (e.g., hypermethylation)
   ■ Corticotropin-releasing factor (CRF$_2$) expression

WEBSITE

Thyroid disease manager. Available at: http://www.thyroidmanager.org

BIBLIOGRAPHY

1. Al-Gahtany M, Horvath E, Kovacs K: Pituitary hyperplasia. Hormones 2:149–158, 2003.

2. Beck-Peccoz P, Brucker-Davis F, Persani L, et al: Thyrotropin-secreting pituitary tumors. Endocr Rev 17:610–638, 1996.

3. Brown RL, Muzzafar T, Wollman R, Weiss RE: A pituitary carcinoma secreting TSH and prolactin: a nonsecreting adenoma gone awry. Eur J Endocrinol 154:639–643, 2006.

4. Buchfelder M: Thyrotroph pituitary adenomas. Endocrinologist 12:117–125, 2002.

5. Burch HB: Abnormal thyroid function test results in euthyroid persons. In Becker KL, editor, *Principles and practice of endocrinology and metabolism*, ed 3, Philadelphia, 2001, Lippincott Williams & Wilkins, pp. 351–360.

6. Caron P, Arlot S, Bauters C, et al: Efficacy of the long-acting octreotide formulation (octreotide-LAR) in patients with thyrotropin-secreting pituitary adenomas. J Clin Endocrinol Metab 86:2849–2853, 2001.

7. Chaidarun SS, Klibanski A: Gonadotropinomas. Semin Reprod Med 20:339–348, 2002.

8. Daousi C, Foy PM, MacFarlane IA: Ablative thyroid treatment for thyrotoxicosis due to thyrotropin-producing pituitary tumours. J Neurol Neurosurg Psychiatry 78:93–95, 2007.

9. Dhillon KS, Cohan P, Kelly DF, et al: Treatment of hyperthyroidism associated with thyrotropin-secreting pituitary adenomas with iopanoic acid. J Clin Endocrinol Metab 89:708–711, 2004.

10. Knoepfelmacher M, Danilovic DLS, Rosa Nasser RHR, Mendonca BB: Effectiveness of treating ovarian hyperstimulation syndrome with cabergoline in two patients with gonadotropin-producing pituitary adenomas. Fertil Steril 86:719 e715–718, 2006.

11. Lamberts SW, Krenning EP, Reubi JC: The role of somatostatin and its analogs in the diagnosis and treatment of tumors. Endocr Rev 12:450–482, 1991.

12. Mannavola D, Persani L, Vannucchi G, et al: Different responses to chronic somatostatin analogues in patients with central hyperthyroidism. Clin Endocrinol 62:176–181, 2005.

13. McGrath GA, Goncalves RJ, Udupa JK, et al: New technique for quantitation of pituitary adenoma size: use in evaluating treatment of gonadotroph adenomas with a gonadotropin-releasing hormone antagonist. J Clin Endocrinol Metab 76:1363–1368, 1993.

14. Refetoff S, Weiss RE, Usala SJ: The syndromes of resistance to thyroid hormone. Endocr Rev 14:348–399, 1993.

15. Reubi JC, Waser B, Vale W, et al: Expression of CRF1 and CRF2 receptors in human cancers. J Clin Endocrinol Metab 88:3312–3320, 2003.

16. Shorts-Cary L, Xu M, Ertel J, Kleinschmidt-Demasters BK, et al: Bone morphogenetic protein and retinoic acid-inducible neural specific protein-3 is expressed in gonadotrope cell pituitary adenomas and induces proliferation, migration, and invasion. Endocrinology 148:967–975, 2007.

17. Simard MF: Pituitary tumor endocrinopathies and their endocrine evaluation. Neurosurg Clin N Am 14:41–54, 2003.

18. Smallridge RC: Thyroid function tests. In Becker KL, editor, *Principles and Practice of Endocrinology and Metabolism*, ed 3, Philadelphia, 2001, Lippincott Williams & Wilkins, pp 329–336.

19. Smallridge RC: Thyrotropin- and gonadotropin-producing tumors. In Korenman SG, Molitch ME, editors, *Atlas of Clinical Endocrinology. Neuroendocrinology and Pituitary Disease*, Philadelphia, 2000, Blackwell Science, pp. 95–113.

20. Smallridge RC: Thyrotropin-secreting pituitary tumors: clinical presentation, investigation, and management. Curr Opin Endocrinol Diabetes 8:253–258, 2001.

21. Smallridge RC, Czervionke LF, Fellows DW, et al: Corticotropin- and thyrotropin-secreting pituitary microadenomas: detection by dynamic magnetic resonance imaging. Mayo Clin Proc 75:521–528, 2000.

22. Snyder PJ: Extensive personal experience: gonadotroph adenomas. J Clin Endocrinol Metab 80:1059–1061, 1995.

23. Socin HV, Chanson P, Delemer B, et al: The changing spectrum of TSH-secreting pituitary adenomas: diagnosis and management in 43 patients. Eur J Endocrinol 148:433–442, 2003.

24. Young WF Jr, Scheithauer BW, Kovacs KT, et al: Gonadotroph adenoma of the pituitary gland: a clinicopathologic analysis of 100 cases. Mayo Clin Proc 71:649–656, 1996.

CHAPTER 23

CUSHING'S SYNDROME

Mary H. Samuels

1. **Describe the normal function of cortisol in healthy people.**
   Cortisol and other glucocorticoids have many effects as physiologic regulators. They increase glucose production, inhibit protein synthesis and increase protein breakdown, stimulate lipolysis, and affect immunologic and inflammatory responses. Glucocorticoids are important for maintenance of blood pressure and form an essential part of the body's response to stress.

2. **How are cortisol levels normally regulated?**
   Adrenal production of cortisol is stimulated by the pituitary hormone adrenocorticotropin (ACTH). ACTH production is stimulated by the hypothalamic hormones corticotropin-releasing hormone (CRH) and vasopressin (ADH). Cortisol feeds back to the pituitary and hypothalamus to suppress levels of ACTH and CRH. Under nonstress conditions, cortisol is secreted with a pronounced circadian rhythm, with higher levels early in the morning and lower levels late in the evening. Under stressful conditions, secretion of CRH, ACTH, and cortisol increases, and the circadian variation is blunted. Because of the wide variation in cortisol levels over 24 hours and appropriate elevations during stressful conditions, it may be difficult to distinguish normal secretion from abnormal secretion. For this reason, the evaluation of a patient with suspected Cushing's disease is often complex and confusing.

3. **What are the clinical symptoms of excessive levels of cortisol?**
   1. Obesity, especially central (truncal) obesity, with wasting of the extremities, moon facies, supraclavicular fat pads, and buffalo hump
   2. Thinning of the skin, with facial plethora, easy bruising, and violaceous striae
   3. Muscular weakness, especially proximal muscle weakness, and atrophy
   4. Hypertension, atherosclerosis, congestive heart failure, and edema
   5. Gonadal dysfunction and menstrual irregularities
   6. Psychologic disturbances (e.g., depression, emotional lability, irritability, sleep disturbances)
   7. Osteoporosis and fractures
   8. Increased rate of infections and poor wound healing

4. **All of my clinic patients look like they have cushing's syndrome. Are some clinical findings more specific for cushing's syndrome than others?**
   Some manifestations of Cushing's syndrome are common but nonspecific, whereas others are less common but quite specific. The clinical findings are listed in Table 23-1, with the more specific findings listed first. The sensitivity and specificity for the diagnosis are listed separately.

5. **A patient presents with a history of obesity, hypertension, irregular menses, and depression. Does she have excessive production of cortisol?**
   Excessive cortisol is highly unlikely. Although the listed findings are consistent with glucocorticoid excess, they are nonspecific; most patients with such findings do not have Cushing's syndrome (see Table 23-1).

TABLE 23-1. SYMPTOMS AND SIGNS OF CUSHING'S SYNDROME

Sign/Symptom	Sensitivity (%)	Specificity (%)
Hypokalemia (K' <3.6)	25	96
Ecchymoses	53	94
Osteoporosis	26	94
Weakness	65	93
Diastolic blood pressure (>105 mm Hg)	39	83
Red or violaceous striae	46	78
Acne	52	76
Central obesity	90	71
Hirsutism	50	71
Plethora	82	69
Oligomenorrhea	72	49
Generalized obesity	3	38
Abnormal glucose tolerance	88	23

6. **The patient also complains of excessive hair growth and has increased terminal hair on the chin, along the upper lip, and on the upper back. Is this finding relevant?**
   Hirsutism is a common, nonspecific finding in many female patients. However, it is also consistent with Cushing's syndrome. If it is due to Cushing's syndrome, hirsutism is a complication not of excessive glucocorticoids but of excessive production of androgen by the adrenal glands under ACTH stimulation. Thus hirsutism in a patient with Cushing's syndrome is a clue that the disorder is due to excessive production of ACTH. (The only other condition associated with excessive production of glucocorticoids and androgen is a malignant adrenal tumor, which is usually obvious on presentation.)

7. **The patient also has increased pigmentation of the areolae, palmar creases, and an old surgical scar. Are these findings relevant?**
   Hyperpigmentation is a sign of elevated production of ACTH and related peptides by the pituitary gland. It is uncommon (but possible) in Cushing's syndrome due to benign pituitary tumors because levels of ACTH do not usually rise high enough to cause hyperpigmentation. It is more common in the ectopic ACTH syndrome because ectopic tumors produce more ACTH and other peptides. The combination of Cushing's syndrome and hyperpigmentation may be bad news.

8. **What is the cause of death in patients with Cushing's syndrome?**
   Patients with Cushing's syndrome have a markedly increased mortality rate, usually from cardiovascular disease or infections.

9. **What causes Cushing's syndrome?**
   Cushing's syndrome is a nonspecific name for any source of excessive glucocorticoids. There are four main causes, which are further detailed in Table 23-2:
   1. Exogenous glucocorticoids (ACTH-independent)
   2. Pituitary Cushing's syndrome (ACTH-dependent)
   3. Ectopic production of ACTH (ACTH-dependent)
   4. Adrenal tumors (ACTH-independent)

TABLE 23-2. CAUSES OF CUSHING'S SYNDROME AND THEIR RELATIVE FREQUENCY	
ACTH-Dependent (80%)	ACTH-Independent (20%)
Pituitary (85%)	Adrenal tumors
Corticotroph adenoma	Adrenal adenoma (>50%)
Corticotroph hyperplasia (rare)	Adrenal carcinoma (<50%)
Ectopic ACTH syndrome (15%)	Micronodular hyperplasia (rare)
Oat-cell carcinoma (50%)	Macronodular hyperplasia (rare)
Foregut tumors (35%)	Exogenous glucocorticoids (common)
Bronchial carcinoid	Therapeutic (common)
Thymic carcinoid	Factitious (rare)
Medullary thyroid carcinoma	
Islet-cell tumors	
Pheochromocytoma	
Other tumors (10%)	
Ectopic CRH (<1%)	

ACTH, adrenocorticotropin; CRH, corticotropin-releasing hormone.

10. **Of the various types of Cushing's syndrome, which is the most common?**
Overall, exogenous Cushing's syndrome is most common. It rarely presents a diagnostic dilemma, because the physician usually knows that the patient is receiving glucocorticoids. Of the endogenous causes of Cushing's syndrome, pituitary Cushing's disease accounts for at least 70% of cases. Ectopic secretion of ACTH and adrenal tumors cause approximately 15% of cases each (see Table 23-1 for frequencies).

11. **Do age and gender matter in the differential diagnosis of Cushing's syndrome?**
Of patients with Cushing's disease (pituitary tumors), 80% are women, whereas the ectopic ACTH syndrome is more common in men. Therefore, in a male patient with Cushing's syndrome, the risk of an extrapituitary tumor is increased. The age range in Cushing's disease is most frequently 20 to 40 years, whereas ectopic ACTH syndrome has a peak incidence at 40 to 60 years. Therefore, the risk of an extrapituitary tumor in an older patient with Cushing's syndrome is increased. Children with Cushing's syndrome have a higher risk of malignant adrenal tumors.

12. **The patient with obesity, hypertension, irregular menses, depression, and hirsutism looks like she may have Cushing's syndrome. What should I do?**
A widely used screening test for Cushing's syndrome is the overnight low-dose dexamethasone suppression test. The patient takes 1 mg of dexamethasone at 11 p.m. and measures her serum cortisol level at 8 a.m. the next morning. In healthy unstressed subjects, dexamethasone (a potent glucocorticoid that does not react with the cortisol assay) suppresses production of CRH, ACTH, and cortisol. Patients with Cushing's syndrome of any cause should not suppress cortisol production (serum cortisol remains >5 mg/dL) when given 1 mg of dexamethasone.
More recently, measurement of cortisol in a nightime saliva sample has been developed as an alternative screening test for Cushing's syndrome. This test appears to be comparable or superior to the standard overnight dexamethasone and 24-hour urine cortisol tests and is much easier to perform.

13. **The patient had a cortisol level drawn after a 1-mg dose of dexamethasone. The level is 12 mg/dL. Does she have Cushing's syndrome?**
    Unfortunately the overnight dexamethasone suppression test is not foolproof. Occasional patients with Cushing's disease suppress cortisol levels with dexamethasone, and many patients without Cushing's syndrome do not. Acute or chronic illnesses, depression, and alcohol abuse all activate the hypothalamic-pituitary-adrenal axis because of stress and make the patient resistant to dexamethasone suppression. In fact, because Cushing's syndrome is so rare, a nonsuppressed cortisol level after dexamethasone is more likely to be a false-positive result, rather than truly indicating the presence of Cushing's syndrome. A more accurate screening test is a 24-hour urine sample for free cortisol levels, which should be ordered in this case.

14. **The patient has an elevated 24-hour urinary level of free cortisol, and serum cortisol levels are not suppressed after overnight 1-mg dexamethasone administration. What should I do?**
    It looks like the patient has Cushing's syndrome. However, it is still possible that the patient has other reasons for her symptoms and elevated cortisol levels. It can be difficult to distinguish mild or moderate Cushing's syndrome from stress-induced hypercortisolism, especially in patients who have active medical or psychiatric illnesses. The distinction between true Cushing's syndrome and pseudo-Cushing's syndrome (stress-induced hypercortisolemia) depends on the clinical suspicion and degree of elevation of the cortisol levels. In general, a 24-hour urine free cortisol level of greater than 3 times normal levels is diagnostic of true Cushing's syndrome in the absence of severe stress. Lesser elevations of urine free cortisol may require confirmatory tests for the presence of Cushing's syndrome.

15. **I am not convinced that the patient has Cushing's syndrome. How can I confirm it?**
    The best confirmatory test is controversial, but two commonly used tests are loss of diurnal variation in plasma cortisol levels and the dexamethasone-CRH test (Fig. 23-1). These tests are best administered and interpreted by experienced endocrinologists because the results can be skewed if the tests are not performed properly.

16. **The patient has elevated cortisol levels at night and an abnormal dexamethasone-CRH test. Now I am convinced that she has Cushing's syndrome. What should I do next?**
    After you have made the biochemical diagnosis of Cushing's syndrome, the next step is to determine whether she has ACTH-dependent or ACTH-independent disease (Fig. 23-2). This distinction is made by measuring plasma levels of ACTH. Measurements should be repeated a number of times because secretion of ACTH is variable.

17. **The patient's ACTH level is "normal." Was the original suspicion of Cushing's syndrome incorrect?**
    No. Normal levels of ACTH are a common finding in pituitary-dependent Cushing's disease. A normal or slightly elevated ACTH level is the usual finding in ACTH-secreting pituitary adenomas. More marked elevations of ACTH levels suggest ectopic secretion of ACTH, although small carcinoid tumors also have normal or mildly elevated levels of ACTH. Suppressed ACTH levels, in contrast, suggest an adrenal tumor.

18. **What happened to the 2-day low-dose and high-dose dexamethasone tests for the differential diagnosis of Cushing's syndrome?**
    The 2-day low-dose and high-dose dexamethasone suppression tests were once widely used in attempts to distinguish pituitary, ectopic, and adrenal causes of Cushing's syndrome. Although they are still performed, the results are often confusing, and rates of both false-positive and false-negative results are high. Therefore these tests have been abandoned by many endocrinologists and supplanted by more accurate ACTH assays, the overnight high-dose dexamethasone test, CRH stimulation tests, and inferior petrosal sinus sampling (IPSS).

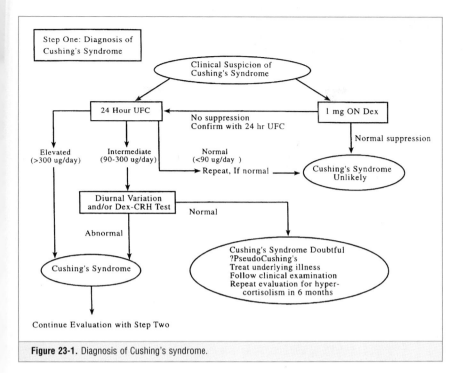

Step One: Diagnosis of
Cushing's Syndrome

Clinical Suspicion of
Cushing's Syndrome

24 Hour UFC ← No suppression
Confirm with 24 hr UFC
1 mg ON Dex

Normal suppression

Elevated
(>300 ug/day)

Intermediate
(90-300 ug/day)

Normal
(<90 ug/day)
Repeat, If normal →

Cushing's Syndrome
Unlikely

Diurnal Variation
and/or Dex-CRH Test

Normal

Abnormal

Cushing's Syndrome

Cushing's Syndrome Doubtful
?PseudoCushing's
Treat underlying illness
Follow clinical examination
Repeat evaluation for hyper-
cortisolism in 6 months

Continue Evaluation with Step Two

Figure 23-1. Diagnosis of Cushing's syndrome.

19. **After diagnosis of ACTH-dependent cushing's syndrome, what is the next step?**
Because the most common site of excessive secretion of ACTH is a pituitary tumor, radiologic imaging of the pituitary gland is the next step. The best study is high-resolution magnetic resonance imaging (MRI) with thin cuts through the pituitary gland. A chest radiograph should also be obtained at this point in case the patient has a carcinoid tumor large enough to be seen on plain film.

20. **The pituitary MRI in the patient with ACTH-dependent cushing's syndrome is normal. Is the next step a search for carcinoid tumor, under the assumption that the pituitary is not the source of excessive ACTH?**
Not so fast. At least half of pituitary MRI or computed tomography (CT) scans are negative in proven pituitary-dependent Cushing's syndrome because most corticotroph adenomas are tiny and may not be visible on MRI or CT.

21. **The pituitary MRI shows a 3-mm hypodense area in the lateral aspect of the pituitary gland. Is it time to call the neurosurgeon?**
Again, not so fast. This finding is nonspecific and occurs in many healthy people. It may or may not be related to Cushing's syndrome. The odds are good that the patient has a pituitary tumor, but the MRI does not prove this. The MRI is diagnostic in Cushing's syndrome only if it shows a large tumor.

22. **So what is the next step?**
One option is to proceed directly to pituitary surgery because a patient with an abnormal MRI has a 90% chance of having an ACTH-secreting pituitary tumor. To achieve more diagnostic certainty, one has to perform bilateral simultaneous IPSS for ACTH levels (Fig. 23-3). Catheters

Figure 23-2. Distinguishing adrenocorticotropin (ACTH)-dependent from ACTH-independent disease.

are advanced through the femoral veins into the inferior petrosal sinuses, which drain the pituitary gland. Blood samples are obtained through the catheters for ACTH levels. If ACTH levels in the petrosal sinuses are significantly higher than those in peripheral samples, the pituitary gland is the source of excessive ACTH. If there is no gradient between petrosal sinus and peripheral levels of ACTH, the patient probably has a carcinoid tumor somewhere. The accuracy of the test is further increased if ACTH responses to injection of exogenous CRH are measured. Bilateral IPSS should be performed by experienced radiologists at referral centers.

23. **IPSS shows no gradient in ACTH levels. Now what?**
    Start the search for a carcinoid tumor. Because the most likely location is the lung, a CT scan of the lungs should be ordered. If the results are negative, a CT scan of the abdomen should be ordered because carcinoids also occur in the pancreas, intestinal tract, and adrenal glands.

24. **IPSS shows a marked central-to-peripheral gradient in ACTH levels. Now what?**
    Transsphenoidal surgery (TSS) should be scheduled with an experienced neurosurgeon who is comfortable examining the pituitary for small adenomas. ACTH levels from the right and left petrosal sinuses obtained during the sampling study may tell the neurosurgeon in which side of the pituitary gland the tumor is likely to be found, but this information is not 100% accurate.

25. **What if surgery is unsuccessful?**
    If TSS does not cure a patient with Cushing's disease, alternative therapies must be tried because patients with inadequately treated hypercortisolism have increased morbidity and mortality rates. Of the various options after failed surgery, none is ideal. Patients may require

Figure 23-3. Distinguishing primary Cushing's syndrome from ectopic adrenocorticotropin syndrome. TSS, transsphenoidal surgery.

repeat pituitary surgery, radiation therapy, medical therapy to block cortisol secretion, bilateral adrenalectomy, or a combination of these. These decisions should be made in consultation with an experienced endocrinologist.

26. **Why not just take out the patient's adrenal glands?**
    One drawback is the extensive nature of the surgery. This problem has been addressed recently by performing adrenalectomy using a laparoscopic approach, which is easier on the patient. Another drawback is lifelong adrenal insufficiency and dependence on exogenous glucocorticoids and mineralocorticoids. However, the main drawback is the development of Nelson's syndrome in up to 30% of patients after adrenalectomy. Nelson's syndrome is the appearance, sometimes years after adrenalectomy, of an aggressive corticotroph pituitary tumor.

27. **What are the correct diagnostic and treatment options for patients with ACTH-independent (adrenal) Cushing's syndrome?**
    Such patients usually have either an adrenal adenoma or an adrenal carcinoma. After consistent suppression of ACTH levels is confirmed, an adrenal CT scan should be ordered. A mass is almost always present, and surgery should be planned. If the mass is obviously cancer, surgery may still help in debulking the tumor and improving the metabolic consequences of hypercortisolemia. If there are multiple adrenal nodules, the patient may have a rare form of Cushing's syndrome and should be evaluated by an experienced endocrinologist.

28. **What happens to the hypothalamic-pituitary-adrenal axis after a patient undergoes successful removal of an ACTH-secreting pituitary adenoma or a cortisol-secreting adrenal adenoma?**
The axis is suppressed, and the patient develops clinical adrenal insufficiency, unless he or she is given gradually decreasing doses of exogenous glucocorticoids for a time after surgery.

29. **What would be the most likely diagnosis if the original patient had all the signs of Cushing's syndrome but *low* urinary and serum levels of cortisol?**
The most likely scenario is that the patient is surreptitiously or accidentally ingesting a glucocorticoid that gives all the findings of glucocorticoid excess but is not measured in the cortisol assay. The patient and family members should be questioned about possible access to medications, and special assays can measure the various synthetic glucocorticoids.

30. **Do tumors ever cause Cushing's syndrome by making excessive CRH?**
Yes. Occasionally patients who undergo TSS for a presumed corticotroph adenoma have corticotroph hyperplasia instead. At least some of these cases are secondary to ectopic production of CRH from a carcinoid tumor in the lung, abdomen, or other location. Therefore levels of serum CRH should be measured in patients with Cushing's syndrome and corticotroph hyperplasia. If the levels are elevated, a careful search should be performed for possible ectopic sources of CRH.

KEY POINTS: CUSHING'S SYNDROME

1. The clinical manifestations of Cushing's syndrome can be subtle or nonspecific.

2. Most patients who look like they might have Cushing's syndrome do not.

3. Screening biochemical tests for Cushing's syndrome can be misleading, and repeated testing or more extensive confirmatory testing is often necessary.

4. Most patients with Cushing's syndrome have a small pituitary tumor producing adrenocorticotropin.

5. Patients with pituitary tumors causing Cushing's syndrome should undergo pituitary surgery by an experienced neurosurgeon because none of the other treatment options are ideal.

BIBLIOGRAPHY

1. Arnaldi G, Angeli A, Atkinson AB, et al: Diagnosis and complications of Cushing' syndrome: a consensus statement. J Clin Endocrinol Metab 88:5593–5602, 2003.
2. Findling JW, Raff H: Diagnosis and differential diagnosis of Cushing's syndrome. Endocrinol Metab Clin N Am 30:729–747, 2001.
3. Morris D, Grossman A: The medical management of Cushing's syndrome. Ann N Y Acad Sci 970:119–133, 2002.
4. Nieman LK: Diagnostic tests for Cushing's syndrome. Ann N Y Acad Sci 970:112–118, 2002.
5. Raff H, Findling JW: A physiologic approach to diagnosis of the Cushing syndrome. Ann Intern Med 138:980–991, 2003.
6. Viardot A, Huber P, Puder JJ, et al: Reproducibility of nighttime salivary cortisol and its use in the diagnosis of hypercortisolism compared with urinary free cortisol and overnight dexamethasone suppression test. J Clin Endocrinol Metab 90:5730–5736, 2005.

CHAPTER 24

WATER METABOLISM

Leonard R. Sanders

1. **What is the water composition of the human body?**

   Water composition of the body depends on age, sex, muscle mass, body habitus, and fat content. Various body tissues have the following water percentages: lungs, heart, and kidneys (80%); skeletal muscle and brain (75%); skin and liver (70%); bone (20%); and adipose tissue (10%). Clearly, people with more muscle than fat will have more water. Generally, thin people have less fat and more water. Men are 60% and women 50% water by weight. Older people have more fat and less muscle. The average man and woman older than 60 years are made up of 50% and 45% water, respectively (see Table 24-1). Most discussions of total body water (TBW) consider a man who is 60% water, weighs 70 kg, and is 69 inches (175 cm) tall.

TABLE 24-1.	WATER AS A PERCENT OF BODY WEIGHT		
Body Habitus	**Infant**	**Man**	**Woman**
Thin	80	65	55
Medium	70	60	50
Obese	65	55	45

2. **Where is water located within the body?**

   TBW equals water located inside the cells (intracellular fluid [ICF]) and outside the cells (extracellular fluid [ECF]). TBW is 60% of body weight; ICF and ECF water are 40% and 20%, respectively, of body weight. ECF contains both interstitial (15%) and intravascular water (5%). Thus in a 70-kg man, TBW = 42 L, ICF water = 28 L, and ECF water = 14 L. The interstitial fluid (ISF) is 10.5 L, and intravascular (plasma) fluid (IVF) is 3.5 L. Therefore, of the TBW, two thirds is ICF and one third is ECF. Of the ECF, approximately one quarter is IVF and three quarters is ISF. Tight regulation of the relatively small volume of IVF (plasma) maintains blood pressure and avoids symptomatic hypovolemia and congestive heart failure. Normal plasma is 93% water and 7% proteins and lipids. Total blood volume (TBV) is only a small portion of the ECF, and arterial volume is only 15% of TBV. Although arterial volume is small, its integrity is most important for maintaining the effective circulation and preventing abnormalities of water balance (Fig. 24-1).

3. **What is transcellular water (TCW)? What is its importance?**

   TCW is water formed by cellular transport activities and located in various ducts and spaces throughout the body. This water includes cerebrospinal fluid (CSF) and aqueous humor; secretions in the sweat, salivary, and lacrimal glands; secretions in pancreas, liver, biliary, gastrointestinal, and respiratory tracts; and peritoneal, pleural, and synovial fluids.

4. **Explain the significance of TCW.**

   TCW carries secretions to specific sites for enzymatic and lubricant activity and is normally quite small, 1.5% of body weight. In disease states, excess or deficiency of TCW can cause

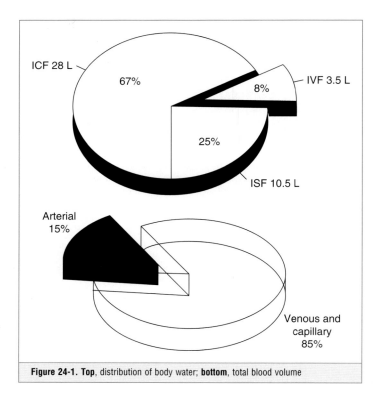

Figure 24-1. Top, distribution of body water; **bottom**, total blood volume

dysfunction. Marked excess TCW formation—third spacing—may decrease effective circulating volume (ECV), stimulate antidiuretic hormone (ADH) and aldosterone release, increase retention of salt and water, and cause hyponatremia.

5. **What controls distribution of body water?**
   With few exceptions (e.g., ascending loop of Henle [LOH] and distal nephron), water moves freely across cell membranes, depending on tonicity. Because tonicity depends on impermeable solutes, such as sodium (Na), disorders of water metabolism are reflected by changes in solute concentrations. In addition to changes in water distribution, changes in TBW, blood volume, and ECV also affect overall water balance. A thorough understanding of disorders of water metabolism requires a clear understanding of changes in plasma Na concentration (P_{Na}), plasma osmolality (P_{osm}), and ECV.

KEY POINTS: WATER METABOLISM

1. Rapid changes in body water or distribution can cause severe neurologic dysfunction and are reflected clinically by hyponatremia or hypernatremia.

2. Treatment requires a clear understanding of changes in plasma sodium, plasma osmolality, and effective circulating volume.

3. Water always moves across cell membranes from lower to higher osmolality.

4. This movement is determined by the concentration of effective osmotic solute in the intracellular or extracellular fluid and is responsible for neurologic symptoms and signs.

5. Water content of the body is a balance of input and output.

6. Balance is controlled by thirst, access to water, solute intake, antidiuretic hormone, cortisol, aldosterone, natriuretic peptides, renal receptors for hormone action, renal water channels called aquaporins, level of kidney function, and drugs.

6. **What is ECV?**
ECV is the arterial volume required to maintain normal baroreceptor pressure that is appropriate for a given level of vascular resistance. ECV is also called effective arterial blood volume (EABV). By inducing changes in baroreceptor tone, alterations in ECV have a major impact on water balance. Low ECV causes renal salt and water retention, whereas high ECV causes renal salt and water loss. Depending on the patient's water intake, these changes may produce significant hyponatremia. Maintaining normal ECV preserves circulatory homeostasis.

7. **How do baroreceptors affect ECV?**
Baroreceptors are the major sensors of changes in ECV (Fig. 24-2). However, their main role is to maintain normal pressure (not volume) at the level of the baroreceptor sensors located primarily in the carotid sinus, aortic arch, atria, pulmonary veins, and afferent renal arterioles. These anatomic locations are important because perfusion to these areas affects the three main effectors of circulatory homeostasis and ECV: brain, heart, and kidneys.

Figure 24-2. Components of effective circulation.

8. **How does vascular pressure as sensed by the baroreceptors relate to ECV and hyponatremia?**
Baroreceptors normally have tonic inhibition of vasoconstrictor nerves and natriuretic hormone release but tonic stimulation of vagal cardiac nerves. A drop in ECV decreases effective vascular pressure (EVP), baroreceptor tone, tonic inhibition, and tonic stimulation. This causes vasoconstriction; increases heart rate; and increases renin, aldosterone, angiotensin II, and ADH secretion. It decreases atrial natriuretic peptide (ANP), brain natriuretic peptide (BNP; atrial and ventricle), and urodilatin (kidney). These alterations enhance renal Na and water retention. If the patient receives free water, these changes may lead to hyponatremia. Hyponatremia cannot

develop unless the patient retains more water than is excreted. Decreased ECV/EVP predisposes to water retention, but the patient must receive free water to develop hyponatremia. The venous system, through atrial stretch receptors, has similar effects but responds to changes in ECV earlier than the arterial system.

9. **Define osmolality and tonicity and outline their effects on water movement.**
Osmolality is the concentration of the substance in 1 L of water divided by its molecular weight. Tonicity is effective osmolality—the osmotic pressure caused by dissolved particles restricted to one side of the cell membrane. Because Na and glucose are partially restricted to the ECF, they are effective osmols and account for normal tonicity. Mannitol, sorbitol, glycerol, and glycine are also effective osmols. Urea freely crosses cell membranes and distributes evenly in TBW, and therefore it changes osmolality but not tonicity. Thus except during early and rapid solute and water changes, urea is an ineffective osmol. Ethanol and methanol are other ineffective osmols. Water always moves across cell membranes from lower osmolality to higher osmolality until osmolality on both sides is equal. At equilibrium, the following is always true:

$$\text{ICF osmolality} = \text{ECF osmolality} = P_{osm}.$$

10. **What formulas are useful in evaluating osmolality and tonicity?**

$$\text{ECF osmolality} = 2P_{Na} + \text{glucose}/18 + \text{blood urea nitrogen (blood urea nitrogen[BUN])}/2.8$$
$$\text{normal osmolality} = 2(140) + 90/18 + 14/2.8 = 280 + 5 + 5 = 290 \text{ mOsm/kg}$$
$$\text{ECF tonicity (effective osmolality)} = 2P_{Na} + \text{glucose}/18$$
$$\text{normal tonicity} = 2(140) + 90/18 = 280 + 5 = 285 \text{ mOsm/kg}$$

The normal range for P_{osm} of 275 to 295 mOsm/kg varies with the normal ranges for plasma Na, urea, and glucose. Correction factors for other effective solutes (osmols) are mannitol/18, sorbitol/18, and glycerol/9. Correction factors for other ineffective solutes (osmols) are ethanol/4.6 and methanol/3.2.

11. **How does P_{Na} relate to TBW?**
The following formulas are useful in understanding the relationship of P_{Na}, plasma potassium (P_K), total body sodium and potassium $[Na^+ + K^+]$, and TBW. $[Na^+ + K^+]$ estimates total body solute:
1. $P_{Na} \cong \text{total body } [Na^+ + K^+]/\text{TBW}$
2. $\text{TBW} \cong [Na^+ + K^+]/P_{Na}$
3. $P_{Na} \cong P_{osm} \cong [\text{total body osmolality}] \cong [\text{total body solutes}] \cong 1/\text{TBW}$

Thus P_{Na} is proportional to $[Na^+ + K^+]$ and inversely proportional to TBW. An increase or decrease in total plasma Na particles can proportionately change the P_{Na}. However, in clinical medicine, changes in P_{Na} usually reflect changes in plasma water. When P_{Na} is high, plasma water is low. When P_{Na} is low, plasma water is high.

12. **How does P_K relate to P_{Na} and TBW?**
Although 98% of K^+ is intracellular, a K^+ infusion increases P_{Na}. This occurs as follows. In hypokalemia, infused K^+ enters cells. To preserve electroneutrality, Na^+ leaves cells or chloride (Cl^-) enters. ECF water follows K^+ and Cl^- into cells because of increased ICF osmolality. Both mechanisms increase P_{Na}. Hypokalemic patients infused with equal amounts of KCl or NaCl will have equal increases in P_{Na}. Thus addition of KCl to isotonic saline makes hypertonic saline, and infusion of saline with KCl may correct hyponatremia too rapidly (see questions 36 and 44).

13. **Describe the input and output of water.**
TBW is a balance of input (including endogenous production) and output. In an average adult, input approximates 1600 mL (liquids), 700 mL (foods), and 200 mL (metabolic oxidation of carbohydrate and fat) for a total of 2500 mL/day. Average water losses are 1500 mL (kidneys), 500 mL (skin [400 mL evaporation and 100 mL perspiration]), 300 mL (lung—respiration), and

200 mL from the gastrointestinal tract (stool) for a total of 2500 mL/day. Large losses of water (increased output) occur with excessive sweating, respiration (exercise), burns, diarrhea, vomiting, and diuresis. Decreased water input occurs when defects in thirst and altered mental or physical function (especially in the elderly) prevent access to water.

14. **What are the normal limits of urine output?**
Water intake and osmotic products of metabolism determine the usual daily output of urine. On a normal diet, a normal adult must excrete 800 to 1000 mOsm of solute per day. The range of normal renal concentrating function is 50 to 1200 mOsm/kg. On this basis, the obligate water excretion varies from 0.8 to 20 L/day. The calculations are as follows:

$$1000 \text{ mOsm}/1200 \text{ mOsm/kg} = 0.8 \text{ L/day at maximal concentration}$$
$$1000 \text{ mOsm}/50 \text{ mOsm/kg} = 20 \text{ L/day at maximal dilution}$$

Note that higher solute loads (e.g., dietary) require more water excretion. For example, body builders on high protein and carbohydrate diets with 1400 mOsm solute/day require a urine output of (1400/1200) to (1400/50) or 1.2 to 28 L/day. Alternatively, a low solute intake (starvation) with high water intake predisposes to water retention and water intoxication. This combination exists in binge beer drinkers, in whom the solute load may be only 300 mOsm/day. Low solute intake may also occur in starvation and the elderly on a "tea and toast diet." The range of urine output would drop to (300/1200) − (300/50) or 0.25 to 6 L/day in such patients.

15. **What are the main factors controlling water metabolism?**
Thirst, hormonal, and renal mechanisms are tightly integrated for control of water metabolism.

16. **What are the stimuli of thirst?**
Osmoreceptors in the organum vasculosum of the anterior hypothalamus control thirst. Increasing plasma tonicity stimulates thirst at a threshold about 5 mOsm/kg higher than that which stimulates ADH release. However, oropharyngeal receptors are also important in thirst regulation. A dry mouth increases thirst. Drinking and swallowing water decrease thirst even without changing P_{osm}. Volume depletion changes afferent baroreceptor input and increases angiotensin II—both changes increase thirst. An unusual idiosyncratic effect of angiotensin-converting enzyme inhibitors causes central polydipsia, increased ADH release, and propensity to hyponatremia.

17. **What hormonal mechanisms are involved in control of body water?**
Although natriuretic peptides, aldosterone, prostaglandins, angiotensin II, and neurohumoral changes affect renal water retention and excretion, ADH is most important. ADH is also called AVP or arginine vasopressin. Supraoptic and paraventricular nuclei in the hypothalamus secrete ADH in response to increased osmolality and decreased volume. ADH attaches to vasopressin 2 (V2) receptors on the basolateral membrane of collecting tubular cells. This activates cyclic adenosine monophosphate and protein kinase, causing intracellular water channels called aquaporins (AQPs) to insert into the luminal membrane. Water moves down osmotic gradients from tubular lumen through AQP channels into the cell and interstitium. At least six AQP isoforms are present in the kidney. The collecting duct has high concentrations of AQP2 that serve as the major target for ADH-mediated water reabsorption. Abnormalities of the V2 receptor cause most cases of nephrogenic diabetes insipidus (DI), but some are caused by abnormalities of AQP2. Increased AQP2 may cause water retention in conditions such as pregnancy and congestive heart failure. Twenty percent of ADH receptors in the collecting tubular cells are vasopressin 1 (V1) receptors. ADH activates V1 receptors only at very high levels. This increases prostaglandin E_2 and prostacyclin that opposes the antidiuretic effects of excessive ADH.

18. **What are the major conditions that influence ADH secretion?**
ADH functions to maintain osmotic and volume homeostasis. Secretion starts at an osmotic threshold of 280 mOsm/kg and increases proportionately to further rises in tonicity. A 1% to 2%

increase in osmolality stimulates ADH secretion, whereas a 10% drop in vascular volume is required for the same effect. By action on baroreceptors, increased ECV raises the osmotic threshold for ADH secretion and decreased ECV lowers this threshold. Severe volume depletion and hypotension may completely override the hypo-osmotic inhibition of ADH secretion. This finding has been called the law of circulating volume. In severe volume depletion and hypotension, ADH secretion continues despite low osmolality, thereby worsening the hyponatremia. Nausea, pain, and stress (as seen postoperatively) are also potent stimuli of ADH release and may produce life-threatening hyponatremia if hypotonic fluid is given. This is particularly true if associated with drugs that potentiate release or action of ADH.

19. **What are the major causes of ADH secretion?**
Major causes of ADH secretion include hyperosmolality, hypovolemia, nausea, pain, stress, human chorionic gonadotropin as in pregnancy (reset osmostat), hypoglycemia, corticotropin-releasing hormone (CRH)/ADH release, central nervous system (CNS) infections, CNS tumors, vascular catastrophes (thrombosis, hemorrhage), and ectopic ADH of malignancy (carcinomas of lung [primarily small cell], duodenum, pancreas, ureter, bladder, and prostate, and lymphoma). ADH secretion may be increased by any major pulmonary disorder, including pneumonia, tuberculosis, asthma, atelectasis, cystic fibrosis, positive pressure ventilation, and adult respiratory distress syndrome. HIV infection may have the multifactorial role of causing CNS dysfunction, pulmonary disease, and malignancy. Excessive exogenous ADH or desmopressin acetate (DDAVP) in patients with DI directly increases ADH effect. Oxytocin also has significant ADH activity in the large dosages used to induce labor. Other drugs that affect ADH secretion and action are listed in Table 24-2.

TABLE 24-2.	DRUGS THAT AFFECT ADH SECRETION AND ACTION*			
Increase ADH Secretion	Increase ADH Effect	Decrease ADH Secretion	Decrease ADH Effect	SIADH Unknown
Bromocriptine	Acetaminophen	Ethanol	Demeclocycline	Amitriptyline
Carbamazepine	Carbamazepine	Phenytoin	Lithium	Fluphenazine
Chlorpropamide	Chlorpropamide		Acetohexamide	Haloperidol
Clofibrate	Cyclophosphamide		Tolazamide	SSRIs
Cyclophosphamide	NSAIDs		Glyburide	Fluoxetine
Ifosfamide	Tolbutamide		Methoxflurane	MAOIs§
Morphine			Propoxyphene	Phenothiazines
Nicotine			Colchicine	Butyrophenones
Thioridazine			Amphotericin	Ecstasy
Vincristine			Vinblastine	
			PGE2	
			Prostacyclin	

ADH, antidiuretic hormone; MAOI, monoamine oxidase inhibitors; NSAID, nonsteroidal anti-inflammatory drugs; PGE2, prostaglandin E_2; SSRIs, selective serotonin reuptake inhibitors.
* Because psychosis itself may cause syndrome of inappropriate secretion of ADH (SIADH), one must question the true ADH stimulatory effect of the antipsychotic drugs. Changes in ADH secretion may be direct or indirect.

KEY POINTS: SYNDROMES AND TREATMENT OF WATER ✓ DYSFUNCTION

1. Clinical syndromes of water dysfunction include syndrome of inappropriate antidiuretic hormone, diabetes insipidus, and changes in effective circulating volume that can cause marked retention of salt and water, pulmonary and peripheral edema, and severe neurologic dysfunction.

2. Effective correction of water problems requires a thorough assessment of volume and neurologic symptoms.

3. If symptoms are present, correction must be rapid; if absent, there is no urgency and correction should occur more slowly.

4. Depending on the water disturbance, treatment includes water restriction or administration; hypertonic, isotonic, or hypotonic saline; sodium; diuretics; antidiuretic hormone; and other medications.

20. **How does the kidney handle salt and water?**
To control excess or deficiency of water intake, there must be adequate glomerular filtration rate (GFR) and delivery of filtrate to the LOH and distal nephron. Solute is separated from water in the ascending limb of the LOH, distal convoluted tubule (DCT), and cortical connecting segment; normal action of ADH allows controlled reabsorption of water in the cortical and medullary collecting tubules. The proximal convoluted tubule reabsorbs 65% and the descending limb of the LOH 25% of filtered solute and water isotonically. The ascending limb is impermeable to water but removes solute that dilutes the luminal filtrate, concentrates the interstitium (important for ADH action), and delivers 10% of the filtrate to the cortical collecting tubules with osmolality of 100 mOsm/kg. In the absence of ADH, this fluid ($\approx$18 L/day) would be lost in the urine and cause marked dehydration. In the presence of ADH, the collecting duct becomes permeable to water and reabsorbs all but 1% of the filtrate. Thus the final urine volume is only 1.5 to 2.0 L/day. Because normal GFR is 125 mL/min, the normal kidneys filter 180 L of plasma each day and reabsorb 99%. In normal adults, 99% of all Na and H_2O filtered is reabsorbed.

21. **What are the consequences and causes of decreased renal excretion of water?**
Any reduction in water excretion predisposes to hyponatremia and hypo-osmolality. Conditions that impair GFR, delivery of tubular fluid to the distal nephron, ability of the distal nephron to separate solute from water, or that increase the permeability of the collecting tubule to water will impair water excretion. Such conditions include renal failure, decreased ECV, diuretics (thiazides and loop), and excessive ADH or ADH action.

22. **How do hypothyroidism and adrenal insufficiency cause hyponatremia?**
Hypothyroidism and adrenal insufficiency decrease cardiac output and thereby decrease ECV and increase ADH release. Hypothyroidism associated decreased ECV causes reduced renal blood flow, glomerular filtration, and maximal solute-free water excretion. Failure to dilute the urine maximally results from increased ADH-mediated AQP2 receptors and nonosmotic ADH release. The main effect of glucocorticoid deficiency is altered systemic hemodynamics, not salt and water loss. Decreased cortisol decreases cardiac output and the systemic vascular response to catecholamines, causing both decreased blood pressure and ECV. The resulting drop in absolute and effective vascular filling pressure decreases stretch on the arterial baroreceptors and thereby decreases tonic vagal and glossopharyngeal inhibition of ADH release. These baroreceptor changes override the hypoosmotic inhibition of ADH release and increase ADH

secretion. The decreased ECV also lowers GFR, which reduces delivery of filtrate to the distal nephron and enhances proximal tubular water reabsorption. Normally, CRH and ADH are cosecreted from the same neurons in the paraventricular nuclei of the hypothalamus, and both hormones work synergistically to release ACTH from the anterior pituitary. Cortisol then feeds back negatively at the hypothalamus and pituitary to inhibit the release of both CRH and ADH. Cortisol deficiency decreases this negative feedback and increases ADH release to further enhance water reabsorption. Unlike secondary adrenal insufficiency, mineralocorticoid deficiency associated with primary adrenal insufficiency has an associated hyperkalemic nonanion gap metabolic acidosis. This is due to retention of K^+ and H^+ that is normally excreted under aldosterone influence. The deficiency of aldosterone also causes renal loss of NaCl and associated volume (ECF) depletion. Thus there is decreased TBV- and ECV-stimulated ADH release. There is also upregulation of collecting duct AQP2 and AQP3, enhancing ADH action. A high sodium diet compensates for the mineralocorticoid deficiency and improves the hyponatremia. Although hyponatremia may occur with both primary and secondary adrenal insufficiency, it occurs more commonly in primary adrenal insufficiency. This emphasizes the importance of aldosterone deficiency on renal salt wasting, volume depletion, and ADH secretion. All of these events combined with continued water intake synergistically contribute to hyponatremia.

23. **What P_{Na} concentrations are causes for concern?**
The severity of hyponatremia or hypernatremia depends on the rapidity of development. Normal P_{Na} ranges from 136 to 145 mEq/L. Patients with a P_{Na} of 115 or 165 mEq/L may not show any clinical abnormalities if they develop the problem over days to weeks. However, both conditions may produce major neurologic dysfunction if they develop over hours to days. As a rule, however, Na concentrations of 120 to 155 mEq/L are not usually associated with symptoms. P_{Na} outside these limits and occasionally rapidly developing disturbances within these limits may be of major concern. With appropriate care, patients with P_{Na} as low as 85 mEq/L and as high as 274 mEq/L have survived without permanent sequelae.

24. **What causes the symptoms and signs of increased or decreased TBW?**
The main symptoms and signs of too much (decreased P_{Na}) or too little (increased P_{Na}) TBW result from brain swelling or contraction. If changes in TBW occur more rapidly than the brain can adapt, symptoms and signs will occur. The severity of the symptoms and signs depends on the degree and rapidity of the TBW change. After adaptation occurs, correcting the disturbance in body water too rapidly may be more deleterious than the initial disturbance.

25. **What are the symptoms and signs of hyponatremia and hypernatremia?**
Hyponatremia: Headache, confusion, muscle cramps, weakness, lethargy, confusion, apathy, agitation, nausea, vomiting, anorexia, altered levels of consciousness, seizures, depressed deep tendon reflexes, hypothermia, Cheyne-Stokes respiration, respiratory depression, coma, and death.
　　Hypernatremia: Weakness, irritability, lethargy, confusion, somnolence, muscle twitching, seizures, respiratory depression, paralysis, and death.

26. **How does the brain adapt to hyponatremia?**
Because ICF and ECF osmolality must always be equal, developing hyponatremia immediately shifts water into the brain, increasing intracranial pressure (ICP). The increased ICP causes loss of NaCl into the CSF. Over the next several hours, there is also loss of intracellular K and, over the next few days, loss of organic solute. These changes return the brain volume to normal. However, if severe hyponatremia occurs too rapidly, there is not enough time for cerebral adaptation. Brain edema occurs, further increasing ICP; the brain herniates, and the patient dies.

27. How does the brain adapt to hypernatremia?

With acute hypernatremia and increased P_{osm}, water immediately shifts out of the brain and decreases ICP. The decreased ICP promotes movement of CSF with NaCl into the brain ICF, partially correcting volume. Within hours, further brain adaptation occurs, increasing brain ICF K^+, Na^+, and Cl^-. The resulting increase in osmolality pulls water from the ECF and restores about 60% of the brain volume. Over the next several days, the brain accumulates organic solutes (osmolites), previously called idiogenic osmoles, that return the brain volume to a near-normal level. These solutes include glutamine, taurine, glutamate, myoinositol, and phosphocreatine. If the brain has no time to adapt to rapidly developing hypernatremia, it will shrink, retract from the dura, and tear vessels, causing intracranial hemorrhage, increased ICP, compressive injury, herniation, and death.

28. How should you approach the patient with hyponatremia?

Hyponatremia occurs in 1% of outpatients, more than 4% of general hospitalized patients, 18% of elderly nursing home residents, and nearly 30% of intensive care patients. Hyponatremia always means too much ECF water relative to Na. Measure serum osmolality (reflective of P_{osm}) and assess volume status. With hyponatremia, the osmolality should be low. If P_{osm} is high (hypertonic hyponatremia) the ECF is high in an osmotically active substance such as glucose (uncontrolled diabetes) or mannitol (treatment of increased ICP). When the P_{osm} is normal (isotonic hyponatremia), there may be displacement of H_2O by excess lipid (hypertriglyceridemia) or protein (multiple myeloma) as in pseudohyponatremia. Large-volume bladder irrigation with mannitol and glycine sometimes cause this as well. Lastly, when P_{osm} is appropriately low (hypotonic hyponatremia), look for an appropriate cause of hyponatremia such as those listed in Table 25-3. Remember to obtain a U_{osm} and, if less than 100 mOsm/kg, primary polydipsia, beer potomania, or malnutrition may be present (see question 48). If the Uosm is greater than 100 mOsm//kg, there is usually an ADH effect (appropriate or not). Because total body volume is proportional to total body Na, a thorough assessment of the patient's volume status helps determine ECV and therapy. Patients with flat neck veins and postural changes in blood pressure and pulse (standing blood pressure decreases greater than 20/10 mm Hg and pulse increases greater than 20 beats/min) are hypovolemic and invariably saline (NaCl and H_2O) depleted. Patients with distended neck veins and edema are volume (saline) overloaded. Hyponatremic patients with no postural changes and no edema are clinically euvolemic but volume may be subclinically increased. If possible, always direct treatment to correct the underlying disorder (Tables 24-3 and 24-4). If patients have lost saline, give them saline. If they have retained too much water, restrict their water. If they have retained too much salt and water but more water than salt, restrict their salt and water but water more than salt. It sounds simple, and it is in concept. However, sometimes it is difficult to determine the subtle changes in volume status that are key to this assessment (see question 29). Carefully use loop diuretics in hypervolemic patients and 3% saline in acutely symptomatic patients (see question 47).

TABLE 24-3. CAUSES OF HYPONATREMIA	
Pathophysiology	**Associated Conditions**
Renal saline loss and decreased ECV $U_{Na} > 20$ mEq/L	Diuretics
	Osmotic diuresis (glucose, urea, mannitol)
	Primary adrenal insufficiency
	Renal tubular acidosis ($NaHCO_3$ loss)
	Salt-losing nephritis
	Ketonuria
	Cerebral salt wasting

(Continued)

TABLE 24-3. CAUSES OF HYPONATREMIA (CONTINUED)

Pathophysiology	Associated Conditions
Nonrenal saline loss and decreased ECV U_{Na} <20 mEq/L	Vomiting
	Diarrhea
	Pancreatitis, rhabdomyolysis, burns
	Peritonitis, bowel obstruction
Water excess U_{Na} >20 mEq/L	SIADH
	Secondary adrenal insufficiency
	Hypothyroidism
Na and H_2O excess with decreased ECV U_{Na} <20 mEq/L	Congestive heart failure
	Cirrhosis
	Nephrotic syndrome
Na and H_2O excess with increased ECV U_{Na} >20 mEq/L	Acute renal failure
	Chronic renal failure

ECV, effective circulating volume; SIADH, syndrome of inappropriate antidiuretic hormone. Hyponatremia always means too much plasma water relative to Na. Thorough volume assessment is crucial. Volume loss (renal or nonrenal) usually means saline (salt > H_2O) loss, and is associated with decreased ECV. Volume excess (hypervolemic) usually means saline (H_2O > salt) excess with associated edema and may be associated with decreased or increased ECV. Water excess usually causes mild excess of volume that affects baroreceptor activity. U_{Na} reflects renal perfusion, tubular integrity, and hormonal status. When U_{Na} > 20, the kidney contributes to Na loss and, if < 20, the kidney is conserving Na.

TABLE 24-4. APPROACH TO HYPONATREMIA

Condition	Postural Signs	Edema	U_{Na}	Treatment
Renal saline loss	Yes	No	>20	Give isotonic saline
Nonrenal saline loss	Yes	No	<20	Give isotonic saline
Water excess	No	No	>20	Restrict water
Na and water excess	No	Yes	<20	Restrict water > salt
Na and water excess	No	Yes	>20	Restrict water > salt

U_{Na} is measured in mEq/L. Because P_{Na} is usually measured with ion-selective electrodes, artifactual lowering of the P_{Na} is now unusual. If your lab does not use ion-selective electrodes, marked hyperlipidemia or hyperproteinemia may produce pseudohyponatremia. Notwithstanding, measured P_{osm} will differentiate these disorders. Because P_{osm} measures the osmotic activity of plasma water and because plasma water excludes lipids and proteins, they contribute little to P_{osm}. Thus the measured P_{osm} will be essentially normal in pseudohyponatremia. Carefully use loop diuretics to treat edema and 3% saline for symptomatic acute hyponatremia.

29. **What is the importance of an initial thorough volume assessment in patients with hyponatremia?**
Perform an initial thorough volume assessment to help determine the underlying cause of the hyponatremia (Table 25-3) and guide treatment (Table 25-4). Assess the patient's volume by looking at neck veins, postural signs, and edema. At times, the best clinician cannot get a good assessment of ECV, but central monitoring with a Swan-Ganz catheter is rarely necessary. Urinary Na and edema are clues to ECV. Get an initial weight and assess weight daily. Continue assessment of postural signs as necessary. Initially, obtain P_{osm}, general chemistry panel (Na, K, Cl, CO_2, Cr, BUN, glucose, albumin, Ca, Mg); urinary Na, Cl, Cr; and fractional excretion of Na. The presence or absence of edema and the U_{Na} are most helpful.

30. **How should you characterize and diagnose the patient with syndrome of inappropriate antidiuretic hormone?**
Syndrome of inappropriate antidiuretic hormone (SIADH) has recently been called SIAD or syndrome of inappropriate antidiuresis because many of these patients do not have measurable ADH levels. Clinical euvolemia, hypotonic plasma, and less than maximally dilute urine are the clues to SIADH. Approach the patient as in question 28. It is important to establish normovolemia by physical examination. Then measure P_{osm}, U_{osm}, P_{Na}, U_{Na}, and U_K. Finally, exclude pituitary, adrenal, and thyroid dysfunction before diagnosis. Confirmatory criteria of SIADH include low P_{Na} (<135 mEq/L), low P_{osm} (<280 mOsm/kg), U_{osm} greater than 100 mOsm/kg, U_{Na} greater than 40 mEq/L, and [U_{Na} + U_K] greater than P_{Na}. Patients with SIADH are usually said to have normal volume status. However, they actually have excessive TBW. Unlike excessive saline, which is limited to ECF, excessive water distributes two thirds to the ICF and one third to the ECF. Thus the ECF excess is minor and not usually perceptible by clinical examination. Nonetheless, patients with SIADH have mildly increased ECV, which is sensed by the kidney. The kidney increases GFR, which causes a low uric acid, BUN, and creatinine. The increased ECV also increases ANP and, along with increased GFR, promotes natriuresis. These are the classic findings in SIADH. Obviously, SIADH does not protect against dehydration and other conditions that can obscure the classic presentation. For example, a patient with ectopic ADH from lung cancer may present with dehydration from diarrhea and lack of water intake from debilitation. In this instance, the U_{Na} and U_{Cl} may be less than 20 mEq/L.

31. **How do you treat the patient with SIADH?**
Initially, treat SIADH with water restriction. If the patient has marked symptoms, treat for symptomatic hyponatremia (see question 40). Also, attempt to correct the underlying abnormality (see questions 18 and 19). If the patient has unresectable cancer and water restriction (500–1500 mL/day) is not tolerated, give demeclocycline, 600–1200 mg/day, or lithium carbonate, 600 to 1200 mg/day, in two to four divided dosages. Because lithium carbonate can cause neurologic, cardiovascular, and other toxicities, avoid it unless there are no other therapeutic options. Demeclocycline may cause severe renal failure in patients with cirrhosis. Thus it is contraindicated in patients with cirrhosis and severe liver disease. A high Na diet (4–8 gm) may be necessary in addition to water restriction to correct the hyponatremia.

32. **What are the four patterns of SIADH?**
The four patterns of SIADH are distinguished according to responses of ADH to P_{osm}:
Type I—erratic ADH secretion with no predictable response to P_{osm} (20% of cases)
Type II—reset osmostat with normal relationship of ADH to P_{osm} but a lower threshold for ADH release (e.g., 250–260 mOsm/kg; 35% of cases)
Type III—ADH leak with selective loss of ADH suppression and continued secretion when P_{osm} is low but normal suppression and secretion when P_{osm} is normal (35% of cases)
Type IV—ADH-dissociated antidiuresis at low P_{osm} with appropriately low or undetectable ADH (possibly from increased renal sensitivity to ADH or unknown ADH-like substance; 10% of cases)

33. **Define polyuria and list the main causes.**
Polyuria is a urine output greater than 3.0 L/day. Four main disorders cause polyuria: psychogenic polydipsia (psychosis), dipsogenic DI (defect in thirst center), central neurogenic DI (defect in ADH secretion), and nephrogenic DI (defect in ADH action on the kidney). All forms of DI may be partial or complete. Polyuria also may occur from osmotic diuresis in such conditions as diabetes mellitus (glucose), recovery from renal failure (urea), and intravenous infusions (saline, mannitol). See Table 25-2 for drugs and conditions that decrease ADH secretion and action. Causes of acquired nephrogenic DI include chronic renal disease, electrolyte abnormalities (hypokalemia and hypercalcemia), drugs (lithium, demeclocycline), sickle-cell disease (damaged medullary interstitium), diet (increased water and decreased solute—beer, starvation), inflammatory or infiltrative renal disease (multiple myeloma, amyloidosis, sarcoidosis), and others. DI may be associated with specific genetic abnormalities. Hereditary central DI is usually autosomal dominant and expresses itself in childhood rather than at birth. Wolfram's syndrome results from a familial defect on the short arm of chromosome 4 and has associated central DI, diabetes mellitus, optic atrophy, and deafness (DIDMOAD). Congenital nephrogenic DI results from abnormalities of the V2 receptor or AQP2 channels and symptoms of polyuria and dehydration appear in the first week of life. Most cases of nephrogenic DI related to abnormalities of the V2 receptors are X-linked and therefore almost always limited to expression in males. More than 150 mutations are noted to cause DI related to V2 receptor abnormalities. Nephrogenic DI related to abnormalities of AQP2 may be autosomal dominant or recessive. When recessive and occurring a female, the DI is likely due to a mutation on chromosome 12.

34. **How do you distinguish polyuric patients with the various forms of DI from excessive water drinking?**
In excessive water drinking, the P_{Na}, BUN, and uric acid are relatively low. In DI, the P_{Na} and uric acid are relatively high, and the BUN is relatively low. Central DI often has an abrupt onset due to a loss of a critical amount of arginine vasopressin (AVP) resulting from destruction of more than 80% to 90% of the ADH-secreting hypothalamic neurons at a critical point in time. However, the diagnosis of polyuria is not always clear from the history and lab tests. In that case, perform a water restriction test (WRT). Other names for the WRT are dehydration test and water deprivation test. The test may take 6 to 18 hours depending on the initial state of hydration.

35. **How is the WRT performed?**
    1. Office testing is acceptable unless the patient cannot be watched closely, in which case hospitalization may be required.
    2. Measure baseline weight, P_{osm}, P_{Na}, P_{BUN}, $P_{glucose}$, U_{volume}, U_{osm}, U_{Na}, and U_K. Measure hourly weight and U_{osm}.
    3. Allow no food or water.
    4. Watch the patient closely for signs of dehydration and surreptitious water drinking.
    5. End the WRT when U_{osm} has not increased more than 30 mOsm/kg for 3 consecutive hours, P_{osm} has reached 295 to 300 mOsm/kg, or the patient has lost 3% to 5% of body weight. If weight loss exceeds 3% to 5% of body weight, further dehydration is unsafe.
    6. At P_{osm} of 295 to 300 mOsm/kg, endogenous ADH levels should be 5 pg/mL or greater, and the kidney should respond with maximal urinary concentration.
    7. Repeat all baseline tests toward and at the end of the WRT.
    8. Give 5 units of aqueous AVP or 2 μg of DDAVP subcutaneously.
    9. Repeat the baseline tests at 30, 60, and 120 minutes.
    10. Calculate U_{osm}/P_{osm} and $[U_{Na} + U_K]/P_{Na}$ as a check on measured U_{osm}/P_{osm}.

36. **How do you interpret the results of the WRT?**
Table 24-5 summarizes the expected results of the WRT. The WRT stimulates maximal endogenous release of ADH by increasing P_{osm} and evaluates the concentrating ability of the kidney by measuring U_{osm}. Giving exogenous ADH allows evaluation of the renal concentrating response to ADH if dehydration-induced ADH production was impaired. Save frozen baseline

and end-test plasma to measure ADH if results are equivocal. Expected normal values for P_{ADH} are 0.5 pg/mL for P_{osm} 280 mOsm/kg or less and 5 pg/mL or greater for P_{osm} 295 mOsm/kg.

TABLE 24-5. VALUES BEFORE AND AFTER WATER RESTRICTION

	Pre P_{osm}	Pre P_{Na}	Post U_{osm}/P_{osm}	Post U_{osm}/P_{osm} + ADH	Post P_{ADH}
Normals	NL	NL	>1	>1 (<10%)	↑
PPD/DDI	↓	↓	>1	>1 (<10%)	↑ on NL
CCDI	↑	↑	<1	>1 (>50%)	—
PCDI	↑	↑	>1	>1(10–50%)	↓
CNDI	↑	↑	<1	<1 (<10%)	↑↑
PNDI	↑	↑	>1	>1 (<10%)	↑↑

ADH, antidiuretic hormone; CCDI, complete central DI; PCDI, partial central DI; CNDI, complete nephrogenic DI; PNDI, partial nephrogenic DI; PPD/DDI, psychogenic polydipsia/dipsogenic DI. Relative to the normal range, the down and up arrows, respectively, mean low or low normal and high or high normal values for P_{osm}, P_{Na}, and P_{ADH}. Recall that when $U_{osm} > P_{osm}$, there is antidiuresis, and the kidney is retaining free water. The same is true when $[U_{Na} + U_K] > P_{Na}$, and these tests are more easily obtainable. When $U_{osm} < P_{osm}$ or $[U_{Na} + U_K] < P_{Na}$, there is net loss of free water with little net clinical ADH effect. The value in parentheses indicates the percentage change in U_{osm} (not the U_{osm}/P_{osm} ratio) after 5 units of subcutaneous aqueous vasopressin or 2 μg of desmopressin acetate.

37. **What are the expected plasma ADH concentrations and urinary osmolality in polyuric patients after water restriction?**
See Table 24-6.

TABLE 24-6. EXPECTED VALUES FOR ADH AND U_{OSM} AFTER WATER RESTRICTION

Cause of Polyuria	ADH (pg/mL)	U_{osm} (mOsm/kg)
Normal	>2	>800
Primary polydipsia	<5	>500
Complete central DI	Undetectable	<300
Partial central DI	<1.5	300–800
Nephrogenic DI	>5	300–500

ADH, antidiuretic hormone; DI, diabetes insipidus.

38. **How should you approach the patient with hypernatremia?**
Problems of hypernatremia are uncommon compared with hyponatremia and occur in less than 1% of general hospitalized patients. Indeed, unless patients have an abnormality of thirst or do not have access to water, they usually maintain near-normal P_{Na} by drinking water in proportion to losses. However, as many as 5% to 10% of intensive care unit (ICU) patients may have some degree of hypernatremia. Loss of water is the usual cause of hypernatremia, and almost all patients require water for treatment (Table 24-7). As in questions 28 and 29, assess the patient's volume status. After lab studies are obtained, approach the patient according to Table 24-8. If the patient has polyuria, also include the approach in questions 33 and 34.

TABLE 24-7. CAUSES OF HYPERNATREMIA	
Pathophysiology	**Associated Condition**
Renal H_2O loss >Na loss	Osmotic diuretics
U_{Na} >20 mEq/L	Loop diuretics
	Renal disease
	Postobstructive diuresis
Nonrenal H_2O loss >Na loss	Osmotic diarrhea
U_{Na} <20 mEq/L	Vomiting
	Sweating
	Diarrhea
	Burns
Excess Na >H_2O	Hyperaldosteronism
U_{Na} >20 mEq/L	Cushing's syndrome
	Primary hyperaldosteronism
	Excessive intake of NaCl or $NaHCO_3$
	Hypertonic saline and bicarbonate
	Hypertonic dialysis
Renal H_2O loss	Central DI
U_{Na} >20 mEq/L	Nephrogenic DI
Nonrenal H_2O loss	Increased sensible loss
U_{Na} <20 mEq/L	No access to H_2O

DI, diabetes insipidus.
Hypernatremia always means too little plasma water relative to Na. With access to water, hypernatremia usually does not occur or is mild. However, unattended patients who are too old, too young, or too sick may not have adequate access to water, and hypernatremia may be severe. Thorough volume assessment is crucial. Volume loss (hypovolemic) usually means renal or nonrenal saline (H_2O > salt) loss and is usually treated with 0.9% to 0.45% saline to correct the volume deficit followed by water. Volume excess (hypervolemic) usually means saline (salt > H_2O) excess with high total body Na and is treated with water and restricting salt. A loop diuretic may also be necessary to treat volume overload. Euvolemic hypernatremia results from water loss and is treated with free water replacement, and vasopressin is used if water loss is caused by DI.

39. **How should you diagnose and manage the patient with DI?**
    DI is a syndrome of excessive water loss by the kidney due to decreased ADH (central DI) or renal unresponsiveness to ADH (nephrogenic DI). Therefore, the hallmark of DI is polyuria. Mild hypernatremia, a low BUN, and a relatively high uric acid are suggestive of DI. In idiopathic central DI, magnetic resonance imaging (MRI) of the pituitary shows absence of the normal pituitary bright spot. However, the pituitary bright spot decreases with age and may be absent in a majority of the elderly without DI. An abrupt onset of polyuria is also suggestive of central DI because 80% to 90% of the ADH-secreting neurons must be lost before polyuria and little ADH is necessary to have some urinary concentration. As in questions 33 and 34, first distinguish primary polydipsia from DI and identify the DI as central or nephrogenic. Then give water to prevent dehydration until the evaluation suggests definitive therapy. Mild cases of DI require no

TABLE 24-8.   APPROACH TO HYPERNATREMIA

Condition	Postural Signs	Edema	U_{Na}	U_{osm}	Treatment
Renal H_2O > Na loss	Yes	No	>20	$\downarrow-$	0.9%–0.45% saline
Nonrenal H_2O > Na loss	Yes	No	<20	$\uparrow$	0.9%–0.45% saline
Na excess	No	Yes/No	>20	$\uparrow-$	Free H_2O/Diuretics
Renal H_2O loss	No	No	>20	$\downarrow\uparrow-$	Free H_2O
Nonrenal H_2O loss	No	No	<20	$\uparrow$	Free H_2O

VAR, variable; $\uparrow$, hypertonic; $\downarrow$, hypotonic; $-$, isosmotic. Free $H_2O = 5\%$ dextrose in water infusion or water orally. Infuse saline to restore the volume deficit when patients show signs of severe volume depletion such as hypotension or postural changes in blood pressure and pulse. This is appropriate when isotonic (0.9%) saline with an osmolality of 308 mOsm/kg is lower than plasma osmolality. This corrects both the volume deficit and the hypernatremia. After the volume deficit has improved, switch to 0.45% saline and eventually 5% dextrose in water. Loop diuretics are used to treat Na excess.

treatment other than adequate fluid intake. A patient with DI will probably self-treat with water unless there is a thirst deficit or the patient has no access to water. Treat central DI with DDAVP as a nasal spray or oral tablet. DDAVP is available for oral use (0.1 or 0.2 mg tablets) with a starting dosage of 0. 05 mg once or twice daily and increased to a maximum of 0.4 mg every 8 hours as necessary. The tablet is 5% absorbed with absorption further decreased as much as 50% with meals. At least one dose should be given at bedtime. Oral desmopressin is preferred for patients with sinusitis from the nasal preparation. The nasal preparation (100 mcg/mL solution) is given every 12 to 24 hours as needed for thirst and polyuria. It may be administered by metered-dose nasal inhaler (0.1 mL/spray) or by a plastic calibrated tube. The starting dosage is 0.05 to 0.1 mL once or twice daily, and the dosage is titrated to an acceptable urine output. Parenteral desmopressin (4 mcg/mL) may be given intravenously, intramuscularly, or subcutaneously at 1 to 2 mcg every 12 to 24 hours to hospitalized patients. Nephrogenic DI may be partial or complete and therefore may respond to DDAVP. If possible, correct or ameliorate the underlying cause, such as lithium use and hypercalcemia (see question 33).

Without compromising nutritional needs, provide a low sodium and low protein diet. Emphasize regular voiding to avoid overdistending the bladder and bladder dysfunction. Both central and nephrogenic diabetes insipidus respond partially to hydrochlorothiazide (50–100 mg daily). Amiloride or potassium supplementation may be necessary. Nephrogenic DI may respond to combination therapy if one does not work. These include indomethacin with hydrochlorothiazide, indomethacin with DDAVP, or indomethacin with amiloride. Although indomethacin at 50 mg orally every 8 hours has been effective, other NSAIDs or lower dose may also be effective.

40. **How quickly should you correct states of water excess or deficiency?**
The main concern of therapy for abnormal TBW is to prevent devastating neurologic complications. Understanding brain adaptation to changes in TBW, as outlined in questions 25 and 26, emphasizes the need for urgent therapy only in the symptomatic patient. There are three useful rules in treating disturbances of water (measured by changes in P_{Na}):
   1. Return the P_{Na} to normal at the relative speed that it became abnormal. If the change in P_{Na} was slow (days), correct it slowly (days). If the change was rapid (minutes to hours), correct it rapidly (minutes to hours).

2. If there are no symptoms of water or Na imbalance (see question 24), there is no immediate urgency. If there are symptoms, there is urgency. Questions 25 and 26 outline the brain adaptations to altered tonicity that may cause devastating changes in brain volume. These adaptations also cause the patient's symptoms. Thus symptoms should drive the clinician to correct the altered tonicity rapidly.

3. The degree of rapid P_{Na} correction should be toward normal (until symptoms abate) not to normal.

These concepts of speed, symptoms, and degree of P_{Na} correction apply for both hyponatremia and hypernatremia (see question 47).

41. **How do frequent measurements of urinary Na and K help with hyponatremia therapy?**

Initial assessments for Na repletion, as outlined in question 47, do not account for urinary water and electrolyte losses that may alter the expected P_{Na} response to therapy. Therefore, replace urinary losses for more accurate correction of P_{Na}. Initially, measure the U_{Na} and U_K and urine volume every 1 to 2 hours, and replace urine volume with saline of appropriate strength. For example, if the urinary volume was 100 mL/h, the $U_{Na} = 43$ mEq/L and the $U_K = 35$ mEq/L, the sum of U_{Na} $U_K = 78$ mEq/L at 100 mL/h. In this case, replacing urinary losses with 0.45% saline (77 mEq/L NaCl) IV at 100 mL/h will prevent major deviations in P_{Na} from the value calculated. Give this replacement fluid in addition to that calculated to correct the P_{Na}. KCl replacement depends on serum K. Replace K to correct the serum K to normal, remembering that K replacement will increase P_{Na}. Therefore decrease the replacement Na by the amount of K given. Some evidence also suggests that hypokalemia may predispose to osmotic demyelination. Correcting serum K may decrease this risk.

42. **What are vasopressin receptor antagonists, and when would you use them for hyponatremia therapy?**

The conventional treatment of hyponatremia is water restriction or saline administration and still is appropriate therapy for most patients with hyponatremia. On December 30, 2005, the Food and Drug Administration approved conivaptan (Vaprisol), a first-in-class vasopressin receptor antagonist (VRA) for treatment of hospitalized patients with hyponatremia and normal extracellular fluid volume (SIADH). Conivaptan prevents AVP binding to V1a and V2 receptors located within the vasculature and renal tubules, respectively. Blocking the V2 receptor decreases free water reabsorption and increases excretion. Blocking the V1a receptor may cause vasodilatation reducing afterload in CHF. Conivaptan is available in 20 mg/5 mL glass ampules. The recommended dosage is a 20-mg loading dose administered intravenously over 30 minutes followed by 20 mg infused continuously over 24 hours for an additional 1 to 3 days. If the serum sodium fails to rise at the desired rate, increase the dosage to 40 mg/day by continuous infusion. Do not exceed 4 days in duration.

Other VRA, like conivaptan, produce a selective water diuresis with no effect on Na and K excretion. The term "aquaretic drugs" (aquaretics) has been coined for these medications to highlight their different mechanisms of action compared with the saliuretic diuretic furosemide. They are proven to be beneficial in SIADH and in hyponatremic patients with CHF and cirrhosis. By blocking ADH effect, rapid correction of hyponatremia may occur; therefore, judicious monitoring of P_{Na} changes is important to prevent excessively rapid correction of P_{Na}. Two oral VRA drugs that are effective in clinical trials include lixivaptan and tolvaptan.

43. **What is the appropriate P_{Na} correction factor for hyperglycemia?**

The standard correction factor is a 1.6-mEq/L decrease in P_{Na} for each 100-mg/dL increase in plasma glucose concentration above 100 mg/dL. For glucose values greater than 400 mg/dL, recent data suggest a correction factor as high as a 4.0-mEq/L decrease in P_{Na} for each 100 mg/dL increase in plasma glucose and an average correction factor of 2.4 mEq/L.

CLINICAL PROBLEMS IN WATER METABOLISM

44. **A 75-year-old woman presents with confusion but no focal neurologic signs. She has type 2 diabetes mellitus. Blood pressure is 110/54 mm Hg. Pulse is 96 beats/min. Neck veins are not visualized in the supine position. $P_{glucose}$ = 900 mg/dL, P_{Na} = 135 mEq/L, plasma creatinine = 3.0 mg/dL, BUN = 50 mg/dL, U_{Na} = 40 mEq/L, urine glucose is 4+ and ketones 3+. Describe her fluid and volume status and treatment.**

Glucose remains in the ECF because of insulin deficiency and increases ECF tonicity. Increased tonicity pulls water from the ICF to the ECF, concentrating the ICF and diluting the ECF until ICF and ECF osmolalities are equal. The osmotic pressure of 900 mg/dL glucose (900/18 = 50 mOsm/kg) is the driving force for water movement from ICF to ECF. Water movement from ICF to ECF dilutes the ECF and decreases P_{Na}. Each 100-mg/dL rise in $P_{glucose}$ above 100 mg/dL decreases the P_{Na} by 1.6 mEq/L. In this patient, the predicted decrease in P_{Na} = (90 − 100)/100 × 1.6 = 13 mEq/L. The predicted P_{Na} would be 140 − 13 = 127 mEq/L. However, a more accurate correction factor for the elevated glucose would be 2.4 mEq/L (see question 43). Thus the predicted decrease in P_{Na} would be (90 − 100)/100 × 2.4 = 19 mEq/L. The predicted P_{Na} would be 140 − 19 = 121 mEq/L. P_{Na} of 135 mEq/L suggests further water loss from osmotic diuresis and significant dehydration. The P_{osm} of 2 (135) + 900/18 + 56/2.8 = 340 mOsm/kg is compatible with hyperosmolar coma. Because this woman has decreased TBW and volume, you might expect her to be prerenal, the U_{Na} to be low, and the U_{osm} high. However, osmotic diuresis caused by urine glucose, ketones, and urea increases urinary Na and water, making U_{Na} and U_{osm} less useful markers of dehydration. Flat neck veins in the supine position are usually due to intravascular volume depletion. Rapid lowering of her glucose to 100 mg/dL will rapidly decrease P_{osm}, shift water to the ICF, increase P_{Na} by 13–19 mEq/L, and potentially cause cardiovascular collapse and cerebral edema. Thus therapy is normal saline to replace volume and judicious lowering of $P_{glucose}$ with IV insulin.

45. **You admit a 35-year-old schizophrenic because of a change in mental function and excessive urine output. U_{osm} = 70 mOsm/kg. P_{osm} = 280 mOsm/kg. 24-hour urine output = 12 L/day. How much free water is being excreted each day?**

Free water clearance (C_{H_2O}) is the amount of solute free water excreted per day. Osmolar clearance is the amount of urine excreted per day that contains all the solute that is isosmotic to plasma. When the urine is hypotonic to plasma, the total urine volume consists of two components: one part free of solute (C_{H_2O}) and the other, all of the solution that is isosmotic to plasma (C_{osm}). To measure how much of the urine is pure (free) water, calculate the free water clearance. To do so, you need to know the osmolar clearance (C_{osm}) and the urine volume (V). The formula for clearance of any substance (including osmols) is always the same:

$$C = UV/P,$$

where C is the volume of plasma cleared of the substance per unit time, U is the urinary concentration of the substance, P is the plasma concentration of the substance, and V is the total urinary volume per unit time. The calculations for this patient follow:

1. $V = C_{osm} + C_{H_2O}$
2. $C_{H_2O} = V - C_{osm}$
3. $C_{osm} = U_{osm} V/P_{osm}$
4. $C_{osm} = (70 \text{ mOsm/kg} \times 12 \text{ L/day})/280 \text{ mOsm/kg} = 3.0 \text{ L/day}$
5. $C_{H_2O} = V - C_{osm} = 12 \text{ L/day} - 3 \text{ L/day} = 9 \text{ L/day}$

By manipulating formula (2), another means of calculating free water clearance follows:

1. $C_{H_2O} = V(1 - U_{osm}/P_{osm})$
2. $C_{H_2O} = 12 \text{ L/day} (1 - 70/280) = 9 \text{ L/day}$

Thus the patient's daily urine output contains 9 L/day of pure (free) water and 3 L/day that is isotonic to plasma. This information does not distinguish primary polydipsia from DI. However, the low P_{osm} of 280 suggests primary polydipsia.

46. **A 45-year-old-man with a 30-pack-year history of smoking presents with cough, dyspnea, fatigue, and a 15-lb weight loss. Chest x-ray shows mediastinal adenopathy and right atelectasis with pleural effusion. $P_{osm} = 270$ mOsm/kg, $P_{Na} = 125$ mEq/L, $U_{osm} = 470$ mOsm/kg, $U_{Na} = 130$ mEq/L, $U_K = 60$ mEq/L, and urine volume $= 1$ L/day. How much free water is being excreted each day? What is the likely pulmonary lesion?**

Urine is hypertonic to plasma if the $U_{osm} > P_{osm}$ or the $U_{[Na+K]} > P_{Na}$. Urine hypertonic to plasma contains two parts: the volume that would be required to contain all solute and remain isosmotic to plasma is the osmolar clearance (C_{osm}); the volume of free water that was removed from the isotonic glomerular filtrate to make $U_{osm} > P_{osm}$ or the $U_{Na+K} > P_{Na}$ is the negative free water clearance (T^{CH_2O}). There are two ways to calculate free water clearance: one method uses osmolality as in question 14; the other uses electrolytes (Na and K). Electrolyte free water clearance more accurately estimates free water clearance and negative free water clearance, especially when urine contains large numbers of nonelectrolyte osmolites, such as urea, that increase osmolality unrelated to free water clearance. To calculate electrolyte free water clearance, use the urinary concentrations of Na and K and the plasma Na. Because $[U_{NA} + U_K] > P_{Na}[(130 + 60) > 130]$, the net urinary excretion of free water is negative, and therefore free water clearance is negative. Calculations for osmolar and electrolyte free water clearance in this patient follow:

Calculations for classic osmolar (negative) free water clearance:
1. $V = C_{osm} - T^{CH_2O}$
2. $T^{CH_2O} = C_{osm} - V$
3. $C_{osm} = 1$ L/day [470/270] $= 1.74$ L/day
4. $T^{CH_2O} = 1.74$ L/day $- 1$ L/day $= 0.74$ L/day

By manipulating formula (2), another means of calculating negative free water clearance follows:
1. $T^{CH_2O} = V[U_{osm}/P_{osm} - 1]$
2. $T^{CH2O} = 1$ L/day [470/270 $- 1$] $= 0.74$ L/day

Calculations for electrolyte (negative) free water clearance:
1. $T^{CH_2O} = C_{[Na + K]} - V$
2. $C_{[Na + K]} = [U_{[Na + K]} /P_{Na} \times V]$
3. $C_{[Na + K]} = [190$ mEq/L/125 mEq/L $\times 1$ L/day] $= 1.52$ L/day
4. $T^{CH_2O} = 1.52$ L/day $- 1$ L/day $= 0.52$ L/day

Thus the patient's kidneys add (by water reabsorption) a net of 520 to 740 mL of free water to plasma each day. With a low P_{osm}, it is usually inappropriate to retain water in excess of output. This finding suggests SIADH. One must exclude volume depletion, adrenal insufficiency, and hypothyroidism before making the diagnosis of SIADH. This patient had small cell carcinoma of the lung with ectopic ADH secretion. Fifteen percent of patients with small cell carcinoma of the lung develop SIADH. This tumor is highly associated with smoking and accounts for 15% to 25% of lung cancer. Other lung cancers rarely secrete ADH.

47. **A 34-year-old, 60-kg woman presents 12 hours after discharge following cholecystectomy. She has headache, confusion, muscle cramps, weakness, lethargy, agitation, nausea, and vomiting. She had no symptoms at discharge. P_{Na} was 110 mEq/L. What has caused the hyponatremia? How quickly should you treat it?**

By this history, hyponatremia developed rapidly and was symptomatic. Treatment is ICU admission and administration of 3% saline and furosemide at rates sufficient to increase P_{Na} 1.5 to 2.0 mEq/L/h for 2 to 4 hours on the basis of symptom resolution. Measure hourly P_{Na}, U_{Na}, and U_K to follow progress and guide therapy. After serious signs and symptoms improve, decrease the rate of correction to 0.5 to 1.0 mEq/h until symptoms further improve or the P_{Na} is 120 mEq/L. Avoid a net increase in P_{Na} greater than 12 mEq/L in the first 24 hours and 18 to 20 mEq/L over 48 hours. For chronic hyponatremia without symptoms, the appropriate rate of correction is 0.5 mEq/L/h with similar net daily increases in P_{Na}. Acute symptomatic hyponatremia requires expeditious correction of the P_{Na} because the symptomatic patient has cerebral edema caused by "normal" brain-cell solute content that pulls water into the brain. Acutely raising P_{Na} increases ECF tonicity, pulls water out of the swollen brain, and reduces the brain volume toward normal. The brain has no room in the skull to swell more than 8% to 10% before herniation. Therefore there is no benefit to acutely correcting the Na more than 8%; in this case to a P_{Na} greater than 119 mEq/L. Conversely, the patient with chronic asymptomatic hyponatremia has adapted by loss of brain solute and has near-normal brain volume. Increasing this patient's P_{Na} too rapidly (>0.5 mEq/L/h) will shrink the brain and predispose to the osmotic demyelination syndrome (previously called central pontine myelinolysis). The risks of not correcting acute symptomatic hyponatremia include increased cerebral edema, seizures, coma, and death. Outlined now are the calculations of water excess. Calculations for 3% saline necessary to correct the P_{Na} to 120 mEq/L are also shown.

$$
\begin{aligned}
\text{Water excess} &= [(\text{normal } P_{Na} - \text{observed } P_{Na})/\text{normal } P_{Na}] \times \text{TBW} \\
&= [(140 - 110)/140] \times 0.5 \times 60 \text{ kg} \\
&= 0.21 \times 30 \text{ L} \\
&= 6.3 \quad \text{L excess in TBW} \\
\text{Na deficit} &= (\text{desired } P_{Na} - \text{observed } P_{Na}) \times \text{TBW} \\
&= (120 - 110) \times 0.5 \times 60 \text{ kg} \\
&= 10 \text{ mEq/L} \times 30 \text{ L} \\
&= 300 \text{ mEq Na}
\end{aligned}
$$

Knowing the Na deficit is useful clinically because it can be replaced at a controlled rate to improve the hyponatremia. The Na in 3% saline is 513 mEq/L:

$$300 \text{ mEq Na}/513 \text{ mEq/L} = 0.585 \text{ L}$$

Thus assuming no Na or water loss, giving 585 mL of 3% saline will correct the P_{Na} to 120 mEq/L. Make a similar calculation for 3% saline to infuse over 3 to 4 hours to increase the P_{Na} by 6 mEq/L. The answer is 350 mL. However, one must also measure P_{Na}, U_{Na}, and U_K frequently to estimate loss and gain of Na and water during therapy and replace those losses. Empiric rate of 3% saline infusion for rapid treatment of symptomatic hyponatremia is 2 mL/kg/h. Use ideal body weight unless the patient is below ideal body weight, and in that case use actual weight. In this patient, 3% saline infusion would be 60 kg $\times$ 2 mL/kg/h or 120 mL/h $\times$ 4 h = 480 mL.

48. **An 80-year-old woman who rarely leaves her home is brought to the hospital after being found confused. Three weeks ago, she saw her physician, who started a diuretic for systolic hypertension. On arrival, her P_{Na} is 110 mEq/L. What is the cause of her hyponatremia?**

As a consequence of aging, elderly patients lose GFR, concentrating ability, and diluting ability. Thus an 80-year-old woman may have a normal (for age) renal-concentrating range of 100 to 700 mOsm/kg. However, maximal U_{osm} in the elderly may be as low as 350 mOsm/kg. This woman's average diet may generate only 600 mOsm/day. Her normal range of urine output would then be 0.9 to 6.0 L/day. If her dietary intake fell to 300 mOsm/day, her maximal urine output would fall to 3 L/day:

$$300 \text{ mOsm/day} \div 100 \text{ mOsm/kg} = 3 \text{L/day}$$

Given free access to water and a thiazide diuretic, which impairs urinary dilution, she could easily become water intoxicated and hyponatremic. The mechanism of hyponatremia in beer potomania and the "tea-and-toast diet" is low total osmolar intake and relatively increased water intake. The decreased osmotic load for excretion limits the amount of water excreted. This patient's hyponatremia is probably chronic; however, she is symptomatic. Thus it is not clear whether the hyponatremia is truly chronic or acute. Therefore how to proceed with therapy in this severely hyponatremic patient is unclear. Computed tomography (CT) scan or MRI may help by showing the presence or absence of cerebral edema. If cerebral edema is present, treat for acute hyponatremia. If cerebral edema is absent, treat judiciously for chronic hyponatremia. Perform frequent reassessment of P_{Na}, symptoms, and signs. Remember, elderly women taking thiazide diuretics; alcoholics; and malnourished, hypokalemic, and burned patients are at particular risk for the demyelination syndrome.

49. **A 35-year-old female marathon runner collapses, unable to finish a 42-km race averaging 5 mph. She water-loaded before the race and drank as much as possible to maintain hydration during the race. She is brought to you confused, afebrile, and tachypneic. Physical examination shows BP 120/60, pulse 110 beats/min and regular, lungs with bilateral crackles, continued confusion, and involuntary twitching during your examination. Laboratory studies show a P_{Na} of 112 mEq/L, and the remainder of the screening laboratory test results are normal. What is the cause of exercise-induced hyponatremia, and how would you treat it?**

Exertional hyponatremia may occur in 20% of ultra-endurance sports participants and be symptomatic in 20% to 30% of these athletes. Excess water intake is the primary cause, and this is suggested by the clinical history. Loss of sweat with Na concentrations of 40 to 80 mEq/L and replacement with hypotonic fluids also contributes to the hyponatremia. In addition, the pain and stress of exercise are known stimulants to ADH secretion. This patient with symptoms and signs of pulmonary and cerebral edema requires urgent treatment as outlined in question 47.

A consensus conference recommended that experienced medical personnel documenting severe symptomatic exertional hyponatremia in the field give 100 mL of 3% saline over 10 minutes. This should safely raise the serum sodium concentration 2 to 3 mEq/L. This recommendation is only for athletes with severe hyponatremia and associated symptoms and signs (confusion, vomiting, respiratory insufficiency) as in this patient. The patient should then always be immediately transported to the hospital for further monitoring, evaluation, and treatment.

50. **A 67-year-old man with longstanding hypertension presents to the ER alert, somewhat confused, and with sudden onset of a severe headache he describes as 10/10 pain. CT scan showed Stage 3 subarachnoid hemorrhage. You see the patient in the ICU 2 days later with hyponatremia, continued headache, irritability, and worsening confusion. He has no focal neurological signs. BP 130/70, P 95 supine, and the patient has no edema. Na 122, K 3.7, BUN 10, Creatinine 1.0, $P_{osm} = 262$, $U_{osm} = 480$, $U_{Na} = 142$, and $U_K = 48$. Thyroid and adrenal function are normal. What is the cause of the hyponatremia and how would you treat it?**

Hyponatremia following subarachnoid hemorrhage may be due to SIADH or to cerebral salt-wasting (CSW). The distinction between the two is controversial and clinically often unclear. The main differentiating feature is volume status. In SIADH, volume is normal or slightly increased. In CSW, volume is low due to excessive urinary sodium loss with resulting decreased ECV, appropriate increase in ADH, and water retention. The cause of the increased urinary sodium excretion and volume loss in the face of deceased ECV is not clear. However, it may be related to increased sympathetic nervous system activity and to excess natriuretic peptides, such as BNP, ANP, and a digoxin-like peptide. Because of his worsening confusion, treat this patient with 3% saline as outlined in question 47 and discontinue any hypotonic fluids. However, if hyponatremia was present with no neurological signs, the approach would be more controversial. Because SAH and other CNS-related hyponatremia is reported more often with SIADH than CSW, water restriction may be considered in the asymptomatic patient. However, if there is any suspicion of decreased volume (as might be in this patient with BP that is relatively low for a hypertensive patient), one must suspect CSW. Treatment of hyponatremia caused by CSW in an asymptomatic patient is infusion of normal saline. Nevertheless, infusion of normal saline in SIADH may worsen hyponatremia, because the water will be retained and the excess sodium excreted. Because true volume status is so difficult to assess in many patients, some experts recommend treating all patients with CNS related hyponatremia with 3% saline. Others do not. Whatever treatment is selected, monitor the patient carefully, and correct the sodium judiciously as outlined in questions 40, 41, and 47.

51. **A 23-year-old woman presents to your clinic with morning nausea and mild headache. She has a normal examination with exception of midline fullness just above the pubic symphysis. Basic labs were also normal except sodium of 132 mEq/L. How might you evaluate her hyponatremia?**
Further history revealed she had never been pregnant, her last menstrual period was 3 months prior, and her pregnancy test was positive. An appointment was made for obstetrical follow-up. Early in pregnancy, there is a 40% expansion of the ECF with more water retained than sodium, causing a 10 mOsm/kg decrease in plasma osmolality and mild hyponatremia. As with many causes of hyponatremia, there is an initial decrease in ECV resulting from systemic arterial vasodilation that occurs early in the first trimester. Normal pregnancy-related increases in estrogen and hCG stimulate increases in nitric oxide and relaxin felt to be responsible for the vasodilation. The prospective mother compensates with an increase in thirst, cardiac output, activation of the renin-angiotensin-aldosterone system, and the activation of arterial baroreceptors. There is a resulting nonosmotic AVP release, upregulation of renal medullary AQP2 receptors, and renal retention of salt and water (water > salt). Nausea may also increase AVP release. The net result of these changes is an expanded ECF with mild hyponatremia commonly seen in normal pregnancy. Because AVP changes to osmolality and volume respond normally around a new set point of about 270 mOsm/kg, hyponatremia of pregnancy is felt related mostly to resetting of the hypothalamic osmostat. However, because there is clearly volume expansion, the pathophysiology is more complex. Nevertheless, hyponatremia of pregnancy is mild, usually asymptomatic, and returns to normal within 1 to 2 months of delivery. Thus no treatment or further evaluation is needed.

WEBSITES

1. American Academy of Family Physicians: Hyponatremia and hypernatremia in the elderly. Available at: http://www.aafp.org/afp/20000615/3623.html

2. British Medical Journal: Exercise-induced hyponatremia. Available at: http://bmj. bmjjournals.com/cgi/content/full/327/7407/113#REF3

3. EMedcine: SIADH review. Available at: http://www.emedicine.com/ped/topic2190.htm

4. EMedicine: Lithium nephropathy review. Available at: http://www.emedicine.com/med/topic1313.htm

5. EMedicine: Diabetes insipidus review. Available at: http://www.emedicine.com/med/topic543.htm

6. EMedicine: Diabetes insipidus review. Available at: http://master.emedicine.com/ped/topic580.htm

7. EMedicine: Hyponatremia review. Available at: http://www.emedicine.com/med/topic1130.htm

8. Postgraduate Medicine: Hyponatremia and hypernatremia. Available at: http://www.postgradmed.com/issues/2000/05_00/fall.htm

9. Quarterly Journal of Medicine: Primary polydipsia review. Available at: http://qjmed.oupjournals.org/cgi/content/full/96/7/531

10. UCLA Endocrinology: SIADH. Available at: http://www.endocrinology.med.ucla.edu/siadh.htm

BIBLIOGRAPHY

1. Adrogue HJ, Madias NE: Hypernatremia. N Engl J Med 342:1493–1499, 2000.

2. Adrogue HJ, Madias NE: Hyponatremia. N Engl J Med 342:1581–1589, 2000.

3. Ayus JC, Varon J, Arieff AI: Hyponatremia, cerebral edema, and noncardiogenic pulmonary edema in marathon runners. Ann Intern Med 132:711–714, 2000.

4. Berendes E, Walter M, Cullen P, et al: Secretion of brain natriuretic peptide in patients with aneurysmal subarachnoid haemorrhage. Lancet 349:245–249, 1997.

5. Berl T, Schrier RW: Disorders of water metabolism. In Schrier RW, editor, *Renal and electrolyte disorders*, ed 6, Philadelphia, 2003, Lippincott Williams & Wilkins, 2003, pp. 1–63.

6. Ellison DH, Berl T: The syndrome of inappropriate antidiuresis. N Engl J Med 356:2064–2072, 2007.

7. Fall PJ: Hyponatremia and hypernatremia: a systematic approach to causes and their correction. Postgrad Med 107:75–82, 179, 2000.

8. Gross P, Reimann D, Henschkowski J, et al: Treatment of severe hyponatremia: conventional and novel aspects. J Am Soc Nephrol 12:S10–S14, 2001.

9. Gutierrez OM, Lin HY: Refractory hyponatremia. Kidney Int 71:79–82, 2007.

10. Hillier TA, Abbott RD, Barrett EJ: Hyponatremia: evaluating the correction factor for hyperglycemia. Am J Med 106:399–403, 1999.

11. Kugler JP, Hustead T: Hyponatremia and hypernatremia in the elderly. Am Fam Physician 61:3623–3630, 2000.

12. Mayinger B, Hensen J: Nonpeptide vasopressin antagonists: a new group of hormone blockers entering the scene. Exp Clin Endocrinol Diabetes 107:157–165, 1999.

13. Moritz ML, Ayus JC: Prevention of hospital-acquired hyponatremia: a case for using isotonic saline. Pediatrics 111:227–230, 2003.

14. Nielsen S, Kwon TH, Christensen BM, et al: Physiology and pathophysiology of renal aquaporins. J Am Soc Nephrol 10:647–663, 1999.

15. Oster JR, Singer I: Hyponatremia, hypo-osmolality, and hypotonicity: tables and fables. Arch Intern Med 159:333–336, 1999.

16. Palmer BF, Gates JR, Malcolm L: Causes and management of hyponatremia. Ann Pharmacother 37:1694–1702, 2003.

17. Rosner MH, Kirven J: In-depth review. Exercise-associated hyponatremia. Clin J Am Soc Nephrol 2:151–161, 2007.

18. Sanghvi SR, Kellerman PS, Nanovic L: Beer potomania: An unusual cause of hyponatremia at high risk of complications from rapid correction. Am J Kidney Dis 50:673–680, 2007.

19. Schrier, RW: Review. Body water homeostasis: clinical disorders of urinary dilution and concentration. J Am Soc Nephrol 17:1820–1832, 2006.

20. Shea AM, Hammill BG, Curtis LH, et al: Medical costs of abnormal serum sodium Levels. J Am Soc Nephrol 19:764–770, 2008.

21. Sherlock M, O'Sullivan E, Agha A, et al: The incidence and pathophysiology of hyponatraemia after subarachnoid haemorrhage. Clin Endocrinol (Oxf) 64:250–254, 2006.

22. Singer I, Oster JR, Fishman LM: The management of diabetes insipidus in adults. Arch Intern Med 157:1293–1301, 1997.

CHAPTER 25

DISORDERS OF GROWTH

Philip S. Zeitler

1. **Summarize normal growth velocity for children until the pubertal growth spurt.**
   - First 6 months: 16 to 17 cm
   - Second 6 months: approximately 8 cm
   - Second year: just over 10 cm
   - Third year: approximately 8 cm
   - Fourth year: 7 cm
   - Later childhood until puberty (5 to 10 years): growth averages 5 to 6 cm/year

2. **Summarize growth velocity during the pubertal growth spurt.**
   Maximum growth rate is 11 to 13 cm/year.
   In girls, growth spurt occurs early in puberty (breast Tanner stage II).
   Growth spurt is later in boys (pubic hair Tanner stage III–IV, testicular volume 12–15 mL).
   Some children may experience a transient period of slow growth just before the onset of puberty.

3. **How is height measured accurately?**
   - The most essential tool for the detection of growth abnormalities is the ability to obtain accurate and reproducible measurements. This requires the availability of appropriate equipment, as well as proper positioning of the patient.
   - At all ages, children should be measured at full stretch with a straight spine, because this is the only position that will be reproducible.
   - Children should be shoeless, and hair decorations or braids may need to be removed.
   - Scales with floppy arms are unreliable.

4. **What technique is used for infants up to 2 years of age?**
   The supine length of infants. Accurate measurement requires a supine stadiometer, a boxlike structure with a headboard and movable footplate. Two people are needed, with one holding the infant's head against the headboard while the other straightens the legs and places the ankles at 90 degrees against the movable footplate. The length is read from the attached measuring device, or marks are made for measurement by tape measure.

5. **Describe the technique for children 2 years of age and older.**
   - Standing height is measured. Accurate measurement requires a stadiometer with a rigid headboard, footplate, and backboard.
   - The child stands against the backboard, with heels, buttocks, thoracic spine, and head touching.
   - The measurer exerts upward pressure on the patient at the angle of the jaw to bring the spine into full stretch, and the headboard is lowered until it touches the top of the head. A counter reads the measurement.

- If a stadiometer is not available, the child should stand against a wall in the same position as used for a stadiometer. A rigid right angle is moved downward to touch the top of the head, and a mark is made and measured.
- Weight and head circumference (when appropriate) should be recorded.

6. **How is height recorded?**
The second critical tool for evaluation of growth is the standardized growth curve, and all measurements should be plotted rather than just recorded in the chart. A carefully constructed and up-to-date growth curve is critical to the recognition of growth abnormalities. Furthermore, the more points that are plotted on the curve, the greater the understanding of the child's growth. Thus efforts should be made to obtain growth measurements at all patient contacts, including illness visits, because well-child visits are infrequent during the middle childhood years when growth abnormalities are most common.

7. **List the common errors in plotting growth charts.**
Errors in plotting of growth points are a frequent cause of apparent growth abnormalities. Common errors include:
- Plotting the wrong height
- Not plotting the patient's height at the exact chronologic age (Height should be plotted to the nearest month or decimal age.)
- Use of an inappropriate growth chart

8. **What is meant by appropriate growth chart?**
A number of growth charts are available, and careful consideration should be given to the appropriate chart for a particular patient at a particular time. Commonly available growth charts include:
- Charts for plotting supine length (the 0- to 36-month charts in common use)
- Charts for plotting stature (i.e., standing height) (2- to 18-year charts)
Other specific growth charts include:
- Ethnic-specific charts
- Growth charts specific for common syndromes (e.g., Turner's syndrome, Down syndrome, achondroplasia) should be used when appropriate

9. **How do age and position affect growth measurements?**
- A patient measured supine is slightly longer than the same patient measured standing up.
- Charting of a standing patient on a supine chart gives the erroneous impression of decreased growth velocity. This is a common cause of apparent growth abnormality in children aged 2 to 3 years who are measured standing up for the first time.

10. **What historic information is necessary for interpreting a growth chart?**
- Birth history and birth weight
- Attainment of developmental milestones
- History of chronic illnesses
- Long-term medication use
- History of surgery or trauma
- Current symptoms
- Height of biological parents and family history of significant short stature
- Timing of parental puberty and family history of significant pubertal delay

11. **What physical examination findings help interpret a growth chart?**
    - Signs of chronic illness
    - Stigmata of a syndrome
    - Specific signs of hormonal abnormality (thyroid deficiency, growth hormone [GH] deficiency, glucocorticoid excess)

KEY POINTS: GENERAL GROWTH

1. Proper evaluation of growth depends on accurate measurement of height and correct plotting of measurements on the appropriate growth curve.

2. Common errors in plotting include plotting the wrong height, not plotting the patient's height at the exact chronologic age, and use of an inappropriate growth chart.

3. An abnormal growth velocity for age generally distinguishes growth abnormalities from normal growth variants.

4. Apparent abnormalities in growth are most frequently due to normal growth variants. Poor growth secondary to chronic medical illness is the next most frequent cause. Hormonal causes are less frequent.

12. **How does radiologic imaging help interpret a growth chart?**
    - A bone-age film can provide important information about skeletal maturity.
    - A radiograph of the left hand and wrist is obtained in children aged over 2 years, and maturation of epiphyseal centers is compared with available standards.

13. **Explain the significance of parental target height or "midparental height."**
    Parental height helps determine expected adult height based on genetic potential. Add the parents' heights in centimeters; add 13 cm if the child is male, and subtract 13 cm if the child is female; then divide by two. The resulting midparental height ±5 cm gives the 10th to 90th percentile for offspring of those parents.

14. **What is the most important factor in identifying an abnormal growth curve?**
    An abnormal growth velocity for age generally distinguishes growth abnormalities from normal growth variants. Although there are many causes of short stature, including genetic, short normal children grow normally, whereas children with a problem almost always have an abnormal growth velocity. For example, a fifth percentile child growing with a normal growth velocity is less worrisome than the child who has fallen from the 90th to the 75th percentile, even though the latter is taller than the former. Growth velocity abnormalities may, however, be subtle.

15. **What causes abnormal growth in children?**
    Abnormalities in growth are most frequently due to either normal growth variants (familial short stature or constitutional delay of growth and puberty) or underlying chronic medical illness, either recognized or unrecognized. Hormonal causes are less frequent.

16. **Which syndromes are associated with abnormal growth?**
    - Down syndrome
    - Prader-Willi syndrome
    - Turner's syndrome
    - Noonan's syndrome
    - Other chromosomal abnormalities

17. **List nonendocrine diseases and treatments that may be associated with poor growth.**
   - Malnutrition
   - Pulmonary disease (cystic fibrosis, asthma)
   - Cardiac disease
   - Rheumatologic disease
   - Gastrointestinal disease (Crohn's disease, inflammatory bowel disease)
   - Neurologic disease (ketogenic diet, stimulant medications)
   - Renal disease
   - Anemia
   - Neoplasia
   - Chronic glucocorticoid use

18. **Using the tools of growth curve, bone age, and height, how does one distinguish between familial (genetic) short stature and other causes?**
   Children with familial short stature grow at a normal velocity for age but with stature below the normal curve. They also grow within the expected target height percentile (i.e., they are as tall as expected for their genetic potential). If the child's projected height (by extrapolation of the growth curve) falls within the target range, the likelihood is high that current height is explained by genetic factors. Children with familial short stature also have a bone age approximately equal to chronologic age.

19. **Give an example of familial short stature versus other causes of short stature.**
   A 5-year-old whose height is below the third percentile, whose growth has traced a line parallel to the third percentile, whose height projects within the parental target range, and whose bone age is also 5 years is likely to have familial short stature. However, if the growth velocity is abnormal or projected height falls below the predicted range, other factors may be involved in the short stature (Figs. 25-1 and 25-2).

20. **Other than familial short stature, what is the most common cause of short stature?**
   Constitutional delay of growth (constitutional short stature), which affects up to 2% of children, is characterized by short stature and delayed bone age and represents a normal growth pattern simply shifted to a later age. Affected children typically have a period of subnormal growth between 18 and 30 months of age, followed by normal growth velocity throughout the remainder of childhood. In accord with the delayed developmental pattern, bone age is delayed. The continuing growth delay also results in a delay in pubertal development and physical maturity. Such children (usually boys) often have a family history of a similar growth pattern and may have a more dramatic deceleration of growth velocity before entering puberty than normal children. They complete their growth at a later age, reaching an adult height within the expected genetic potential (Fig. 25-3).

21. **How is the diagnosis of constitutional delay of growth made?**
   The diagnosis of constitutional delay of growth based on the following criteria does not require further laboratory support:
   - Period of slowed growth in the second year of life with downward crossing of percentiles
   - Normal growth velocity during childhood but with stature below the expected percentile for family
   - Delayed bone age
   - Height prediction appropriate for family (Plot the current height at the patient's bone age and follow the resulting percentile to adult height. In constitutional delay, this generally leads to a projected height within the parental target range.)
   - Positive family history, delayed dentition, and delayed puberty in adolescence

Girls: 2–18 years
Physical growth

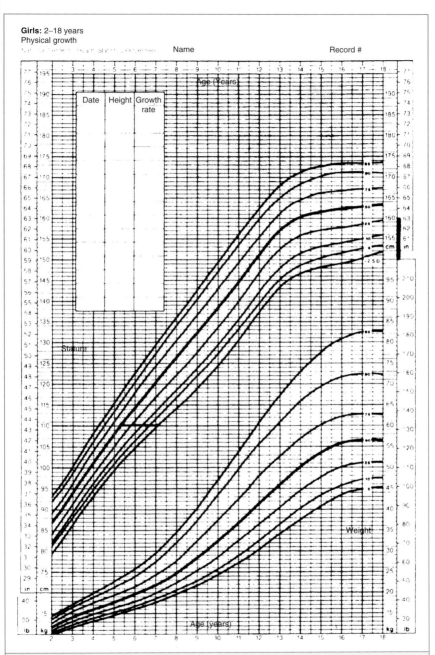

Figure 25-1. A 7-year-old girl with a height of 110 cm. Height age = 5 years, 3 months; bone age = 7 years; father's height = 65 inches (165 cm); mother's height = 62 inches (157 cm); corrected midparental height (± 1 SD) = 155 ± 5 cm; predicted adult height = 60 inches. The child has a predicted adult height within genetic potential and a bone age equal to chronologic age. She has genetic or familial short stature.

Girls: 2–18 years
Physical growth

Name   Record #

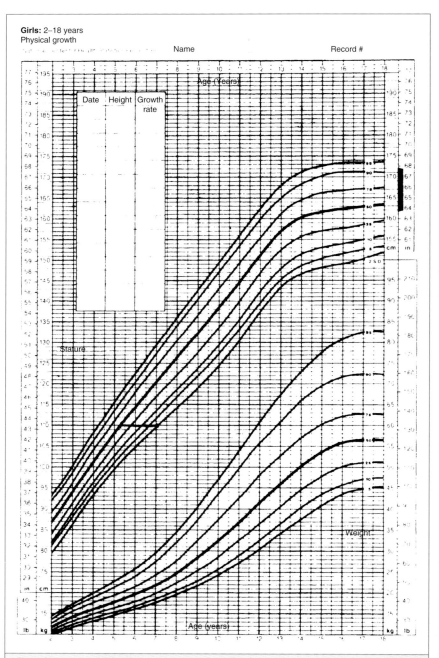

Figure 25-2. A 7-year-old girl with a height of 110 cm. Height age = 5 years, 3 months; bone age = 5 years; father's height = 70 inches (178 cm); mother's height = 66 inches (168 cm); corrected midparental height (± 1 SD) = 167. 5 ± 5 cm. The child is growing below the fifth percentile, but extrapolation of her growth curve to adult height gives a final height below genetic potential. Clearly her height cannot be attributed to genetic short stature alone.

Figure 25-3. Constitutional delay of growth. Subnormal velocity during second year of life followed by normal velocity through childhood and a prolonged growth period with eventual achievement of normal adult height.

22. **What is the effect of testosterone therapy on boys with constitutional delay of growth?**

Short-term testosterone therapy for boys with constitutional delay (75–100 mg of long-acting testosterone esters given once a month for 6 months) accelerates growth and stimulates pubertal development without compromising final adult height or advancing bone age. Clinically the boys experience pubertal changes, including genital enlargement (but not testicular growth), growth of pubic and axillary hair, deepening of voice, body odor, and acne. There may be personality changes characteristic of early puberty as well.

23. **List the endocrine causes for short stature in children in order of prevalence.**
    - Hypothyroidism: congenital or acquired
    - GH deficiency
    - Glucocorticoid excess: iatrogenic or endogenous (less common)
    - Pseudohypoparathyroidism

24. **What laboratory measures should be considered in evaluating a patient for short stature?**

Laboratory tests should be designed to achieve two goals: (1) exclusion of undiagnosed chronic illness and (2) exclusion of specific disorders associated with poor growth.

25. **Which laboratory tests help to exclude undiagnosed chronic illness?**
    - Electrolytes
    - Blood urea nitrogen/creatinine

- Liver transaminases
- Complete blood count
- Erythrocyte sedimentation rate (ESR)

26. **Which laboratory tests help to exclude gastrointestinal disorders associated with poor growth?**
Because symptoms may be limited, the following tests are recommended:
   - Celiac antibody (anti-tissue transglutaminase)
   - Inflammatory bowel disease screen if elevated ESR or anemia

27. **List the laboratory tests for genetic disorders associated with poor growth.**
   - Karyotype (Turner's syndrome): consider in all short girls
   - FISH for Prader Willi
   - PTPN11 mutation for Noonan's syndrome

28. **Which hormonal disorders should be excluded by laboratory results?**
   - Thyroid deficiency (thyroid-stimulating hormone [TSH] and total or free T4)
   - GH deficiency (see question 30)

29. **Describe the causes of GH deficiency.**
Most cases of GH deficiency are isolated and idiopathic. Idiopathic GH deficiency affects as many as 1:10000 to 1:15000 children. It is sporadic in the great majority of cases, but an increasing number of specific gene mutations involved in the synthesis of GH or the regulation of its secretion are being reported. The other important underlying causes are listed in the following sections.

30. **How is GH deficiency diagnosed?**
The diagnosis of GH deficiency is primarily a clinical one, aided by laboratory support, rather than a diagnosis based on definitive testing. Most important is choosing the appropriate patient. Children with subnormal growth should be evaluated for GH deficiency only after a thorough search fails to reveal any other cause for growth delay.

31. **List the components of the laboratory evaluation for GH deficiency.**
   - Serum levels of insulin-like growth factor 1 (IGF-1)
   - IGF-binding protein 3 may be useful in specific clinical situations (minimal variation with age, less affected by nutritional state)
   - GH testing

32. **Why are serum levels of IGF-1 important?**
IGF-1 is a GH-dependent protein that is produced in target tissues in response to GH. Serum levels of IGF-1 reflect production of the protein by the liver and give an indirect indication of GH secretion. The following characteristics of IGF-1 should be kept in mind when serum levels are assessed:
   - Concentrations of IGF-1 remain constant during the day, unlike levels of GH.
   - Concentrations of IGF-1 vary with age, and values must be compared with appropriate age-specific and pubertal stage—specific norms available from performing laboratories.
   - Low serum levels of IGF-1 (>2 SD below the mean for age) are 70% to 80% predictive of failing more rigorous tests of GH secretion.

33. **Do normal levels of IGF-1 exclude GH deficiency?**
Normal levels of IGF-1 are reassuring but do not rule out partial GH deficiency in the appropriate clinical context.

34. Do low serum levels of IGF-1 confirm the diagnosis of GH deficiency?
No. Poor nutrition, chronic disease, and hypothyroidism suppress IGF-1 concentrations.
In addition, before the age of 6 years, values are low, and the overlap between normal and
GH-deficient levels renders the test highly insensitive.

35. How is GH testing done?
Because secretion of GH is episodic, random levels are not helpful for the diagnosis of GH
deficiency. GH must be formally measured in response to a series of stimuli. Various
pharmacologic agents are used, but there is no consensus about which agents are optimal.
The child must have fasted overnight, be euthyroid, and have no underlying chronic disease or
psychosocial deviation. In addition, at least two tests are generally performed using different
stimulating agents.

36. How are the results of GH testing interpreted?
Normal children respond to stimulation with GH concentrations above 10 ng/mL. Failure to
respond to all tests with a value greater than 10 ng/mL is consistent with the diagnosis of classic
GH deficiency.
    Criteria for the diagnosis of partial GH deficiency and neurosecretory dysfunction (normal
pituitary response to stimuli, but low IGF-1, suggesting that endogenous GH secretion is
impaired) are less well established.

37. How is idiopathic GH deficiency diagnosed?
GH deficiency can be isolated or associated with other pituitary hormone deficiencies. It can be
congenital or result from trauma or an intracranial neoplasm. All patients diagnosed with GH
deficiency should have cranial imaging, unless the cause of the deficiency is previously known.
Isolated GH deficiency without identifiable etiology is considered idiopathic.

38. How is idiopathic GH deficiency treated?
GH is available through recombinant DNA technology, and the majority of children are treated
with 6 or 7 daily shots per week at a total weekly dose of approximately 0.30 mg/kg
administered subcutaneously. Because the effect of GH wanes after several years of therapy, it is
common to see dramatic catch-up growth ($\approx$10–12 cm/year) in the first or second year of
therapy, followed by velocities ranging from normal to 1.5 times normal in subsequent years.

**39. What is the prognosis for adult height in treated children with idiopathic
GH deficiency?**
Although nearly all treated children reach an adult height significantly better than predicted
before therapy is initiated, many do not reach their predicted genetic potential. Children
diagnosed and treated at an earlier age have a better height prognosis than those whose therapy
is initiated later. Similarly, the more mature the skeleton at diagnosis, the poorer the final
outcome.

40. When is GH therapy discontinued?
In children with idiopathic GH deficiency, the point of diminishing benefit of therapy correlates
with skeletal maturity rather than chronologic age or duration of therapy. Therapy often is
discontinued at a bone age of 15 years (96% of growth) to 16 years (98% of growth) in boys and
14 years (98% of growth) in girls. However, given what is now known about the effects of GH
deficiency in adulthood, some patients with severe deficiencies may require lifelong hormonal
replacement.

41. What other syndromes are considered indications for GH therapy?
GH is now U.S. Food and Drug Administration (FDA)–approved for the treatment of short stature
in a number of conditions in addition to GH deficiency:

1. Chronic renal insufficiency before transplant
2. Turner's syndrome (45 XO or mosaic variants)
3. AIDS wasting syndrome
4. Prader-Willi syndrome
5. Short stature due to intrauterine growth retardation in the absence of "catch-up" growth
6. Idiopathic short stature in boys with predicted adult height less than 63 inches and girls with predicted height less than 59 inches (normal GH secretion)

Indications 2 through 6 do not require demonstration of GH deficiency. The use of GH for treatment of idiopathic short stature remains controversial among pediatric endocrinologists.

42. **What is the prognosis for girls with Turner's syndrome treated with GH?**
Girls with Turner's syndrome generally demonstrate a significant increase in predicted adult height, with an average increase of 8.8 cm. The overall effectiveness of therapy, like that in GH deficiency, depends on chronologic age at initiation, bone age at initiation, and duration of treatment. Because GH therapy in Turner's syndrome normalizes height in younger girls, estrogen replacement therapy can be initiated at an age similar to the age of puberty of the patient's peers.

43. **What are the potential risks of human GH therapy?**
The side effects of GH therapy can be divided into three categories: (1) common but clinically unimportant, (2) uncommon with potential clinical importance, and (3) rare or theoretical.

44. **List the common but clinically unimportant side effects of GH therapy.**
- Acute correction of body water deficit after initiation of GH in deficient patients may lead to transient peripheral edema, headache, and joint aches and stiffness
- Increased average glucose concentration
- Increased systolic blood pressure

45. **List the uncommon side effects with potential clinical importance.**
- Pseudotumor cerebri
- Slipped capital femoral epiphysis
- Glucose intolerance
- Worsening of underlying scoliosis

46. **What rare or theoretical side effects may be associated with GH therapy?**
- Increased recurrence of brain tumors: not currently considered a concern.
- Increased incidence of leukemia: not currently considered to be a real concern
- Increased risk for development of a secondary neoplasm: recent reports suggest a small increase in the long-term risk of secondary development of meningioma in childhood cancer survivors treated with GH

47. **Should children with idiopathic short stature (without GH deficiency) be treated with GH?**
The FDA has approved the use of GH in children with idiopathic short stature with a predicted adult height less than 63 inches for boys and less than 59 inches for girls. However, the use of GH in children in whom no secretory abnormality can be demonstrated continues to be intensely controversial among pediatric endocrinologists. Short-term studies involving small cohorts have demonstrated a consistent increase in growth velocity with GH therapy in such children. Several studies that followed children to final height disagreed about the overall effectiveness of therapy. However, most studies agree that the increase in final adult height is limited and can be obtained only at significant financial cost. The decision to use GH in such children should be carefully considered and requires a thoughtful dialogue among child, family, and an experienced pediatric endocrinologist who knows the child well.

48. **How does the pattern of growth in children with excessive glucocorticoids differ from the pattern in children with exogenous obesity?**
    Glucocorticoid excess, whether iatrogenic (common) or intrinsic (rare), results in impairment of linear growth. The mechanism reflects increased protein catabolism, increased lipolysis, and a decline in collagen synthesis. Glucocorticoids also suppress the pulsatile release of GH from the pituitary gland and the production of IGF-1 at the target organ. The net result is that children with steroid excess are frequently short. They also have an increased weight/height ratio and appear obese. Children with exogenous obesity, on the other hand, generally show accelerated linear growth; thus they are not only obese but also tall for age.

49. **What conditions are associated with excessive growth in childhood?**
    Relatively few conditions result in overgrowth during childhood. These include familial tall stature (stature appropriate for parental target), constitutional advanced growth, hormonal causes, and genetic syndromes.

50. **Explain constitutional advanced growth.**
    Constitutional advanced growth is associated with advanced bone age, accelerated growth, and early puberty, with predicted adult height appropriate for parental target (see question 21). Obesity and familial factors may be involved.

51. **List the hormonal causes of excessive growth.**
    - Hyperthyroidism
    - Androgen excess
    - GH excess (pituitary gigantism)
    - Estrogen excess

52. **Summarize the characteristics of GH excess in childhood.**
    GH excess is rare in children, in whom it causes tall stature rather than the bony overgrowth seen in adults (acromegaly). Diagnosis is based on the following laboratory results:
    - Elevated random levels of GH
    - Lack of suppression of GH during a standard glucose tolerance test
    - Extremely high levels of IGF-1

53. **With what findings is androgen excess associated?**
    - Precocious puberty
    - Congenital adrenal hyperplasia
    - Androgen-producing tumor

54. **With what findings is estrogen excess associated?**
    - Precocious puberty
    - Estrogen-producing tumor

55. **List the genetic syndromes associated with excessive growth.**
    - Klinefelter's syndrome (47 XXY): tall stature, small testes, delay of puberty
    - Connective tissue disorders:
        - Marfan's syndrome: tall stature, arachnodactyly, joint laxity, lens displacement
        - Stickler's syndrome
    - Sotos's syndrome (cerebral gigantism): macrocephaly, progressive macrosomia, dilatated ventricles, retardation, advanced bone age
    - Beckwith-Wiedemann syndrome: macroglossia, umbilical hernia, hypoglycemia, macrosomia in infancy
    - Homocystinuria: arachnodactyly, retardation, homocystine in urine

KEY POINTS: GROWTH VARIANTS

1. Children with familial short stature grow at a normal velocity for age and within their expected target height percentile and have a bone age approximately equal to chronologic age.

2. Children with constitutional delay of growth have a period of slow growth in the second year of life but then grow with a normal growth velocity.

3. Children with constitutional delay of growth also have delayed bone age, height prediction appropriate for family, and delayed entry into puberty.

4. The diagnosis of a growth variant does not require laboratory confirmation, but growth should be followed over time to confirm the initial impression.

KEY POINTS: GROWTH HORMONE DEFICIENCY

1. Growth hormone deficiency is a clinical diagnosis.

2. Other causes of poor growth should be excluded.

3. Laboratory testing is supportive and confirmatory.

4. Laboratory measures include measurement of serum IGF-1 and growth hormone stimulation testing.

BIBLIOGRAPHY

1. Carel JC: Management of short stature with GnRH agonist and co-treatment with growth hormone: a controversial issue. Mol Cell Endocrinol 254–255:226–233, 2006.

2. Clayton PE, Cianfarani S, Czernichow P, et al: Management of the child born small for gestational age through to adulthood: a consensus statement of the International Societies of Pediatric Endocrinology and the Growth Hormone Research Society. J Clin Endocrinol Metab 92:804–810, 2007.

3. Cytrynbaum CS, Smith AC, Rubin T, Weksberg R: Advances in overgrowth syndromes: clinical classification to molecular delineation in Sotos syndrome and Beckwith-Wiedemann syndrome. Curr Opin Pediatr 17:740–746, 2005.

4. Davenport ML: Evidence for early initiation of growth hormone and transdermal estradiol therapies in girls with Turner syndrome. Growth Horm IGF Res 16:591–597, 2006.

5. Lee MM: Clinical Practice. Idiopathic short stature. N Engl J Med 354:2576–2582, 2006.

6. Myers SE, Carrel AL, Whitman BY, Allen DB: Sustained benefit after 2 years of growth hormone on body composition, fat utilization, physical strength and agility, and growth in Prader-Willi syndrome. J Pediatr 137:42–49, 2000.

7. Quigley CA. Growth hormone treatment of non-growth hormone deficient disorders. Endocrinol Metab Clin North AM 36:131–186, 2007.

8. Rosenbloom AL, Connor EL: Hypopituitarism and other disorders of the growth hormone-insulin like growth factor-1 axis. In Lifshitz F, editor, *Pediatric endocrinology*, New York, 2007, Informa Healthcare, Volume 2, pp. 65–100.

9. Zeitler PS, Meacham LR, Allen DB, et al, editors, *Principles and Practice of Pediatric Endocrinology*, Springfield IL, 2005, Charles C Thomas, pp. 857–910.

CHAPTER 26

GROWTH HORMONE AND INSULIN USE AND ABUSE

Kurt J. Reyes and Homer J. LeMar, Jr.

Marion Jones, Andy Pettitte, Jose Conseco, and Sean Merriman are only some of the major athletes who have admitted or been caught using performance-enhancing substances. Their admissions and the Mitchell Report have renewed the public's interest in performance-enhancing substances such as growth hormone and anabolic-androgenic steroids. This chapter and chapter 51 will cover the most recent evidence about the use, effect, and detection of these substances.

1. **What is growth hormone?**
   Growth hormone (GH) is a single-chain peptide hormone produced and secreted by somatotroph cells in the anterior pituitary gland. It is the most abundant hormone in the human pituitary. GH production increases at puberty and decreases with aging at an average rate of 14% per decade beyond age 40.

2. **How is the release of GH regulated?**
   GH secretion is stimulated by GH-releasing hormone (GH-RH) and inhibited by somatostatin, both from the hypothalamus. Another major regulator of GH production is insulin-like growth factor-1 (IGF-1), which acts at the pituitary to directly inhibit GH production and at the hypothalamus to inhibit the production of GH-RH and to stimulate somatostatin.

3. **List the actions of GH**
   As the name implies, GH stimulates both linear growth and growth of internal organs (Table 26-1).

4. **Does GH exert all of its effects directly?**
   No. Many of the effects are mediated by IGF-1, which is also called somatomedin C. GH stimulates the production of IGF-1 in peripheral tissues, particularly the liver.

5. **What causes excessive GH secretion, and what are the consequences?**
   The only significant cause of excessive GH secretion is a GH-producing pituitary tumor. GH excess during childhood results in gigantism. Robert Wadlow, the "Alton giant," reached a height of just over 8 feet 11 inches and wore size 37AA shoes. GH excess after epiphyseal closure results in acromegaly.

6. **What conditions are associated with a deficiency of GH?**
   GH deficiency can be congenital (genetic mutations) or may result from damage to the pituitary gland from intracranial tumors, surgery, radiation therapy, trauma, and a variety of infiltrative and infectious diseases. GH deficiency in adults, frequently overlooked in the past, has been more thoroughly studied and more frequently diagnosed in recent years.

7. **What are some common signs and symptoms of GH deficiency?**
   Deficient GH production in childhood results in short stature. GH deficiency in adults can result in increased adiposity, decreased lean body mass, decreased bone density, decreased

TABLE 26-1. ACTIONS OF GROWTH HORMONE AT SPECIFIC SITES	
Target System	**Actions**
Liver and muscle	Increases nitrogen retention, amino acid uptake, and protein synthesis
Cardiovascular	Increases cardiac muscle mass and increases cardiac output at rest and during maximal exercise
Hematologic	Increases plasma volume and red cell mass
Skeletal tissue	Increases bone mineral density and bone turnover
Connective tissue	Increases collagen turnover at nonskeletal sites, including tendons
Metabolism	Increases rates of sweating and thermal dispersion during exercise
Endocrine	
Acute action	Increases the uptake and utilization of glucose by muscle; antagonizes the lipolytic effect of catecholamines on adipose tissue
Chronic action	Reduces glucose utilization, enhances lipolysis, and increases lean body mass

extracellular water, reduced cardiac function, decreased muscle force and strength, and diminished exercise performance. Patients have reduced aerobic capacity and strength levels and often complain of lethargy and fatigue. Their quality of life is diminished, manifested by depression, anxiety, mental fatigue, and decreased self-esteem and life fulfillment. Excessive intra-abdominal fat is associated with an increased risk of cardiovascular disease, which is the predominant cause of mortality in these patients.

8. **Where do we get the GH used therapeutically?**
   From 1958 to 1985, GH was available only from the pituitaries of human cadavers. Since 1985, biosynthetic GH preparations have allowed production of much larger quantities of GH and markedly improved availability. A requirement for bioassays has become a U.S. Food and Drug Administration (FDA) requisite to substantiate biological activity among different preparations. The bioassays could soon be replaced by in vitro binding assays using GH receptors derived from molecular techniques.

9. **Besides availability, what problem was associated with GH derived from human cadavers?**
   Creutzfeldt-Jakob disease, an uncommon, rapidly progressive, and fatal spongiform encephalopathy, has been reported to result from iatrogenic transmission through human cadaver pituitary tissue. More than 30 young adults who had received human cadaver pituitary products have died of this disease, and at least 60 to 70 cases of Creutzfeldt-Jakob disease have been identified in recipients.

10. **List the FDA-approved uses of GH.**
    For several years, the only approved indication for GH therapy was treatment of short stature in children with GH deficiency. Currently, GH is also approved for treatment of short stature associated with Turner's syndrome, Prader-Willi syndrome and progressive chronic renal insufficiency in children, for wasting in patients with AIDS, and for replacement therapy in GH-deficient adults.

11. List the potential uses of GH.

GH has other potential uses: (1) Noonan's syndrome, (2) Russell-Silver syndrome, (3) intrauterine growth retardation (IUGR), (4) chondrodysplasia in children, (5) steroid-induced growth suppression, (6) short stature associated with myelomeningocele, (7) any severe wasting state (e.g., wounds, burns, cancer), (8) normal aging, (9) nonislet-cell tumor hypoglycemia, (10) gonadal dysgenesis, (11) Down syndrome, (12) short stature associated with neurofibromatosis, (13) osteoporosis, and (14) congestive heart failure.

12. How does GH help GH-deficient adults?

The reported beneficial effects in GH-deficient adults are an increase in muscle mass and function, reduction of total body fat mass, and increased plasma volume and improved peripheral blood flow. Reductions in serum total and low-density lipoprotein (LDL) cholesterol, reduction in diastolic blood pressure, a trend toward reduction in systolic blood pressure, and beneficial effects on bone metabolism and skeletal mass have also been documented. In addition, an improvement in psychological well-being and quality of life can occur with GH replacement.

13. What are the therapeutic doses of GH? How is it administered?

The recommended doses in North America for children are 0.175 to 0.35 mg/k/week in GH deficiency, 0.35 mg/k/week for impaired growth of chronic renal insufficiency, and 0.375 mg/k/week for Turner's syndrome. The dose can be divided into twice-weekly, thrice-weekly, or daily regimens. Daily injections appear to give greater growth velocity than less frequent administration. Currently, the appropriate adult replacement dose appears to be 0.006 mg/k/day with a maximal dose of 0.0125 mg/k/day. GH is administered by subcutaneous injection.

14. Why is GH used as an ergogenic aid by athletes?

Athletes have used GH in an effort to improve performance. Supraphysiologic doses of GH have been reported to increase lean body mass and reduce body fat in trained athletes. However, most data available suggest that GH administration has no beneficial effects on muscle strength, growth, or exercise performance in non-GH-deficient adults. In addition, some athletes using GH have reportedly been disappointed with the results.

15. How is abuse detected?

To date, there is no reliable way to detect GH use by athletes. During the 2000 Summer Olympics in Sydney, Australia, commentators discussed the use of drugs among athletes and noted the difficulty in detecting GH.

16. Why is GH abuse so difficult to detect?

Detection presents a number of unique problems. Endogenous GH is secreted naturally in a pulsatile manner; therefore, an increased level detected on random testing could simply reflect a spontaneous peak, especially because GH secretion is stimulated by acute exercise. Furthermore, GH release can also be affected by the nutritional supplements frequently used by athletes. Finally, exogenous GH is not distinguishable from endogenous GH by biochemical testing.

17. What is currently being tried to detect GH?

The International Olympic Committee and the European Union have established a collaborative study group to examine the possibility of developing a test to differentiate exogenous GH from endogenous GH secretion in athletes. Currently, these studies are evaluating the use of serum bone turnover markers, changes in GH-related peptides, serum concentrations of mixed GH isomers, and concentrations of IGF-1 and related peptides.

18. How prevalent is GH use among athletes?

The prevalence is not known because abuse is currently undetectable, but there has been an increase in reported GH abuse by athletes over the past decade. There have been several reported recent seizures of GH found in athletes' luggage. The well-publicized seizures of recombinant GH from Tour de France cyclists in 1998 suggest use at an elite level. Use is probably not as extensive as with anabolic-androgenic steroids. One limiting factor is the expense. Even a 1-month supply may cost several thousand dollars, depending on dosages.

19. What are the adverse effects of the therapeutic use of GH in adults?

Fluid retention causing edema and carpal tunnel syndrome are common in adults but not in children. Arthralgias, myalgias, paresthesias, and worsening glucose tolerance are also common and may be present in up to one third of patients taking GH. Other potential side effects include gynecomastia, pancreatitis, behavioral changes, worsening of neurofibromatosis, scoliosis and kyphosis, and hypertrophy of tonsils and adenoids.

20. What are the adverse effects of GH in children?

Pseudotumor cerebri has been reported in children; this is most common in children with renal disease, although it has also been observed in children with GH deficiency and in girls with Turner's syndrome. GH therapy is associated with an increased risk of slipped capital femoral epiphysis in the same three groups of children. Children with GH deficiency due to deletion of the GH gene may develop antibodies to GH with secondary growth deceleration. This phenomenon is rare in other children.

21. What malignancy has been linked to GH use?

None. More than 50 cases of leukemia have been reported in GH-treated patients; however, all such patients had risk factors or syndromes associated with the development of leukemia. No data support an increased risk of nonleukemic extracranial neoplasms with therapeutic GH use. Nevertheless, GH must be used cautiously in patients with known malignancy or benign tumors given the theoretical risk of potential growth in these lesions.

22. What adverse effects occur in athletes using GH?

Little is known about side effects of GH use in athletes. Chronic abuse of supraphysiologic GH doses may lead to features of acromegaly, osteoarthritis, irreversible bone and joint deformities, increased vascular, respiratory and cardiac abnormalities, hypertrophy of other organs, hypogonadism, diabetes mellitus, abnormal lipid metabolism, increased risk of breast and colon cancer, and muscle weakness due to myopathy. Current studies also suggest that GH use in combination with anabolic androgenic steroids may increase left ventricular mass and cause concentric myocardial remodeling. Clearly, in this scenario, the risk to athletes is potentially high.

23. GH is the proverbial fountain of youth. True or false?

False. However, alternative medicine companies promote products alleged to stimulate increased production of GH in hopes of reversing normal aging. This theory has been sustained through the years due to a study that suggested diminished secretion of GH is responsible for the effects of aging, including increased adipose tissue, decreased lean body mass, and thinning of the skin. Although GH replacement has a role in deficient individuals, no data prove that supplemental GH can reverse physiological aging. Nevertheless, many "antiaging" compounds that reportedly stimulate GH release are being marketed to the public with increasing popularity.

KEY POINTS: GROWTH HORMONE USE AND ABUSE

1. Common side effects of therapeutic growth hormone use are fluid retention, carpal tunnel syndrome, arthralgias, myalgias, paresthesias, and worsening glucose tolerance.

2. To date, there is no reliable way to detect growth hormone use by athletes because of the pulsatile manner of its release and the inability of current assays to distinguish exogenous hormone from endogenous hormone.

3. Chronic abuse of supraphysiologic doses of growth hormone may lead to features of acromegaly; osteoarthritis; irreversible bone and joint deformities; increased vascular, respiratory, and cardiac abnormalities; hypogonadism; diabetes mellitus; and abnormal lipid metabolism.

4. Athletes use growth hormone in an effort to improve performance; however, most available data suggest that the use of growth hormone does not have any effect on muscle strength, growth, or exercise performance in non–growth-hormone-deficient adults.

WEBSITES

1. Human Growth Foundation. Available at: http://www.hgfound.org/index.htm

2. Non-medical, commercial website about GH. Available at: http://www.steroid.com/Human-Growth-Hormone.php

3. Mayo Clinic Article about performance-enhancing medications. Avaiable at: http://www.mayoclinic.com/health/performance-enhancing-drugs/HQ01105

BIBLIOGRAPHY

1. Bildlingmaier M, Wu Z, Strasburger C: Doping with growth hormone. J Pediatr Endocrinol Metab14:1077–1083, 2001.

2. Blackman M, Sorkin J, Munzer T, et al: Growth hormone and sex steroid administration in healthy aged women and men: a randomized controlled trial. JAMA 288:2282–2292, 2002.

3. Blethen SL: Monitoring growth hormone NE treatment: safety considerations. Endocrinologist 6:369–374, 1996.

4. Bouillanne O, Raenfray M, Tissandier O, et al: Growth hormone therapy in elderly people: an age delaying drug? Fundam Clin Pharmacol 10:416–430, 1996.

5. Consensus guidelines for the diagnosis and treatment of adults with growth hormone deficiency: summary statement of the Growth Hormone Research Society Workshop on Adult Growth Hormone Deficiency. J Clin Endocrinol Metab 83:379,1998.

6. Cummings DE, Merriam GR: Growth hormone therapy in adults. Annu Rev Med 54:513–533, 2003.

7. Dean H: Does exogenous growth hormone improve athletic performance? Clin J Sport Med 12:250–253, 2002.

8. Hurel SJ, Koppiker N, Newkirk J, et al: Relationship of physical exercise and ageing to growth hormone production. Clin Endocrinol 51:687–691, 1999.

9. Jenkins PJ: Growth hormone and exercise. Clin Endocrinol 50:683–689, 1999.

10. Karila TA, Karjalainen JE, Mantysarri MJ, et al: Anabolic androgenic steroids produce dose-dependent increase in left ventricular mass in power athletes, and this effect is potentiated by concomitant use of growth hormone. Int J Sports Med 24:337–343, 2003.

11. Murray RD, Skillicorn CJ, Howell SJ, et al: Influences on quality of life in growth hormone-deficient adults and their effect on response to treatment. Clin Endocrinol 51:565–573, 1999.

12. Reiter EO, Rosenfeld RG: Normal and aberrant growth. In Wilson JD, Foster DW, editors, *Williams textbook of endocrinology*, ed 10, Philadelphia, 2003, W.B. Saunders, pp. 1427–1507.

13. Rodrigues-Arnao J, Jabbar J, Fulcher K, et al: Effects of growth hormone replacement on physical performance and body composition in growth hormone-deficient adults. Clin Endocrinol 51:53–60, 1999.

14. Rudman D, Feller A, Nagraj H, et al: Effects of growth hormone in men 60 years old. N Engl J Med. 323:1–6, 1990.

15. Melmed S, Kleinberg D: Anterior pituitary. In Wilson JD, Foster DW, editors, *Williams textbook of endocrinology*, ed 10, Philadelphia, 2003, pp. 219–242.

16. Wallace JD, Cuneo RC: Growth hormone abuse in athletes: a review. Endocrinologist 10:175–184, 2000.

17. Weber MM: Effects of growth hormone on skeletal muscle. Hormone Res 58(Suppl 3):43–48, 2002.

18. Zachwieja JJ, Yarasheski EK: Does growth hormone therapy in conjunction with resistance exercise increase muscle force production and muscle mass in men and women aged 60 years or older? Phys Ther 79:76–81, 1999.

PRIMARY ALDOSTERONISM

Arnold A. Asp

CHAPTER 27

1. **Define primary aldosteronism.**

   Primary aldosteronism is a generic term for a group of disorders, in which excessive production of aldosterone by the zona glomerulosa of the adrenal cortex occurs independently of normal renin-angiotensin stimulation. These primary disorders of the adrenal system are distinct from forms of secondary hyperaldosteronism due to excessive renin, such as renal artery stenosis. The five clinical entities comprising primary aldosteronism include bilateral hyperplasia of the zona glomerulosa (also known as idiopathic hyperaldosteronism [IHA]), solitary aldosterone-producing adenoma (APA), primary adrenal hyperplasia (PAH), adrenal carcinoma, and glucocorticoid-remediable aldosteronism. IHA and APA are the most important causes of primary aldosteronism.

2. **How common are these disorders?**

   The most common manifestation of hyperaldosteronism is hypertension. It is estimated that 0.05% to 12% of the hypertensive population may have primary aldosteronism. Excessive aldosterone secretion is associated with increased risk of cardiovascular disease.

3. **What are the common clinical manifestations of primary aldosteronism?**

   Aldosterone normally acts at the renal distal convoluted tubule to stimulate reabsorption of sodium ions (Na), as well as secretion of potassium (K) and hydrogen ions (H), and at the cortical and medullary collecting ducts to cause direct secretion of H. Excess secretion of aldosterone in primary aldosteronism results in hypertension, hypokalemia, and metabolic alkalosis; hypomagnesemia may occur (Fig. 27-1). Spontaneous hypokalemia (K <3.5 mEq/L) occurs in 80% of cases of primary aldosteronism; the remaining patients develop hypokalemia within 3 to 5 days of initiation of liberal sodium intake (150 mEq/day). Most symptoms are manifestations of hypokalemia: weakness, muscle cramping, paresthesias, headaches, palpitations, polyuria, and polydipsia. Hyperglycemia due to insulinopenia occurs in approximately 25% of patients.

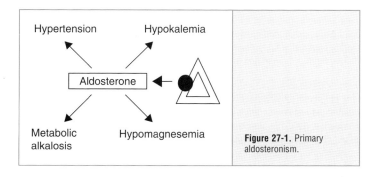

Figure 27-1. Primary aldosteronism.

4. **When and in whom is primary aldosteronism most common?**
   This group of disorders affects more women than men and occurs most commonly in the third through fifth decades of life.

5. **What is the most common form of primary aldosteronism?**
   Of the five causes mentioned in question 1, IHA is most common, accounting for up to 70% of cases in most series. IHA, also known as bilateral adrenal glomerulosa hyperplasia, is characterized by bilateral hyperplasia (diffuse and focal) of the zona glomerulosa layer of both adrenal glands. The most likely cause is supranormal sensitivity of the zona glomerulosa in affected adrenal glands to physiologic concentrations of angiotensin II.

6. **What is the second most common cause of primary aldosteronism?**
   APAs comprise 30% of primary aldosterone cases. APAs are small (<2 cm), occur more commonly in the left adrenal gland, and are composed of zona glomerulosa cells, zona reticularis cells, and hybrid cells with characteristics of both layers. APAs are also known as Conn's syndrome.

7. **How do adenomas produce symptoms of hyperaldosteronism?**
   Adenomas produce greater amounts of aldosterone than do other forms of aldosteronism; consequently, the degree of hypertension and the extent of biochemical abnormalities tend to be more severe. APAs also secrete excess 18-hydroxycorticosterone (18-OHB), an immediate precursor of aldosterone produced by hydroxylation of corticosterone; this facilitates the biochemical diagnosis. APAs demonstrate partial autonomy of function, secreting aldosterone in response to stimulation by corticotropin (adrenocorticotropic hormone [ACTH]) but not by angiotensin II. Aldosterone synthesis by these tumors, therefore, parallels the normal circadian rhythm of ACTH secretion, with the highest serum aldosterone concentrations occurring in the mornings and the lowest in the evenings.

8. **How do symptoms of IHA differ from symptoms of APAs?**
   Aldosterone is produced in smaller amounts in IHA than in APA; therefore the degree of hypertension, hypokalemia, hypomagnesemia, and metabolic alkalosis is less dramatic. Serum aldosterone levels tend to increase during upright posture, perhaps owing to increased sensitivity to angiotensin II.

9. **How commonly does adrenal cancer cause primary aldosteronism?**
   Adrenal carcinoma as a cause of aldosteronism is extremely rare. The tumors are very large (>6 cm) and metastatic at the time of diagnosis.

10. **What is PAH?**
    Primary adrenal hyperplasia, in which the zona glomerulosa of one adrenal gland becomes hyperplastic and histopathologically resembles unilateral IHA. Biochemically, however, such cases more closely resemble APA and respond to surgical resection.

11. **What is glucocorticoid-remediable aldosteronism?**
    In this rare cause of aldosteronism, production of mineralocorticoid is stimulated solely by ACTH. The disorder is inherited in an autosomal-dominant fashion.

12. **How is aldosterone synthesis regulated in the human body?**
    Humans possess two mitochondrial 11 b-hydroxylase isoenzymes that are responsible for cortisol and aldosterone synthesis (designated CYP11B1 and CYP11B2). Both are encoded on chromosome 8. CYP11B1, which is responsible for conversion of 11-deoxycortisol to cortisol, is expressed only in the zona reticularis. CYP11B2, which is responsible for the conversion of corticosterone to aldosterone, is expressed only in the zona glomerulosa. CYP11B1 activity is stimulated by ACTH, whereas CYP11B2 is stimulated by angiotensin II or hypokalemia.

13. **Explain the genetic basis of glucocorticoid-remediable aldosteronism.**
    Glucocorticoid-remediable aldosteronism results from a heritable mutation that causes the fusion of the promoter region of the CYP11B1 gene with the structural region of the CYP11B2 gene. The resulting chimeric gene responds to ACTH with overproduction of aldosterone, as well as precursors 18-hydroxycortisol and 18-oxocortisol. These metabolites of the cortisol C-18 oxidation pathway are biochemical markers that facilitate identification of affected kindreds. Excessive secretion of aldosterone may be inhibited by administration of glucocorticoids that suppress secretion of ACTH by the pituitary.

14. **How is primary aldosteronism diagnosed?**
    The diagnosis of primary aldosteronism is based on the demonstration of inappropriately elevated levels of plasma aldosterone (PA) with concomitantly suppressed plasma renin activity (PRA). Hypokalemia (K <3.5 mEq/L) is often the first clue.

15. **How are patients screened for primary aldosteronism?**
    The most sensitive screening test is the aldosterone/renin ratio (ARR). Concomitant PA and PRA values are obtained in the office (PA in ng/dL; PRA in ng/mL/h). ARR greater than 20 with PA exceeding 15 raises the possibility of primary aldosteronism. Most antihypertensive agents do not affect the PA/PRA ratio; spironolactone and eplrenone, however, must be discontinued for 6 weeks before screening.

16. **How is the diagnosis of primary aldosteronism confirmed?**
    In most centers, a 24-hour urine collection for aldosterone is used to confirm hyperaldosteronism. The patient must be sodium-replete to potentiate aldosterone excretion. Ample potassium supplements are given to ensure a serum potassium level greater than 3.5 mEq/L. The patient should consume 150 to 500 mEq of sodium and excrete at least 200 mEq of sodium a day. Urinary excretion of aldosterone (18-monogluconide) that exceeds 12 mg/day confirms primary aldosteronism.

17. **After confirmation of primary aldosteronism, why is it important to differentiate APA from IHA?**
    APA is amenable to surgical resection of the involved adrenal gland, whereas IHA is usually treated medically.

18. **Does computed tomography or magnetic resonance imaging aid in differentiation?**
    To a limited extent, both localizing procedures may aid in identifying the cause of primary aldosteronism. A large APA may be discernible on high-resolution computed tomography (CT), which at some institutions can identify adenomas as small as 5 mm. Magnetic resonance imaging (MRI) at present performs as well as CT in identifying APA but involves higher cost and longer scan time. The diagnostic accuracy of MRI or CT in preoperatively localizing an APA has been reported to be 70% to 85%, but accuracy declines in older populations in which incidental hormonally inactive adrenal masses are more common. Some experts believe that biochemically silent adrenal masses are so rare in patients younger than 40 that no further evaluation is necessary. In patients over 40 years, adrenal venous sampling (AVS) must be performed to verify unilateral aldosterone production (see question 19). Adrenal carcinoma, a rare cause of excessive aldosterone, is easily identified with either CT or MRI.

19. **Which localizing test is required if CT or MRI identify an APA in a patient aged over 40 years?**
    A more invasive localizing procedure to differentiate a normal adrenal gland from one containing an adenoma is AVS. Many institutions feel AVS should be performed before surgical intervention for an APA is considered. In this procedure, catheters are introduced into the left and right adrenal veins and the inferior vena cava. Levels of PA are determined from these sites, along

with concomitant levels of cortisol following infusion of cosyntropin (synthetic ACTH). Cortisol levels are determined to ensure that the adrenal veins are properly catheterized. PA/cortisol is referred to as "cortisol-corrected" aldosterone. APAs produce large amounts of aldosterone; the normal adrenal vein concentration of PA is 100 to 400 ng/dL, whereas APAs may generate concentrations of 1000 to 10,000 ng/dL. The ratio of PA/cortisol produced on the affected side versus the unaffected side always exceeds 4:1. When compared with CT scan results, discordant AVS results are found in up 30% of cases.

20. **Explain the difficulty with adrenal venous sampling.**
Collection of aldosterone and cortisol from the left adrenal gland is relatively simple, because the venous effluent drains directly into the left renal vein. The venous flow from the right adrenal, however, flows directly into the inferior vena cava. Catheterization of the right adrenal vein is difficult because of the few angiographic landmarks. Contrast material used to localize the right adrenal gland can cause corticomedullary hemorrhage during the procedure.

21. **How accurate is adrenal venous sampling?**
Overall, the procedure is 90% accurate in localizing APA.

22. **How is the patient with APA managed?**
The patient undergoes screening tests, as described in question 15. The diagnosis of primary aldosteronism is confirmed with 24 hour urine aldosterone collection salt loading, as described in question 16. AVS reveals a 4:1 gradient between the adenoma and the "normal" adrenal and surgical resection of the affected adrenal is considered.

23. **What should be done after the APA is localized?**
After the APA is localized, unilateral adrenalectomy is performed. Laparoscopic resection is now widely available and is preferable to the open posterior approach. One year postoperatively, 70% of patients are normotensive. By the fifth postoperative year, only 53% remain normotensive. Normal potassium balance tends to be permanent.

24. **Do all patients with APA require surgery?**
No. Although surgical resection is preferred, patients who have other comorbid conditions that preclude surgery may be successfully treated medically as described in question 28.

25. **How is a patient with IHA managed?**
The patient undergoes screening and confirmatory tests, as described in questions 15 and 16. CT fails to reveal unilateral enlargement of the adrenals. AVS fails to lateralize. After the diagnosis of IHA is made, the patient is scrupulously sequestered from surgical colleagues.

KEY POINTS: PRIMARY ALDOSTERONISM

1. Spontaneous hypokalemia in a hypertensive patient should suggest the possibility of primary or secondary hyperaldosteronism.

2. Primary hyperaldosteronism may be due to bilateral hyperplasia or a small adenoma.

3. The best screen for primary hyperaldosteronism is a PA/PRA ratio greater than 20, with PA greater than 15 ng/dL.

4. Because computed tomography and magnetic resonance imaging are often unable to distinguish adenomas from hyperplasia, adrenal venous sampling may be necessary to localize the lesion.

5. Adenomas are treated surgically; bilateral hyperplasia is treated pharmacologically.

26. **What is the agent of choice for pharmacologic treatment of IHA?**
Pharmacologic therapy is effective. The agent of choice is spironolactone (50–200 mg b.i.d.), a competitive inhibitor of aldosterone. Hypokalemia corrects dramatically, whereas hypertension responds after 4 to 8 weeks. Unfortunately, spironolactone also inhibits synthesis of testosterone and peripheral action of androgens, causing decreased libido, impotence, and gynecomastia in men. Eplerenone (50 mg b.i.d.) is a selective aldosterone antagonist without many of the side effects of spironolactone; it is more costly and there are fewer long-term data available for this agent.

27. **What other pharmacological options are available?**
In patients intolerant of the agents in question 26, amiloride (5–15 mg b.i.d.) corrects hypokalemia within several days. A concomitant antihypertensive agent is usually necessary to reduce blood pressure. Success also has been reported in cases of IHA treated with calcium channel blockers (calcium is involved in the final common pathway for production of aldosterone) and angiotensin-converting enzyme inhibitors (IHA appears to be sensitive to low concentrations of angiotensin II).

28. **Describe the management of a patient with PAH.**
During evaluation, these rare cases appear to be APA. Screening and confirmatory tests, as described in questions 15 and 16, seemingly indicate an APA. Localizing tests are consistent with APA, and patients usually undergo surgical resection of a nodular hyperplastic gland. The diagnosis is made retrospectively, but surgery is curative.

29. **How is a patient with glucocorticoid-remediable aldosteronism managed?**
This disorder is discussed in questions 11 and 13. Therapy with low dosages of dexamethasone (0.75 mg/day) or any of the agents used for therapy of IHA (see questions 25 and 26) may be effective.

BIBLIOGRAPHY

1. Artega E, Klein R, Biglieri EG: Use of the saline infusion test to diagnose the cause of primary aldosteronism. Am J Med 79:722–728, 1985.

2. Blumenfeld JD, Sealey JE, Schlussel Y, et al: Diagnosis and treatment of primary hyperaldosteronism. Ann Intern Med 121:877–885, 1994.

3. Bornstein SR (moderator): Adrenocortical tumors: recent advances in basic concepts and clinical management. Ann Intern Med 130:759–771, 1999.

4. Dluhy RG, Lifton RP: Glucocorticoid-remediable aldosteronism. J Clin Endocrinol Metab 84:4341–4344, 1999.

5. Fardella CE, Mosso L, Gomez-Sanchez C, et al: Primary hyperaldosteronism in essential hypertensives: prevalence, biochemical profile, and molecular biology. J Clin Endocrinol Metab 85:1863–1867, 2000.

6. Ghose RP, Hall PM, Bravo EL: Medical management of aldosterone-producing adenomas. Ann Intern Med 131:105–108, 1999.

7. Harper R, Ferrett CG, McKnight JA, et al: Accuracy of CT scanning and adrenal vein sampling in the pre-operative localization of aldosterone-secreting adrenal adenomas. Q J Med 92:643–650, 1999.

8. Jossart GH, Burpee SE, Gagner M: Surgery of the adrenal glands. Endocrinol Metab North Am 29:57–68, 2000.

9. Liftin RP, Dluhy RG, Powers M, et al: A chimaeric 11-hydroxylase/aldosterone synthetase gene causes glucocorticoid-remediable aldosteronism and human hypertension. Nature 355:262–265, 1992.

10. Lim PO, Young WF, MacDonald TM. A review of the medical treatment of primary aldosteronism. J Hyperens 19:353–361, 2001.

11. Magill SB, Raff H, Shaker JL, et al: Comparison of adrenal vein sampling and computed tomography in the differentiation of primary aldosteronism. J Clin Endocrinol Metab 86:1066–1071, 2001.

12. Milliez P, Girerd X, Plouin PF, et al. Evidence for an increased rate of cardiovascular events in patients with primary aldosteronism. J Am Coll Cardiol 45:1243–1248, 2005.

13. Mulatero P, Rabbia F, Milan A et al. Drug effects on aldosterone/plasma renin activity ratio in primary aldosteronism. Hypertension 40:897–902, 2002.

14. Mulatero P, Stowasser M, Loh K, et al: Increased diagnoses of primary aldosteronism, including surgically correctable forms, in centers from five continents. J Clin Endocrinol Metab 89:1045–1050, 2004.

15. Sohaib SA, Peppercorn PD, Allen C, et al: Primary hyperaldosteronism (Conn syndrome): MR imaging findings. Radiology 214:527–531, 2000.

16. Tanabe A, Naruse M, Takagi S, et al: Variability in the renin/aldosterone profile under random and standardized sampling conditions in primary aldosteronism. J Clin Endocrinol Metab 88:2489–2492, 2003.

17. Tiu SC, Choi CH, Shek CC, et al. The use of aldosterone-renin ratio as a diagnostic test for primary hyperaldosteronism and its test characteristics under different conditions of blood sampling. J Clin Endocrinol Metab 90:72–78, 2005.

18. White PC: Disorders of aldosterone biosynthesis and action. N Engl J Med 331:250–258, 1994.

19. Young WF: Pheochromocytoma and primary aldosteronism: diagnostic approaches. Endocrinol Metab N Am 26:801–827, 1997.

20. Funder JW, Carey RM, Fardella C, et al: Case detection, diagnosis, and treatment of patients with primary aldosteronism: an Endocrine Society clinical practice guideline. J Clin Endocrinol Metab 93: 3266–3281, 2008.

CHAPTER 28

PHEOCHROMOCYTOMA

Arnold A. Asp

1. What is a pheochromocytoma?

A pheochromocytoma is an adrenal medullary tumor composed of chromaffin cells and capable of secreting biogenic amines and peptides, including epinephrine (EPI), norepinephrine (NE), and dopamine. These tumors arise from neural crest–derived cells, which also give rise to portions of the central nervous system and the sympathetic (paraganglion) system. Because of this common origin, neoplasms of the sympathetic ganglia, such as neuroblastomas, paragangliomas, and ganglioneuromas, may produce similar amines and peptides.

2. How common are pheochromocytomas?

Pheochromocytomas are relatively rare. Data from the Mayo Clinic indicate that pheochromocytomas occur in 2 to 8/1 million people/year; autopsy data from the same institution reflect an incidence of 0.3% (3/1000 autopsies), indicating that many pheochromocytomas go undetected during life. The incidence of pheochromocytoma from other countries, such as Japan, is lower: 0.4 cases/1 million people/year.

3. Where are pheochromocytomas located?

Nearly 90% of tumors arise within the adrenal glands, whereas approximately 10% are extra-adrenal and therefore classified as paragangliomas. Sporadic, solitary pheochromocytomas are located more commonly in the right adrenal gland, whereas familial forms (10% of all pheochromocytomas) are bilateral and multicentric. Bilateral adrenal tumors raise the possibility of multiple endocrine neoplasia 2A or 2B (MEN 2A or MEN 2B) syndromes (see Chapter 53).

4. Where are paragangliomas found?

Paragangliomas occur most commonly within the abdomen but also have been described along the entire sympathetic paraganglia chain from the base of the brain to the testicles. The most common locations for paragangliomas are the organ of Zuckerkandl, the aortic bifurcation, and the bladder wall; the mediastinum, heart, carotid arteries, and glomus jugulare bodies are less common locations.

5. Can pheochromocytomas metastasize?

Yes. Demonstration of a metastatic focus in tissue normally devoid of chromaffin cells is the only accepted indication that a pheochromocytoma is malignant. Metastasis occurs in 3% to 14% of cases. The most common sites of metastases include regional lymph nodes, liver, bone, lung, and muscle.

6. What is the rule of 10s for pheochromocytomas?

Approximately 10% are extra-adrenal, 10% bilateral, 10% familial, and 10% malignant.

7. What are the common clinical features of a pheochromocytoma?

The signs and symptoms of a pheochromocytoma are variable. The classic triad of sudden severe headaches, diaphoresis, and palpitations carries a high degree of specificity (94%) and sensitivity (91%) for pheochromocytoma in a hypertensive population. The absence of all three symptoms reliably excludes the condition. Hypertension occurs in 90% to 95% of cases and is paroxysmal in 25% to 50% of these (Fig. 28-1). Orthostatic hypotension occurs in 40% because of hypovolemia and impaired arterial and venous constriction responses. Tremor, pallor, and anxiety also may be accompanying signs, whereas flushing is uncommon.

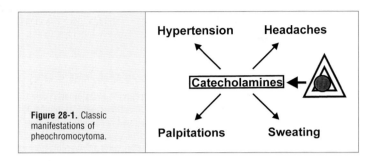

Figure 28-1. Classic manifestations of pheochromocytoma.

8. **What are some of the nonclassic manifestations of pheochromocytomas?**
Signs and symptoms of other endocrine disorders may dominate the presentation of a pheochromocytoma. Tumors may elaborate corticotropin (adrenocorticotropic hormone) with resultant manifestations of Cushing's syndrome and hypokalemic alkalosis. Vasoactive intestinal peptide may be produced, resulting in severe diarrhea. Hyperglycemia, resulting from catecholamine-associated antagonism of insulin release, and hypercalcemia, resulting from adrenergic stimulation of the parathyroid glands or elaboration of parathyroid hormone-related peptide, also have been encountered. Lactic acidosis may occur as a result of catecholamine-associated decrements in tissue oxygen delivery.

9. **Discuss the cardiovascular manifestations of pheochromocytomas.**
Cardiovascular manifestations of pheochromocytomas include arrhythmias and catecholamine-induced congestive cardiomyopathy. Atrial and ventricular fibrillations commonly result from precipitous release of catecholamines during surgery or from therapy with tricyclic antidepressants, phenothiazines, metoclopramide, and naloxone. Although cardiogenic pulmonary edema may result from cardiomyopathy, noncardiogenic pulmonary edema also may occur as a result of transient pulmonary vasoconstriction and increased capillary permeability.

10. **Describe the intracerebral symptoms related to pheochromocytoma.**
Seizures, altered mental status, and cerebral infarctions may occur as a result of intracerebral hemorrhage or embolization.

11. **What do pheochromocytomas elaborate?**
Most pheochromocytomas secrete NE. Tumors that produce EPI are more commonly intra-adrenal, because the extra-adrenal sympathetic ganglia do not contain phenylethanolamine-N methyltransferase (PNMT), which converts NE to EPI. Dopamine is most commonly associated with malignant tumors.

12. **Why is the blood pressure response among patients with pheochromocytomas so variable?**
    1. The tumors elaborate different biogenic amines. EPI, a beta-adrenergic stimulatory vasodilator that causes hypotension, is secreted by some intra-adrenal tumors, whereas NE, an alpha stimulatory vasoconstrictor that causes hypertension, is produced by most intra-adrenal and all extra-adrenal tumors.

2. Tumor size indirectly correlates with concentrations of plasma catecholamines. Large tumors (>50 g) manifest slow turnover rates and release catecholamine degradation products, whereas small tumors (<50 g) with rapid turnover rates elaborate active catecholamines.

3. Tissue responsiveness to ambient concentrations of catecholamines does not remain constant. Prolonged exposure of tissue to increased plasma catecholamines causes downregulation of $alpha_1$-receptors and tachyphylaxis. Plasma catecholamine levels therefore do not correlate with mean arterial pressure.

13. **How is a pheochromocytoma diagnosed?**
The diagnosis depends on the demonstration of excessive amounts of catecholamines in plasma or urine or degradation products in urine. The best screening test is measurement of plasma-free metanephrines (MNs). Plasma-free MNs may be drawn with the patient supine for 15 minutes following an overnight fast. Labetalol may alter results and should be withdrawn before assessment.

14. **How is pheochromocytoma differentiated from essential hypertension?**
Confirmation of elevated plasma-free MNs involves measurement of urinary MN, normetanephrine (NMN), vanillylmandelic acid (VMA), and free catecholamines produced in a 24-hour period. The ability of such tests to differentiate pheochromocytomas from essential hypertension varies among institutions: for VMA, sensitivity is 28% to 56% and specificity is 98%; for MN and NMN, sensitivity is 67% to 91% and specificity is 100%; and for free catecholamines, sensitivity is 100% and specificity is 98%. Many groups advocate 24-hour urinary levels of MN and catecholamines as good screening tests. Yield is improved when urine is collected after a paroxysmal episode of symptoms.

15. **What conditions may alter the diagnostic tests discussed earlier?**
Older assays for VMA were sensitive to dietary vanillin and phenolic acids, requiring patients to restrict their intake of such substances. High-pressure liquid chromatography assays have eliminated most false-positive results due to diet and drugs that alter the metabolism of catecholamines.

16. **Which drugs alter the metabolism of catecholamines?**
- Drugs that reduce plasma and urine concentrations: $alpha_2$ agonists, calcium channel blockers (chronic), angiotensin-converting enzyme inhibitors, bromocriptine
- Drugs that decrease VMA and increase catecholamines and MN: methyldopa, monoamine oxidase inhibitors
- Drugs that increase plasma or urine catecholamines: $alpha_1$ blockers, beta-blockers, labetalol
- Drugs that produce variable changes in any test: phenothiazines, tricyclic antidepressants, levodopa

17. **What other medications may interfere with test results?**
- Methylglucamine in radiocontrast agents (decreases MN)
- Methenamine mandelate (decreases urinary catecholamines)
- Clofibrate (decreases VMA)
- Nalidixic acid (increases VMA)

18. **List two other conditions that may interfere with test results.**
- Stimulation of endogenous catecholamines: physiologic stress (ischemia, exercise), drug withdrawal (alcohol, clonidine), vasodilator therapy (nitroglycerin, acute administration of calcium channel blockers)
- Administration of exogenous catecholamines: appetite suppressants, decongestants

19. **What other biochemical tests are available?**
Cases in which screening tests are equivocal may warrant a clonidine suppression test. This test employs a centrally acting $alpha_2$ agonist that, in patients without a pheochromocytoma,

suppresses neurogenically mediated release of catecholamines through the sympathetic nervous system. Blood samples to assess plasma catecholamines (NE and EPI) are drawn through an indwelling venous catheter; clonidine, 0.3 mg, is administered orally; plasma catecholamines are sampled again at 1, 2, and 3 hours. Plasma catecholamines decrease to less than 500 pg/mL in patients with essential hypertension but exceed this level in patients with pheochromocytomas.

20. **Compare computed tomography and magnetic resonance imaging (MRI) for localization of pheochromocytomas.**
The majority of tumors are larger than 3 cm, rendering them detectable by computed tomography (CT) or magnetic resonance imaging (MRI). CT, with special attention to the adrenal glands and pelvis, is advocated as the initial localizing procedure (97% are intra-abdominal). CT is the most cost-effective means of localization. Many also recommend MRI as an adjunctive localizing modality. Advantages of MRI include the lack of radiation exposure and the characteristic hyperintense image on T_2-weighted scans. The hyperintense image allows definition of tumor size, differentiation from vascular structures, and identification of unsuspected metastases.

KEY POINTS: PHEOCHROMOCYTOMA

1. Episodic headache, diaphoresis, and palpitations in a hypertensive patient suggest pheochromocytoma.

2. 10% of pheochromocytomas are bilateral, 10% extra-adrenal, 10% familial, and 10% malignant.

3. The best screening assay for pheochromocytoma is plasma-free metanephrines.

4. Confirmation of the diagnosis of pheochromocytoma is elevated 24-hour urine levels of metanephrines and catecholamines.

5. Localization of tumor is accomplished with computed tomography (most cost-effective) or magnetic resonance imaging (T_2-weighted phase).

6. Therapy is surgical resection after administration of alpha blockade followed by beta blockade.

21. **What other modalities are useful for localization of pheochromocytomas?**
Scintigraphic localization with m-(^{123}I) iodobenzylguanidine (MIBG) may also reveal unsuspected metastases. MIBG is actively concentrated by sympathomedullary tissue and is subject to interference by drugs that block reuptake of catecholamines (tricyclic antidepressants, guanethidine, labetalol).

22. **Summarize the performance criteria of each localizing procedure.**

	CT (%)	MRI (%)	MIBG (%)
Sensitivity	98	100	78
Specificity	70	67	100
Positive predictive value	69	83	100
Negative predictive value	98	100	87

23. **How are pheochromocytomas treated?**
Surgical resection is the only definitive therapy.

24. **Why is preoperative preparation with alpha blockade recommended?**
Alpha blockade reduces the incidence of intraoperative hypertensive crisis and postoperative hypotension. The most commonly used agent is phenoxybenzamine, a long-acting, noncompetitive antagonist (10–20 mg 2–3 times/day, advanced to 80–100 mg/day), or prazosin, a short-acting antagonist (1 mg t.i.d., advanced to 5 mg t.i.d.). Therapy may be limited by hypotension, tachycardia, and dizziness. Goals of therapy include blood pressure less than 160/90, an electrocardiogram (ECG) free of ST- or T-wave changes over 2 weeks before surgery, and no more than one premature ventricular contraction within 15 minutes. Opinions about the duration of preparation vary between 7 and 28 days before surgery.

25. **Discuss the role of beta-blocker and other agents in the preoperative period.**
Beta blockade to control tachycardia is added only after alpha-adrenergic blockade has been instituted to prevent unopposed alpha stimulation. Other agents used in the preoperative period include labetalol or calcium channel blockers. Intraoperative hypertension associated with tumor manipulation may be controlled with either phentolamine or nitroprusside. Postoperative hypotension may be minimized by preoperative volume expansion with crystalloid.

26. **How are malignant pheochromocytomas treated?**
Although evidence of malignancy may be discovered at the time of surgery, metastases from slow-growing pheochromocytomas may remain inapparent for several years. Therapy is rarely curative, because the tumors respond poorly to radiation therapy and chemotherapy; treatment is therefore palliative. Surgical debulking is the therapy of choice, followed by use of alpha-methyltyrosine. This drug is a "false" catecholamine precursor that inhibits tyrosine hydroxylase (the rate-limiting enzyme in catecholamine synthesis) and reduces excessive production of catecholamines.

27. **Discuss the role of combination chemotherapy and MIBG ablation.**
Combination chemotherapy with cyclophosphamide, vincristine, and adriamycin may slow tumor growth, as may ablation with MIBG. Unfortunately, neither of these therapeutic measures has resulted in prolonged survival.

28. **What is the prognosis for patients with malignant pheochromocytoma?**
Prognosis is not dismal. Cases of 20-year survival have been reported, and the 5-year survival rate with malignant pheochromocytomas is 44%.

29. **Which medical conditions are associated with pheochromocytomas?**
   - MEN 2A: hyperparathyroidism, medullary carcinoma of the thyroid, pheochromocytoma
   - MEN 2B: medullary carcinoma of the thyroid, marfanoid habitus, pheochromocytoma
   - Carney's triad: paragangliomas, gastric epithelial leiomyosarcomas, benign pulmonary chondromas (females), and Leydig's cell tumors (males)
   - Neurofibromatosis: café-au-lait spots in 5% of patients with pheochromocytoma; 1% of patients with neurofibromatosis have pheochromocytomas
   - von Hippel-Lindau syndrome: retinal and cerebellar hemangioblastomas; as many as 10% may have pheochromocytomas

BIBLIOGRAPHY

1. Bravo EL: Evolving concepts in the pathophysiology, diagnosis and treatment of pheochromocytoma. Endocrine Rev 15:356–368, 1994.

2. Eisenhofer G: Editorial: Biochemical diagnosis of pheochromocytoma—Is it time to switch to plasma-free metanephrines? J Clin Endocrinol Metab 88:550–552, 2003.

3. Francis IR, Gross MD, Shapiro B, et al: Integrated imaging of adrenal disease. Radiology 187:1–13, 1992.

4. Golub MS, Tuck ML: Diagnostic and therapeutic strategies in pheochromocytoma. Endocrinologist 2:101–105, 1992.

5. Jossart GH, Burpee SE, Gagner M: Surgery of the adrenal glands. Endocrinol Metab Clin North Am 29:57–68, 2000.

6. Krane NK: Clinically unsuspected pheochromocytomas: experience at Henry Ford Hospital and a review of the literature. Arch Intern Med 146:54–57, 1986.

7. Kudva YC, Sawka AM, Young WF: The laboratory diagnosis of adrenal pheochromocytoma: the Mayo Clinic experience. J Clin Endocrinol Metab 88:4533–4539, 2003.

8. Lenders JW, Pacak K, Walther MM, et al. Biochemical diagnosis of pheochromocytoma: which test is best? JAMA 287: 1427–1434, 2002.

9. Prys-Roberts C: Phaeochromocytoma—recent progress in management. Br J Anaesth 85:44–57, 2000.

10. Sawka AM, Jaeschke R, Singh RJ, et al: A comparison of biochemical tests for pheochromocytoma: measurement of fractionated plasma metanephrines compared with the combination of 24-hour urinary metanephrines and catecholamines. J Clin Endocrinol Metab 88:553–558, 2003.

11. Sheps SG, Jiang N, Klee GG, van Heerden JA: Recent developments in the diagnosis and treatment of pheochromocytoma. Mayo Clin Proc 65:88–95, 1990.

12. Ulchaker JC, Goldfarb DA, Bravo EL, et al: Successful outcomes in pheochromocytoma surgery in the modern era. J Urol 161:764–767, 1999.

13. Wittles RM, Kaplan EL, Roizen MF: Sensitivity of diagnostic and localization tests for pheochromocytoma in clinical practice. Arch Intern Med 160:2521–2524, 2000.

14. Young WF: Pheochromocytoma and primary aldosteronism: diagnostic approaches. Endocrinol Metab Clin N Am 26:801–827, 1997.

15. Pacak K: Preoperative management of the pheochromocytoma patient. J Clin Endocrinol Metab 92: 4069–4079, 2007.

CHAPTER 29

ADRENAL MALIGNANCIES

Michael T. McDermott

1. **What types of cancer occur in the adrenal glands?**
   Carcinomas may arise in the adrenal cortex (adrenocortical carcinomas) or the adrenal medulla (malignant pheochromocytomas). They also may metastasize to the adrenals from other primary sites.

2. **Do adrenocortical carcinomas produce hormones?**
   Approximately 60% secrete steroid hormones; about 40% are nonfunctioning.

3. **What are the clinical features of functioning adrenocortical carcinomas?**
   Functioning adrenocortical carcinomas secrete cortisol, aldosterone, or androgens—alone or in combination. Cortisol overproduction, the most common of these, results in Cushing's syndrome. Excessive aldosterone causes hypertension and hypokalemia (Conn's syndrome). Excessive androgen secretion causes hirsutism and virilization in women and precocious puberty in children but is often asymptomatic in men (Fig. 29-1).

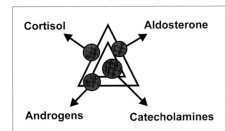

Figure 29-1. Functioning adrenal tumors.

4. **What are the clinical features of nonfunctioning adrenocortical carcinomas?**
   Nonfunctioning adrenocortical carcinomas present clinically as abdominal or flank pain or as an adrenal mass discovered incidentally during an imaging procedure.

5. **What clues are most suggestive that an adrenocortical tumor is malignant?**
   Malignancy is strongly suggested by tumor size greater than 6 cm, evidence of locally invasive or metastatic disease to the liver or lungs, and elevated urinary 17-ketosteroid excretion. The diagnosis of malignancy is often not suspected, however, until histologic examination after tumor removal.

6. **Describe the initial treatment for an adrenocortical carcinoma.**
   The initial treatment of choice is surgery. Adjuvant radiation therapy of the adrenal bed has been reported to significantly reduce the risk of local recurrence. Adjuvant chemotherapy with mitotane, an adrenal cytotoxic agent, has been shown to improve disease-free survival. Because of the high recurrence rates and poor survival rates associated with this malignancy, adjuvant tumor bed radiation therapy, mitotane therapy, or both should be considered after initial surgery in patients with adrenal cortical carcinoma.

7. **What studies are most commonly used to identify recurrent or metastatic adrenal cortical carcinoma?**
Computed tomography (CT) scanning of the chest, abdomen, and pelvis, F18-fluorodeoxyglucose positron emission tomography (FDG-PET) and PET/CT fusion scanning are the most effective modalities for identifiying recurrent and metastatic disease.

8. **What measures show the most promise for the treatment of metastatic adrenal cortical carcinoma?**
Mitotane, etoposide, and doxorubicin are the most effective individual chemotherapy agents, and cisplatin and streptozotocin in combination with mitotane show additional promise. An international phase III trial using these agents is currently underway (http://www.firm-act.org). Targeted therapies with antiangiogenesis agents and tyrosine kinase inhibitors are also under investigation.

9. **What is the prognosis for patients with adrenocortical carcinoma?**
The mean survival is 15 months. The 5-year survival rate is less than 30%. Prognosis is improved by young age, small tumor size, localized disease, complete tumor resection, and nonfunctioning tumors.

10. **How often are pheochromocytomas malignant?**
Approximately 10% to 15% of pheochromocytomas are malignant.

11. **What are the clinical features of a malignant pheochromocytoma?**
Most pheochromocytomas, whether benign or malignant, cause hypertension, headaches, sweating, and palpitations. They are diagnosed biochemically by the finding of increased levels of metanephrine or catecholamines in the plasma or urine. Malignant pheochromocytomas usually do not differ clinically at presentation from those that are benign.

12. **What clues suggest that a pheochromocytoma is malignant?**
Malignancy is most strongly suggested by tumor size greater than 6 cm, evidence of extra-adrenal spread (usually to the lymph nodes, liver, lungs, or bones) and by disproportionately increased plasma or urine levels of dopamine and/or homovanillic acid (HVA). The malignant character of some tumors may be missed, even histologically, and not become apparent until metastatic disease appears.

KEY POINTS: ADRENAL MALIGNANCIES

1. Adrenal cortical carcinomas present with features of cortisol, aldosterone, or androgen excess; with abdominal or flank pain; or as an incidentally discovered adrenal mass.

2. Malignant pheochromocytomas often present with features similar to those of benign pheochromocytomas (hypertension, headaches, palpitations, sweating).

3. Features suggesting that an adrenal tumor is malignant are size greater than 6 cm, evidence of local invasion or metastases to the liver or lung, and high levels of urinary 17 ketosteroids, homovanillic acid, or plasma dopamine.

4. Surgery is the treatment of choice for malignant adrenal tumors; tumor bed radiation therapy and mitotane chemotherapy are useful adjuvant therapies for adrenocortical carcinomas.

5. Incidentally discovered adrenal masses should be evaluated for evidence of malignancy (size >6 cm or progressive growth) and excess hormone secretion (cortisol, aldosterone, androgens, catecholamines).

13. **What is the treatment for a malignant pheochromocytoma?**
    Surgery is the treatment of choice. Alpha-adrenergic blocking agents (phenoxybenzamine, prazosin) or calcium channel blockers are given preoperatively to control blood pressure and replete intravascular volume. Beta-blockers may then be added for reflex tachycardia or persistent hypertension. These drugs and alpha-methyltyrosine, an inhibitor of catecholamine synthesis, are also effective chronic therapy for patients with unresectable tumors. Cyclophosphamide, vincristine, dacarbazine, and m-(^{131}I) iodobenzylguanidine may cause partial regression of residual tumors.

14. **What is the prognosis for malignant pheochromocytoma?**
    The 5-year survival rate for malignant pheochromocytoma is about 40%.

15. **What tumors metastasize to the adrenal glands?**
    The vascular adrenal glands are a frequent site of bilateral metastatic spread from cancers of the lung, breast, stomach, pancreas, colon, and kidney, and from melanomas and lymphomas.

16. **What is the clinical significance of metastatic disease to the adrenal glands?**
    Acute adrenal crises are rare. However, up to 33% of patients may have subtle adrenal insufficiency manifested by nonspecific symptoms and an inadequate response (peak cortisol level <20 mcg/dL) to a 250-mcg cosyntropin stimulation test. These patients may experience improvement in well-being when given physiologic glucocorticoid replacement.

17. **How should the incidentally discovered adrenal mass be evaluated?**
    Malignancy and excess hormone secretion are the main concerns. The best predictor of cancer is size; 25% of masses greater than 6 cm in size are malignant, whereas less than 2% of those that are under 4 cm in size are malignant. Subclinical Cushing's syndrome is the most common hormone disorder; the most risky is pheochromocytoma. Accordingly, the recommended hormone evaluation is a 1-mg overnight dexamethasone suppression test and measurement of plasma free metanephrines or fractionated urinary catecholamines and metanephrines. Patients with hypertension should also have measurements of plasma aldosterone and renin levels.

18. **How should the incidentally discovered adrenal mass be managed?**
    Surgery is often recommended for tumors greater than 4 cm in size, for those showing significant growth on follow-up, and for those with evidence of excessive cortisol, catecholamine, or aldosterone secretion. Nonfunctioning adrenal masses less than 4 cm in size should be reassessed in 6 months and then annually.

BIBLIOGRAPHY

1. Abiven G, Coste J, Groussin L, et al: Clinical and biological features in the prognosis of adrenocortical cancer: poor outcome of cortisol-secreting tumors in a series of 202 consecutive patients. J Clin Endocrinol Metab 91:2650–2655, 2006.

2. Allolio B, Fassnacht M: Clinical Review: Adrenocortical carcinoma: clinical update. J Clin Endocrinol Metab 91:2027–2037, 2006.

3. Assie G, Antoni G, Tissier F, et al: Prognostic parameters of metastatic adrenocortical carcinoma. J Clin Endocrinol Metab 92:148–154, 2007.

4. Berruti A, Terzolo M, Pia A, et al: Mitotane associated with etoposide, doxorubicin, and cisplatin in the treatment of advanced adrenocortical carcinoma. Cancer 83:2194–2200, 1998.

5. Beuschlein F, Looyenga BD, Reincke M, et al: Clinical impact of recent advances in the biology of adrenal cortical cancer. Endocrinologist 13:470–478, 2003.

6. Bornstein SR, Stratakis CA, Chrousos GP: Adrenocortical tumors: recent advances in basic concepts and clinical management. Ann Intern Med 130:759–771, 1999.

7. Fassnacht M, Hahner S, Polat B, et al: Efficacy of adjuvant radiotherapy of the tumor bed on local recurrence of adrenocortical carcinoma. J Clin Endocrinol Metab 91:4501–4504, 2006.

8. Kirschner LS: Review: Emerging treatment strategies for adrenocortical carcinoma: a new hope. J Clin Endocrinol Metab 91:14–21, 2006.

9. Leboulleux S, Dromain G, Bonniaud G, et al: Diagnostic and prognostic value of 18-fluorodeoxyglucose positron emission tomography in adrenocortical carcinoma: a prospective comparison with computed tomography. J Clin Endocrinol Metab 91:920–925, 2006.

10. Mackie GC, Shulkin BL, Ribiero RC, et al: Use of [F18] fluorodeoxyglucose positron emission tomography in evaluating locally recurrent and metastatic adrenocortical carcinoma. J Clin Endocrinol Metab 91: 2665–2671, 2006.

11. Terzolo M, Angeli A, Fassnacht M, et al: Adjuvant mitotane treatment for adrenocortical carcinoma. N Engl J Med 356:2372–2380, 2007.

12. Tritos NA, Cushing GW, Heatley G, Libertino JA: Clinical features and prognostic factors associated with adrenocortical carcinoma: Lahey Clinic Medical Center experience. Am Surg 66:73–79, 2000.

13. Williamson SK, Lew D, Miller GJ, et al: Phase II evaluation of cisplatin and etoposide followed by mitotane at disease progression in patients with locally advanced or metastatic adrenocortical carcinoma: a Southwest Oncology Group Study. Cancer 88:1159–1165, 2000.

14. Young WF: The incidentally discovered adrenal mass. N Engl J Med 356: 601–610, 2007.

CHAPTER 30

ADRENAL INSUFFICIENCY

Cecilia C. L. Wang, Marissa Grotzke, and Robert E. Jones

1. **What is adrenal insufficiency, and how is it categorized?**

   Adrenal insufficiency is the term used to describe inadequate production of glucocorticoids, mineralocorticoids, or both by the adrenal glands. This can occur because of dysfunction or complete destruction of the adrenal cortex (primary adrenal insufficiency), inadequate adrenocorticotropic hormone (ACTH) production by the pituitary (secondary adrenal insufficiency), or inadequate corticotropin-releasing hormone (CRH) production by the hypothalamus (tertiary adrenal insufficiency).

2. **What are common causes of adrenal insufficiency?**

   Autoimmune adrenalitis (Addison's disease) is the most common cause of primary adrenal insufficiency. This can occur in isolation or in combination with other endocrine deficiencies as part of an autoimmune polyglandular syndrome.

   Adrenal insufficiency occurring as part of panhypopituitarism is probably the most common cause of secondary adrenal insufficiency. Large pituitary tumors can compress and interfere with the function of pituitary corticotrophs (ACTH-producing cells in the pituitary). Radiation therapy for pituitary tumors also destroys corticotrophs.

   Another common cause for central (secondary/tertiary) adrenal insufficiency is withdrawal of glucocorticoids after long-term use or discontinuation after large doses are used. Prednisone is used to treat many chronic inflammatory diseases such as rheumatoid arthritis and systemic lupus erythematosis, as well as for exacerbations and maintenance of many common diseases such as chronic obstructive pulmonary disease and asthma. Therefore many individuals are at risk for developing temporary adrenal insufficiency from suppression of the hypothalamic-pituitary-adrenal axis by exogenous glucocorticoids and subsequent discontinuation of glucocorticoid therapy.

3. **What are other causes of adrenal insufficiency?**

   See Table 30-1.

4. **What are common symptoms of adrenal insufficiency?**

   Most patients report nonspecific symptoms such as weakness, fatigue, and anorexia. Many also complain of gastrointestinal symptoms such as nausea, vomiting, vague abdominal pain, or constipation. Symptoms of orthostatic hypotension, arthralgias, myalgias, and salt craving are also reported. Psychiatric symptoms can range from mild cognitive deficits to psychosis.

5. **How does adrenal insufficiency usually present clinically?**

   Weight loss is a common presenting sign. Hyperpigmentation, particularly of the buccal mucosa and gums, is noted in most patients with primary adrenal insufficiency. Patients should be examined for darkening of the palmar creases, nail beds, and scars forming after onset of ACTH excess, as well as increased numbers of freckles. Hyperpigmentation occurs because there is increased ACTH production in response to primary adrenal failure with subsequently increased binding of ACTH to the melanocyte-stimulating hormone receptor. Hypotension is common in

TABLE 30-1. CAUSES OF ADRENAL INSUFFICIENCY

Primary	Secondary	Tertiary
■ Autoimmune ■ Bilateral adrenal hemorrhage or thrombosis: coagulopathy, meningococcal sepsis ■ Metastases: lymphoma, lung, breast, renal, gastrointestinal ■ Infectious: tuberculosis, HIV, CMV, fungal (Histo, Cocci) ■ Adrenoleukodystrophy and other congenital disorders ■ After adrenalectomy ■ Infiltrative: hemochromatosis, amyloidosis ■ Congenital adrenal hyperplasia ■ Adrenal enzyme deficiency ■ Drugs: etomidate, ketoconazole, metyrapone, aminoglutethimide, rifampin	■ Pituitary tumors including craniopharyngioma ■ Metastases to the pituitary ■ Pituitary surgery or irradiation ■ Lymphocytic hypophysitis ■ Infiltrative diseases: sarcoidosis, histiocytosis X ■ Infection: e.g., tuberculosis, histoplasmosis ■ Sheehan's syndrome (massive blood loss leading to shock in the peripartum period) ■ Severe head trauma disrupting the pituitary stalk or otherwise affecting the pituitary	■ Withdrawal of long-term suppressive glucocorticoid therapy ■ Hypothalamic tumors ■ Infiltrative diseases affecting the hypothalamus ■ Cranial irradiation

CMV, cytomegalovirus.

both primary and secondary adrenal insufficiency. Loss of adrenal androgen secretion can cause loss of axillary and pubic hair that is more noticeable in women.

6. **What laboratory abnormalities can be found in adrenal insufficiency?**
   The classic laboratory abnormalities are hyponatremia and hyperkalemia. The hyperkalemia is from mineralocorticoid deficiency, whereas the hyponatremia mostly occurs because of glucocorticoid deficiency. Hyponatremia is the result of elevated vasopressin levels with free water retention, shift of extracellular sodium into cells, and decreased delivery of filtrate to the diluting segments of the nephron because of decreased glomerular filtration rate. Azotemia can be seen because of hypovolemia, with increased blood urea nitrogen and creatinine. Patients often develop a normocytic normochromic anemia and may have eosinophilia and a lymphocytosis. Mild to moderate hypercalcemia may occur in up to 6% of patients. Fasting blood glucose is usually low-normal, but occasionally patients can develop fasting or even postprandial hypoglycemia.

7. **How do the clinical presentations of primary and central adrenal insufficiency differ?**
   The clinical presentations of primary and secondary/tertiary adrenal insufficiency are similar with two key exceptions: hyperpigmentation and hyperkalemia are not observed in secondary/

tertiary adrenal insufficiency. The former is not seen because hyperpigmentation occurs as a result of increased ACTH production, and by definition there is insufficient ACTH production in central adrenal insufficiency. Hyperkalemia does not occur in central adrenal insufficiency because the adrenal zona glomerulosa remains responsive to the renin-angiotensin system, and aldosterone secretion remains intact. Therefore severe volume depletion is uncommon, and hyperkalemia is not encountered with loss of ACTH production alone. However, cortisol is important for free water clearance, so cortisol deficiency from any cause may cause hyponatremia.

8. **How is adrenal insufficiency usually diagnosed biochemically?**
   In the outpatient setting, a low morning cortisol (<3 μg/dL) is sufficient to diagnose adrenal insufficiency, and a high morning cortisol (>20 μg/dL) excludes the diagnosis.

   In most instances, the presence or absence of adrenal insufficiency is also evaluated using a dynamic test, the cosyntropin stimulation test. This test determines whether the adrenals are able to respond to maximal stimulation by synthetic ACTH, and is most useful for evaluating primary adrenal insufficiency. However, because there is loss of ACTH and/or CRH stimulation of the adrenal cortex in secondary/tertiary adrenal insufficiency resulting in adrenal atrophy and inability to produce cortisol normally in response to ACTH, this test is also useful in diagnosing secondary/tertiary adrenal insufficiency after the adrenal cortex has atrophied in response to lack of ACTH stimulation.

   The standard cosyntropin test is performed by drawing a baseline serum cortisol level, administering 250 μg of cosyntropin (brand name Cortrosyn) intravenously (IV) or intramuscularly (IM), then drawing serum cortisol 30 and 60 minutes later. An abnormal result seen in adrenal insufficiency is defined as a stimulated cortisol (at either 30 or 60 minutes) of less than 20 μg/dL (500 nmol/L). This test can be performed at any time during the day. If an individual is receiving hydrocortisone or prednisone, this should be held for 24 hours before the test is performed.

9. **What other methods are available for testing for adrenal insufficiency?**
   Other dynamic testing includes the insulin tolerance test and the metyrapone test. The insulin tolerance test evaluates the hypothalamic-pituitary-adrenal axis in response to insulin-induced hypoglycemia (blood glucose of <40 mg/dL). This test should only be performed in experienced centers with trained staff, and should not be performed if the individual has significant coronary artery disease or uncontrolled seizure disorder.

   Metyrapone is not generally available but can be obtained by contacting the manufacturer. Metyrapone blocks 11-beta hydroxylase and results in the inhibition of conversion of 11-deoxycortisol to cortisol. Thus administering metyrapone in the presence of a normally functioning hypothalamic-pituitary-adrenal (HPA) axis causes serum cortisol to decrease and 11-deoxycortisol to increase. Metyrapone is administered at midnight, and serum 11-deoxycortisol is measured the next morning. 11-deoxycortisol metabolites 17-hydroxycorticosteroids can also be measured in the urine. This test will be abnormal in any form of adrenal insufficiency (primary or secondary).

10. **What about the low dose cosyntropin stimulation test?**
    It has been argued that mild cases of primary adrenal insufficiency may be missed with the standard dose cosyntropin stimulation test because the dose of ACTH administered in this test is so supraphysiologic. Several studies have been published examining the potential role of low-dose cosyntropin stimulation testing, in which 1 μg cosyntropin is administered instead. However, these data do not clearly establish that the low-dose test is better than the standard test. Furthermore, there are several potential problems with performing the test, including false-positive testing as a result of inaccurate or irreproducible dilution of cosyntropin, the need for IV administration, and the need for carefully timed sampling for serum cortisol levels. A key question is whether abnormal results from this test are clinically relevant.

The standard test can be performed by administering cosyntropin intramuscularly with a single postdose cortisol determination, the exact timing of which is not very important. Therefore the standard dose test should be used in most instances because it is much easier to perform and has an accuracy similar to the low-dose test.

11. **What testing can be used to distinguish primary from secondary/tertiary adrenal insufficiency?**
Measuring serum ACTH and cortisol simultaneously helps to distinguish primary from secondary or tertiary adrenal insufficiency. In primary adrenal insufficiency, ACTH is elevated, whereas ACTH is "abnormally normal" (i.e., not elevated in response to low cortisol as would be expected) or frankly low in secondary or tertiary adrenal insufficiency.

12. **When can the results of the ACTH stimulation test be misleading?**
Partial ACTH deficiency and recent ACTH deficiency are situations that may lead to false-negative results of the cosyntropin stimulation test. Unfortunately the low-dose cosyntropin stimulation test is not consistently better than the standard dose test at distinguishing these individuals from those with normal adrenal axis function. Insulin-induced hypoglycemia (insulin tolerance testing) and metyrapone testing may be used in this situation.
    Clinical judgment must be used regarding whether the patient should receive empiric glucocorticoid replacement while testing is being performed and how to interpret results of the testing in the setting of exogenous glucocorticoids. In the acute setting, dexamethasone can be used for replacement because it cross-reacts less with the cortisol assay; however, this must be balanced with suppression of the HPA axis that can occur with longer-tem administration of exogenous glucocorticoids.

13. **When are imaging tests appropriate?**
After biochemical diagnosis of adrenal insufficiency, imaging may be performed in certain instances to help determine the cause. In cases of central adrenal insufficiency, imaging of the pituitary and hypothalamus would be indicated. Isolated central adrenal insufficiency is rare, but if panhypopituitarism is suspected with evidence for hypogonadism and possibly even central hypothyroidism, a pituitary MRI may be performed to search for a destructive process such as a pituitary macroadenoma or hypothalamic tumor. If a primary adrenal process is suspected such as bilateral adrenal hemorrhage or metastasis, an abdominal CT scan can be performed with thin cuts through the adrenals. Imaging should not be performed before a biochemical diagnosis is made because of the high incidence of incidental findings without clinical significance.

14. **When should the diagnosis of adrenal crisis be considered?**
Adrenal crisis should be suspected in patients with unexplained catecholamine-resistant hypotension or other signs or symptoms consistent with adrenal insufficiency. Acute adrenal hemorrhage should be suspected if there is a constellation of abdominal/flank pain, hypotension/shock, fever, and hypoglycemia in a deteriorating patient.

15. **How is adrenal crisis managed?**
If adrenal crisis is suspected, it should be treated aggressively. If left untreated, adrenal crisis is fatal. Formal diagnosis of adrenal insufficiency can be performed later. However, the patient can be treated with a dose of dexamethasone initially while the cosyntropin stimulation test is performed, then empirically treated with IV Solu-Medrol or hydrocortisone.
    Please see Table 30-2 for management of adrenal crisis.

16. **How is adrenal insufficiency diagnosed in the critical care setting?**
Because the diurnal rhythm of ACTH and cortisol secretion is disrupted in acute illness, and because severe stress should stimulate cortisol production, a random cortisol can be drawn to

TABLE 30-2.	MANAGEMENT OF ADRENAL CRISIS
The Five S's	
Salt	Normal saline
Sugar	5% dextrose added to normal saline
Steroids	Dexamethasone 4 mg initially then hydrocortisone 100 mg IV every 8 hours or just hydrocortisone IV (draw cortisol and ACTH first). Taper to maintenance levels 1–3 days after precipitating event or illness is under control
Support	In an intensive care unit setting
Search for precipitating illness	Draw serum cortisol and ACTH before giving hydrocortisone, or this can be done soon after a dose of dexamethasone

ACTH, adrenocorticotropic hormone; IV, intravenously.

diagnose adrenal insufficiency in the critical care setting. Patients who are hemodynamically unstable and unresponsive to pressors despite adequate fluid resuscitation, and patients with signs or symptoms suggestive of adrenal insufficiency should have a random cortisol level drawn and a cosyntropin stimulation test performed immediately afterward.

The cortisol level at which adrenal insufficiency should be diagnosed (<20 μg/dL as in the outpatient setting, some other value such as <25 μg/dL, and/or an increment of 9 μg/dL) is controversial. This is because of a concern about the existence of a cortisol resistant state in critically ill patients due to inflammatory cytokines, a reduction in binding affinity to cortisol binding globulin, and pro-inflammatory transcription factors. Therefore the thought is that a cortisol level that is adequate in an ambulatory setting or in routine uncomplicated anesthesia or surgical procedures may not be adequate in the setting of severe stress or prolonged or complicated surgical procedures. More studies are necessary to define the best approach to diagnosis and treatment in this setting.

17. **When and how should glucocorticoids be used in the critical care setting?**
Stress-dose steroids should be used empirically until results of the random cortisol and cosyntropin stimulation testing are available. Diagnostic testing for adrenal insufficiency must be performed to confirm the diagnosis, and patients should not be assumed to have adrenal insufficiency merely because of prolonged hypotension and response to glucocorticoids. Clinical studies have been mixed regarding which criteria to use and whether there is benefit of administering glucocorticoids unless adrenal insufficiency has been clearly demonstrated. However the benefit of stress-dose steroids in septic shock has been shown more consistently in clinical trials. There are also data that show benefit of stress-dose steroids in acute respiratory distress syndrome and in early bacterial meningitis.

Empiric therapy with hydrocortisone dosages ranging from 50 mg IV every 6 hours to 100 mg IV every 8 hours can be administered until results of cosyntropin stimulation testing available. These dosages should be tapered quickly as the patient's clinical status improves and the underlying illness resolves.

18. **How do I manage chronic adrenal insufficiency, and when should I consider prescribing fludrocortisone?**
Patients with chronic adrenal insufficiency require replacement with glucocorticoids, and occasionally with mineralocorticoid. Hydrocortisone and cortisone are the most frequently used

replacement glucocorticoids in primary adrenal insufficiency because these are synthetic forms of cortisol and have some mineralocorticoid activity. The usual dosage of hydrocortisone is 15 to 20 mg every morning and 5 to 10 mg in the afternoon. For cortisone, the usual dosage is 25 mg every morning and 12.5 mg in the afternoon. If additional mineralocorticoid effect is necessary for persistent hyperkalemia and/or orthostatic hypotension, fludrocortisone 0.05 to 0.2 mg once a day or in divided doses can be added.

Prednisone is most often used in secondary adrenal insufficiency and is usually given as a single dose of 5 mg every morning, but this can range from 2.5 to 7.5 mg every morning.

19. **Should I recommend dehydroepiandrosterone replacement for my adrenally insufficient patient?**
Dehydroepiandrosterone (DHEA) and dehydroepiandrosterone sulfate (DHEA-S) are the main androgens produced by the adrenals. Both are weak androgens, but in women they are converted to the more potent androgens testosterone and 5α-dihydrotestosterone (DHT) peripherally. This peripheral conversion is a significant source of androgens in women, and women with adrenal insufficiency have very low levels of circulating DHEA-S. Oral DHEA supplementation using 25 to 50 mg/day normalizes circulating levels of androgens in women with adrenal insufficiency. The impact on well-being, libido, and sexual function is variable in clinical trials, and larger trials are needed to examine this issue. Meanwhile, a trial of DHEA therapy in individual patients with adrenal insufficiency and impaired well-being may be justified.

A recent study showed that despite standard therapy, patients with adrenal insufficiency have significantly impaired subjective health status irrespective of the cause of the adrenal insufficiency or concomitant illnesses. Future studies will need to confirm these observations, and strategies may need to be developed to better replace glucocorticoids and possibly adrenal androgens to further improve the quality of life for patients with adrenal insufficiency.

20. **What are the relative potencies of available glucocorticoids?**
See Table 30-3.

TABLE 30-3. RELATIVE POTENCIES OF AVAILABLE STEROID FORMULATIONS				
Compound	Physiologic Replacement Dose, mg	Glucocorticoid Activity	Mineralocorticoid Activity	Duration of Action
Hydrocortisone*	20–25	1.0	1.0	Short
Cortisone	20–25	0.7	0.7	Short
Prednisone	5	4.0	0.7	Longer
Methylprednisolone	4	5.0	0.5	Short
Dexamethasone	0.5–0.75	30.0	0.0	Long

* Hydrocortisone is the synthetic form of cortisol.

21. **How is treatment for chronic adrenal insufficiency monitored?**
Adequate treatment for chronic adrenal insufficiency is monitored by taking a focused history regarding overall well-being and symptoms suggestive of orthostasis, and periodically evaluating blood pressure, electrolytes, and serial weights. It is important to avoid having patients on excessive dosages of replacement glucocorticoids, leading to iatrogenic Cushing's

syndrome, which can result in needless weight gain, osteoporosis, glaucoma, or avascular necrosis. The goal should be to use the smallest replacement dosage of glucocorticoids possible while maintaining normal electrolytes and good quality of life.

22. **When do individuals with chronic adrenal insufficiency require "stress-dose" glucocorticoids?**

Any medical stress including febrile illnesses, trauma, and diagnostic or surgical procedures can precipitate an acute adrenal crisis in patients with chronic adrenal insufficiency. Supplemental steroids should be used judiciously to prevent adrenal crisis, but care should be taken to avoid unnecessary supplemental doses of glucocorticoids.

The usual replacement dose should be doubled or tripled for mild to moderate infections, and during labor and delivery. Doses should also be doubled or tripled for approximately 24 hours for dental surgeries, minor surgeries (cataract, laparoscopic), and invasive diagnostic procedures. Patients who are unable to take their oral glucocorticoids or who develop symptoms suggestive of adrenal crisis should be hospitalized. Higher doses of IV or IM steroids are required for more severe infections, severe acute illnesses, and major surgeries. Patients who have had moderate-severe trauma should also receive stress dose glucocorticoids.

Planning ahead for situations in which patients will be in a remote area or otherwise far from medical care can help prevent morbidity and mortality from untreated adrenal crisis. Patients with adrenal insufficiency should wear a medical alert bracelet or necklace identifying them as individuals with adrenal insufficiency in case they are incapable of providing an adequate history. An alternative form of hydrocortisone or dexamethasone can be provided so that patients will still be able to receive glucocorticoids intramuscularly (hydrocortisone or dexamethasone) or per rectum (hydrocortisone) in an emergency situation.

23. **What are recommended stress doses of glucocorticoids?**

Stress doses of hydrocortisone should be tailored to the degree of stress. For moderate surgical stress, this should be 50 to 75 mg/day in divided doses for 1 or 2 days. Patients undergoing major surgery should receive 300 to 400 mg/day in divided doses for 2 to 3 days. The doses should be divided and given every 6 to 8 hours.

24. **How should glucocorticoids be tapered after stress dosing?**

The stress dose can be tapered over 1 to 2 days and the previous replacement dosage of glucocorticoids resumed after the underlying stress has resolved.

25. **What are some unusual causes of exogenous Cushing's syndrome?**

Glucocorticoids are used to treat a wide variety of disorders, so pharmacologic doses are used widely, and exogenous Cushing's syndrome is common. However, not all cases of exogenous Cushing's are a result of prescribed glucocorticoids. Cases have been reported involving surreptitious use of glucocorticoids. Cushing's syndrome resulting from herbal or complementary/alternative therapies containing glucocorticoids has also been reported. Glucocorticoids may also be prescribed for questionable diagnoses, and Cushing's has also been reported to result from a failure to stop glucocorticoid therapy after the illness being treated had resolved.

Megestrol acetate has sufficient glucocorticoid activity to cause Cushing's syndrome. It is a progestational agent used to treat AIDS cachexia and cancer cachexia. Megestrol and medroxyprogesterone are two nonglucocorticoid medications with enough glucocorticoid activity to cause Cushing's syndrome.

26. **What is the difference between adrenal suppression and adrenal insufficiency in patients on exogenous glucocorticoids?**

Adrenal suppression is caused by administration of exogenous glucocorticoids resulting in abnormal adrenal function. In 2001, more than 34 million prescriptions were written for the most commonly prescribed oral glucocorticoids in the United States (prednisone, methylprednisolone, prednisolone, and dexamethasone). Patients are also at risk for developing adrenal suppression from topical, inhaled, or intra-articular glucocorticoids. Factors that increase the risk for adrenal suppression with topical steroids include: use of highly potent class I glucocorticoids, application over a large skin surface area, prolonged period of administration, and use with an occlusive dressing. Inhaled glucocorticoids are more likely to cause adrenal suppression with greater dosage, longer duration of use, and use of a more potent agent such as fluticasone.

Adrenal suppression, which most often occurs without hypotension, is common, and these patients are at risk for developing overt adrenal insufficiency under stresses such as surgery and critical illness. However, secondary adrenal insufficiency induced by ACTH deficiency in this setting is much less common. Whether adrenal suppression occurs with a particular dosage, duration, or type of steroid varies widely among patients and is difficult to predict reliably.

Keep in mind that hypotension in acute illness can be due to a number of other causes including hypovolemia, sepsis, myocardial infarction, other disease processes, anesthesia per se, or other medications.

27. **How should steroids be tapered in patients on pharmacologic dosages of steroids to treat nonadrenal diseases?**
Patients may be placed on glucocorticoids to treat a variety of autoimmune, neoplastic, or inflammatory disorders. Discontinuing glucocorticoid therapy can be challenging for a number of reasons: (1) worsening of the disorder for which the glucocorticoid is being used, (2) suppression of the HPA axis with resulting secondary adrenal insufficiency upon discontinuation of the glucocorticoid, and (3) steroid withdrawal syndrome.

The initial tapering of glucocorticoids from pharmacologic to physiologic doses depends on the underlying illness for which the steroids are being used. If the illness worsens during this period of tapering, the dosage needs to be increased and continued until the symptoms stabilize before another attempt at more gradual tapering. When the patient is on a near-physiological dosage, she or he can be switched to a shorter-acting glucocorticoid such as hydrocortisone, and tapering continued to below-physiological dosages and alternate-day therapy in certain instances.

Testing should be performed when patients are at physiological doses or below, to ensure that adrenal suppression has resolved and that normal responsiveness of the HPA axis has returned. A morning cortisol should be drawn 24 hours after the last dose of glucocorticoid. A plasma cortisol level less than 3 μg/dL is consistent with adrenal insufficiency, so the glucocorticoid should be continued for 4 to 6 weeks before retesting. A level greater than 20 μg/dL is consistent with return of adrenal function, and glucocorticoids can be discontinued. A level between 3 and 20 μg/dL is equivocal, and further testing is necessary, usually using a cosyntropin stimulation test. It takes approximately 9 months and up to 12 months for the axis to respond normally to ACTH.

Adrenal suppression and resulting secondary adrenal insufficiency should be suspected in individuals with a clinical presentation suggestive of adrenal insufficiency and who have received the equivalent of 20 mg prednisone for 5 days or physiological dosages of glucocorticoid for at least 30 days in the past 12 months. These patients should receive stress doses of glucocorticoids during moderate to severe illness or surgeries.

28. **How long can it take for patients who have had successful resection of the tumor causing Cushing's syndrome to be tapered off glucocorticoids?**
It generally takes at least 6 months and often 9 months for the HPA axis to recover fully after removal of a tumor causing Cushing's syndrome. In some patients this recovery period lasts as long as 18 months. Patients can be very symptomatic. They can also develop symptoms that have been termed "steroid withdrawal syndrome," which is manifested by difficulty decreasing or discontinuing glucocorticoids because of significant symptoms despite a normal HPA axis with usual biochemical testing. Steroid withdrawal syndrome is not well understood. Symptoms

may include malaise, lethargy, anorexia, myalgias, headache, fever, and possibly desquamation of the skin. The syndrome is rare, and the etiology is unknown. However, patients do not appear to be at risk for acute adrenal crisis, and the decision of whether to continue glucocorticoids with those associated risks is up to the physician and the patient.

BIBLIOGRAPHY

1. Allolio B, Arlt W, Hahner S. DHEA: why, when, and how much—DHEA replacement in adrenal insufficiency. Ann Endocrinol 68:268–273, 2007.

2. Arafah BM. Hypothalamic pituitary adrenal function during critical illness: limitations of current assessment methods. J Clin Endocrinol Metab 91:3725–3745, 2006.

3. Aron DC, Findling JW, Tyrrell JB. Glucocorticoids and adrenal androgens. In Gardner DG, Shoback D, editors, *Greenspan's basic and clinical endocrinology*, ed 8. McGraw-Hill Medical, 2007, Chicago, Chapter 10. pp. 346–395,

4. Axelrod L. Perioperative management of patients treated with glucocorticoids. Endocrinol Metab Clin N Am 32:367–383, 2003.

5. Bouillon R. Acute adrenal insufficiency. Endocrinol Metab Clin N Am 35:767–775, 2006.

6. Dickstein G, Shechner C, Nicholson WE, et al. Adrenocorticotropin stimulation test: effects of basal cortisol level, time of day, and suggested new sensitive low dose test. J Clin Endocrinol Metab 72:773–778, 1991.

7. Dorin RI, Qualls CR, Crapo LM. Diagnosis of adrenal insufficiency. Ann Intern Med 139:194–204, 2003.

8. Hahner S, Loeffler M, Fassnacht M, et al. Impaired subjective health status in 256 patients with adrenal insufficiency on standard therapy based on cross-sectional analysis. J Clin Endocrinol Metab 92:3912–3922, 2007.

9. Hopkins RL, Leinung MC. Exogenous Cushing's syndrome and glucocorticoid withdrawal. Endocrinol Metab Clin N Am 34:371–384, 2005.

10. Merenich JA, McDermott MT, Asp AA, et al. Evidence of endocrine involvement early in the course of human immunodeficiency virus infection. J Clin Endocrinol Metab 70:566–571, 1990.

11. Schuetz P, Müller B. The hypothalamic-pituitary-adrenal axis in critical illness. Endocrinol Metab Clin N Am 35:823–838, 2006.

12. Thomas Z, Fraser GL. An update on the diagnosis of adrenal insufficiency and the use of corticotherapy in critical illness. Ann Pharmacother 41:1456–1465, 2007.

CHAPTER 31

CONGENITAL ADRENAL HYPERPLASIA

Jeannie A. Baquero and Robert A. Vigersky

1. **Define congenital adrenal hyperplasia.**
   Congenital adrenal hyperplasia (CAH) is a group of several autosomal recessive disorders that involve a deficiency or relative defect in cortisol synthesis, aldosterone synthesis, or both, resulting in some degree of cortisol deficiency, aldosterone deficiency, or both.

2. **What enzyme defects can lead to CAH?**
   Defects in any of the five enzymes required for the synthesis of cortisol from cholesterol in the adrenal cortex can lead to CAH, including steroidogenic acute regulatory (StAR) protein, which is essential in transporting cholesterol to the mitochondria; 3 β-hydroxysteroid dehydrogenase, which is responsible for cholesterol side-chain cleavage; and three hydroxylases, CYP 17 (17 α-hydroxylase), CYP21A2 (21-hydroxylase), and CYP11B1 (11 β-hydroxylase).

3. **Describe the functions of the three hydroxylases.**
   - CYP 17 (17 α-hydroxylase) is essential in converting progesterone to 17-hydroxyprogesterone (17-OHP) and pregnenolone to 17-hydroxypregnenolone.
   - CYP21A2 (21-hydroxylase) converts progesterone to deoxycorticosterone (DOC) and 17-OHP to 11 deoxycortisol.
   - CYP11B1 (11 β-hydroxylase) converts DOC to corticosterone (which then goes on to aldosterone) and 11 deoxycortisol to cortisol.

4. **How is CAH inherited?**
   All of the enzyme defects leading to CAH are autosomal recessive disorders, that is, both copies of the involved gene must be abnormal for the condition to occur.

5. **What is the most common form of CAH?**
   By far the most common form is 21-hydroxylase deficiency CYP21A2, which accounts for 90% of cases and leads to deficiencies of the salt-retaining hormones DOC and aldosterone in both sexes, as well as virilization of genetic females. Both of these are considered "classic" CAH.

6. **Which genes encode for 21-hydroxylase?**
   Two genes encode for 21-hydroxylase: CYP21A1 (pseudogene) and CYP21A2, both of which are located in a 35-kb region on the long arm of chromosome 6 (6p21.3). Both genes are located downstream of the gene coding for complement factor 4 (C4A and C4B). CYP21A1 and CYP21A2 genes have 98% nucleotide sequence identity; the former has accumulated several mutations that totally inactivate its gene product. CYP21A1 is thus an inactive pseudogene, whereas the CYP21A2 gene codes for the active 21-hydroxylase enzyme.

7. **What causes most of the genetic events responsible for *CYP21A2* deficiencies?**
   Most of the genetic events responsible for CYP21A2 deficiencies result from the similarity between CYP21A1 and CYP21A2 and are due to two types of recombination events between CYP21A2 and the pseudogene. Seventy-five percent represent deleterious mutations found in the pseudogene that are transferred to the CYP21A2 during mitosis; this process is termed

gene conversion. Twenty percent are meiotic recombinations producing a nonfunctional chimeric pseudogene. More than 60 additional mutations account for the remaining 5%.

8. **What determines the patient's phenotype?**

Clinical manifestations of the disease are related to the degree of cortisol deficiency, aldosterone deficiency, or both and the accumulation of precursor hormones. The patient's phenotype is generally based on the specific genetic alteration of the CYP21A2 gene and can be grouped into four categories:

- Patients with no enzyme activity typically have large deletions or nonsense mutations and predominantly have the salt-wasting form of the disorder.
- Patients with low but detectable enzyme activity have missense mutations, yielding enyzymes with 1% to 2% of normal activity, and typically have the simple virilizing form of the disease.
- Patients with 20% to 60% of normal enzyme activity have conservative amino acid substitutions and most often have the nonclassic form of the disease.
- Patients who are heterozygotes have mild abnormalities but no clinically important endocrine disorder.

9. **What is the second most common cause of CAH?**

The second most common cause of CAH (7% of all cases) is deficiency of the 11 β-hydroxylase enzyme (CYP11B), which is also an autosomal recessive defect caused by a mutation on the short arm of chromosome 8 (8q24.3). The result of this deficiency is an increased level of DOC, which causes hypertension due to sodium retention, hypokalemic alkalosis, and increased androgen and androgen precursors, which cause ambiguous genitalia in genetic females.

10. **Summarize the rarer forms of CAH.**

The rarer forms of CAH are 17 α-hydroxylase and 3 β-hydroxysteroid dehydrogenase deficiency. There have been fewer than 200 cases of 17 α-hydroxylase with 40 described mutations of CYP17 that span an 8.7-kb region on the short arm of chromosome 10 (10q24.3). The consequence of this deficiency is hypertension due to sodium retention and hypokalemia due to DOC excess (associated with suppressed renin and aldosterone), along with deficiency of androgens and androgen precursors, which causes pseudohermaphroditism in genetic males and delayed puberty in both sexes (see questions 16 and 21).

11. **How common is CAH?**

CAH is one of the most common inherited diseases. The most common form of CAH, 21-hydroxylase deficiency, occurs in about 1/16,000 in most populations. The prevalence of this disorder varies greatly among ethnic groups and is highest among the Ashkenazi Jewish population of Eastern Europe. The nonclassic 21-hydroxylase deficiency occurs in approximately 0.2% of the general white population but more frequently, 1% to 2%, in certain populations such as Jews of Eastern European origin.

12. **What percentage of the population at large are heterozygote carriers of the 12-hydroxylase defect?**

Fewer than 2% of the population at large are heterozygote carriers of the 21-hydroxylase defect; that is, one of the two copies of the 21-hydroxylase gene is abnormal. Such heterozygote carriers appear normal in all respects but may have elevated 17-OHP with adrenocorticotropic hormone (ACTH) stimulation testing.

13. **How common is 11-hydroxylase deficiency?**

The 11-hydroxylase deficiency, the second most frequent form of CAH, occurs in 1/100,000 births in the general population but in 1/5000 births in Jews of Moroccan decent. CAH due to defects of the other enzymes listed here is extremely rare.

14. **Explain why adrenal hyperplasia develops.**

The process of adrenal hyperplasia begins in utero. Reduced production of cortisol in the fetus, due to decreased activity of one of the enzymes necessary for cortisol synthesis, results in lowered levels of serum cortisol. Cortisol normally acts through a negative feedback loop to inhibit the secretion of ACTH by the pituitary gland and corticotropin-releasing hormone (CRH) by the hypothalamus. Thus the low serum cortisol levels that occur in a person with CAH increase the secretion of ACTH and CRH in an attempt to stimulate the adrenal glands to overcome the enzyme block and to return the serum cortisol level to normal. As this process continues over time, the elevated levels of serum ACTH stimulate growth of the adrenal glands, leading to hyperplasia.

15. **What is the most serious clinical consequence of CAH?**

Adrenal crisis in the newborn period is the most serious consequence of CAH. It usually occurs with genetic defects that result in severe reductions in enzyme activity of both aldosterone and cortisol. It is especially insidious in genetic males who do not have ambiguous genitalia as a clue to the diagnosis. Overall, about two thirds of patients with 21-hydroxylase deficiency have the salt-wasting form. These patients have decreased production of DOC and aldosterone but an increased level of progesterone and 17-OHP, which may act as mineralocorticoid antagonists exacerbating the effects of aldosterone deficiency. Aldosterone deficiency leads to hypotension, volume depletion, hyponatremia, hyperkalemia, and increased renin activity. Cortisol deficiency contributes to poor cardiac function, poor vascular response to catecholamines, decreased glomerular filtration rate, and increased secretion of antidiuretic hormone. Both deficiencies lead to hyponatremia, dehydration, and shock.

16. **What are other clinical consequences of CAH in females?**

Many of the precursors and metabolites that build up behind the blocked enzymes 21-hydroxylase, 11 β-hydroxylase, or 3β-hydroxysteroid dehydrogenase, are androgens. They may cause the following:

- Masculinization of the external genitalia of a genetic female fetus, leading to ambiguous genitalia at birth (female pseudohermaphroditism).
- Behaviors more typical of boys during childhood in terms of toy preference, rough play, and aggressiveness. (However, most females are heterosexual, and their sexual identity is invariably female.)
- Rapid growth during early childhood with ultimate short stature as an adult due to early closure of epiphyses.
- Twenty percent of females with simple virilizing disease and approximately 40% of females with salt-wasting disease are infertile.
- Forty-five percent of women with salt wasting have osteopenia as young adults.

17. **What are other clinical consequences of CAH in males?**

- No overt signs
- Short stature
- Variable and subtle hyperpigmentation
- Variable and subtle penile enlargement
- Development of testicular adrenal rests, which produce adrenal-specific hormones
- Oligospermia, infertility, or both

18. **How do patients with 17 α-hydroxylase deficiency present?**

In 17 α-hydroxylase deficiency, the enzyme defect blocks synthesis of androgens, thus precluding masculinization or ambiguity of the external genitalia. Patients present at puberty with the following:

- Primary (or rarely secondary) amenorrhea
- Hypertension
- Hypokalemia (because of increased mineralocorticoid production)

19. **How do patients with nonclassic CAH present?**

Patients with nonclassic CAH (also called late-onset CAH) produce normal amounts of cortisol and aldosterone at the expense of mild to moderate overproduction of sex hormone precursors. Usually they are asymptomatic and have normal external genitalia but later present with the following:

- Premature puberty
- Severe cystic acne—occurring in 33% of patients
- Hirsutism—the most common symptom, occurring in 60% of symptomatic females
- Oligomenorrhea and polycystic ovaries—second most common, occuring in 54% of patients
- Infertility—occurring in 13% of patients

20. **Summarize the relationship between adrenal "incidentalomas" and CAH.**

Adrenal incidentalomas are more common in patients with CAH and in heterozygotes. Conversely, 60% of patients with incidentalomas have exaggerated 17-OH progesterone responses to ACTH.

21. **How do the manifestations of CAH differ in males?**

Newborn males with CAH due to deficiency of 21-hydroxylase or 11 β-hydroxylase do not have ambiguous genitalia. Because of their typical normal physical appearance, it is often difficult to detect affected males, especially when symptoms of salt wasting occur after the first week of life. Later in childhood or early adulthood, males can present with the following:

- Premature puberty
- Advanced height in early childhood with ultimate short stature
- Acne
- Testicular enlargement due to adrenal rests

22. **Describe the presentation of males with CAD due to deficiency of other enzyme activity.**

Males with CAH due to deficient activity of 3 β-hydroxysteroid dehydrogenase, 17 α-hydroxylase, or cholesterol side-chain cleavage enzymes are unable to produce androgens during fetal development that are necessary for the formation of male external genitalia. As a consequence, they may have the following:

- External genitalia at birth that are only partially masculinized
- Normal female appearance (male pseudohermaphroditism)

23. **Describe the clinical features that suggest the possibility of CAH.**

Adrenal crisis or severe salt wasting in the newborn period suggests the possibility of CAH. CAH also must be considered prominently in the differential diagnosis of any newborn with ambiguous genitalia. Because adrenal crisis and salt loss in CAH may be fatal if not treated, the finding of ambiguous genitalia in a newborn should trigger a rapid attempt to confirm or exclude CAH. Most males with CAH do not have ambiguous genitalia; consequently, many cases go unrecognized at birth, unless there is a documented family history of the disorder.

24. **What clinical clues help to support or refute the diagnosis of CAH in a newborn with ambiguous genitalia?**

The overwhelming majority of genetic males with CAH have unambiguous external genitalia at birth; conversely, CAH is an uncommon cause of ambiguous genitalia in a genetic male. Thus determination that the infant with ambiguous genitalia is a genetic male makes CAH unlikely and decreases the diagnostic urgency because the disorders giving rise to ambiguous genitalia in genetic males are rarely associated with a fatal outcome. For example, the finding of palpable gonads in the scrotal or inguinal area suggests that the infant is a genetic male because such palpable gonads are almost always testes. Conversely, the detection of a uterus in an infant with ambiguous genitalia, either by physical examination or by ultrasound, strongly suggests that the infant is a genetic female, thus heightening the possibility of CAH.

25. Discuss the role of molecular biology techniques in the diagnosis of CAH.
Molecular biology techniques can rapidly confirm the genetic sex of a newborn without the prolonged wait for a traditional chromosome analysis. Because of the potentially severe consequences of CAH, it is probably prudent to assume that any genetic female with ambiguous genitalia has CAH until proved otherwise. Furthermore, it is probably best to wait to assign gender until molecular testing is performed, because gender misassignment may cause long-term psychological problems for the families of such children. Early diagnosis and appropriate therapy also allow one to avoid the progressive effects of excess adrenal androgens, which will cause short stature, gender confusion in girls, and psychosexual disturbances in both boys and girls.

26. How is the diagnosis of CAH confirmed?
Because one does not know which enzyme is deficient in a newborn with suspected CAH (unless the family has a documented history of a particular enzyme defect), serum levels of all steroids that may be in the affected biosynthetic pathway can be measured before and after the administration of 250 μg of synthetic ACTH. Urinary measurement of these steroids by gas chromatography/mass spectroscopy has recently become economically feasible. Plasma renin activity and aldosterone levels should also be measured to assess the adequacy of aldosterone synthesis. Determination of which steroid levels are supranormal and which are low facilitates localization of the exact enzyme block.

KEY POINTS: CONGENITAL ADRENAL HYPERPLASIA

1. Congenital adrenal hyperplasia (CAH), the most common inherited disease, is a group of autosomal recessive disorders, the most frequent of which is 21-hydroxylase deficiency.

2. The most serious consequences of CAH are ambiguous genitalia in females at birth, neonatal salt wasting, short stature, and premature puberty.

3. CAH is diagnosed through measurement of cortisol precursors before and 1 hour after the intravenous administration of 250 μg of synthetic ACTH.

4. Predicted adult height can be achieved through early diagnosis, lower doses of corticosteroids in the first year of life and during puberty, and the use of fludrocortisone even in those who are salt wasters genetically but not clinically.

5. CAH is a rare cause of ambiguous genitalia in a genetic male.

6. The most common symptom in nonclassic CAH in females is hirsutism.

27. How are specific genetic defects confirmed?
Specific genetic defects may be confirmed with molecular genetic testing. Polymerase chain reaction (PCR) amplification for the rapid simultaneous detection of the 10 mutations that are found in approximately 95% of 21-hydroxylase deficiency alleles is used for rapid results. Molecular genetic analysis of CYP21 is not essential for diagnosis but may be helpful in the following circumstances:
- To confirm the basis of the defect
- To aid in genetic counseling
- To establish the disease in certain cases

28. What should be done when nonclassic CAH is suspected in older patients?

When nonclassic CAH is suspected in the preteen, teenage, or adult patient, ACTH stimulation testing should be performed with 250 μg (not 1 μg) of synthetic ACTH; measurement of 17-OHP, 17-OH pregnenolone, and cortisol should be performed before and 60 minutes after injection. Hyperandrogenism can be assessed in women by measuring serum levels of testosterone, androstenedione, and 3 α-androstanediol glucuronide.

29. Describe the classic test used for newborn screening.

Newborn screening programs for CAH focus on the rapid detection of classic 21-hydroxylase deficiency on Guthrie cards (filter paper on which blood samples are collected, dried, and transported) measured by radioimmunoassay. This screening method measures 17-OHP. Basal 17-OHP usually exceeds 10,000 ng/dL in affected infants, whereas the levels in normal infants are below 100 ng/dL. This large difference makes it possible to screen newborns. If elevated, this test can be used for genotyping. As stated previously, genotyping can be helpful to determine severity of the disease. In the United States, testing for 21-hydroxylase deficiency is mandatory in 47 of 50 states.

30. What other tests may be used?

If CAH is suspected and newborn filter paper screening is not available, ACTH stimulation with steroid precursor measurements should be performed after the first 24 hours of life. Adrenal ultrasonography can also be used as a potential screening test for CAH neonates with ambiguous genitalia, salt-losing crisis, or both by detecting less than 4 mm adrenal limb width.

31. How is CAH treated in neonates?

The most important goal of treatment is to prevent salt loss and adrenal crisis in the newborn period. This goal requires the prompt administration of glucocorticoids and, in many cases, mineralocorticoids, as well as careful monitoring of salt intake. This treatment not only replaces the deficient hormones but also suppresses elevated serum ACTH levels, thereby reducing adrenal production of androgenic precursors and metabolites. Such treatment may be given presumptively while awaiting the results of definitive laboratory tests and then discontinued if the tests are not confirmatory.

32. When is surgical correction of ambiguous genitalia carried out?

Surgical correction of ambiguous genitalia in girls consists of genitoplasty of the clitoris and labia and vaginoplasty. Single-stage surgery is now implemented between 2 and 6 months of life. There may be variable degrees of impairment of psychosexual functioning in adults depending on the method, timing, and underlying mutation.

33. Describe the treatment of CAH in children.

The preferred glucocorticoid for chronic replacement is hydrocortisone in dosages of 10–18 mg/m^2/day in three divided doses. Hydrocortisone is preferred because of its short half-life, which minimizes growth suppression. It is sometimes extremely difficult or impossible to find a dosage of glucocorticoid that normalizes production of androgen and maintains normal growth and weight gain. In such situations, mineralocorticoids (fludrocortisone) or spironolactone/flutamide (androgen receptor blockers that prevent virilization) (or both) in combination with the aromatase inhibitor testolactone (which prevents estrogen-induced epiphyseal fusion) may be useful adjunctive therapy in combination with nonsuppressive replacement doses of glucocorticoids. Rarely, adrenalectomy has been used for difficult-to-control patients because treatment of adrenal insufficiency is relatively much simpler.

34. How is CAH treated in adolescents and adults?

The use of a combination of growth hormone and gonadotropin-releasing hormone analog has been demonstrated to improve final height in children as they enter puberty. Prednisone

(5–7 mg daily in two divided doses) or dexamethasone (0.25–0.5 mg in one or two doses/day) may be used after growth has been completed. Patients should be monitored carefully for signs of iatrogenic Cushing's syndrome and sonography used in males to detect testicular adrenal rests.

35. **What factors favor the achievement of predicted adult height?**
   - Early diagnosis
   - Lower doses of hydrocortisone in the first year of life
   - Use of hydrocortisone rather than prednisone or dexamethasone during the pubertal growth spurt
   - Mineralocorticoid treatment in all patients who are genetically determined to be salt wasters even if they are not so clinically

36. **What changes in therapy are necessary as a result of medically significant stress?**
   Patients with CAH who have been on steroid therapy should wear a medical alert bracelet or necklace and should be provided with an emergency kit of hydrocortisone or dexamethasone for intramuscular use. For medically significant stress, the following measures are recommended:
   - Triple the oral dose of glucocorticoids.
   - Use intramuscular (or intravenous) steroid if the patient is unable to consume oral medications.
   - Sodium chloride, 1 to 3 g/day, may be necessary in infants.
   - Fludrocortisone acetate should be used in patients with salt wasting (infants: 70 $\mu g/m^2/$ day; adults: 0.05–0.3 mg/day).

37. **What changes in therapy are necessary during pregnancy?**
   - Use hydrocortisone or prednisone instead of dexamethasone, which passes through the placenta unmetabolized.
   - Adjust steroid dosage according to the clinical status.
   - Keep testosterone and free testosterone in the normal range for pregnancy.
   - Use stress doses of steroids during labor and delivery.

38. **How is treatment monitored?**
   The goals of treatment are to prevent symptoms of adrenal insufficiency and to suppress ACTH and adrenal androgen production. For the second goal, it is most appropriate to monitor the levels of the key precursors immediately behind the blocked enzyme (e.g., 17-OHP and androstenedione in the case of 21-hydroxylase deficiency). The goal is not to normalize the 17-OHP level, because this will lead to iatrogenic Cushing's syndrome. This should be done every 3 months initially and then every 4 to 12 months. The levels of 17-OHP can be kept between 400 and 1200 ng/dL (normal is <150 in children), and the androstenedione level should be appropriate for the patient's age and sex.

39. **What other monitoring tools may be beneficial?**
   Androgen levels should be monitored during treatment. These include testosterone, androstenedione, and 3--androstanediol glucuronide. In addition, plasma renin activity should be monitored in patients with salt-wasting CAH. Children must have annual bone age determinations, and their height should be carefully monitored.

40. **What genetic counseling is appropriate for a couple who previously had a child with CAH?**
   Because all forms of CAH are autosomal recessive disorders, both parents of a child with CAH are obligate heterozygote carriers of the gene defect. Consequently, the chance that another child of the same couple will have CAH is one in four; 50% of the children will be heterozygote

carriers. Modern genetic techniques and chorionic villus sampling of fetal DNA at 9 weeks of gestation allow the diagnosis of CAH during the first trimester of pregnancy. The other use for genotypic identification includes the prediction of the phenotype (i.e., severity of the disease). There appears to be a good relationship between genotype and phenotype in classic but not in nonclassic CAH.

41. Are any prenatal treatments available for the fetus with CAH?

Preliminary evidence suggests that prenatal treatment of female fetuses with 21-hydroxylase deficiency in the fifth to seventh week of gestation by giving relatively high dosages of dexamethasone (0.5–2.0 mg/day) to the mother may ameliorate the masculinization of genitalia and have no effect on subsequent cognitive or motor development. By contrast, male fetuses with 21-hydroxylase deficiencies do not develop ambiguous genitalia and do not require steroid treatment until after birth.

WEBSITE

http://www.hormone.org/public/cah.cfm

BIBLIOGRAPHY

1. Balsamo A, Cicognani A, Baldazzi L, et al: CYP21 genotype, adult height, and pubertal development in 55 patients treated for 21-hydroxylase deficiency. J Clin Endocrinol Metab 88:5680–5688, 2003.

2. Cabrera MS, Vogiatzi MG, New MI: Long term outcome in adult males with classic congenital adrenal hyperplasia. J Clin Endocrinol Metab 86: 3070–3078, 2001.

3. Chrousos GP, Loriaux DL, Mann DL, et al: Late-onset 21-hydroxylase deficiency mimicking idiopathic hirsutism or polycystic ovarian disease: an allelic variant of congenital virilizing adrenal hyperplasia with a milder enzymatic defect. Ann Intern Med 96:1–43, 1982.

4. Claahsen-van der Grinten HL, Otten BJ, Sweep FCGJ, et al: Testicular tumors in patients with congenital adrenal hyperplasia due to 21-hydroxylase deficiency show functional features of adrenocortical tissue. J Clin Endocrinol Metab 92: 2674–3680, 2007.

5. Deneux C, Veronique T, Dib A, et al: Phenotype–genotype correlation in 56 women with nonclassical congenital adrenal hyperplasia due to 21-hydroxylase deficiency. J Clin Endocrinol Metab 86:207–213, 2001.

6. Forest MG, Betuel H, David M: Prenatal treatment in congenital adrenal hyperplasia due to 21-hydroxylase deficiency: update 88 of the French multicenter study. Endocr Res 15:277, 1989.

7. Hirvikoski T, et al: Cognitive functions in children at risk for congenital adrenal hyperplasia treated prenatally with dexamethasone. J Clin Endocrinol Metab 92:542–548, 2007.

8. King JA, Wisniewski AB, Bankowski BJ, et al: Long-term corticosteroid replacement and bone mineral density in adult women with classical congenital adrenal hyperplasia. J Clin Enocrinol Metabl 91: 865–869, 2006.

9. Levine LS: Congenital adrenal hyperplasia. Pediatric Rev 21:159–171, 2000.

10. Lin-Su K, Vogiatzi MG, Marshall I, et al: Treatment with growth hormone and luteinizing hormone releasing hormone analog improves final adult height in children with congenital adrenal hyperplasia. J Clin Endocrinol Metab 90:3318–3325, 2005.

11. Linder B, Esteban NV, Yergey AL, et al: Cortisol production rate in childhood and adolescence. J Pediatr 117:892, 1991.

12. Lo JC, Schwitzgebel VM, Tyrrell JB, et al: Normal female infants born of mothers with classic congenital adrenal hyperplasia due to 21-hydroxylase deficiency. J Clin Endocrinol Metab 84:930–936, 1999.

13. Merke DP, Bornstein DP. Congenital adrenal hyperplasia. Lancet 365:2125–2136, 2005.

14. Merke DP, Keil MF, Jones JV, et al: Flutamide, testolactone, and reduced hydrocortisone dose maintain normal growth velocity and bone maturation despite elevated androgen levels in children with congenital adrenal hyperplasia. J Clin Endocrinol Metab 85:1114–1120, 2000.

15. Mulaikal RM, Migeon CJ, Rock JA: Fertility rates in female patients with congenital adrenal hyperplasia due to 21-hydroxylase deficiency. N Engl J Med 316:178, 1987.

16. New MI, Carlson A, Obeid J, et al: Prenatal diagnosis for congenital adrenal hyperplasia in 532 pregnancies, J Clin Endocrinol Metab 86:5651–5657, 2001.

17. Nordenskjold A, Holmdahl G, Frisen L, et al: Type of metation and surgical procedure affect long-term quality of life for women with congenital adrenal hyperplasia. J Clin Endocrinol Metab 93:380–386, 2008.

18. Nordenström A, Servin A, Bohlin G, et al: Sex-typed toy play behavior correlates with the degree of prenatal androgen exposure assessed by CYP21 genotype in girls with congenital adrenal hyperplasia. J Clin Endocrinol Metab 87:5119–5124, 2002.

19. Pang S: Congenital adrenal hyperplasia. Endocrinol Metab Clin N Am 26:853–891, 1997.

20. Sherman SL, Aston CE, Morton NE, et al: A segregation and linkage study of classical and nonclassical 21-hydroxylase deficiency. Am J Hum Genet 42:830, 1988.

21. Speiser PW, White PC: Congenital adrenal hyperplasia. N Engl J Med 349:776, 2003.

22. Therrell BL Jr, Berenbaum SA, Manter-Kapanke V, Simmank J: Results of screening 1.9 million Texas newborns for 21-hydroxylase-deficient congenital adrenal hyperplasia. Pediatrics 101:583, 1998.

23. Urban MD, Lee PA, Migeon CJ: Adult height and fertility in men with congenital virilizing adrenal hyperplasia. N Engl J Med 299:1392, 1978.

24. Van Wyk JJ, Ritzen EM: The role of bilateral adrenalectomy in the treatment of congenital adrenal hyperplasia. J Clin Endocrinol Metab 88: 2993–2998, 2003.

25. Wedell A: Molecular genetics of congenital adrenal hyperplasia (21-hydroxylase deficiency): implications for diagnosis, prognosis and treatment. Acta Paediatr 87:159–164, 1998.

26. White PC, New MI, Dupont B: Structure of the human 21-hydroxylase gene. Proc Natl Acad Sci USA 83:5111, 1986.

27. White PC, Spieser PW: Congenital adrenal hyperplasia due to 21-hydroxylase deficiency. Endocr Rev 21:245–291, 2000.

THYROID TESTING

Michael T. McDermott

1. **What is the single best test to screen for abnormal function of the thyroid gland?**

   The serum thyroid-stimulating hormone (TSH) level is the best test for assessing thyroid function. This is true because the vast majority of thyroid dysfunction is due to primary thyroid disease. TSH levels are misleading, however, when thyroid dysfunction is secondary to hypothalamic or pituitary disease and in patients with nonthyroidal illnesses. Measurement of serum thyroxine (T_4) and triiodothyronine (T_3) are mainly useful when the TSH is outside the reference range.

2. **How do you interpret the serum TSH level in the evaluation of suspected thyroid disease?**

   When TSH is elevated, the patient has primary hypothyroidism; when TSH is low, the patient has primary hyperthyroidism. The main exceptions to these rules are in patients who have pituitary-hypothalamic disorders or nonthyroidal illnesses. Abnormal serum TSH values can detect mild thyroid dysfunction long before serum T_4 and T_3 levels are outside their reference ranges. Measurement of serum free T_4 should be performed whenever the TSH is high; both free T4 and total T_3 (or free T_3 by equilibrium dialysis) are often informative when the TSH is low.

3. **Explain how the serum TSH is used to manage patients on thyroid hormone therapy.**

   Thyroid hormone therapy is usually given to patients for one of two purposes: replacement therapy for hypothyroidism or suppression therapy for thyroid cancer. When replacement is the goal, the dosage should be adjusted to maintain the serum TSH level within the reference range. When suppression is the goal, the dosage should be adjusted to maintain the serum TSH level in the low normal or slightly low range for most patients and in the undetectable range for those with aggressive or metastatic thyroid cancer.

4. **Discuss the advantages of free thyroid hormone assays.**

   Free T_4 and T_3 assays determine the amounts of unbound, bioactive thyroid hormones in the circulation. Free thyroid hormone tests fall into two main categories: equilibrium dialysis and analog assays. Equilibrium dialysis methods are not affected by abnormalities of serum thyroid hormone-binding proteins. Analog methods are variably affected by protein binding but still give a more accurate assessment of biologically active thyroid hormone levels than do total T_4 and T_3 assays. Analog assays are used by most commercial laboratories. Currently free T_4 assays are considered far more accurate than free T_3 assays. This is why many experts still prefer total T_3 measurements.

5. **What do total T_4 and T_3 assays measure?**

   These assays measure the total T_4 and T_3 concentrations in the circulation. More than 99% of circulating T_4 and approximately 98% of T_3 are bound to proteins, such as thyroxine-binding globulin (TBG), thyroxine-binding prealbumin (TBPA or transthyretin), and albumin.

Consequently, serum total T_4 and T_3 levels can be altered by protein binding disorders just as they can by thyroid disease.

6. **Name the major disorders of thyroid hormone-binding proteins.**
Pregnancy, estrogen use, congenital TBG excess, and familial dysalbuminemic hyperthyroxinemia (FDH) are the most common. FDH is an inherited disorder, in which albumin has enhanced affinity for T_4, resulting in increased levels of total T_4 but not T_3. Protein binding of T_4 and T_3 is reduced by androgens and congenital TBG deficiency.

A T_3 resin uptake (T_3RU) measurement helps distinguish protein-binding disorders from true thyroid diseases. The T_3RU is inversely proportional to the protein-bound T_4; accordingly, T_3RU is low when T_4 protein binding is increased and high when protein binding is reduced.

Table 32-1 indicates how these tests are used to make the correct diagnosis.

TABLE 32-1. DIAGNOSIS OF DISORDERS OF THYROID HORMONE-BINDING PROTEINS

	Total T_4	Total T_3	T_3RU
Hyperthyroidism	↑	↑	↑
Increased protein-binding state	↑	↑	↓
Hypothyroidism	↓	↓	↓
Decreased protein-binding state	↓	↓	↑

T_4, thyroxin; T_3, triiodothyronine; T_3RU, triiodothyronine resin uptake.

7. **What antithyroid antibody measurements are clinically useful?**
Antibodies against thyroid peroxidase (TPO) and thyroglobulin are present in the serum of most patients with Hashimoto's thyroiditis. Either test can establish a diagnosis of Hashimoto's disease, but the TPO antibodies are more sensitive. Thyroid-stimulating immunoglobulins (TSI) and TSH receptor antibodies (TRAb) are present in the serum of most patients with Graves' disease; their measurement is not necessary in patients with obvious Graves' disease but may be helpful when the diagnosis is in question.

8. **How useful are thyroglobulin measurements?**
Thyroglobulin (TG) is the major iodoprotein constituent of thyroid follicles. Serum TG levels are mildly increased in many thyroid diseases, but marked elevations suggest the presence of destructive thyroiditis (subacute, postpartum, or silent thyroiditis), in which TG leaks from the damaged thyroid gland into the circulation. TG measurements are also useful in monitoring patients with thyroid cancer. When a patient has been treated and is cancer-free, the serum TG should be undetectable. Normal or elevated serum TG levels in such patients suggest the presence of residual or metastatic thyroid cancer. Most TG assays are not reliable in patients who have positive anti-TG antibodies because these antibodies interfere with the method of TG measurement.

9. **Under what circumstances should a serum calcitonin level be measured?**
Calcitonin is made by thyroid parafollicular C cells rather than by follicular cells. Serum calcitonin is elevated in medullary carcinoma of the thyroid (MCT) and in its familial precursor lesion, C-cell hyperplasia. Because MCT is an uncommon thyroid neoplasm, serum calcitonin

measurements should not be used in the routine evaluation of most thyroid nodules. They are indicated, however, if a patient exhibits a feature, such as familial occurrence or associated diarrhea, that is characteristic of MCT.

10. **Discuss the utility and interpretation of the radioactive iodine uptake (RAIU) test.**
    Thyroid follicular cells have iodine symporters or pumps that bring iodine into the cells for thyroid hormone synthesis. The activity of these iodine pumps can be assessed by measuring the radioactive iodine uptake (RAIU). The normal 24-hour RAIU is approximately 10% to 25% in the United States, but this value varies according to location because of geographic differences in dietary iodine intake. The RAIU is most useful in the differential diagnosis of thyrotoxicosis by separating cases into two distinct categories: high-RAIU thyrotoxicosis and low-RAIU thyrotoxicosis. See Table 32-2.

TABLE 32-2. HIGH–RAIU THYROTOXICOSIS AND LOW–RAIU THYROTOXICOSIS CATEGORIES

High-RAIU Thyrotoxicosis	Low-RAIU Thyrotoxicosis
Graves' disease	Factitious thyrotoxicosis
Toxic multinodular goiter	Iodine-induced thyrotoxicosis
Solitary toxic adenoma	
Human chorionic gonadotropin (HCG)-induced thyrotoxicosis	Subacute thyroiditis
TSH-secreting tumor	Postpartum thyroiditis
	Silent thyroiditis

RAIU, radioactive iodine uptake; TSH, thyroid-stimulating hormone.

11. **When and why should a thyroid scan be ordered?**
    The thyroid scan helps to distinguish the three types of high-RAIU thyrotoxicosis. Graves' disease is characterized by diffuse tracer uptake; toxic multinodular goiter, by multiple discrete areas of increased uptake; and the solitary toxic adenoma, by a single area of intense uptake. The scan is not helpful in low-RAIU thyrotoxicosis.
    The thyroid scan is also sometimes used in the evaluation of thyroid nodules, although its cost efficiency in this workup is doubtful. According to the scan, thyroid nodules may be divided into those that are hot (hyperfunctioning), warm (eufunctioning), and cold (nonfunctioning). Cold nodules have a 20% risk of being a carcinoma, whereas malignancy is rare in hot nodules.

12. **What is Thyrogen? How is it used?**
    Thyrogen is recombinant human TSH. It can be used to stimulate neoplastic thyroid tissue to absorb radioiodine for an imaging procedure. Thyroid cancer tissue ordinarily traps iodine poorly and can be imaged only if the serum TSH is elevated. This can be accomplished either by stopping levothyroxine treatment for 3 to 6 weeks or by giving Thyrogen injections. After the serum TSH level has been increased by either method, serum TG is measured and radioiodine (I-131 or I-123) is given for whole-body scanning. A positive scan or detectable TG level indicates the presence of residual or metastatic thyroid cancer. A Thyrogen-stimulated scan and TG measurement has the same accuracy as a levothyroxine withdrawal scan and has the advantage of not causing symptoms of hypothyroidism.

13. **How can heterophile antimouse antibodies interfere with assessment of thyroid function?**

Heterophile antimouse antibodies (HAMA) sometimes develop in people who are regularly exposed to rodents, such as laboratory workers, farm workers, and other people who spend a lot of time outdoors, including homeless people. HAMA can interfere with the measurement of several hormones, including TSH and thyroglobulin. When TSH or thyroglobulin values are not consistent with the clinical picture, interference by HAMA should be suspected and the patient questioned about possible exposure to rodents. When a laboratory is alerted to the possibility of HAMA interference, assay conditions can be altered to minimize or eliminate the misleading results.

KEY POINTS: THYROID TESTING

1. Serum thyroid-stimulating hormone (TSH) measurement is the best overall test to screen and evaluate patients for thyroid disease and to monitor thyroid hormone replacement therapy.

2. Serum free thyroxin (T_4) should be measured in all patients whose TSH is elevated, and serum free T_4 and total triiodothyronine (T_3) or free T_3 should be measured in patients whose TSH is suppressed.

3. Antithyroperoxidase (TPO) antibodies are the most accurate test to establish a diagnosis of chronic lymphocytic thyroiditis (Hashimoto's disease).

4. Serum thyroglobulin (TG) is useful for assisting in the diagnosis of destructive thyroiditis and for monitoring for recurrence of differentiated thyroid cancer.

5. RAIU is used primarily to determine whether patients with thyrotoxicosis have a high RAIU or a low RAIU disorder.

6. A thyroid scan is used mainly to distinguish among the three types of high-RAIU thyrotoxicosis and to determine whether thyroid nodules are nonfunctioning (cold), eufunctioning (warm), or hyperfunctioning (hot).

BIBLIOGRAPHY

1. Andersen S, Pedersen KM, Bruun NH, Laurberg P: Narrow individual variations in serum T4 and T3 in normal subjects: a clue to the understanding of subclinical thyroid disease. J Clin Endocrinol Metab 87:1068–1072, 2002.

2. Cavaleri R: Thyroid radioiodine uptake: indications and interpretation. Endocrinologist 2:341, 1992.

3. Demers LM, Spencer CA: Laboratory medicine practice guidelines: laboratory support for the diagnosis and monitoring of thyroid disease. Thyroid 13(1):2–126, 2003.

4. Haugen BR, Pacin F, Reiners C, et al: A comparison of recombinant human thyrotropin and thyroid hormone withdrawal for the detection of thyroid remnant or cancer. J Clin Endocrinol Metab 84:3877–3885, 1999.

5. Nelson JC, Wang R, Asher DT, Wilcox RB: The nature of analogue-based free thyroxine estimates. Thyroid 14:1030–1036, 2004.

6. Nicoloff JT, Spencer CA: The use and misuse of the sensitive thyrotropin assays. J Clin Endocrinol Metab 71:553–558, 1990.

7. Preissner CM, Dodge LA, O'Kane DJ, et al: Prevalence of heterophilic antibody interference in eight automated tumor marker immunoassays. Clin Chem 51:208–210, 2005.

8. Preissner CM, O'Kane DJ, Singh RJ, Morris JC, Grebe SK. Phantoms in the assay tube: heterophile antibody interference with serum thyroglobulin assays. J Clin Endocrinol Metab 88:3069–3074, 2003.

9. Smith SA: Commonly asked questions about thyroid function. Mayo Clin Proc 70:573–577, 1995.

10. Wang R, Nelson JC Weiss RM, Wilcox RB: Accuracy of free thyroxine measurements across natural ranges of thyroxine binding to serum proteins. Thyroid 10:31–39, 2000.

CHAPTER 33

HYPERTHYROIDISM

Amanda M. Bell and Henry B. Burch

1. **What is the difference between thyrotoxicosis and hyperthyroidism?**
   Thyrotoxicosis is the general term for the presence of increased levels of thyroxine (T_4), triiodothyronine (T_3), or both from any cause. It does not imply that a patient is markedly symptomatic or "toxic." Hyperthyroidism refers to causes of thyrotoxicosis in which the thyroid overproduces thyroid hormone.

2. **Define the term "autonomy" as it applies to thyroid hyperfunction.**
   Thyroid autonomy refers to the spontaneous synthesis and release of thyroid hormone independent of thyroid-stimulating hormone (TSH).

3. **What is subclinical thyrotoxicosis?**
   Subclinical thyrotoxicosis refers to elevation of T_4, T_3, or both within the normal range, leading to suppression of pituitary TSH secretion into the subnormal range. Clinical symptoms and signs are frequently absent or nonspecific.

4. **What are the long-term consequences of subclinical thyrotoxicosis?**
   Some studies have linked subclinical thyrotoxicosis to accelerated bone loss in postmenopausal women and a higher incidence of atrial dysrhythmia, including atrial fibrillation. A TSH below the lower limit of normal but above 0.1 mIU/L is less likely to result in such complications.

5. **List the three most common causes of hyperthyroidism.**
   - Graves' disease
   - Toxic multinodular goiter (TMNG)
   - Toxic adenomas or autonomously functioning thyroid nodules (AFTNs)

6. **Define Graves' disease.**
   Graves' disease is an autoimmune disorder in which antibodies directed against the TSH receptor result in continuous stimulation of the thyroid gland to produce and secrete thyroid hormone. Extrathyroidal manifestations of Graves' disease include ophthalmopathy, pretibial myxedema, and thyroid acropachy.

7. **Explain TMNG.**
   TMNG generally arises in the setting of a longstanding multinodular goiter in which certain individual nodules have developed autonomous function.

8. **What are AFTNs?**
   Toxic adenomas or autonomously functioning thyroid nodules (AFTNs) are benign tumors that have constitutive activation of the TSH receptor or its signal-transduction apparatus. These tumors frequently produce subclinical thyrotoxicosis and have a predilection for spontaneous hemorrhage. AFTNs generally must be larger than 3 cm in diameter before attaining sufficient secretory capacity to produce overt hyperthyroidism. Often, inefficient iodine processing leads to an excess of T_3 relative to T_4 in AFTNs.

9. **What is the Jod-Basedow phenomenon?**

The Jod-Basedow phenomenon is induction of thyrotoxicosis in patients previously euthyroid as a result of exposure to large quantities of iodine (dietary, in the iodine-containing drug amiodarone, or in iodinated radiographic contrast material). It was first described in patients with underlying iodine-deficiency but can also be seen in patients with subclinical thyroid autonomy, usually from a multinodular goiter.

10. **What are some rarer causes of hyperthyroidism?**

Rarer causes of hyperthyroidism include TSH-secreting pituitary adenomas; stimulation of the TSH receptor by extremely high levels of human chorionic gonadotropin (hCG), such as those found in choriocarcinomas in women or germ cell tumors in men; struma ovarii (ectopic thyroid hormone production in thyroid tissue–containing ovarian teratomas); and thyroid hormone resistance. Thyroiditis and ingestion of excessive exogenous thyroid hormone (iatrogenic, inadvertent, or surreptitious) are causes of thyrotoxicosis but not hyperthyroidism (see question 1).

11. **How do thyrotoxic patients present clinically?**

Common symptoms include palpitations, shakiness, insomnia, difficulty with concentrating, irritability or emotional lability, weight loss, heat intolerance, exertional dyspnea, fatigue, hyperdefecation, menses with lighter flow or shorter duration, and brittle hair. Occasionally patients may experience weight gain rather than loss during thyrotoxicosis, presumably owing to polyphagia beyond that necessary to support their increased metabolism.

12. **What is apathetic hyperthyroidism?**

Older patients with hyperthyroidism may lack typical adrenergic features and present instead with depression or apathy, weight loss, atrial fibrillation, worsening angina pectoris, or congestive heart failure.

13. **Describe the physical signs of thyrotoxicosis.**

Tremors, tachycardia, flow murmurs, warm and moist skin, hyperreflexia with rapid relaxation phases, and a goiter (with a bruit in patients with Graves' disease) may be found in hyperthyroid patients. Eye findings in thyrotoxicosis are discussed in question 14.

14. **How does hyperthyroidism cause eye disease?**

Lid retraction and stare can be seen with any cause of thyrotoxicosis and are due to increased adrenergic tone. True ophthalmopathy is unique to Graves' disease and is thought to be caused by thyroid autoantibodies that cross-react with antigens in fibroblasts, adipocytes, and preadipocytes behind the eyes. Common manifestations of ophthalmopathy include proptosis, diplopia, and inflammatory changes such as conjunctival injection and periorbital edema.

15. **What laboratory testing should be performed to confirm thyrotoxicosis?**

Measurement of serum TSH with a second- or third-generation assay is the most sensitive test for detecting thyrotoxicosis. Because a low TSH also may be seen in central hypothyroidism, a free T_4 level should be measured to confirm thyrotoxicosis. If the free T_4 level is normal, a T_3 level should be determined to rule out T_3 toxicosis. Other associated laboratory findings may include mild leukopenia, normocytic anemia, elevations of hepatic transaminases and bone alkaline phosphatase, mild hypercalcemia and hyperphosphatemia, and low levels of albumin and cholesterol.

16. **When is thyroid antibody testing necessary for the diagnosis of hyperthyroidism?**

The cause of hyperthyroidism usually can be determined with history, physical examination, and radionuclide studies. Testing for TSH receptor antibodies is useful in pregnant women with Graves' disease to determine the risk of neonatal thyroid dysfunction due to transplacental passage of stimulating or blocking antibodies. It is also useful in euthyroid patients suspected of having euthyroid Graves' ophthalmopathy and in patients with alternating periods of hyper- and hypothyroidism as a result of fluctuations in blocking and stimulating TSH receptor antibodies.

17. **What is the difference between a thyroid scan and an uptake?**
A radioactive iodine uptake (RAIU) uses ^{131}I or I^{123} to assess quantitatively the functional status of the thyroid gland. A small dose of radioactive iodine is given orally followed by measurement of radioactivity in the area of the thyroid in 4 to 24 hours. Often 2 measurements are taken, at 4 to 6 hours and at 24 hours. A high uptake confirms hyperthyroidism. A scan provides a two-dimensional image depicting the distribution of iodine trapping within the thyroid gland. Uniform distribution in a hyperthyroid patient suggests Graves' disease, patchy distribution suggests TMNG, and unifocal activity corresponding to a nodule, with suppression of the rest of the thyroid, suggests a toxic adenoma.

18. **How should hyperthyroidism be treated?**
The three main treatment options are antithyroid drugs (ATDs), including methimazole (MMI) and propylthiouracil (PTU); radioiodine (^{131}I) ablation; and surgery. Unless contraindicated, most patients should receive beta-blockers for heart rate control and symptomatic relief. Most thyroidologists in the United States prefer ^{131}I over surgery or prolonged courses of ATDs. Patients scheduled to receive ^{131}I should be advised to avoid pregnancy and should be cautioned that oral contraceptives may not be fully protective in the hyperthyroid state because of increased levels of sex hormone–binding globulin and increased clearance of the contraceptive.

19. **When is surgery indicated for hyperthyroidism?**
Surgery is generally not the treatment of choice for hyperthyroidism. It is most often used when a cold nodule is present in a patient with Graves' disease, in pregnant patients allergic to or intolerant of antithyroid drugs (^{131}I is contraindicated in pregnancy), or in patients with extremely large goiters who are less likely to respond to ATDs or ^{131}I. Surgery may also be the preferred modality when patients have other serious medical problems that make the rapid attainment of normal thyroid levels crucial, or have significant eye involvement with Graves' disease. Patients should be euthyroid before surgery to decrease the risk of arrhythmias during induction of anesthesia and the risk of postoperative thyroid storm.

20. **What is the role of iodine in the treatment of hyperthyroidism? What is the Wolff-Chaikoff effect?**
Inorganic iodine acutely reduces the synthesis and release of T_4 and T_3. The inhibition of thyroid hormone synthesis by iodine is known as the Wolff-Chaikoff effect. However, because escape from this effect generally occurs after 10 to 14 days, iodine is used only to prepare a patient rapidly for surgery or as an adjunctive measure in patients with thyroid storm after ATDs have been administered. Typical doses are Lugol's solution, 8 drops 4 times/day, or saturated solution of potassium iodide (SSKI), 5 drop 4 times/day.

21. **Are other treatments available to lower thyroid hormone levels?**
Yes. Two iodine-containing oral cholecystographic agents, ipodate and iopanoic acid, cause dramatic reductions in serum T_3 and T_4 through inhibition of T4 5' deiodinase. Unfortunately, both of these agents are no longer available in the United States. Other agents occasionally used to treat hyperthyroidism include lithium, which decreases thyroid hormone release, and potassium perchlorate, which inhibits thyroid uptake of iodine.

22. **Which medications block peripheral conversion of T_4 to T_3?**
PTU, propranolol, glucocorticoids, iopanoic acid, and amiodarone inhibit the peripheral conversion of T_4 to T_3.

23. **How effective are ATDs?**
Ninety percent of patients taking ATDs become euthyroid without significant side effects. Approximately half of patients attain a remission from Graves' disease after a treatment course of 12 to 18 months. However, only 30% maintain long-term remission; the remainder experience recurrence within 1 to 2 years after the drugs are withdrawn. TMNG and AFTNs are not autoimmune diseases; therefore, they do not go into remission. The role of ATDs in these two disorders is only to render a patient euthyroid before surgery or when pretreatment is necessary before radioiodine therapy (see question 27). The usual starting dosages for moderate thyrotoxicosis are methimazole, 30 mg/day, or PTU, 100 mg 3 times/day. MMI is generally prefered over PTU for several reasons (longer half-life allowing for less frequent dosing, higher success rate, faster response time). PTU, however, is the preferred treatment in thyroid storm, pregnancy, and lactation.

24. **What side effects are associated with ATDs?**
    1. Agranulocytosis is a rare but life-threatening complication of ATD therapy, occurring in approximately 1 in every 200 to 500 patients treated with ATDs. Patients should be instructed to report promptly fever, sore throat, or minor infections that do not resolve quickly. Agranulocytosis appears to be dose-related with methimazole but not with PTU. Patients developing agranulocytosis on one antithyroid drug should not be exposed to another.
    2. Hepatotoxicity can progress to fulminant hepatitis with necrosis with PTU, and cholestatic jaundice has been reported with methimazole. Patients should report right upper quadrant pain, anorexia, nausea, and new pruritus.
    3. Rashes can range from limited erythema to an exfoliative dermatitis. Dermatologic reaction to one ATD does not preclude the use of another, although cross-sensitivity occurs in approximately 50% of cases.

25. **What lab tests should be monitored in patients taking ATDs?**
Thyroid hormone levels should be monitored to determine when ATD doses can be reduced from the initial high dosages to maintenance dosages (usually 25%–50% of initial doses). TSH may remain suppressed for several months; in this situation, free T_4 levels are more reliable for assessing thyroid hormone status. Hepatic enzymes and complete blood count with differential should be checked every 1 to 3 months. Because transaminase elevation and mild granulocytopenia can be seen in untreated Graves' disease, it is important to check these parameters before initiating ATD therapy. Many cases of agranulocytosis appear to arise without preceding granulocytopenia; thus a high index of suspicion is required even if recent testing is normal.

26. **How does radioactive iodine work?**
Thyroid cells trap and concentrate iodine and use it to make thyroid hormone. ^{131}I is organified in the same manner as organic iodine. Because ^{131}I emits locally destructive beta particles, cellular damage and death occur over a period of several months after treatment. Dosages of ^{131}I should be high enough to result in permanent hypothyroidism to decrease the recurrence rate. A typical dose for Graves' disease is 15 milliCuries (mCi); for TMNG, higher doses of 25 to 30 mCi are given. These doses are effective in 90% to 95% of patients.

27. **When is pretreatment with ATDs indicated before ^{131}I ablation?**
Elderly patients and patients with underlying systemic illnesses are often pretreated with ATDs in an effort to deplete the thyroid of preformed hormones and thereby theoretically reduce the risk of ^{131}I-induced thyroid storm. When pretreatment with ATDs is used, the drugs are generally stopped 4 to 7 days before ^{131}I is given. However, pretreatment with antithyroid drugs is associated with a rapid increase in thyroid hormone levels upon ATD discontinuation. Most nonpretreated patients experience a rapid decrease in thyroid hormone levels after radioiodine.

Therefore most patients do not require or benefit from ATD pretreatment. If pretreatment is given, MMI should be used preferentially over PTU because the latter has radioprotective effects that diminish the effectiveness of radioiodine ablation.

28. **How long after ^{131}I treatment should women wait before becoming pregnant or resuming breast-feeding?**
Pregnancy should be deferred for at least 6 months after ^{131}I ablation because of an increased risk of pregnancy loss. In addition, patients should be on a stable dose of thyroid hormone replacement and free of active ophthalmopathy. Breast milk radioactivity, measured in one study after an 8.3-mCi therapeutic dose of ^{131}I, remained unacceptably high for 45 days. If ^{99m}Technetium or ^{123}I is used for diagnostic studies, breast-feeding may be resumed in 2 to 3 days, with pumping and disposal of breast milk in the interim.

29. **Does ^{131}I cause or worsen ophthalmopathy in Graves' disease?**
This is an area of ongoing controversy. The natural history of Graves' disease is such that 15% to 20% of patients develop significant ophthalmopathy. The majority of cases arise in the period from 18 months before to 18 months after the onset of thyrotoxicosis. Thus a fair number of new cases can be expected to coincide with the timing of ^{131}I ablation. Two prospective randomized trials have shown that ^{131}I is more likely to worsen ophthalmopathy than other treatment modalities. Patients with preexisting eye disease and those who smoke cigarettes are more likely to experience worsening. As a result, it is prudent to avoid ^{131}I in patients with active moderate-to-severe Graves' ophthalmopathy, or to treat these patients with a course of oral corticosteroids immediately after the dose of ^{131}I.

30. **How is thyrotoxicosis managed in pregnancy?**
Caution must be used in interpreting thyroid laboratory results during pregnancy, because low TSH values are not uncommon in the first trimester, and total T_4 levels are elevated by increased thyroxine-binding globulin (TBG) levels. Free T_4 levels using equilibrium dialysis or an assay with pregnancy-specific normal ranges are the best indicator of thyroid function during pregnancy. Nuclear medicine testing with RAIU or thyroid scanning is contraindicated in pregnancy because of concerns about fetal exposure to isotopes. Because ^{131}I therapy is also contraindicated during pregnancy, treatment options are limited to ATDs or surgery in the second trimester. PTU is generally the preferred ATD during pregnancy because it crosses the placenta to a lesser extent than methimazole, and the use of the latter has been associated with a rare neonatal scalp disorder known as aplasia cutis as well as choanal and esophogeal atresia. Pregnant patients with Graves' disease require close follow-up to ensure adequate control and to prevent hypothyroidism because the disorder frequently remits during the course of pregnancy. TSH receptor antibodies, which are able to cross the placenta after 26 weeks, should be measured in the third trimester to assess the risk of neonatal thyroid dysfunction. If TSH receptor antibodies are elevated or the mother is on ATDs, fetal ultrasound should be performed around 32 weeks' gestation to look for evidence of fetal thyroid dysfunction that could include growth restriction, hydrops, goiter, or fetal tachycardia.

KEY POINTS: HYPERTHYROIDISM

1. The three most common causes of hyperthyroidism are Graves' disease, toxic multi-nodular goiter, and toxic adenoma.

2. Thyroiditis can cause severe thyrotoxicosis but resolves without intervention and may be followed by a hypothyroid phase.

3. Routine diagnostic testing for hyperthyroidism includes thyroid-stimulating hormone (TSH), free thyroxine (T_4), $\pm$ free triiodothyronine (T_3), radioactive iodine uptake (RAIU), and thyroid scanning with I^{123} or ^{99m}technetium.

4. The major treatment choices for hyperthyroidism are radioiodine, antithyroid drugs (methimazole, propylthiouracil), and thyroidectomy. Beta-blockers can significantly improve adrengic symptoms of thyrotoxicosis and do not interfere with testing or later treatment.

5. Treatment is generally indicated when TSH is less than 0.1 mIU/L. Asymptomatic patients with a suppressed TSH higher than 0.1 mIU/L may be followed closely.

TOP SECRETS

1. The three most common causes of hyperthyroidism are Graves' disease, toxic multi-nodular goiter, and toxic adenoma.

2. Routine diagnostic testing for hyperthyroidism includes thyroid-stimulating hormone (TSH), free thyroxine (T_4), $\pm$ free triiodothyronine (T_3), radioactive iodine uptake (RAIU), and thyroid scanning with I^{123} or ^{99m}technetium.

3. The major treatment choices for hyperthyroidism are radioiodine, antithyroid drugs (methimazole, propylthiouracil), and thyroidectomy.

BIBLIOGRAPHY

1. Abalovich M, Amino N, Barbour LA, et al: Management of thyroid dysfunction during pregnancy and postpartum: an endocrine society clinical practice guideline. J Clin Endocrinol Metab Supplement 92:s1–s7, 2007.

2. Bartalena L, Marcocci C, Bogazzi F, et al: Relation between therapy for hyperthyroidism and the course of Graves' ophthalmopathy. N Engl J Med 338:73–78, 1998.

3. Biondi B, Fazio S, Carella C, et al: Cardiac effects of long term thyrotropin-suppressive therapy with levothyroxine. J Clin Endocrinol Metab 77:334–338, 1993.

4. Bonnema SJ, Bennedbæk FN, Veje A, et al: Propylthiouracil before ^{131}I therapy of hyperthyroid diseases: effect on cure rate evaluated by a randomized cinical trial. J Clin Endocrinol Metab 89:4439–4444, 2004.

5. Burch HB, Shakir F, Fitzsimmons TR, et al: Diagnosis and management of the autonomously functioning thyroid nodule: The Walter Reed Army Medical Center experience, 1975–1996. Thyroid 8:871–880, 1998.

6. Burch HB, Solomon BL, Cooper DS, Ferguson P, Walpert N, Howard R: The effect of antithyroid drug pretreatment on acute changes in thyroid hormone levels after ^{131}I ablation for Graves' disease. J Clin Endocrinol Metab. 86:3016–3021, 2001.

7. Burch HB, Wartofsky L: Graves' ophthalmopathy: current concepts regarding pathogenesis and management. Endocr Rev 14:747–793, 1993.

8. Burrow GN: Thyroid function and hyperfunction during gestation. Endocr Rev 14:194–202, 1993.

9. Col NF, Surks MI, Daniels GH: Subclinical thyroid disease: clinical applications. JAMA 291:239–243, 2004.

10. Cooper DS: Antithyroid drugs in the management of patients with Graves' disease: an evidence-based approach to therapeutic controversies. J Clin Endocrinol Metab 88:3474–3481, 2003.

11. Cooper DS: Antithyroid drugs. N Engl J Med 352:905–917, 2005.

12. Cooper DS: Hyperthyroidism. Lancet 362:459–468, 2003.

13. Kahaly GJ, Nieswandt J, Mohr-Kahaly S: Cardiac risks of hyperthyroidism in the elderly. Thyroid 8:1165–1169, 1998.

14. Luton D, Le Gac I, Vuillard E, et al: Management of Graves' disease during pregnancy: the key role of fetal thyroid gland monitoring. J Clin Endocrinol Metab 90:6093–6098, 2005.

15. McDermott MT, Ridgway EC: Central hyperthyroidism. Endocrinol Metab Clin North Am 27:187–203, 1998.

16. McDermott MT, Ridgway EC: Thyroid hormone resistance syndromes. Am J Med 94:424–432, 1993.

17. Sawin CT, Geller A, Wolf PA, et al: Low serum thyrotropin concentration as a risk factor for atrial fibrillation in older persons. N Engl J Med 331:1249–1252, 1994.

18. Singer PA, Cooper DS, Levy EG, et al: Treatment guidelines for patients with hyperthyroidism and hypothyroidism. Standards of Care Committee, American Thyroid Association. JAMA 273:808–812, 1995.

19. Surks MI, Ortiz E, Daniels GH, et al: Subclinical thyroid disease: scientific review and guidelines for diagnosis and management. JAMA 291:228–239, 2004.

20. Uzzan B, Campos J, Cucherat M, et al: Effects on bone mass of long term treatment with thyroid hormones: a meta-analysis. J Clin Endocrinol Metab 81:4278, 1996.

CHAPTER 34

HYPOTHYROIDISM

Katherine Weber and Bryan R. Haugen

1. **How common is hypothyroidism?**
   Hypothyroidism is relatively common with a prevalence of 4% to 8% in the general population. The mean age at diagnosis is the mid-50s. Hypothyroidism is much more common in women, with a female-to-male ratio of 3:1. Postpartum hypothyroidism, a transient hypothyroid phase after pregnancy, is found in 5% to 10% of women.

2. **What is subclinical hypothyroidism?**
   Subclinical hypothyroidism (now called mild thyroid failure) is a mild and much more common form of hypothyroidism, often with few or no symptoms. Hypercholesterolemia and subtle cardiac abnormalities have been associated. Biochemically, the levels of thyroxine (T_4) or free T_4 are normal, whereas the level of thyroid-stimulating hormone (TSH) is mildly elevated. As many as 10% to 20% of women older than 50 years have mild thyroid failure.

3. **How is subclinical hypothyroidism treated?**
   When patients are treated with T_4, they have an improved sense of well-being (compared with placebo) and the cardiac and lipid abnormalities improve. Therefore treatment is generally recommended, especially for patients with a persistent TSH > 10 mU/L. Thyroid antibodies, an indicator of autoimmune thyroid disease, may help to predict which patients will progress to clinical hypothyroidism; testing is recommended for patients with a minimally elevated TSH level.

4. **What are the two most common causes of hypothyroidism?**
   Although many disorders can cause hypothyroidism, the two most common causes are chronic lymphocytic thyroiditis (Hashimoto's disease), an autoimmune form of thyroid destruction, and radioiodine-induced hypothyroidism after treatment of Graves' disease (autoimmune hyperthyroidism).

5. **How common is postpartum thyroiditis?**
   Postpartum thyroiditis occurs in approximately 10% of women, two thirds of whom experience a transient hypothyroid phase (6–12 months) that requires treatment.

6. **List the less common causes of hypothyroidism.**
   - Subacute thyroiditis
   - External irradiation to the neck
   - Medications (antithyroid drugs, amiodarone, lithium, bexarotene, sunitinib, and interferon)
   - Infiltrative diseases
   - Central (pituitary/hypothalamic) hypothyroidism (Fig. 34-1)
   - Congenital defects
   - Endemic (iodine-deficient) goiter, which is fairly common outside the United States

7. **List the symptoms commonly associated with hypothyroidism.**
   Hypothyroidism commonly presents with nonspecific symptoms, such as fatigue, cold intolerance, depression, weight gain, weakness, joint aches, constipation, dry skin, hair loss, and menstrual irregularities.

Hypothalamus

TRH

(−)

Pituitary

TSH

Thyroid

T_4/T_3

Peripheral effects

Figure 34-1. Hypothalamic-pituitary-thyroid axis.

8. **What findings on physical examination are consistent with hypothyroidism?**
   Physical examination may be normal with mild thyroid failure and should not deter further workup if clinical suspicions are high. Common signs of moderate-to-severe hypothyroidism include:
   - Hypertension (diastolic hypertension is a clue)
   - Bradycardia
   - Coarse hair
   - Periorbital swelling
   - Yellow skin (due to elevated levels of beta-carotene)
   - Carpal tunnel syndrome
   - Delayed relaxation of the deep tendon reflexes

9. **What does palpation of the thyroid reveal?**
   The thyroid may be enlarged, normal, or small, but thyroid consistency is usually firm.

10. **Summarize unusual presentation of hypothyroidism.**
    Unusual presentations of hypothyroidism include megacolon, cardiomegaly, pericardial effusion, and congestive heart failure (CHF). Severe CHF in one reported patient scheduled for cardiac transplant resolved with thyroid hormone replacement alone.

11. **Describe the laboratory tests that may show abnormal results during hypothyroidism.**
    Laboratory clues to hypothyroidism include normochromic, normocytic anemia (menstruating women may also have iron deficiency anemia due to excessive bleeding from irregular menses), hyponatremia, hypercholesterolemia, and elevated levels of creatine phosphokinase.

12. **What tests best confirm the diagnosis of hypothyroidism in the outpatient setting?**

Many thyroid function tests are available to the clinician, including assessments of TSH, T_4, triiodothyronine (T_3), resin uptake, free T_4, free T_3, and reverse T_3. In the outpatient setting only one test is usually necessary: assessment of TSH. TSH, which is synthesized and secreted from the anterior pituitary gland, is the most sensitive indicator of thyroid function in the nonstressed state. Basically, if the TSH is normal (range: 0.5–5 mU/L), the patient is euthyroid; if the TSH is elevated (>5 mU/L), the patient has primary gland failure.

13. **How should total T_4 levels be interpreted?**

Care must be taken in interpreting T_4 levels (occasionally performed on health-screening panels). Many conditions unrelated to thyroid disease cause low or elevated levels of total T_4 because more than 99% of T_4 is protein-bound, and total T_4 levels depend on the amount of thyroid-binding proteins, which may vary greatly. Total T_4 levels must always be compared with the T_3 resin uptake (T_3RU), which reflects the amount of thyroid hormone-binding protein.

KEY POINTS: HYPOTHYROIDISM

1. Thyroid-stimulating hormone (TSH) level is the best screening test for primary hypothyroidism in the outpatient setting.

2. Levothyroxine (LT_4) is the preferred initial treatment for hypothyroidism and in healthy young patients can be started at a dose of 1.6 µg/k/day.

3. The goal TSH for treatment of primary hypothyroidism is between 0.5 and 2.0 mU/L.

4. Subclinical hypothyroidism (elevated TSH but normal thyroxine/triiodothyronine [T_4/T_3]) is common, and treatment can alleviate symptoms, as well as cardiac and lipid abnormalities.

14. **Explain why thyroid function tests are more difficult to interpret in acutely ill inpatients.**

Interpretation of thyroid function tests in acutely ill inpatients is more difficult when hypothyroidism is suspected. Acute nonthyroidal illness may cause suppression of the T_4 and T_3 levels, and TSH may be elevated in the recovery phase (see Chapter 40). Medications, such as dopamine and glucocorticoids, may suppress the TSH. Severe illness may even cause low levels of free T_4.

15. **How do you diagnose hypothyroidism in acutely ill inpatients?**

When hypothyroidism is suspected in the stressed, hospitalized patient, a combination of clinical signs (inappropriate bradycardia, puffy facies, dry skin, and delayed relaxation of deep tendon reflexes) and laboratory tests (TSH and free T_4 levels) is necessary to exclude or confirm the diagnosis of hypothyroidism. If these tests are equivocal, a reverse T_3 level, which is normal or elevated in nonthyroidal illness and low in hypothyroidism, may prove helpful. Inpatient TSH testing also may be confounded by normal diurnal variations in TSH. TSH levels in euthyroid people may exceed the normal range at night, when patients are frequently admitted. A morning test may help to clarify the significance of a mildly elevated TSH.

16. **Which thyroid hormone preparation should you use?**

Since 1891, when sheep thyroid extract was first used to treat myxedema, many preparations have been developed and are still available. Currently the best replacement regimen is L-thyroxine (LT_4). Brand-name LT_4 (Synthroid, Levothroid, and Levoxyl) is preferred over the generic preparations because cost is a minor issue (generic LT_4 costs $6/month, whereas brand names cost about $10/month) and because generic LT_4 may vary 15% to 20% in bioavailability.

17. **What other thyroid hormone preparations are available?**
Other thyroid hormone preparations include L-triiodothyronine (LT_3), which is reserved for special cases because of its potency and short half-life, and desiccated thyroid and thyroglobulin, which give unpredictable concentrations of serum thyroid hormone because of varied content and bioavailability.

18. **What is the recommended dose of LT_4 for replacement therapy in a hypothyroid patient?**
Otherwise healthy, young patients may be started on full replacement doses of LT_4 (1.6 μg/k/day). Elderly patients and patients with known or suspected cardiac disease should be started on low doses of LT_4 (25 μg/day), which are increased by 25 μg/day every 2 to 3 months until the TSH is normal. In patients with subclinical hypothyroidism, consider starting the patient on 50% to 75% of the predicted full replacement dose.

19. **What is the appropriate goal for TSH in the treatment of primary hypothyroidism?**
The target TSH in treated hypothyroid patients should be between 0.5 and 2.0 mU/L, which represents the lower end of the normal range reported by most laboratories. When the usual reference ranges for TSH were developed, they included subjects with antithyroid antibodies suggestive of occult autoimmune thyroid disease. The "normal" ranges are therefore thought to be skewed toward higher TSH values. When normal subjects with no antithyroid antibodies are evaluated, most have TSH values below 2.5 mU/L.

20. **Discuss the evidence supporting combination T_4/T_3 therapy.**
The medical and lay literature has taken a renewed interest in combination therapy. A recent placebo-controlled study suggested that patients taking combination therapy had improved cognitive function and mood scores compared with when they took LT_4 alone. Studies in thyroidectomized animals have shown that T_4 therapy alone does not restore tissue levels of T_4 and T_3 to euthyroid levels, even when the TSH is normalized. Although these studies are provocative and intriguing, most experts agree that more information is needed before we can recommend combination T_4/T_3 therapy in most patients. Our current approach is to discuss this information openly with inquiring patients.

21. **When should you consider combination T_4/T_3 therapy?**
The authors suggest a trial of LT_4 alone to normalize TSH within the low normal range (0.5–2.0 mU/L) for a period of 2 to 4 months. Many patients do extremely well with this approach. Patients who have low-normal TSH while taking LT_4 and still feel "hypothyroid" require further evaluation before considering T_3 therapy. We generally exclude anemia and vitamin B_{12} deficiency (associated with Hashimoto's thyroiditis) and inquire about sleep apnea. If this assessment is negative, we decrease the LT_4 by 12 to 25 μg and add 5 μg of Cytomel (T_3) in the morning. The goal is to see whether the patient's symptoms improve without persistent suppression of the serum TSH (measured in the morning before taking medication). No data clearly support or refute this position; we believe it is a position of "good" medical practice.

22. **How should the clinician approach surgery in the hypothyroid patient?**
There are two broad categories to consider: emergent/cardiac surgery and elective surgery. Hypothyroidism is associated with minor postoperative complications—gastrointestinal (prolonged constipation, ileus), as well as neuropsychiatric (confusion, psychosis); in addition, the incidence of fever with infections is lower. Patients scheduled for elective surgery should wait until TSH is normalized because of the postoperative complications associated with

hypothyroidism. However, rates of mortality and major complications (blood loss, arrhythmias, and impaired wound healing) are similar to the rates in euthyroid patients.

23. **Summarize the current recommendations for emergent surgery.**
Current recommendations are to proceed with emergent surgery in the hypothyroid patient and to monitor for potential postoperative complications while giving replacement therapy with LT_4. Patients with ischemic coronary artery disease requiring surgery should proceed without LT_4 replacement because T_4 increases myocardial oxygen demands and may precipitate worsening cardiac symptoms if given before surgery. Postoperatively the patient should receive replacement therapy with LT_4 at a slow rate and be followed for CHF (increased in hypothyroid patients undergoing cardiac surgery).

24. **How does myxedema differ from hypothyroidism?**
Myxedema is a severe, uncompensated form of prolonged hypothyroidism. Complications include hypoventilation, cardiac failure, fluid and electrolyte abnormalities, and coma (see Chapter 39). Myxedema coma is frequently precipitated by an intercurrent systemic illness, surgery, or narcotic/hypnotic drugs. Patients with myxedema coma should receive replacement therapy with 300 to 500 μg of intravenous LT_4 followed by 50 to 100 μg each day. Because conversion of T_4 to T_3 (active hormone) is decreased with severe illness, patients with profound cardiac failure that requires pressors or patients unresponsive to 1 to 2 days of LT_4 therapy should be given LT_3 at 12.5 μg intravenously every 6 hours.

WEBSITE

http://www.nacb.org

BIBLIOGRAPHY

1. Arem R, Patsch W: Lipoprotein and apolipoprotein levels in subclinical hypothyroidism. Arch Intern Med 150:2097–2100, 1990.
2. Bunevicius R, Kazanavicius G, Zalinkevicius R, Prange AJ: Effects of thyroxine as compared with thyroxine plus triiodothyronine in patients with hypothyroidism. N Engl J Med 340:424–429, 1998.
3. Canaris GJ, Manowitz NR, Mayor G, Ridgway EC: The Colorado thyroid disease prevalence study. Arch Intern Med 104:526–534, 2000.
4. Cooper DS, Halpern R, Wood LC, et al: L-thyroxine therapy in subclinical hypothyroidism. Ann Intern Med 101:18–24, 1984.
5. Demers LM, Spencer CA: Laboratory medicine practice guidelines: laboratory support for the diagnosis and monitoring of thyroid disease. Thyroid 13:45–56, 2003.
6. Elder J, McLelland A, O'Reilly SJ, et al: The relationship between serum cholesterol and serum thyrotropin, thyroxine, and tri-iodothyronine concentrations in suspected hypothyroidism. Ann Clin Biochem 27:110–113, 1990.
7. Hay ID, Duick DS, Vliestra RE, et al: Thyroxine therapy in hypothyroid patients undergoing coronary revascularization: a retrospective analysis. Ann Intern Med 95:456–457, 1981.
8. Hollowell JG, Staehling NW, Flanders WD, et al: Serum TSH, T_4, and thyroid antibodies in the United States population (1988 to 1994): National Health and Nutrition Examination Survey (NHANES III). J Clin Endocrinol Metab 87:489–499, 2002.
9. Ladenson PW: Recognition and management of cardiovascular disease related to thyroid dysfunction. Am J Med 88:638–641, 1990.
10. Ladenson PW, Levin AA, Ridgway EC, Daniels GH: Complications of surgery in hypothyroid patients. Am J Med 77:262–266, 1984.

11. Mandel SJ, Brent GA, Larsen PR: Levothyroxine therapy in patients with thyroid disease. Ann Intern Med 119:492–502, 1993.

12. Patel R, Hughes RW: An unusual case of myxedema megacolon with features of ischemic and pseudomembranous colitis. Mayo Clin Proc 67:369–372, 1992.

13. Rosenthal MJ, Hunt WC, Garry PJ, Goodwin JS: Thyroid failure in the elderly: microsomal antibodies as discriminant for therapy. JAMA 258:209–213, 1987.

14. Roti E, Minelli R, Gardini E, Braverman LE: The use and misuse of thyroid hormone. Endocr Rev 14:401–423, 1993.

CHAPTER 35

THYROIDITIS

Robert C. Smallridge

1. **Give the differential diagnosis for thyroiditis.**
   1. Infectious
      a. Acute (suppurative)
      b. Subacute (granulomatous; de Quervain's)
   2. Autoimmune
      a. Chronic lymphocytic (Hashimoto's disease)
      b. Atrophic (primary myxedema)
      c. Juvenile
      d. Postpartum
   3. Painless (nonpostpartum)
   4. Drug induced
   5. Riedel's struma
   6. Radiation-induced
   7. Traumatic
   8. Tumor embolization

2. **What causes acute thyroiditis?**
   This rare disease is infectious and usually bacterial; at times, however, fungal, tuberculous, parasitic, or syphilitic infections have been reported. *Pneumocystis carinii* has been observed in patients with AIDS. Patients may develop hyperthyroid symptoms.

3. **How is acute thyroiditis managed?**
   Treatment involves incision and drainage of the abscess and antibiotics. Children often have a pyriform sinus fistula, which should be surgically repaired.

4. **Describe the four stages of subacute thyroiditis.**
   - Stage I: Patients have a painful (unilateral or bilateral) tender thyroid and may have systemic symptoms (fatigue, malaise, fever). Inflammatory destruction of thyroid follicles permits release of thyroxine (T_4) and triiodothyronine (T_3) into the blood, and thyrotoxicosis may ensue.
   - Stage II: A transitory period (several weeks) of euthyroidism occurs after the T_4 is cleared from the body.
   - Stage III: With severe disease, patients may become hypothyroid until the thyroid gland repairs itself.
   - Stage IV: Euthyroid state returns.

5. **Summarize the natural history of subacute thyroiditis.**
   Subacute thyroiditis is probably viral in origin. Histologically, the inflammation is granulomatous. Although patients almost always recover clinically, serum thyroglobulin levels remain elevated, and intrathyroidal iodine content is low for many months (Fig. 35-1). Patients requiring steroids are more likely to become hypothyroid at a later time. Such findings suggest

persistent subclinical abnormalities after an episode of subacute thyroiditis. Approximately 2% of patients have a second episode many years later.

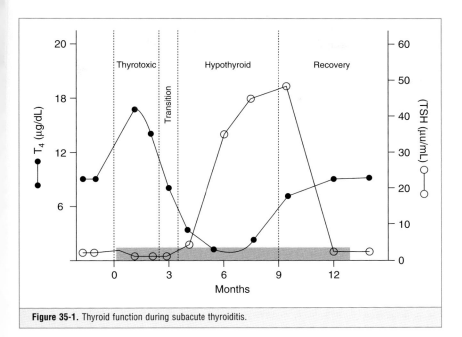

Figure 35-1. Thyroid function during subacute thyroiditis.

6. **What is the most common cause of thyroiditis?**
   Autoimmune thyroid disease, which is recognized by the presence of thyroid peroxidase (TPO) antibodies and, less frequently, thyroglobulin antibodies in serum.

7. **Give the clinical characteristics of autoimmune thyroid disease.**
   Chronic lymphocytic thyroiditis (Hashimoto's disease) usually presents as a euthyroid goiter that progresses to hypothyroidism in middle-aged and older persons, especially women. Atrophic thyroiditis is characterized by a very small thyroid gland in a hypothyroid patient. Some evidence suggests that thyroid growth inhibitory antibodies may account for the lack of a goiter. Two thirds of adolescents with goiter have autoimmune (juvenile) thyroiditis.

8. **Does postpartum thyroiditis follow a different clinical course from other types of autoimmune thyroiditis?**
   Yes. Postpartum disease develops in women between the third and ninth month after delivery. It typically follows the stages seen in patients with subacute thyroiditis, although histologically patients have lymphocytic infiltration.

9. **How common is postpartum thyroiditis?**
   After delivery, 5% to 10% of women develop biochemical evidence of thyroid dysfunction. Approximately one third of affected women develop symptoms (either hyperthyroidism, hypothyroidism, or both) and benefit from 6 to 12 months of therapy with L-thyroxine (LT_4) if hypothyroid. The frequency of each clinical presentation is depicted in Fig. 35-2.

Figure 35-2. Frequency of clinical presentations of postpartum thyroiditis.

10. **Summarize the differences between subacute and postpartum thyroiditis.**
    See Table 35-1.

TABLE 35-1. SUBACUTE VERSUS POSTPARTUM THYROIDITIS		
	Subacute Thyroiditis	**Postpartum Thyroiditis**
Thyroid pain	Yes	No
Sedimentation rate	Increased	Normal
TPO antibody	Transient increase only	Positive
HLA status	B-35	DR3, DR5
Histology	Giant cells, granulomas	Lymphocytes

HLA, human eucocyte antigen; TPO, thyroid peroxidase.

11. **Why do women develop postpartum thyroiditis?**
    Women who develop postpartum thyroiditis have underlying, usually asymptomatic,
    autoimmune thyroiditis. During pregnancy, the maternal immune system is partially suppressed,
    with a dramatic rebound rise in thyroid antibodies after delivery. Although TPO antibodies are
    not believed to be cytotoxic, they are currently the most reliable marker of susceptibility to
    postpartum disease.

12. **Does thyroid function in patients with postpartum thyroiditis return to normal,
    as it does in subacute thyroiditis?**
    Not always. Approximately 20% of women become permanently hypothyroid, and a similar
    number have persistent mild abnormalities. An annual TSH test is therefore recommended.

13. **Do any factors identify women at increased risk for developing
    postpartum thyroiditis?**
    Women with a higher TPO antibody titer are more likely to develop thyroiditis. Approximately
    25% of women with type 1 diabetes mellitus develop thyroiditis after delivery. For high-risk

patients, screening for thyroid antibodies and careful monitoring of thyroid function at 3 to 6 months postpartum are indicated.

14. **What is painless thyroiditis?**

Both men and nonpostpartum women may present with transient thyrotoxic symptoms. As with subacute thyroiditis, they often experience subsequent hypothyroidism. Unlike subacute disease, this disorder is painless. It has been given a variety of names, including hyperthyroiditis, silent thyroiditis, transient painless thyroiditis with hyperthyroidism, and lymphocytic thyroiditis with spontaneously resolving hyperthyroidism. This disease was first described in the 1970s and reached its peak incidence in the early 1980s. It seems to occur less often now.

15. **What causes painless thyroiditis?**

Some investigators believe that it is a variant of subacute thyroiditis because a small percentage of patients with biopsy-proved subacute disease have had no pain (they may have fever and weight loss and may be mistaken for having systemic disease or malignancy). Others believe that painless thyroiditis is a variant of Hashimoto's disease because the histology of the two is similar. Hashimoto's thyroiditis can occasionally present with thyroid pain; rarely surgery is necessary to relieve symptoms.

KEY POINTS: THYROIDITIS

1. In early subacute thyroiditis, the radioactive iodine uptake (RAIU) is suppressed, and sedimentation rate markedly elevated.

2. Approximately 10% of premenopausal women are TPO-antibody positive; many develop postpartum thyroid dysfunction.

3. Amiodarone-induced thyroid disease (AITD) may be due to iodine-induced hyperthyroidism (type 1 AITD) or destruction-induced thyroiditis (type 2 AITD).

4. Subacute thyroiditis may require analgesics (or steroids) and beta-blockers early and L-thyroxine (LT$_4$) during recovery but usually resolves.

5. Acute infectious thyroiditis requires prompt incision and drainage and antibiotics.

16. **What is destruction-induced thyroiditis?**

Destruction-induced thyroiditis refers to disorders (subacute, postpartum, drug-induced and painless thyroiditis), in which an inflammatory infiltrate destroys thyroid follicles, and excessive amounts of T$_4$ and T$_3$ are released into the circulation.

17. **When a patient presents with hyperthyroid symptoms, an elevated level of T4, and a suppressed level of TSH, what is the next test that should be ordered?**

A 24-hour RAIU should be performed. When the thyroid is overactive (as in Graves' or toxic nodular disease), the RAIU is elevated. In destruction-induced thyroiditis, the RAIU is low, as a result of both suppression of TSH by the acutely increased level of serum T$_4$ and the diminished ability of damaged thyroid follicles to trap and organify iodine.

18. **What is the appropriate therapy for patients with any type of destructive thyroiditis?**

In the thyrotoxic stage, beta-blockers relieve adrenergic symptoms. All forms of antithyroid therapy (drugs, radioactive iodine ablation, and surgery) are absolutely contraindicated.

Analgesics (salicylates or prednisone) provide prompt relief of thyroid pain. Thyroid hormone relieves hypothyroid symptoms and should be continued for 6 to 12 months, depending on the severity of disease. Some patients require no therapy.

19. Which drugs can induce thyroiditis?

Amiodarone, an iodine-containing antiarrhythmic drug, may cause thyroid damage and thyrotoxicosis. Interferon alpha (less commonly, interferon beta) and interleukin-2 can cause thyroiditis, and both hyperthyroidism and hypothyroidism have occurred during therapy.

20. Does amiodarone induce only thyroiditis?

No. Because of the large amount of iodine in this drug, it can cause either iodine-induced hypothyroidism or hyperthyroidism. Distinguishing hyperthyroidism due to iodine excess (type 1 disease) from amiodarone-induced thyroiditis (type 2 disease) can be difficult. Some differentiating features are listed in Table 35-2. Absence of blood flow on Doppler sonography is particularly helpful in confirming type 2 disease.

TABLE 35-2. TYPE 1 VERSUS TYPE 2 THYROIDITIS

	Type 1	Type 2
Thyroid size	Goiter; nodules	Normal
RAIU	↓, normal, ↑	↓↓
Thyroid antibodies	↑, negative	Negative
Interleukin-6	Normal, ↑	↑↑
Ultrasound Doppler flow	↑	↓
Therapy	Antithyroid drugs; potassium perchlorate; thyroidectomy	Antithyroid drugs (?); steroids

RAIU, radioactive iodine uptake.

21. What is Riedel's struma?

Riedel's struma is a rare disorder in which the thyroid becomes densely fibrotic and hard. Local fibrosis of adjacent tissues may produce obstructive symptoms that require surgery. In some cases, fibrosis of other tissues (fibrosing retroperitonitis, orbital fibrosis, or sclerosing cholangitis) may occur.

22. How is Riedel's thyroiditis treated?

Surgical removal of the thyroid isthmus may relieve constrictive symptoms. Glucocorticoids have been helpful, as has tamoxifen (by stimulating transforming growth factor-β, which inhibits fibroblast growth).

23. Are there any other causes of thyroiditis?

Yes. External beam radiotherapy can cause painless thyrotoxic thyroiditis. Various forms of neck trauma (neck surgery, cyst aspiration, seat-belt injury, and tumor emboli) have also been reported.

WEBSITE

http://www.thyroidmanager.org

BIBLIOGRAPHY

1. Abalovich M, Amino N, Barbour LA, et al: Management of thyroid dysfunction during pregnancy and postpartum: an Endocrine Society clinical practice guideline. J Clin Endocrinol Metab 92:s1–7, 2007.

2. Aizawa T, Watanabe T, Suzuki N, et al: Radiation-induced painless thyrotoxic thyroiditis followed by hypothyroidism: a case report and literature review. Thyroid 8:273–275, 1998.

3. Bartalena L, Brogioni S, Grasso L, et al: Treatment of amiodarone-induced thyrotoxicosis, a difficult challenge: results of a prospective study. J Clin Endocrinol Metab 81:2930–2933, 1996.

4. Berger SA, Zonszein J, Villamena P, et al: Infectious diseases of the thyroid gland. Rev Infect Dis 5:108–122, 1983.

5. Bogazzi F, Martino E, Dell'Unto E, et al: Thyroid color flow doppler sonography and radioiodine uptake in 55 consecutive patients with amiodarone-induced thyrotoxicosis. J Endocrinol Invest 26:635–640, 2003.

6. Carella C, Mazziotti G, Amato G, et al: Interferon-α-related thyroid disease: pathophysiological, epidemiological, and clinical aspects. J Clin Endocrinol Metab 89:3656–3661, 2004.

7. de Lange WE, Freling NJ, Molenaar WM, et al: Invasive fibrous thyroiditis (Riedel's struma): a manifestation of multifocal fibrosclerosis? A case report with review of the literature. Q J Med 72:709–717, 1989.

8. Fatourechi V, Aniszewski J, Fatourechi G, et al: Clinical features and outcome of subacute thyroiditis in an incidence cohort: Olmsted County, Minnesota, study. J Clin Endocrinol Metab 88:2100–2105, 2003.

9. Guttler R, Singer PA, Axline SG, et al: Pneumocystis carinii thyroiditis. Report of three cases and review of the literature. Arch Intern Med 153:393–396, 1993.

10. Iitake M, Momotani N, Ishii J, et al: Incidence of subacute thyroiditis recurrences after a prolonged latency: 24-year survey. J Clin Endocrinol Metab 81:466–469, 1996.

11. Kon YC, DeGroot LJ: Painful Hashimoto's thyroiditis as an indication for thyroidectomy: clinical characteristics and outcome in seven patients. J Clin Endocrinol Metab 88:2667–2672, 2003.

12. Meek SE, Smallridge RC: Diagnosis and treatment of thyroiditis and other more unusual forms of hyperthyroidism. In Cooper DS, editor, *Medical management of thyroid disease*, New York, 2001, Marcel Dekker, pp. 93–134.

13. Ross DS: Syndromes of thyrotoxicosis with low radioactive iodine uptake. Endocrinol Metab Clin N Am 27:169–185, 1998.

14. Rotenberg Z, Weinberger I, Fuchs J, et al: Euthyroid atypical subacute thyroiditis simulating systemic or malignant disease. Arch Intern Med 146:105–107, 1986.

15. Roti E, Minelli R, Gardini E, et al: Iodine-induced hypothyroidism in euthyroid subjects with a previous episode of subacute thyroiditis. J Clin Endocrinol Metab 70:1581–1585, 1990.

16. Seminara SB, Daniels GH: Amiodarone and the thyroid. Endocr Pract 4:48–57, 1998.

17. Shigemasa C, Ueta Y, Mitani Y, et al: Chronic thyroiditis with painful tender thyroid enlargement and transient thyrotoxicosis. J Clin Endocrinol Metab 70:385–390, 1990.

18. Smallridge RC: Hypothyroidism and pregnancy. Endocrinologist 12:454–464, 2002.

19. Smallridge RC: Postpartum thyroid disease: a model of immunologic dysfunction. Clin Appl Immunol Rev 1:89–103, 2000.

20. Smallridge RC, De Keyser FM, Van Herle AJ, et al: Thyroid iodine content and serum thyroglobulin: cues to the natural history of destruction-induced thyroiditis. J Clin Endocrinol Metab 62:1213–1219, 1986.

21. Volpé R: The management of subacute (de Quervain's) thyroiditis. Thyroid 3:253–255, 1993.

22. Woolf PD: Transient painless thyroiditis with hyperthyroidism: a variant of lymphocytic thyroiditis? Endocr Rev 1:411–420, 1980.

CHAPTER 36

THYROID NODULES AND GOITER

William J. Georgitis

1. **What is a goiter?**
   Goiter is a visible swelling in front of the neck from an enlarged thyroid gland. The derivation of the term has been traced to the French *goitre,* the Middle French *goitron* or throat, a vulgate Latin term *guttrion,* and the Latin terms *guttrio* and *guttur* for throat.

2. **How does a nontoxic goiter develop?**
   The pathogenesis for euthyroid goiter remains an enigma. Proposed mechanisms include:
   - Thyroid-stimulating hormone (TSH)-dependent thyroid enlargement to compensate for diminished thyroid hormone production due to environmental goitrogens
   - Iodine deficiency
   - Inherited biosynthetic defects

   Regression of goiter after iodine supplementation or thyroxine suppression of TSH supports these mechanisms. However, TSH levels are not elevated in endemic goiter. Important genetic variants may involve thyroglobulin, thyroperoxidase, intracellular signaling pathways affecting cell life cycles, and the sodium/iodine (Na/I^-) symporter.

3. **Describe the natural history of diffuse nontoxic goiter.**
   Simple goiter tends to become multinodular over time. The nodules are heterogenous in both morphology and function. Autonomous function, defined as TSH-independent production and secretion of thyroid hormone, can evolve. Supplementation programs in iodine-deficient populations, although clearly decreasing the incidence of cretinism and goiter, have also caused some people to develop iodine-associated hyperthyroidism. This Jodbasedow hyperthyroidism is more likely to occur in older people with autonomous adenomatous goiters. In the United States, this form of hyperthyroidism usually results from iodine excess due to radiographic contrast agents or medications rich in iodine. It may be transient and not require ablative therapies, such as thyroidectomy or radioiodine treatment.

4. **How does lithium affect thyroid function?**
   Lithium has diverse effects on thyroid function. It inhibits iodine uptake, dampens iodotyrosine coupling, alters thyroglobulin structure, blocks thyroid hormone secretion, and has mitogenic effects. Both goiter and hypothyroidism can appear during prolonged exposure to lithium (Fig. 36-1).

5. **Describe the mechanism by which lithium produces goiter and hypothyroidism.**
   The inhibitory effect of lithium on thyroid hormone release provokes an increase in TSH even in patients free of thyroid disease. Compensatory thyroid enlargement occurs without hypothyroidism except in patients with an underlying decrease in thyroid functional reserve. In this category of patients, thyroid hormone levels may be normal before lithium treatment, but hypothyroidism may appear in patients with chronic lymphocytic thyroiditis, a past history of subacute thyroiditis, or partial thyroidectomy. Because hypothyroid signs and symptoms may be difficult to decipher in the presence of depression or bipolar disorder, TSH testing before and during lithium treatment is recommended.

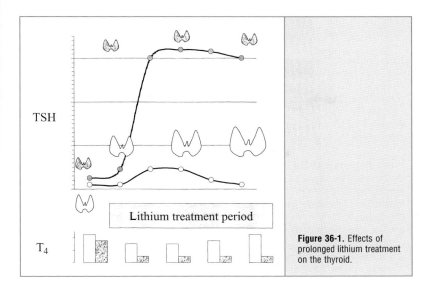

TSH

T₄

Lithium treatment period

Figure 36-1. Effects of prolonged lithium treatment on the thyroid.

6. **How common are thyroid nodules?**
   Thyroid nodules are common. Prevalence increases as a linear function of age. The cumulative lifetime chance of having a palpable thyroid nodule approaches 6%. The prevalence at autopsy in 90-year-olds is about 60%. The vast majority of thyroid nodules are benign. The yield of thyroid cancer in surgical series before the widespread use of fine-needle aspiration (FNA) averaged about 10%.

7. **List the differential diagnosis for a thyroid nodule.**

Adenoma	Carcinoma	Thyroid cyst
Thyroiditis	Thyroid hemiagenesis	Parathyroid cyst
Metastatic cancer	Lymphoma/sarcoma	

8. **Can the nature of a thyroid nodule be determined from the family history?**
   Family history is usually not helpful. An exception is medullary thyroid cancers associated with the multiple endocrine neoplasia syndromes. Inheritance of these tumors is autosomal dominant with almost complete penetrance for the abnormal ret oncogene.

9. **Do personal history and physical examination help to determine the nature of a thyroid nodule?**
   In general, no. Most patients with thyroid nodules have no symptoms and normal thyroid function. Hoarseness, dysphagia, dyspnea, or hemoptysis are rare features that suggest malignancy but also occur in benign thyroid disorders. When a patient with a visible goiter reports any of these symptoms, it suggests either rapid growth or involvement of the recurrent laryngeal nerve. An aggressive form of thyroid malignancy, such as lymphoma or anaplastic thyroid cancer, is a consideration, but fortunately it is rare. Thyroid cancer grows without

causing pain. Other traits of nodules that suggest malignancy include size greater than 3 cm, fixation to adjacent structures, and palpable cervical lymph nodes.

10. **How are most thyroid cancers discovered?**
Most thyroid cancers are discovered by chance. Often the patient is the first to notice a lump. A change in the appearance of the neck may be reported by a family member or during a medical visit for some unrelated matter. Ultrasound, magnetic resonance imaging (MRI), and computed tomography (CT) studies for myriad indications may first detect a thyroid nodule. Because they are recognized incidental to the purpose of the procedure, these nodules are often referred to as thyroid incidentalomas.

11. **What diagnosis should be suspected when a thyroid nodule is first discovered because of neck pain?**
Hemorrhagic degeneration of a benign adenoma. Visceral pain fibers are triggered by acute expansion of the nodule, which stretches the thyroid capsule. The resulting deep, aching pain may radiate to the jaw or ear. Pain may be mistaken for dental abscess, otitis media, or otitis externa. Aspiration of hemorrhagic fluid can relieve the discomfort and confirms the diagnosis.

12. **If a nodule is cancer, what kind is it likely to be?**
A papillary thyroid cancer or variant of papillary is the most common by far (Table 36-1).

TABLE 36-1. FREQUENCY OF THYROID CANCER TYPES	
Papillary	50%–70%
Follicular	10%–15%
Medullary	1%–2%
Anaplastic	Rare
Primary thyroid lymphoma	Rare
Metastatic to thyroid	Rarely diagnosed

13. **How does the appearance of the fluid help in diagnosing thyroid cysts?**
Simple thyroid cysts have yellow-, burgundy-, or chocolate-colored fluid and are generally benign. Complex thyroid nodules with both cystic and solid components contain brown or hemorrhagic fluid. Complex cysts have a higher risk of malignancy than simple cysts. Cytology of cyst fluid is almost always nonspecific and shows histiocytes and crenated erythrocytes. If the fluid removed is crystal-clear like water, the lesion is a parathyroid cyst. Serum calcium should be measured to exclude hyperparathyroidism.

14. **How does the amount of thyroid cyst fluid help guide management?**
One third of cysts reappear days to weeks after aspiration. If the volume on sequential aspirations does not decrease or the aspirated fluid is grossly bloody, surgical removal of the cyst should be considered.

15. **How important is sampling of the solid component of the complex nodule?**
FNA of any solid component palpable after the fluid has been drained or with ultrasound guidance to ensure sampling of the solid component of the complex nodule can provide diagnostic material.

16. **Is the risk of cancer less in multinodular goiter or Hashimoto's disease than in solitary thyroid nodules?**
Although autopsy series indicate that up to 75% of thyroid nodules are multiple and that malignancy is rare, any thyroid nodule can be cancerous. Contrary to old axioms, a palpable nodule in the presence of multinodular goiter or lymphocytic thyroiditis seems to have the same risk of cancer as a solitary palpable nodule. Size does seem to matter. Palpable nodules are generally at least 1 cm in greatest dimension. Nodules smaller than 1 cm are often not palpable and have a low risk of malignancy.

17. **Summarize the role of FNA in the evaluation of thyroid nodules.**
FNA is a safe, outpatient procedure with an accuracy of 90% to 95% in adequate specimens interpreted by experienced cytopathologists. FNA should be performed on all readily palpable solitary thyroid nodules and on dominant nodules in a multinodular goiter. After a serum TSH level is shown to be normal, an FNA is really the next evaluation for a thyroid nodule. Most FNAs return benign diagnoses, including adenomatous hyperplasia (benign multinodular goiter), colloid adenoma, and autoimmune thyroiditis. A reading of papillary thyroid cancer helps guide planning for thyroid resection.

18. **Is FNA helpful in diagnosing follicular neoplasms?**
Follicular neoplasms are more vexing. FNA cannot reliably differentiate adenoma from carcinoma because features of capsular or vascular invasion that define follicular carcinoma can be determined only on surgical pathology. Aspirates are inadequate for interpretation in about 15%. This rate can be reduced by using ultrasound guidance, especially for lesions with a cystic component.

19. **Should an FNA be performed for a palpable nodule if the TSH is low?**
No. A low TSH indicates hyperthyroidism.

20. **If the TSH is found to be low, what is the next step?**
A thyroid scan, to rule in solitary toxic nodule or toxic multinodular goiter, should be the next test. Although the scan is ordered with the anticipation of finding lesions with autonomous function, a photopenic (cold) nodule may sometimes be encountered.

21. **Explain the distinction between cold and hot nodules.**
A cold nodule has diminished uptake of the radioactive agent compared with surrounding normal thyroid tissue. Most cold nodules are benign, but virtually all thyroid cancers are cold on scan. The solitary toxic or hot nodule avidly absorbs tracer, whereas uptake in the remainder of the thyroid is suppressed. Solitary toxic nodules are usually larger than 3 cm in diameter. Most occur in patients older than 40. Toxic adenomas are never cancerous. The majority has gain of function mutations in the thyrotropin receptor.

22. **What is the significance of a warm nodule?**
In contrast, a warm nodule may be malignant. Some hyperfunctional or isofunctional nodules are really cold nodules that appear to concentrate tracer because they are invested by normal thyroid tissue. Other autonomous nodules fail to secrete sufficient thyroid hormone to suppress TSH to dampen tracer uptake by surrounding normal thyroid tissue. Thyroid scanning with the patient taking a TSH-suppressive dose of thyroid hormone can define the autonomous nature of these nodules. Autonomous nodules may be observed, whereas all others deserve FNA to exclude thyroid cancer.

23. **Who invented the incision used for thyroidectomy?**
Theodor Kocher (1841–1917), a Swedish surgeon, devised the incision. He was an innovator, so be cautious when you ask for a "Kocher" in the operating room. Kocher's name is also

associated with a surgical forceps, a wrist operation, and a right subcostal incision for cholecystectomy.

24. **Which treatment was used first for diffuse toxic goiter (Graves' disease): radioactive iodine or antithyroid medications?**
Both were developed in the early 1940s. Thiourea, the first goitrogenic substance to be used, had undesirable toxicities and soon was replaced by methimazole and propylthiouracil. Of the fission products developed during World War II, ^{130}I was used before ^{131}I. Radioiodine became widely available in about 1946.

25. **What goitrous thyroid conditions are treated with radioactive iodine?**
Radioiodine treatment is effective for diffuse toxic goiter, toxic nodular goiter, and solitary toxic nodules. Compressive symptoms from benign multinodular goiters in patients judged to be poor surgical risks can also be relieved by radioactive iodine. Although the goiter shrinks only about 30% or less, relief of symptoms is common.

26. **What does recent evidence reveal about the role of suppression therapy with thyroxine?**
Although thyroxine suppression therapy was widely used in the past in the belief that it reduced the size of thyroid nodules, more recent randomized controlled studies, including some with objective measurements by ultrasound, indicate that suppression therapy is ineffective. For euthyroid patients, thyroid hormone administration to induce regression of thyroid nodules has not proved to be effective except under special circumstances, such as iodine deficiency or prevention of new nodules after lobectomy in radiation-exposed patients. Used in solitary nodules, the apparent reduction in size judged only by palpation may represent regression of surrounding thyroid tissue rather than the nodule itself. Routine treatment with TSH-suppressive doses of thyroid hormone for thyroid nodules or goiter may be associated with more iatrogenic side effects than benefits.

27. **When is suppression therapy with thyroxine useful?**
Suppression therapy may still be of value in selected cases. For example, the patient with an elevated serum TSH and thyroid enlargement may show regression of the goiter with thyroid hormone replacement.

KEY POINTS: THYROID NODULES AND GOITER

1. The cumulative lifetime chance of having a palpable thyroid nodule is about 6%.

2. A thyroid nodule is present in about 60% of 90 year olds.

3. The vast majority of thyroid nodules are benign.

4. Nodules in multinodular goiter are heterogenous in both morphology and function.

5. Fine needle aspiration of the thyroid is a safe outpatient procedure with an accuracy of 90% to 95% in determining malignancy.

TOP SECRETS

1. Aspirating clear watery fluid from an thyroid region nodule indicates the nodule is a parathyroid cyst.

2. When goiter and hypothyroidism appear with lithium therapy, suspect underlying chronic lympocytic thyroiditis.

3. Although thyroid hormone suppression therapy is rarely used because it is not effective for nodule or goiter size reduction, observing a rise in thyroxine blood levels disproportionate to the suppression dose may indicate a nodule or goiter is functioning autonomously helping to rule in benign autonomous nodule or multinodular goiter or even Graves' disease. Consider ordering a scan on suppression therapy to make these diagnoses.

WEBSITE

http://www.thyroidmanager.org/

BIBLIOGRAPHY

1. Bennedbæk FN, Nielsen LK, Hegedüs L: Effect of percutaneous ethanol injection therapy versus suppressive doses of L-thyroxine on benign solitary solid cold thyroid nodules: a randomized trial. J Clin Endocrinol Metab 83:830–835, 1998.

2. Bennedbæk FN, Perrild H, Hegedüs L: Diagnosis and treatment of the solitary thyroid nodule. Results of a European survey. Clin Endocrinol 50:357–363, 1999.

3. Braverman LE, Utiger RD: *Werner and Ingbar's the thyroid: a fundamental and clinical text edition*, ed 8, Philadelphia, 2000, Lippincott, Williams & Wilkins.

4. Cheung PSY, Lee JMH, Boey JH: Thyroxine suppressive therapy of benign solitary thyroid nodules: a prospective randomized study. World J Surg 13:818–822, 1989.

5. Dremier S, Coppee F, Delange F, et al: Thyroid autonomy: mechanism and clinical effects. J Clin Endocrinol Metab 81:4187–4193, 1996.

6. Hegedus L, Nygaard B, Hansen JM: Is routine thyroxine treatment to hinder postoperative recurrence of nontoxic goiter justified? J Clin Endocrinol Metab 84:756–760, 1999.

7. Lazarus JH: The effects of lithium therapy on thyroid and thyrotropin-releasing hormone. Thyroid 8:909–913, 1998.

8. Mazzaferri EL: Management of a solitary thyroid nodule. N Engl J Med 328:553–559, 1993.

9. Mortensen JD: Gross and microscopic findings in clinically normal thyroid glands. J Clin Endocrinol Metab 15:1270–1280, 1955.

10. Ridgway EC: Medical treatment of benign thyroid nodules: have we defined a benefit? Ann Intern Med 128:403–405, 1998.

11. Rojeski MT: Nodular thyroid disease. N Engl J Med 313:428–436, 1985.

12. Ross DS: Evaluation of the thyroid nodule. J Nucl Med 32:2181–2192, 1991.

CHAPTER 37

THYROID CANCER

Arnold A. Asp

1. **Describe the types of thyroid cancer.**
   The thyroid consists predominantly of follicular epithelial cells, which incorporate iodine into thyroid hormone to be stored in follicles, and of smaller numbers of parafollicular cells, which produce calcitonin (CT). Malignant transformation of either type of cell may occur, but the parafollicular malignancy (medullary thyroid carcinoma [MTC]) is much less common than cancers derived from follicular epithelial cells. Malignancies originating from follicular epithelial cells are designated according to their microscopic appearance and include papillary, follicular, and anaplastic carcinomas (Fig. 37-1).

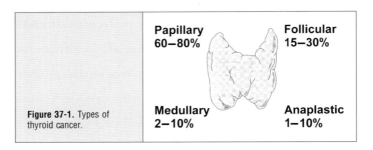

Papillary
60–80%

Follicular
15–30%

Figure 37-1. Types of thyroid cancer.

Medullary
2–10%

Anaplastic
1–10%

2. **Summarize the frequency of each type of thyroid cancer.**
   Papillary carcinoma and its variants comprise approximately 80% of thyroid cancers, whereas follicular carcinoma makes up approximately 11% of primary thyroid malignances. Hürthle cell carcinoma comprises 4% of malignancies. These three forms are frequently referred to as the differentiated thyroid carcinomas (DTCs). MTC accounts for 2% to 10% of thyroid carcinomas, whereas anaplastic forms of thyroid carcinoma account for 1% to 10%.

3. **Describe the histology of the two differentiated forms of thyroid carcinoma.**
   Papillary and follicular carcinomas are histologically distinct. Papillary carcinoma is generally an unencapsulated tumor marked by enlarged cells with dense cytoplasm and overlapping nuclei that have granular, powdery chromatin, nucleoli, and pseudonuclear inclusion bodies (often called "Orphan Annie eyes"), all arranged in papillary fronds. Follicular carcinoma is generally characterized by atypical-appearing thyroid cells with dense, uniform, overlapping nuclei, and a disorganized microfollicular architecture.

4. **How is follicular carcinoma differentiated from benign follicular adenomas?**
   Follicular carcinoma cannot be differentiated reliably from benign follicular adenomas on cytomorphologic criteria alone; follicular cancer must demonstrate invasion of the tumor capsule or blood vessels.

5. **Summarize the types of papillary carcinoma.**
   Tumors that contain histologic elements of both types of carcinoma are classified as mixed papillary-follicular cancer and are considered to be variants of papillary carcinoma. Two additional pathologic variants of papillary carcinoma, tall cell and insular cell, may be slightly more aggressive than other papillary forms.

6. **Distinguish the clinical behavior of papillary and follicular carcinomas.**
   Papillary and follicular carcinomas behave as clinically distinct entities. Most endocrinologists consider follicular carcinoma to be the more aggressive of the differentiated cancers, with a higher rate of metastases, more frequent recurrence after therapy, and an exaggerated mortality rate compared with the relatively indolent papillary carcinoma. This view is not universal. Some authors believe that the sharp dichotomy between the clinical courses of papillary and follicular carcinomas is artificial and attribute the apparent aggressiveness of follicular carcinoma to its occurrence in an older population; they argue that when cases are controlled for age, outcomes of patients with either form of DTC are comparable.

7. **Who gets papillary carcinoma?**
   The disease may occur at any age but has a peak incidence during the fourth decade. Women are more commonly affected than men and account for 62% to 81% of patients in most series.

8. **Describe the clinical course of papillary carcinoma.**
   Papillary carcinoma usually presents as a painless nodule within the thyroid gland or cervical lymphatics. The primary tumor is rarely encapsulated (4%–22% in most series) but is less aggressive if a capsule is present. Papillary carcinoma is more commonly multifocal within the thyroid than is follicular carcinoma; 20–80% of glands have multiple lesions at resection. Extrathyroidal invasion through the capsule of the thyroid occurs in 5% to 16% of cases. Compared with other malignancies, papillary carcinoma is relatively indolent. Cancer-related death occurs in only 4% to 12% of patients during 20-year follow-up. Prognostic factors at the time of diagnosis that augur a poor outcome include male sex, age over 40 years, extrathyroidal invasion, distant metastases, and large primary tumor (>1.5-cm diameter).

9. **Discuss the significance of lymph node metastases of papillary carcinoma.**
   Papillary carcinoma frequently metastasizes to regional cervical and high mediastinal lymphatics. At the time of surgery, 35% to 43% of patients have enlarged regional lymph nodes that harbor cancer. If lymph nodes are systematically harvested and examined for microscopic foci, the prevalence of cervical metastases increases to 90%. Unlike other neoplasms, the presence of papillary carcinoma in regional lymph nodes does not increase mortality; it does, however, increase the likelihood of recurrence after therapy. Up to 20% of recurrent lesions cannot subsequently be eradicated.

10. **How common is metastasis of papillary carcinoma to sites other than lymph nodes?**
    Although lymphatic metastases are common, only 3% to 7% of patients with papillary carcinoma manifest distant metastatic lesions during initial therapy. Distant metastases involve the lung (76% of distant foci), bone (23% of distant foci), and brain (15% of distant foci).

11. **Who gets follicular carcinoma?**
    Follicular carcinoma may occur at any age but has a later peak incidence (fifth decade) than papillary carcinoma. Women outnumber men, accounting for approximately 60% of cases. Follicular carcinoma occurs more commonly in areas of iodine deficiency; the incidence of this malignancy has decreased as iodine supplementation has increased.

12. **Describe the clinical course of follicular carcinoma.**

Follicular carcinoma usually presents as an asymptomatic nodule within the thyroid, but unlike papillary carcinoma, it may present as an isolated metastatic pulmonary or osseous focus without a palpable thyroid lesion. Rarely metastatic foci of follicular carcinoma retain hormonal synthetic capability and overproduce thyroid hormones, causing thyrotoxicosis. The tumor is nearly always encapsulated, and the degree of vascular or capsular invasiveness (minimal to extensive) is indicative of malignant potential. Follicular carcinoma is usually unifocal ($<10\%$ multifocal). Death from follicular carcinoma occurs in 13% to 59% of patients followed for 20 years. Prognostic factors at the time of initial therapy that portend a poor outcome include age greater than 50 years, male sex (in some settings), marked degree of vascular invasion, and distant metastases.

13. **How common are metastases of follicular carcinomas?**

Hematogenous metastases occur in follicular carcinomas; for this reason, cervical and mediastinal lymphatic involvement is less common than in papillary carcinoma (only 6%–13% of patients during initial surgery). In contrast to cases of papillary carcinoma, the presence of cervical metastases indicates advanced disease. Distant metastases to the lung, bone, and central nervous system (in descending order of occurrence) are discovered more commonly in follicular than in papillary carcinoma, occurring in 12% to 33% of cases.

14. **Discuss the relationship between Graves' disease and DTC.**

DTC is discovered in 5% to 10% of the surgical resections performed for the treatment of Graves' disease. In some series of patients with Graves' disease, up to 45% of palpable nodules contain papillary carcinoma. Such data have led to the speculation that the thyroid-stimulating immunoglobulins responsible for thyrotoxicosis may potentiate the growth of neoplastic cells and predispose to aggressive forms of DTC.

15. **How is chronic lymphocytic thyroiditis related to DTC?**

Chronic lymphocytic thyroiditis is found concomitantly with papillary carcinoma in 5% to 10% of cases. Local recurrence and metastatic disease are less common in such cases and may indicate a favorable effect of Hashimoto's disease.

16. **How does metastatic disease affect the prognosis of DTC?**

Distant metastatic disease, as mentioned earlier, occurs more commonly in follicular carcinoma than in papillary cancer. Regardless of the primary type of cancer, the prognosis associated with distant metastases is dismal. Overall, 50% to 66% of patients with pulmonary, osseous, or central nervous system lesions die within 5 years. On rare occasions, pulmonary metastases may be compatible with 10- to 20-year survival in younger patients. Metastases to bone are associated with brief survival, despite aggressive therapy.

17. **How are the DTCs treated?**

Simply stated, therapy for DTC is based on surgical removal of the primary tumor and eradication of all metastatic disease with radioactive iodine (^{131}I). Lifelong suppression of thyroid-stimulating hormone (TSH) with exogenous thyroid hormone subsequently reduces the risk of recurrence.

18. **What factors favor limited surgery?**

Opinions about the extent of initial surgical resection have been tempered by the possible complications of thyroid surgery; recurrent laryngeal nerve damage with resultant hoarseness, iatrogenic hypoparathyroidism, or both may occur in 1% to 5% of thyroid resections. Fear of complications, coupled with the relatively low mortality rate associated with DTC, has prompted some surgeons to remove only the thyroid lobe in which cancer is apparent at the time of exploration if the tumor is smaller than 1.5 cm in diameter.

19. **Why do most surgeons favor more extensive surgery?**

Most surgeons are cognizant of the frequency of clinically inapparent multicentric lesions, the increased recurrence rates in patients treated with simple lobectomy, and the low rate of postsurgical complications; thus they have rejected simple lobectomy and instead prefer near-total thyroidectomy, which entails the removal of the thyroid lobe containing the tumor, the isthmus, and the majority of the contralateral thyroid lobe. The posterior capsule of the contralateral lobe is left undisturbed in an attempt to preserve the underlying parathyroid glands and the recurrent laryngeal nerve. With this procedure, the surgeon is able to remove the primary tumor and the bulk of normal thyroid tissue that may harbor microscopic malignancy.

20. **Are lymph nodes removed surgically?**

Cervical and high mediastinal lymph nodes (compartment VI) that appear to harbor metastatic disease are harvested at the time of surgery. Radical neck dissections do not reduce mortality or rate of recurrence and should be avoided, unless there are direct extensions of the tumor throughout the neck. In the event that a single, small ($<$1.5 cm) papillary or minimally invasive follicular carcinoma is discovered, lobectomy and isthmusectomy may be curative.

21. **How does ^{131}I therapy benefit the patient?**

Most (but not all) differentiated thyroid malignancies retain the ability to trap inorganic iodine when stimulated by TSH. When ^{131}I is concentrated within normal or malignant thyroid tissue, beta irradiation results in cellular damage or death. If a metastatic lesion is capable of concentrating ^{131}I, it becomes visible with a gamma camera; if it absorbs enough ^{131}I to impart 8000 cGy of irradiation, the tumor focus may be eradicated. This is the basis of postsurgical radioiodine scans (^{131}I or ^{123}I) for whole-body surveillance and the therapeutic use of ^{131}I to treat residual, recurrent, and metastatic disease. Patients with one thyroid lobe intact (after lobectomy and isthmusectomy) concentrate the entire scanning dose of radioiodine within the remaining lobe. Metastatic foci outside the thyroid cannot be detected in these patients, and surveillance scans are therefore uninformative and should be avoided.

22. **How can the efficacy of whole-body scans be optimized?**

To optimize the efficacy of whole-body scans and to maximize the concentration of therapeutic radioiodine in metastatic lesions, serum levels of TSH must be elevated. Withdrawal of exogenous L-thyroxine for 6 weeks before the scan allows the protein-bound fraction of the hormone to be exhausted. To alleviate symptoms of hypothyroidism, liothyronine (Cytomel, 25 mg twice daily) is administered for the first 4 weeks of the withdrawal period but discontinued during the 2 weeks before the scan. Liothyronine, with a shorter half-life than thyroxine, is rapidly depleted after withdrawal. During the 2-week period, in which no exogenous thyroid hormone is available, a rapid rise in serum TSH ($>$30 mU/L) ensues. Normal remnant thyroid tissue (on the posterior capsule of the thyroid bed) and malignant tissue are maximally stimulated by elevated levels of TSH and usually concentrate any available radioiodine. A low-iodine diet during the 2 weeks before administration of radioiodine enhances thyroid absorption of radioactive iodine.

23. **How is the whole-body scan performed?**

During the whole-body scan, 2 to 5 mCi of ^{131}I or 200 microCi of ^{123}I is administered orally to the patient, who is subsequently positioned under a gamma camera after the radioiodine is allowed to equilibrate (48–72 hours for ^{131}I; 24 hours for ^{123}I). The resultant image indicates the amount of thyroid tissue remaining in the thyroid bed and the extent of local and distant metastatic diseases. Scanning with ^{123}I (minimal radiation) may prevent "stunning" of residual normal and malignant thyroid tissue. Therapeutic ^{131}I is then administered.

24. **How much ^{131}I is administered to the patient after surgical removal of a single, small papillary tumor without extrathyroidal lesions?**

Generally, in the patient with a single, small papillary tumor (<1.5 cm) free of extrathyroidal metastases at the time of surgery and on subsequent whole-body scan, many endocrinologists consider the resection curative and do not administer radioiodine. In such cases, the use of adjunctive radioiodine does not alter the course of the disease. The author prefers, however, to administer a small dose of ^{131}I (30 mCi) in an attempt to ablate the thyroid bed and thereby to improve the accuracy of future surveillance scans. The procedure is called radioactive remnant ablation. This "small" dose ablates up to 80% of thyroid remnants. Other endocrinologists believe that this dose is insufficient to ablate all residual normal and malignant tissue and prefer a dose of 70 to 150 mCi of radioiodine.

25. **How much ^{131}I is administered to the patient after surgical removal of a large or aggressive tumor or extrathyroidal lesions?**

Patients with large or aggressive tumors, metastatic disease evident during surgery, or extrathyroidal lesions visible on postsurgical whole-body scans usually receive 100 to 200 mCi of ^{131}I in an attempt to eradicate the malignancy. These "large" doses of radioiodine have traditionally been administered only in an approved inpatient facility under the auspices of the Nuclear Regulatory Commission (NRC). Patients remain isolated until ambient levels of radioactivity fall to acceptable levels. Radionuclide is excreted renally, but significant amounts are also present in saliva and sweat. Such wastes must be disposed of appropriately. Currently, the NRC has lifted the absolute requirement for inpatient administration of high-dose ^{131}I, and it is now performed in most centers on an outpatient basis.

26. **Discuss the early complications of ^{131}I therapy.**

Radioiodine is absorbed by the salivary glands, gastric mucosa, and thyroid tissue. Within 72 hours of oral administration of ^{131}I, patients may experience radiation sialadenitis and transient nausea. Such symptoms are self-limited. Thyroid tissue may become edematous and tender but rarely requires corticosteroid therapy. Radioiodine, borne in the blood, causes transient, clinically insignificant suppression of the bone marrow. In some centers, dosimetry is used to determine the maximum dose of ^{131}I that can be safely administered at one time to patients with invasive or metastatic disease.

27. **What are the late complications of ^{131}I therapy?**

Late complications of high-dose radioiodine therapy may include gonadal dysfunction and predisposition to nonthyroidal malignancies. Some studies have demonstrated reduced sperm counts in male patients proportional to the administered dose of ^{131}I. Older women may experience temporary amenorrhea and reduced fertility. Two deaths from bladder cancer and three deaths from leukemia have been reported among patients treated with lifetime cumulative doses of radioiodine exceeding 1000 mCi. Most studies suggest that cumulative doses of ^{131}I less than 700 to 800 mCi, given in increments of 100 to 200 mCi separated by 6 to 12 months, are not leukemogenic.

28. **How are bony and pulmonary metastases treated?**

Radioiodine (^{131}I) is often used to treat bony and pulmonary metastases. Multifocal skeletal metastases from differentiated thyroid cancer are generally treated with 200 mCi of ^{131}I. However, isolated bony lesions are often treated instead with surgical resection or curettage or with external beam radiation therapy. Pulmonary metastases present a therapeutic dilemma, because radiation absorbed by the malignant cells often causes fibrosis of the underlying lung parenchyma. For this reason, pulmonary metastases that absorb more than 50% of the scanning dose of radioiodine are usually treated with no more than 75 to 80 mCi of ^{131}I.

29. **How are patients monitored for recurrent disease?**
Following surgery and radioiodine therapy (if required), all patients are placed on a large enough dosage of exogenous thyroid hormone to render serum TSH levels low or undetectable. In patients who presented with small tumors, without evidence of metastasis, most endocrinologists recommend detection of recurrent disease in the asymptomatic patient by annual ultrasound examination of the thyroid bed and measurement of serum thyroglobulin. Thyroglobulin, manufactured only by normal or malignant thyroid cells, should be undetectable in the serum of a patient who has undergone complete surgical and radioiodine ablation. Sensitivity of thyroglobulin measurement is enhanced if the patient is stimulated with recombinant TSH (see question 31).
   Cervical ultrasound of the thyroid bed is performed annually for 3 to 5 years in conjunction with thyroglobulin measurements to survey for local recurrence.

30. **When is a whole-body scan used?**
Whole-body scans have low sensitivity in detection of recurrent DTC and are not routinely employed for tumor surveillance in patients with low likelihood of recurrent disease. Evidence of recurrent tumor (rising levels of thyroglobulin or radiographic evidence of potential metastasis) may warrant repetition of a whole-body scan. Preparation of the patient is described in Question 22.

31. **Discuss the alternative to withdrawal of thyroid hormone before a whole-body scan.**
Recombinant human TSH (rhTSH; Thyrogen) has been approved for use in scanning patients with DTC. rhTSH acts just as native TSH produced by the pituitary, stimulating iodine uptake and thyroglobulin secretion from remnant thyroid tissue and metastatic foci of cancer. rhTSH (0.9 mg) is administered intramuscularly once daily for 2 consecutive days, followed by a scanning dose of [131]I (4 mCi) given orally on the third day. The patient is then imaged under a gamma camera on the fifth day. Serum thyroglobulin levels are drawn before administration of rhTSH and compared with those obtained on the fifth day.
   rhTSH-stimulated scans, when coupled with concomitant serum thyroglobulin measurements, are generally as accurate as standard whole-body scans and do not cause the significant hypothyroid symptoms that patients experience with levothyroxine withdrawal scans. Unfortunately, rhTSH has not yet been approved for use in raising serum TSH levels before therapeutic ^{131}I administration. Therefore rhTSH scans should be avoided if recurrent or metastatic thyroid cancer requiring ^{131}I treatment is anticipated.

32. **Which malignancy is associated with prior radiation exposure?**
From 1940 through the early 1970s, external irradiation of the head and neck was used in the treatment of acne, enlarged thymus, enlarged tonsils and adenoids, tinea capitis, and asthma. It was recognized belatedly that such radiation exposure caused neoplastic transformation of thyroid cells; after a 10- to 20-year latency period, 33% to 40% of exposed individuals developed benign thyroid nodules, and 5% to 11% developed carcinoma. The carcinomas in irradiated glands mirror those found within the nonirradiated population, with papillary cancer predominating. The tumors are no more aggressive but are more often multicentric (55%) than in nonirradiated individuals (22%).

33. **What is a hürthle cell?**
Hürthle, or Askanazy, cells are large polygonal cells with abundant cytoplasm and compact nuclei; they are found in benign nodules, Hashimoto's disease, and either form of DTC. Hürthle-cell carcinoma, composed solely of these cells, is believed to be a particularly aggressive variant of follicular cancer that is characterized by frequent pulmonary metastases.

34. **What is anaplastic thyroid carcinoma?**
Anaplastic thyroid carcinoma is one of the most aggressive and resistant forms of human cancer. It accounts for only 1% to 10% of all thyroid carcinomas in the Western Hemisphere but

for up to 50% of thyroid carcinomas in some areas of Eastern Europe. Like follicular carcinoma, it is more prevalent in areas of iodine deficiency; the incidence is currently declining throughout North America.

35. Discuss the histologic variants of anaplastic carcinoma.

Four histologic variants of anaplastic carcinoma are currently recognized: giant cell, spindle cell, mixed spindle-giant cell, and small cell carcinoma. True small cell carcinoma is extremely rare, and most "small cell" tumors are actually a malignant form of lymphoma that is more amenable to therapy. Microscopic examination of the anaplastic malignancies reveals bizarre fibrous whorls, primitive follicles, and cartilage and osteoid reminiscent of chondrosarcoma.

36. Who gets anaplastic carcinoma?

Anaplastic carcinoma occurs more commonly in the elderly (peak age: 65–70 years) and affects equal numbers of males and females. These cancers may arise in preexisting DTCs (dedifferentiation), in benign nodules, or, most commonly, de novo. The minuscule number of anaplastic malignancies within large series of patients followed for decades with DTC may discredit the theory of dedifferentiation of established cancers.

37. How does anaplastic carcinoma present?

Anaplastic carcinoma expands rapidly; most patients present with steric symptoms, such as dyspnea, dysphagia, hoarseness, and pain. Nearly half of all patients require tracheostomy as a result of explosive tumor growth.

38. Summarize the prognosis for patients with anaplastic carcinoma.

The type of histologic variant does not appear to affect outcome; prognosis is dismal in most cases. Surgical extirpation has been combined with external beam irradiation (4500–6000 cGy) or chemotherapy (usually doxorubicin or paclitaxel) in an attempt to eradicate the malignancy. Despite vigorous therapy, average survival is approximately 6 to 8 months.

39. What is MTC?

MTC is a neoplasm that arises from the parafollicular cells (or C cells) of the thyroid. Embryologically, these cells originate in the neural crest and migrate to the thyroid, where, despite close proximity, there is no apparent physical or hormonal interaction with the follicular cells.

40. Describe the function of parafollicular cells.

The parafollicular cells elaborate CT, which acts on osteoclasts to modulate release of calcium from skeletal stores. The DNA that contains the genetic code for CT also contains the code for another peptide, CT gene-related peptide (CGRP). Tissue-specific alternative splicing allows parafollicular cells to secrete CT, whereas neural cells produce only CGRP.

41. How does neoplastic transformation affect the parafollicular cells?

Neoplastic transformation of parafollicular cells results in unbridled expression of normal cell products (CT) and abnormal products (CGRP, chromogranin A, carcinoembryonic antigen [CEA], adrenocorticotropin [ACTH]). CT serves as an excellent tumor marker for the malignancy, and the abnormal products mediate the clinical syndromes associated with MTC. Accumulation of massive amounts of procalcitonin within the thyroid is detectable histologically as amyloid (AE type).

42. How common is MTC?

MTC accounts for approximately 2% to 10% of all thyroid malignancies and occurs in sporadic and hereditary forms. Sporadic MTC is the more common form.

43. Describe the presentation of sporadic MTC.

Most patients present in the fourth or fifth decade, with most series reporting nearly equal numbers of men and women. Sporadic MTC is usually unifocal within the thyroid and may originate in any portion of the gland. Half of all patients manifest metastatic disease at the time of presentation; metastatic sites include (in descending order) local lymphatics, lung, liver, and bone.

44. Summarize the forms in which hereditary MTC may occur within kindreds.
The hereditary form of MTC occurs within kindreds as an isolated condition (familial MTC), as a component of multiple endocrine neoplasia (MEN) 2A (MTC, hyperparathyroidism, pheochromocytoma), as a component of the MEN 2B syndrome (MTC, pheochromocytoma, mucosal neuromas), or in conjunction with pheochromocytoma and cutaneous lichen amyloidosis.

45. How does hereditary MTC present?
Hereditary tumors are bilateral and arise in the junction of the upper one third and lower two thirds of the thyroid lobes, where the concentration of C cells is highest. Biochemical screening for MTC to detect early disease within affected kindreds enhances the survival of individuals with hereditary MTC compared with those with the sporadic form. A discussion of the MEN syndromes is included in Chapter 53.

46. Are extrathyroidal manifestations associated with MTC?
The wide array of peptides and prostaglandin products secreted by MTC tumors results in multiple extrathyroidal symptoms. The most common is diarrhea, which occurs in up to 30% of patients with MTC. Although CT, CGRP, prostaglandins, 5-hydroxytryptamine, and vasoactive intestinal peptide have been proposed as the causative secretagogue, none has been convincingly implicated.
    On rare occasions, Cushing's syndrome may occur in MTC and is attributable to the secretion of ACTH, corticotropin-releasing hormone, or both. Successful therapy of the underlying malignancy ameliorates the Cushingoid features. There are no reported cases of hypocalcemia due to the chronic production of CT by MTC.

47. How can CT be used as a clinically useful tumor marker?
CT is secreted by normal parafollicular cells and cells undergoing neoplastic transformation. Most certainly in the hereditary form, and probably in the sporadic form, of MTC, malignant degeneration of the C cells is preceded by a period of "benign" hyperplasia, during which curative resection is theoretically feasible. The serum level of CT is proportional to the mass of hyperplastic or malignant parafollicular cells. Unfortunately, the Kulchitsky cells of the lung, as well as cells of the thymus, pituitary, adrenal glands, and prostate, also secrete small amounts of CT, as do certain malignancies, such as small cell lung cancer and breast cancer.

48. How is CT related to MTC distinguished from CT of non-MTC sources?
The pentagastrin stimulation test is used to distinguish the CT of non-MTC sources from the CT produced by hyperplastic and malignant C cells. Currently, pentagastrin is not available within the United States. The test involves the intravenous administration of pentagastrin (0.5 mg/kg body weight) with the collection of CT at baseline, 1.5, 2, 5, and 10 minutes after injection. Normal subjects demonstrate little or no response to the infusion, whereas subjects with C-cell hyperplasia or MTC manifest an exaggerated response. Absolute values depend on the assay used for determining CT.

49. What test may be used if pentagastrin is not available?
Where pentagastrin is unavailable, a calcium infusion (2 mg/kg over 5 minutes) can similarly be used to stimulate CT secretion. As assays for the MTC gene on chromosome 10 become clinically available (see Chapter 53), screening of kindreds for the hereditary form of MTC with stimulation tests may be unnecessary. The test, however, will remain valuable in elucidating residual disease after therapy.

50. How is MTC treated?

Therapy for MTC remains frustrating. When MTC is discovered on biopsy or suspected as a result of the screening of kindred members, the entire thyroid should be surgically removed, with care to preserve the parathyroids and laryngeal nerves. A dissection of the lymphatics of the central neck also should be undertaken, because 50% to 70% of these nodes contain metastases. Laparoscopic hepatic biopsies reveal 25% to 30% of patients have unsuspected liver metastasis following intial thyroidectomy.

Because parafollicular cells do not accumulate radioiodine, postsurgical radioablation is not warranted. External beam radiotherapy and chemotherapy do not appear to improve survival, although they are sometimes used in desperation against recurrent disease. Residual disease grows slowly, causing obstructive symptoms and the symptoms listed in question 46.

51. What are the survival rates of patients with MTC?

Rates of 10- and 20-year survival in one large series were 63% and 44%, respectively.

52. Summarize the prevalence and detection of thyroid nodules.

The prevalence of nodular thyroid disease increases with age and is approximately 4 times higher in women than in men. By the sixth decade of life, 5% to 10% of the general population in developed nations has one or more palpable thyroid nodules. Detection by palpation is relatively insensitive, however; ultrasonographic or pathologic (autopsy) examination of the population reveals a much higher prevalence of thyroid nodules (20% by 40 years of age, 50% by 70 years of age). Only 8% to 17% of surgically resected nodules are cancerous; the remainder is nonmalignant and mandate excision only for obstructive symptoms or cosmesis.

53. What is the primary responsibility of the internist in regard to thyroid nodules?

The responsibility of the internist is to steer patients with nodules of malignant potential to resection but to stay the hand of the surgeon when excision of a benign nodule is proposed.

54. What is the first test performed on a palpable thyroid nodule?

After a history and physical examination are performed, a serum TSH is obtained to determine whether the patient is thyrotoxic. A suppressed TSH may indicate the presence of an autonomous nodule or Graves' disease with a nonfunctional nodule. Nonfunctional or "cold" nodules in a Graves' gland often contain DTC.

- If a low or suppressed TSH is found, a radionuclide (I-123or Tc-99) scan should be obtained.
- If TSH is normal or high, an ultrasound examination of the thyroid should be obtained to characterize the nodule.

55. Discuss the role of radionuclide scans.

When baseline TSH is low or suppressed, most advocate the performance of a radionuclide scan to determine the metabolic activity of the nodule and to discern the existence of other unsuspected nodules. Such data are potentially valuable; autonomous or "hot" nodules rarely harbor malignancy but may yield cytopathologic specimens that mimic malignancy.

56. How does ultrasound examination contribute to the evaluation?

Ultrasound of examination of the thyroid may help detect other nodules that are difficult to palpate because of their posterior or substernal location. More importantly, sonographic characterization of a dominant nodule or other smaller nodules may direct fine-needle aspiration (FNA) of the most suspicious lesions.

Hypoechoic nodules, nodules containing microcalcifications or hypervascular nodules should be aspirated. Ultrasound guided FNA should be used if the nodule is impalpable or predominantly cystic to ensure representative sampling. Collection of the sample is relatively simple; cytologic interpretation of the sample is the limiting factor in this procedure. The diagnostic accuracy of FNA is reported to range between 70% and 97%.

57. How is the FNA sample interpreted?
Interpretation of the aspiration sample may indicate that the nodule is malignant, benign, or "suspicious for malignancy." The sample also may be judged to have inadequate material for interpretation, requiring reaspiration. Papillary carcinoma may be diagnosed with some certainty from FNA samples, but the diagnosis of follicular carcinoma requires the demonstration of vascular invasion. Some large centers boast cytopathologists who can reliably differentiate follicular carcinoma from follicular adenoma; these uncommon, grizzled old demigods have forsaken the company of mortals for the solace of their microscopes. Most cytopathologists designate such samples as "follicular neoplasm" or "suspicious for malignancy."

58. How do the results of FNA affect further management?
Nodules designated as malignant on FNA should be resected. Those designated as "suspicious for malignancy" or "follicular neoplasm" also should be referred for excision, because up to 20% are malignant. Benign nodules should be observed for change in size or obstructive symptoms; the administration of suppressive amounts of exogenous thyroid hormone is controversial because of the attendant risk for osteoporosis and the lack of data demonstrating unequivocal efficacy of this intervention.

59. Is surgery justified for a nodule judged as benign by FNA?
The internist occasionally encounters a patient who chooses surgical resection of a nodule despite benign results with FNA. This scenario prompts a final word of advice: "Never stand between a ready surgeon and a willing patient who has been thoroughly apprised of the risks of thyroid surgery." False-negative results of FNA range between 1% and 6%, and up to 35% of thyroids in autopsy series contain clinically insignificant papillary carcinomas, either of which, if discovered at a later date, will engender distrust on the part of the patient.

60. Has a molecular defect been associated with thyroid carcinoma?
Mutation of a single protooncogene or tumor suppressor gene has not been associated with thyroid carcinogenesis. Several mutations have been described in thyroid neoplasms; however, none appears to be able to induce malignant changes without concomitant cooperating mutations. Although the practical relevance of these defects is limited at this time, further research may identify these or others as clinical indicators of the malignant potential of individual tumors.

61. Discuss the potential role of the ras protooncogene.
The ras protooncogene code for a family of receptor-associated proteins, named p21, serves as signal transducers between membrane receptors and intracellular effectors. When the receptors are stimulated, p21 becomes complexed with guanosine triphosphate (GTP) and activates MAP kinase. Because excessive kinase activity would be detrimental, native p21 possesses intrinsic GTPase activity, which eventually inactivates the complex and terminates the activity of MAP kinase. Mutation of the ras protooncogene results in p21 that lacks GTPase activity, causing uncontrolled accumulation of kinase activity and prompting disordered cellular growth. Ras oncogene has been described in 10% to 50% of follicular carcinomas in iodine-deficient areas.

62. How may the G-stimulatory (Gs) proteins be related to thyroid cancer?
Closely related to ras-coded p21 are the Gs proteins, which also link transmembrane receptors to intracellular effectors, such as adenyl cyclase. Gs proteins consist of a, b, and g subunits, noncovalently bound together, that become active when GTP complexes to the "a" subunit. Native Gsa possesses intrinsic GTPase activity that functions as a timer, stopping the reaction at an appropriate point. Mutations of the Gsa gene that code for proteins lacking intrinsic GTPase activity have been discerned. These constitutively activated Gs proteins promote both cell growth and function; they have been detected primarily in functioning benign thyroid nodules and rarely in DTCs.

63. **Discuss the potential role of the Ret/ptc oncogene.**
The ret/ptc mutation has been described in DTCs. The ret protooncogene is found on chromosome 10 and normally codes a receptor (ret) with intrinsic tyrosine kinase activity. The ligand for ret is a glial cell derived neurotrophic factor; ret is not normally expressed on thyroid follicular cells. The ret/ptc mutation results in constitutively activated tyrosine kinase, which causes disordered cellular development and is found in 2% to 70% of papillary thyroid carcinomas, depending on the ethnic group. Although tumors expressing this mutation are not larger than other papillary cancers, they may be more likely to metastasize.

64. **How is abnormal protein p53 implicated in thyroid cancer?**
A final mutation associated with up to 25% of anaplastic thyroid carcinomas codes for abnormal protein p53. Normal p53 is found in the cytoplasm, where it forms a complex with heat shock protein-70 (hsp70) and crosses the nuclear membrane to interact with nuclear transcription factors. Mutation of the gene coding for p53 results in translation of a protein that cannot interact with these nuclear proteins. Loss of this tumor suppressor causes unrestricted cell growth and, along with other coexisting mutations, malignant degeneration.

KEY POINTS: THYROID CANCER

1. Papillary and follicular carcinomas comprise the differentiated thyroid carcinomas (DTCs). Mortality rates are low.

2. DTC is diagnosed by fine-needle aspiration (FNA) of a thyroid nodule.

3. Therapy of DTC is based on surgical resection of the primary tumor and removal of all remaining thyroid tissue (bed).

4. Orally administered radioactive iodine is accumulated by thyroid tissue, ablating the thyroid bed and metastatic foci.

5. Thyroglobulin is the most sensitive tumor marker for DTC after surgery and ablation of the remnant have been performed.

6. Elimination of TSH, a DTC growth factor, by suppressive doses of levothyroxine is the most important therapeutic intervention.

WEBSITE

NCCN thyroid carcinoma practice guidelines. Available at: http://www.nccn.org

BIBLIOGRAPHY

1. Baudin E, Cao D, Cailleux AF, et al: Positive predictive value of serum thyroglobulin levels, measured during first year follow-up after thyroid hormone withdrawal, in thyroid cancer patients. J Clin Endocrinol Metab 88:1107–1111, 2003.

2. Brennan MD, Bergstralh EJ, van Heerden JA, McConahey WM: Follicular thyroid cancer treated at the Mayo Clinic, 1946 through 1970: initial manifestations, pathologic findings, therapy, and outcome. Mayo Clin Proc 66:11–22, 1991.

3. Chua EL, Wu WM, Tran KT, et al: Prevalence and distribution of ret/ptc 1, 2, and 3 in papillary thyroid carcinoma in New Caledonia and Australia. J Clin Endocrinol Metab 85:2733–2739, 2000.

4. Cooper DS, Doherty GM, Haugen BR, et al: Management guidelines for patients with thyroid nodules and differentiated thyroid cancer. The American Thyroid Association Guidelines Taskforce. Thyroid 18:1–33, 2006.

5. Dulgeroff AJ, Herschman JM: Medical therapy for differentiated thyroid carcinoma. Endocr Rev 15:500–515, 1994.

6. Farid NR, Shi Y, Zou M: Molecular basis of thyroid cancer. Endocr Rev 15:202–232, 1994.

7. Fogelfeld L, Wiviott MBT, Shore-Freedman E, et al: Recurrence of thyroid nodules after surgical removal in patients irradiated in childhood for benign conditions. N Engl J Med 320:835–840, 1989.

8. Gagel RF, Robinson MF, Donovan DT, Alford BB: Medullary thyroid carcinoma: recent progress. J Clin Endocrinol Metab 76:809–814, 1993.

9. Gharib H: The use of recombinant thyrotropin in patients with thyroid cancer. Endocrinologist 10:255–263, 2000.

10. Gharib H, McConahey WM, Tiegs RD, et al: Medullary thyroid carcinoma: clinicopathologic features and long-term follow-up of 65 patients treated during 1946 through 1970. Mayo Clin Proc 67:934–940, 1992.

11. Hay ID: Management of patients with low-risk papillary thyroid carcinoma. Endocr Pract 13:521–533, 2007.

12. Kebebew E, Clark OH: Differentiated thyroid cancer: "complete" rational approach. World J Surg 24:942–951, 2000.

13. Mazzaferi EL: Management of low-risk differentiated thyroid cancer. Endocri Pract 13: 498–512, 2007.

14. Mazzaferi EL, Robbins RJ, Spencer AC, et al: A consensus report of the role of serum thyroglobulin as a monitoring method for low-risk patients with papillary thyroid carcinoma. J Clin Endocrinol Metab 88:1433–1441, 2003.

15. McConahey WM, Hay ID, Woolner L, et al: Papillary thyroid cancer treated at the Mayo Clinic, 1946 through 1970: initial manifestations, pathologic findings, therapy, and outcome. Mayo Clin Proc 61:978–996, 1986.

16. Nel CJC, van Heerden JA, Goellner JR, et al: Anaplastic carcinoma of the thyroid: a clinico-pathologic study of 82 cases. Mayo Clin Proc 60:51–58, 1985.

17. Pacini F, Capezzone M, Elisei R, et al: Diagnostic 131-iodine whole-body scan may be avoided in thyroid cancer patients who have undetectable stimulated serum Tg levels after initial treatment. J Clin Endocrinol Metab 87:1499–1501, 2002.

18. Robbins J (moderator): Thyroid cancer: a lethal endocrine neoplasm. Ann Intern Med 115:133–147, 1991.

19. Wartofsky L: Editorial: using baseline and recombinant human TSH-stimulated Tg measurements to manage thyroid cancer without diagnostic 131-I scanning. J Clin Endocrinol Metabol 87:1486–1489, 2002.

CHAPTER 38

THYROID EMERGENCIES
Michael T. McDermott

1. **What is thyroid storm?**
   Thyroid storm or crisis is a life-threatening condition characterized by an exaggeration of the manifestations of thyrotoxicosis.

2. **How do patients develop thyroid storm?**
   Thyroid storm usually occurs in patients who have unrecognized or inadequately treated thyrotoxicosis and a superimposed precipitating event, such as thyroid surgery, nonthyroid surgery, infection, or trauma.

3. **What are the clinical manifestations of thyroid storm?**
   Fever (>102°F) is the cardinal manifestation. Tachycardia is usually present, and tachypnea is common, but the blood pressure is variable. Cardiac arrhythmias, congestive heart failure, and ischemic heart symptoms may develop. Nausea, vomiting, diarrhea, and abdominal pain are frequent features (Fig. 38-1). Central nervous system manifestations include hyperkinesis, psychosis, and coma. A goiter is a helpful finding but is not always present.

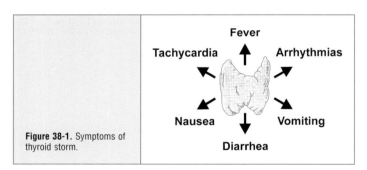

Figure 38-1. Symptoms of thyroid storm.

4. **What laboratory abnormalities are seen in thyroid storm?**
   Serum thyroxine (T_4; total and free T_4) and triiodothyronine (T_3; total and free T_3) are usually significantly elevated, and the serum thyroid-stimulating hormone (TSH) is undetectable. Other common laboratory abnormalities include anemia, leukocytosis, hyperglycemia, azotemia, hypercalcemia, and elevated liver-associated enzymes.

5. **How is the diagnosis of thyroid storm made?**
   The diagnosis must be made on the basis of suspicious but nonspecific clinical findings. Serum thyroid hormone levels are elevated, but if the diagnosis is strongly suspected, waiting for the results of tests may cause a critical delay in the initiation of effective life-saving therapy. Furthermore, thyroid hormone levels do not reliably distinguish patients with thyroid storm from those who have uncomplicated thyrotoxicosis as a coincident disorder. Clinical features are therefore the key. Table 38-1 provides a useful scoring system to aid in diagnosis.

TABLE 38-1. THYROID STORM SCORING SYSTEM (REF: BURCH HD, 1993)

Feature	Score
Fever	
99–99.9	5
100–100.9	10
101–101.9	15
102–102.9	20
103–103.9	25
≥104	30
Central Nervous System	
Absent	0
Mild agitation	10
Moderate	20
Severe	30
Cardiac—Pulse	
99–109	5
110–119	10
120–129	15
130–139	20
≥140	25
Atrial fibrillation	10
Cardiac—Congestive Heart Failure	
Absent	0
Mild (edema)	5
Moderate (rales)	10
Severe (pulmonary edema)	15
Gastrointestinal	
Absent	0
Nausea, vomiting, diarrhea, or pain	10
Jaundice	20
Precipitant History	
Absent	0
Present	10

Score	Thyroid Storm
<25	Unlikely
25–44	Suggestive
≥45	Likely

6. **What other conditions may mimic thyroid storm?**
   Similar presentations may be seen with sepsis, pheochromocytoma, and malignant hyperthermia.

7. **How should patients with thyroid storm be treated?**
   The immediate goals are to decrease thyroid hormone synthesis, to inhibit thyroid hormone release, to reduce the heart rate, to support the circulation, and to treat the precipitating condition. Because beta$_1$-adrenergic receptors are significantly increased in patients with this condition, beta$_1$-selective blockers are the preferred agents for heart rate control.

8. **What drugs are used to decrease thyroid hormone synthesis?**
   - Propylthiouracil, 200 mg every 4 hours (orally, rectally, or via nasogastric [NG] tube)
   - Methimazole, 20 mg every 4 hours (orally, rectally, or via NG tube)

9. **List drugs used to inhibit thyroid hormone release.**
   - Sodium iodide (NaI), 1 g over 24 hours intravenously (IV)
   - Potassium iodide (SSKI), 5 drops every 8 hours orally
   - Lugol's solution, 10 drops every 8 hours orally

10. **What drugs are used to reduce the heart rate?**
    - Esmolol, 500 mg over 1 minute IV, followed by 50 to 100 mg/kg/min infusion
    - Metoprolol, 5 to 10 mg IV every 2 to 4 hours
    - Diltiazem, 60 to 90 mg every 6 to 8 hours orally, or 0.25 mg/kg over 2 min IV, followed by infusion of 10 mg/min

11. **List agents used to support the circulation.**
    - Dexamethasone, 2 mg every 6 hours IV or
    - Hydrocortisone, 100 mg every 8 hours IV
    - Intravenous fluids

12. **What is the prognosis for patients with thyroid storm?**
    When thyroid storm was first described, the acute mortality rate was nearly 100%. Today the prognosis is significantly improved when aggressive therapy, as described earlier, is initiated early; however, the mortality rate continues to be approximately 20%.

13. **Define myxedema coma.**
    Myxedema coma is a life-threatening condition characterized by an exaggeration of the manifestations of hypothyroidism.

14. **How do patients develop myxedema coma?**
    Myxedema coma usually occurs in elderly patients who have inadequately treated or untreated hypothyroidism and a superimposed precipitating event. Important events include prolonged cold exposure, infection, trauma, surgery, myocardial infarction, congestive heart failure, pulmonary embolism, stroke, respiratory failure, gastrointestinal bleeding, and administration of various drugs, particularly those that have a depressive effect on the central nervous system.

15. **What are the clinical manifestations of myxedema coma?**
    Hypothermia, bradycardia, and hypoventilation are common; blood pressure, although generally reduced, is more variable. Pericardial, pleural, and peritoneal effusions are often found. An ileus is present in approximately two thirds of patients, and acute urinary retention also may be seen. Central nervous system manifestations include seizures, stupor, and coma (Fig. 38-2); deep tendon reflexes are absent or exhibit a delayed relaxation phase. Typical hypothyroid skin and hair changes may be apparent. A goiter, although frequently absent, is a helpful finding; a thyroidectomy scar also may be an important clue.

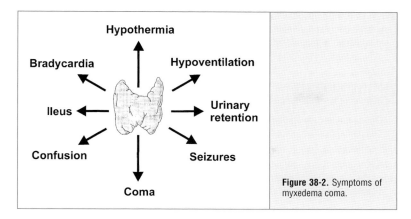

Figure 38-2. Symptoms of myxedema coma.

16. **What laboratory abnormalities are seen in myxedema coma?**
Serum T_4 (total and free T_4) and T_3 (total and free T_3) are usually low, and the TSH is significantly elevated. Other frequent abnormalities include anemia, hyponatremia, hypoglycemia, and elevated serum levels of cholesterol and creatine kinase (CK). Arterial blood gases often reveal carbon dioxide retention and hypoxemia. The electrocardiogram often shows sinus bradycardia, various types and degrees of heart block, low voltage, and T-wave flattening.

17. **How is the diagnosis of myxedema coma made?**
The diagnosis must be made on clinical grounds on the basis of the findings described earlier. Serum levels of thyroid hormones are reduced and the TSH level is elevated, but the delay involved in waiting for test results may unnecessarily postpone the initiation of effective therapy.

18. **How should patients with myxedema coma be treated?**
The goals are to replace rapidly the depleted thyroid hormone pool, to replace glucocorticoids, to support vital functions, and to treat any precipitating conditions. The normal total body pool of T_4 is about 1000 µg (500 µg in the thyroid; 500 µg in the rest of the body).

19. **How are circulating thyroid hormones replaced?**
Whether to use levothyroxine (LT_4), liothyronine (LT_3), or both remains controversial, but the author favors the combination of LT_4 plus LT_3. Regimens for LT_4 alone, LT_3 followed by LT_4, and LT_4 plus LT_3 are listed in the following:
   - LT_4 alone: 200 to 300 µg over 5 minutes IV, followed by 50 to 100 µg /day orally or IV
   - LT_3 followed by LT_4: LT_3, 50 to 100 µg over 5 minutes IV, followed by LT_4, 50 to 100 µg / day orally or IV
   - LT_4 plus LT_3: LT_4, 200 to 300 µg over 5 minutes IV, plus LT_3, 20 to 50 µg over 5 minutes IV, followed by LT_4, 50 to 100 µg /day, and LT_3, 20 to 30 µg /day orally or IV

20. **What agent is used for glucocorticoid replacement?**
Hydrocortisone, 100 mg every 8 hours IV.

21. **What agents and modalities are used to support vital functions?**
   - Oxygen
   - IV fluids
   - Rewarming (blankets or central rewarming)
   - Mechanical ventilation (if necessary)

22. **What is the prognosis for patients with myxedema coma?**
- Myxedema coma originally had a mortality rate of 100%. Today the outlook is much improved for appropriately treated patients, although the mortality rate in recent studies has varied from 0% to 45%.

KEY POINTS: THYROID EMERGENCIES

1. Thyroid storm is a life-threatening form of severe thyrotoxicosis that usually has an identifiable precipitating factor and a high mortality rate if not treated promptly and appropriately.

2. When thyroid storm is diagnosed or suspected, treatment with antithyroid drugs, cold iodine, beta-blockers, and stress doses of glucocorticoids, along with management of any precipitating factors, should be promptly initiated.

3. Myxedema coma is a life-threatening form of severe hypothyroidism that often has a precipitating cause and a high mortality rate if not promptly and adequately treated.

4. When myxedema coma is diagnosed or suspected, management should include rapid repletion of the thyroid hormone deficit, stress doses of glucocorticoids, and treatment of any precipitating causes.

BIBLIOGRAPHY

1. Brooks MH, Waldstein SS: Free thyroxine concentrations in thyroid storm. Ann Intern Med 93:694–697, 1980.

2. Burch HD, Wartofsky L: Life-threatening thyrotoxicosis: thyroid storm. Endocrinol Metab Clin N Am 22:263–278, 1993.

3. Dillmann WH: Thyroid storm. Curr Ther Endocrinol Metab 6:81–85, 1997.

4. Fliers E, Wiersinga WM. Myxedema coma. Rev Endo Metab Dis 4:137–141, 2003.

5. Jordan RM: Myxedema coma. Pathophysiology, therapy, and factors affecting prognosis. Med Clin N Am 79:185–194, 1995.

6. Nicoloff JT: Myxedema coma: a form of decompensated hypothyroidism. Endocrinol Metab Clin N Am 22:279–290, 1993.

7. Pittman CS, Zayed AA: Myxedema coma. Curr Ther Endocrinol Metab 6:98–101, 1997.

8. Rodriguez I, Fluiters E, Perez-Mendez LF, et al: Severe mental impairment and poor physiologic status are associated with mortality in myxedema coma. J Endocrinol 180:347–350, 2004.

9. Sarlis NJ, Gourgiotis L: Thyroid emergencies. Rev Endo Metab Dis 4:129–136, 2003.

10. Tietgens ST, Leinung MC: Thyroid storm. Med Clin N Am 79:169–184, 1995.

11. Tsitouras PD: Myxedema coma. Clin Geriatr Med 11:251–258, 1995.

12. Yamamoto T, Fukuyama J, Fujiyoshi A: Factors associated with mortality of myxedema coma: report of eight cases and literature survey. Thyroid 9:1167–1174, 1999.

13. Yeung S-CJ, Go R, Balasubramanyam A: Rectal administration of iodide and propylthiouracil in the treatment of thyroid storm. Thyroid 5:403–405, 1995.

CHAPTER 39

EUTHYROID SICK SYNDROME

Michael T. McDermott

1. **What is euthyroid sick syndrome?**

   Euthyroid sick syndrome refers to changes in serum thyroid-stimulating hormone (TSH), serum thyroid hormone, and tissue thyroid hormone levels that occur in patients with various types of nonthyroidal illnesses and starvation. It is not a primary thyroid disorder but instead results from changes in TSH secretion, thyroid hormone secretion, transport, and metabolism induced by the nonthyroidal illness.

2. **What hormone changes occur in patients with mild-to-moderate nonthyroidal illnesses?**

   Serum total triiodothyronine (T_3) and free T_3 levels and tissue T_3 levels decrease as a result of reduced thyroxine (T_4) to T_3 conversion in peripheral tissues, predominantly the liver, where decreased hepatic deiodinase type I activity has been demonstrated. Serum free T_4 and TSH levels usually remain within the reference range.

3. **Describe the hormone changes in patients with moderate-to-severe nonthyroidal illnesses.**

   Serum total T_3 and free T_3 levels decrease further; total T_4 also decreases, and T_3 resin uptake (T_3RU) increases. The latter changes result from reduced binding of thyroid hormones to their transport proteins due both to impaired protein synthesis and the presence of circulating inhibitors of protein binding. Free T_4 may be normal, decreased, or increased. Serum TSH levels remain normal or become slightly decreased at this stage.

4. **Describe the hormone changes associated with recovery from nonthyroidal illnesses.**

   Free T_4 decreases and TSH increases. As hepatic protein synthesis improves and circulating inhibitors of protein binding disappear, serum free T_4 levels drop transiently with a compensatory increase in serum TSH levels before complete normalization occurs. Serum T3 levels eventually normalize also.

5. **How can euthyroid sick syndrome be distinguished from hypothyroidism?**

   In the euthyroid sick syndrome, serum T_3 is decreased proportionately more than T_4, the T_3RU tends to be high, and the TSH is normal or mildly decreased and then mildly increased in the recovery phase. In primary hypothyroidism, serum T_4 is reduced proportionately more than T_3, the T_3RU tends to be low, and the TSH is increased. Other tests also may be helpful. In the euthyroid sick syndrome, free T_4 is usually normal and reverse T_3 (RT_3) is increased; in hypothyroidism, both free T_4 and RT_3 are decreased.

6. **What causes euthyroid sick syndrome?**

   Euthyroid sick syndrome is believed to be caused by increased circulating levels of cytokines and other inflammation mediators resulting from the underlying nonthyroidal illness. These mediators can inhibit the thyroid axis at multiple levels, including the pituitary (decreased TSH secretion), the thyroid (decreased T_4 and T_3 responses to TSH), transport proteins (decreased thyroid hormone binding), and peripheral tissues (decreased conversion of T_4 to T_3; decreased responses to T_3).

KEY POINTS: EUTHYROID SICK SYNDROME

1. Euthyroid sick syndrome is not a thyroid disorder but instead is a group of changes in serum TSH and thyroid hormones and tissue thyroid hormone levels that result from cytokines and inflammatory mediators produced in patients with nonthyroidal illnesses.

2. The most common feature of the euthyroid sick syndrome is a decrease in serum triiodothyronine (T_3) levels due to reduced conversion of thyroxine (T_4) to T_3 in the liver and other tissues.

3. Low serum total T_4, increased T_3 resin uptake (T_3RU), and decreased thyroid-stimulating hormone (TSH) develop in patients with more severe nonthyroidal illnesses because of reduced thyroid hormone binding to transport proteins and suppressed pituitary TSH secretion.

4. A transient elevation of serum TSH levels is sometimes seen in patients as they recover from the nonthyroidal illness.

5. Euthyroid sick syndrome appears to be an adaptive response to reduce tissue metabolism and preserve energy during systemic illnesses; therefore treatment with thyroid hormone is not currently recommended.

7. **Is euthyroid sick syndrome an adaptive mechanism, or is it harmful?**
Many experts consider euthyroid sick syndrome to be an adaptive mechanism that may reduce peripheral tissue energy expenditure during the nonthyroidal illness. Conversely, others argue that the alterations in circulating thyroid hormone levels may be harmful and may accentuate the effects of the nonthyroidal illness. This issue is likely to remain controversial for years to come.

8. **Should patients with euthyroid sick syndrome be treated with thyroid hormones?**
Management of euthyroid sick syndrome is also highly controversial. Currently there are no consistent or convincing data demonstrating a recovery or survival benefit from treating euthyroid sick syndrome patients with either levothyroxine (LT_4) or liothyronine (LT_3). Experts continue to debate this issue, however, and agree that large, prospective studies are necessary to answer this question. In the absence of more definitive data, thyroid hormone therapy cannot be recommended at this time.

9. **Does euthyroid sick syndrome have any prognostic significance?**
Low serum T_3 levels have significant prognostic value. The degree of reduction of serum T_3 has been shown to predict a poor prognosis in patients with ischemic heart disease, valvular heart disease, congestive heart failure, meningococcal sepsis, and a variety of illnesses in the intensive care setting. Patients with extremely low serum T_3 levels have a high mortality rate.

10. **Are levels of thyroid hormone ever elevated in patients with nonthyroid diseases?**
The serum T_4 may be transiently elevated in patients with acute psychiatric illnesses and various acute medical illnesses. The mechanisms underlying such elevations of T_4 are not well understood but may be mediated by alterations in neurotransmitters or cytokines. This condition must be distinguished from true thyrotoxicosis.

BIBLIOGRAPHY

1. Adler SM, Wartofsky L: The nonthyroidal illness syndrome. Endocrinol Metab Clin NA 36:657–672, 2007.

2. DeGroot LJ: Dangerous dogmas in medicine: the nonthyroidal illness syndrome. J Clin Endocrinol Metab 84:151–164, 1999.

3. den Brinker M, Joosten KFM, Visser, et al: Euthyroid sick syndrome in meningococcal sepsis: the impact of peripheral thyroid hormone metabolism and binding proteins. J Clin Endocrinol Metab 90:5613–5620, 2005.

4. Iervasi G, Pingitore A, Landi P, et al: Low serum free triiodothyronine values predict mortality in patients with cardiac disease. Circulation 107:708–711, 2003.

5. Kimura T, Kanda T, Kotajima N, et al: Involvement of circulating interleukin-6 and its receptor in the development of euthyroid sick syndrome in patients with acute myocardial infarction. Eur J Endocrinol 143:179–184, 2000.

6. McIver B, Gorman CA: Euthyroid sick syndrome: an overview. Thyroid 7:125–132, 1997.

7. Nagaya T, Fujieda M, Otsuka G, et al: A potential role of activated NF-kappa B in the pathogenesis of euthyroid sick syndrome. J Clin Invest 106:393–402, 2000.

8. Peeters RP, Kester MHA, Wouters PJ, et al: Increased thyroxine sulfate levels in critically ill patients as a result of a decreased hepatic type I deiodinase activity. J Clin Endocrinol Metab 90: 6460–6465, 2005.

9. Peeters RP, van der Geyten S, Wouters PJ, et al: Tissue thyroid hormone levels in critical illness. J Clin Endocrinol Metab 90:6498–6507, 2005.

10. Peeters RP, Wouters PJ, Kaptein E, et al: Reduced activation and increased inactivation of thyroid hormone in tissues of critically ill patients. J Clin Endocrinol Metab 88:3202–3211, 2003.

11. Peeters RP, Wouters PJ, van Toor H, et al: Serum 3, 3′, 5′-triiodothyronine and 3, 5, 3′- triiodothyronine/rT3 are prognostic markers in critically ill patients and are associated with tissue deiodinase activities. J Clin Endocrinol Metab 90:4559–4565, 2005.

12. Pingitore A, Landi P, Taddei MC, et al: Triiodothyronine levels for risk stratification of patients with chronic heart failure. Am J Med 118:132–136, 2005.

13. Plikat K, Langgartner J, Buettner R, et al: Increasing thyroid dysfunction is correlated with degree of illness and mortality in intensive care unit patients. Metabolism 56:239–244, 2007.

14. Vanhorebeek I, Langouche L, Van den Berghe G: Endocrine aspects of acute and prolonged critical illness. Nat Clin Pract Endocrinol Metab 2:20–31, 2006.

CHAPTER 40

THYROID DISEASE IN PREGNANCY

Linda A. Barbour

1. **How does normal pregnancy affect maternal thyroid function?**
   The hormonal changes of pregnancy and the increased metabolic demands of the fetus cause significant changes in maternal thyroid function (Table 40-1).

TABLE 40-1.   THYROID FUNCTION TESTS DURING NORMAL PREGNANCY

	First Trimester	Second Trimester	Third Trimester
Total T_4	1.5 × ↑	1.5 × ↑	1.5 × ↑
Total T_3	1.5 × ↑	1.5 × ↑	1.5 × ↑
T_3RU	↓	↓	↓
Free thyroxine index	Normal	Normal	Normal
TSH	↓ or Normal	Slight ↓ or Normal	Slight ↓ or Normal
Free T_4	Usually normal	Usually normal	Usually normal

T_3, triiodothyronine; T_3RU, T_3 resin uptake; T_4, thyroxine; TSH, thyroid-stimulating hormone.

2. **Why must thyroid function tests be interpreted cautiously in pregnancy?**
   The influence of estrogen and human chorionic gonadotropin (hCG) on circulating thyroid hormone levels requires that thyroid function tests in pregnancy be interpreted cautiously. Estrogen increases thyroid-binding globulin (TBG) by two- to threefold beginning a few weeks after conception. The result is an approximately 50% increase in serum total thyroxine (TT_4) and total triiodothyronine (TT_3) levels because circulating thyroid hormones are highly protein bound. Throughout pregnancy, both hormones should be approximately 1.5 times the nonpregnant range (Soldin 2004). Measurement of the T_3 resin uptake (T_3RU), which is inversely related to serum thyroid binding capacity, is correspondingly low, so that the free T_4 index (FT_4I; calculated by multiplying the total T_4 by the T_3RU) is usually normal. Although the free T_4 and free T_3 are usually normal in pregnancy, they must be interpreted with caution because the reference ranges provided by the manufacturers have been established using pools of nonpregnant sera. These free assays may be influenced by the increase in TBG and albumin unless an equilibrium dialysis method is used which is expensive and is usually not available (Kahric-Janic 2007). A slightly low free T_4 in the late second or third trimester may represent true hypothyroidism or may be falsely low and should be interpreted in the context of a thyroid-stimulating hormone (TSH) and TT_4 (Sapin 2004). If the TSH is less than 3.5 and the TT_4 is 1.5 times elevated, it is unlikely that the patient has true hypothyroidism. If at all possible, pregnancy specific norms for free T_3 and free T_4 should be established by the laboratory. TSH values are also affected by the thyrotropic effect of hCG, and in one large series (Panesar 2001), the 95% confidence limits were as low as 0.03 in the first and second trimester and 0.13 in the third trimester with an upper limit of normal of less than 3.0 in the first trimester and less than 3.5 in

the second and third trimester. Once again, the TSH must be interpreted in the context of the actual thyroid hormone levels. If the TT_4 and TT_3 are less than 1.5 times elevated from the nonpregnancy range and the free T_4 and free T_3 hormones are not increased, the suppressed TSH may be due to the effect of hCG versus subclinical hyperthyroidism from Gave's diseases or a hot nodule, none of which warrant treatment.

3. **What particular effects may be seen during the first trimester?**
During the first trimester, high levels of hCG may stimulate thyroid T_4 secretion sufficiently to suppress the serum TSH into the 0.03 to 0.5 mU/L range in up to 15% of pregnant women. The TSH may be slightly suppressed in the second and third trimester as well but usually increases into the lower limit of the normal range. The beta subunit of hCG has 85% sequence homology in the first 114 amino acids with TSH and can bind to and stimulate the TSH receptor. Levels of hCG above 50,000 IU/L, which may be seen when hCG peaks at the end of the first trimester, can therefore increase the free T_4 level enough to suppress the serum TSH. However, the TSH is usually detectable, the TT_4 is less than 1.5 times elevated above the nonpregnancy range, and free T_4 is usually within the normal range. A TSH in the high-normal range (>3.5) during the first trimester is therefore suspicious for subclinical hypothyroidism. If rechecked and still elevated, treatment with small doses of thyroid hormone should be considered, especially if the patient is found to have positive thyroid peroxidase (TPO) antibodies (Endocrine Society Committee, 2007).

4. **Why must the mother significantly increase thyroid hormone production during pregnancy?**
   - Maternal plasma volume expands 30% to 40%, requiring a concomitant expansion of the thyroid hormone pool.
   - Placental type III deiodinase activity results in increased maternal T_4 metabolism to reverse T_3.
   - Transfer of T_4 across the placenta to the fetus occurs to a limited degree.
   - High TBG levels decrease the levels of free hormone.
   - Gastrointestinal absorption of exogenous thyroid hormone may be impaired by iron in prenatal vitamins.

5. **What factors may compromise maternal ability to increase thyroid hormone production?**
Women with limited thyroid reserve due to thyroiditis, partial ablation, or surgical resection may be unable to increase thyroid hormone production and often develop hypothyroidism. Women with inadequate iodide intake may also develop hypothyroidism and a goiter, because iodine requirements increase by approximately 40% in pregnancy.

6. **What is the "goiter of pregnancy"?**
The goiter of pregnancy has been well described in iodine-deficient areas of the world but does not occur in geographic regions that are iodine-replete. In fact, one of the first pregnancy tests to be developed in these iodine-deficient areas was a loosely braided choker necklace that broke when a woman developed such a goiter. The thyroid gland increased in size with each subsequent pregnancy.

7. **Why do iodine requirements increase in pregnancy?**
Iodine requirements increase markedly during pregnancy as a result of increased urinary iodine losses due to the 50 to 100% increase in glomerular filtration rate (GFR) during pregnancy, diversion of iodine to the fetus for thyroid hormone synthesis, and increased maternal thyroid hormone requirements.

8. **What is the recommended iodine intake during pregnancy and how can it be met?**
The World Health Organization's recommendations for iodine intake are 250 μg/day during pregnancy and 150 μg/day in the nonpregnant state. Iodine insufficiency is an increasing

problem in the United States due to the availability of deiodinated salt and is estimated at 5% to 10%. Because the vast majority of prenatal vitamins do not contain iodine, women of childbearing age should be instructed to use only iodinated salt.

9. **What happens if iodine intake is insufficient?**

If iodine intake is insufficient, thyroid hormone production drops, resulting in increased secretion of TSH, which then stimulates thyroid gland growth. Thyroid volume commonly increases by 30% or more during pregnancy in iodine-deficient regions and often does not completely regress after delivery. Many European and Third World countries with endemic iodine deficiency do not supplement with iodine; therefore women are at risk of iodine-deficiency goiters during pregnancy. When iodine intake is severely deficient, overt hypothyroidism results both in mother and fetus. Endemic cretinism occurs if severe hypothyroidism due to iodine deficiency goes unrecognized and untreated at birth.

10. **What happens to thyroid gland volume in iodine-replete areas during pregnancy?**

In iodine-replete areas, such as the United States, thyroid gland volume may increase by 10% to 15%, primarily as a result of pregnancy-induced vascular swelling of the gland. Although this enlargement can be recognized by ultrasound, it cannot usually be appreciated by palpation. Therefore any goiter found during pregnancy in an iodine-replete area should be evaluated in the same manner as a goiter occurring outside of pregnancy.

11. **Does thyroid hormone cross the placenta?**

Thyroid hormone crosses the placenta poorly but significantly, owing in part to the high placental activity of the type III monodeiodinase that converts T_4 to reverse T_3 (rT_3) and T_3 to T_2. However, it is now clear that some T_4 does cross the placenta, because fetuses with complete thyroid agenesis have approximately 30% of the normal amount of thyroid hormone at birth. This amount of thyroid hormone appears to be protective to the brain, and neurologic development usually progresses normally as long as thyroid supplementation is begun immediately after birth. Significant amounts of thyroid hormone cross in the first trimester and early second trimester before the fetal thyroid begins functioning and appears necessary for normal brain development.

12. **Does iodine cross the placenta?**

Iodine easily crosses the placenta for use by the fetal thyroid, which, after 12 weeks' gestation, takes up iodine even more avidly than the maternal thyroid.

13. **What about thyrotropin-releasing hormone and TSH?**

Thyrotropin-releasing hormone (TRH), but not TSH, also crosses the placenta and has been used in experimental protocols to attempt to accelerate fetal lung maturity.

14. **Summarize the ability of thyroid-related antibodies to cross the placenta.**

Immunoglobulin G (IgG) TSH receptor-stimulating antibodies (thyroid-stimulating immunoglobulin [TSI]) cross the placenta, especially in the third trimester, and can occasionally cause fetal or neonatal hyperthyroidism in infants of women with Graves' disease. Although TPO antibodies and antithyroglobulin (TG) antibodies can also cross, they usually have no clinical significance. In rare cases, they may be associated with thyrotropin receptor-blocking antibodies that can cause transient neonatal hypothyroidism.

15. **List common medications that cross the placenta.**
   - Propylthiouracil (PTU)
   - Methimazole (MMI)
   - Beta-blockers

16. **When does the fetus begin making thyroid hormone?**
At approximately 10 to 12 weeks, the fetal thyroid gland develops and the hypothalamic-pituitary-thyroid axis begins to function. Because little thyroid hormone synthesis occurs until 18 to 20 weeks, the fetus is dependent on maternal thyroid hormone in the first and early second trimester.

17. **Is fetal thyroid hormone production independent of the mother?**
After the first and early second trimester, the fetal hypothalamic-pituitary-thyroid axis is fairly independent of the mother with the exception of its dependence on adequate maternal iodine stores. Antithyroid drugs or high levels of TSI may, however, affect fetal thyroid function or cause goiter development at this stage. Thyroid hormone and TBG levels increase in the fetus and plateau at about 35 to 37 weeks' gestation. High levels of rT_3 and low levels of T_3 are maintained throughout the pregnancy as a result of the high placental activity of type III monodeiodinase. The fetal pituitary-thyroid axis is relatively immature, however, considering the increased fetal TSH levels relative to the low level of T_4 production at birth. At the time of labor and in the early neonatal period, there is a dramatic increase in the levels of T_4 and the capacity of the liver to convert T_4 to T_3.

18. **What is gestational transient thyrotoxicosis or thyrotoxicosis related to hyperemesis gravidarum?**
Gestational transient thyrotoxicosis (GTT) refers to maternal hyperthyroidism caused by elevated levels of hCG, which binds to the TSH receptor and can stimulate thyroid hormone release. Levels greater than 75,000 IU/mL, which may be seen in women with hyperemesis gravidarum, twin gestation, and especially in molar pregnancies, can often cause hyperthyroidism. Posttranslational modification of the sialylation of hCG can change its affinity for the TSH receptor and half-life in the circulation, resulting in elevated thyroid levels in the first half of pregnancy. A woman who presents with hyperthyroidism, vomiting, and a positive pregnancy test should have a fetal ultrasound to exclude a molar pregnancy.
    Women with hyperemesis gravidarum (persistent nausea and vomiting accompanied by electrolyte derangements and at least 5% weight loss) commonly have abnormal thyroid function tests. In one of the largest series yet to be published, half of the 57 women with hyperemesis gravidarum had elevated free T_4.

19. **What are the most common causes of hyperthyroidism in pregnancy? During what period of gestation is hyperthyroidism most likely to occur?**
Hyperthyroidism complicates pregnancy in about 0.2% of women. Graves' disease is the most common cause of hyperthyroidism in pregnancy, accounting for nearly 85% of the cases. Autoimmune thyroid disease is most likely to present in the first trimester or the postpartum period because the immune suppression of pregnancy has been shown to decrease thyroid antibody levels significantly during the second and third trimesters. Other causes include toxic multinodular goiters, solitary toxic adenomas, iodine-induced hyperthyroidism, and subacute thyroiditis. As noted earlier, hCG-induced hyperthyroidism is common in women with hyperemesis gravidarum or hydatidiform moles and also usually presents in the first trimester.

20. **Summarize the diagnostic approach to the pregnant woman with hyperthyroidism.**
Normal pregnancy can produce clinical features that mimic hyperthyroidism, such as heat intolerance, mild tachycardia, increase in cardiac output, a systolic flow murmur, peripheral vasodilatation, and a widened pulse pressure. Weight loss may be obscured by the weight gain of pregnancy. As in the nonpregnant state, hyperthyroidism in pregnancy is usually characterized by low serum TSH levels and increased serum levels of free T_4. However, in interpreting thyroid tests in pregnant women, it is important to realize that serum TSH levels are also frequently low in normal women, especially during the first trimester of pregnancy.

21. **How can the various causes of hyperthyroidism be differentiated with certainty?**
Radioisotope scans are contraindicated during pregnancy; therefore the differential diagnosis of hyperthyroidism in pregnant women must be based on the history, physical examination, and laboratory testing. An obstetric ultrasound may be indicated to exclude a hydatidiform mole or to look for twin pregnancies.

22. **What findings help distinguish between Graves' disease and hyperemesis gravidarum?**
Although a diffusely enlarged thyroid gland with a bruit in a woman with ophthalmopathy and prepregnancy symptoms is strongly suggestive of Graves' disease, the diagnosis is often less clear, because these findings may be absent. If a woman is actively vomiting, the distinction between early Graves' disease and hyperemesis gravidarum may be particularly difficult. It is unusual, however, for women to develop hCG-induced hyperthyroidism at hCG levels less than 50,000 IU/mL. Clues pointing to Graves' disease rather than hCG-induced hyperthyroidism include the presence of a goiter, ophthalmopathy, onycholysis, or preexisting hyperthyroid symptoms antedating the pregnancy. In addition, TSI levels are often positive and T_3 levels are generally higher in Graves' disease because hyperemesis gravidarum results in a compromised nutritional state and decreased conversion of T_4 to T_3 in peripheral tissues.

23. **Why is it important to distinguish GTT from Graves' disease?**
It may be difficult to differentiate GTT from other causes of hyperthyroidism, because autoimmune hyperthyroidism also commonly presents during the first trimester of pregnancy and the biochemical profile of the two conditions is similar. However, it is extremely important to determine whether the thyrotoxicosis is due to Graves' disease or hyperemesis gravidarum because the latter usually resolves without antithyroid treatment by approximately 18 weeks when hCG levels decline. It is rarely necessary to treat with beta-blocker therapy or antithyroid drugs, because the hyperthyroid state is usually self-limited. Hyperthyroidism is probably not the cause of the nausea. Instead it appears that hCG mediates both the hyperthyroidism and perhaps the nausea by different mechanisms.

24. **Why is the woman's original country of residence significant?**
Women who have goiters from endemic areas of iodine deficiency and who move to the United States may develop iodine-induced hyperthyroidism when they suddenly become iodine replete. Hot nodules can also occur and do not improve in later pregnancy with the immune suppression of pregnancy.

25. **What are the risks of Graves' disease to the mother?**
Inadequately treated hyperthyroidism in the mother can result in preeclampsia, weight loss, tachycardia, proximal muscle weakness, anxiety, and atrial fibrillation. Left ventricular dysfunction can occur and is usually reversible but may persist for several weeks after biochemical hyperthyroidism has been corrected. This may place the pregnant woman at risk for the development of congestive heart failure, especially in the presence of superimposed preeclampsia, infection, anemia, or at the time of delivery. Thyroid storm can rarely occur in these women.

26. **What are the risks to the fetus of maternal Graves' disease?**
Inadequately treated maternal hyperthyroidism can result in fetal tachycardia, severe growth restriction, premature births, and a ninefold increased incidence of low birth weight in the infants. Congenital malformations are probably not increased in babies born to mothers with either treated or untreated hyperthyroidism. Inadequately treated maternal hyperthyroidism can cause suppression of the hypothalamic-pituitary-thyroid axis, resulting in temporary central hypothyroidism in the neonate and the inability for the neonate to mount an appropriate TSH response (Kempers 2003).

27. **Describe the possible effects on the fetus of high levels of TSH-receptor-stimulating antibodies and how it manifests in the fetus.**

In about 2 to 5% of cases, fetal or neonatal hyperthyroidism can develop as a result of very high levels of maternal TSH receptor-stimulating antibodies (TSI). Because transplacental passage of IgG is limited, this condition is unusual unless the TSI levels are elevated at least fivefold in the second and third trimesters. Fetal manifestations include goiter, tachycardia, advanced bone age, and growth restriction. (Luton 2005). All women with Graves' disease or a history of Graves' disease should be tested for TSI (functional assay) and TSH-receptor antibodies (radioimmunoassay). If elevated after 24 weeks, the fetus should receive an ultrasound for growth and to rule out a goiter by 28 weeks (Luton 2005; Nachum 2003; Pelag 2002).

28. **How are such effects treated?**

Hyperthyroidism in the fetus should be confirmed by percutaneous umbilical sampling if there is any question in regards to the cause of the goiter given that high doses of maternal PTU can also cause a goiter and render the fetus hypothyroid (Luton 2005; Nachum 2003). Fetal tachycardia is relatively nonspecific, and growth restriction is usually a late sign of fetal Graves' disease. Treatment consists of administering higher doses of PTU to the mother so that a sufficient amount of medication is delivered into the fetal circulation. Occasionally mothers are rendered hypothyroid with these high PTU doses, and maternal T_4 supplementation may be required.

29. **Why is neonatal hyperthyroidism more common than fetal hyperthyroidism?**

Neonatal hyperthyroidism is more common than fetal hyperthyroidism because of the high activity of placental type III monodeiodinase, relatively low serum T_3 levels in utero, and the effects of maternal antithyroid drugs on the fetus. TSH receptor-stimulating antibodies remain at high levels after birth, stimulating the neonatal thyroid to produce excess thyroid hormone.

30. **How does neonatal hyperthyroidism manifest?**

Neonatal hyperthyroidism may manifest as irritability, failure to thrive, hyperkinesis, diarrhea, poor feeding, jaundice, tachycardia, poor weight gain, thrombocytopenia, goiter, and, less commonly, exophthalmos, cardiac failure, hepatosplenomegaly, hyperviscosity syndrome, or craniosynostosis.

31. **What is the mortality rate of neonatal hyperthyroidism?**

The neonatal mortality rate may be as high as 30% if the condition is unrecognized.

32. **How should hyperthyroid infants be treated?**

They may require antithyroid medications until the antibody levels wane, which usually occurs by 12 weeks. If the mother has been receiving antithyroid drugs during pregnancy, it may take 5 to 10 days for the neonate to manifest symptoms because of the residual effects of these medications. Occasionally women who are euthyroid from previous ablative therapy still have high enough levels of TSI to cause their infants to develop fetal or neonatal hyperthyroidism.

33. **How can pregnant women with Graves' disease be safely treated in pregnancy?**

Treatment of overt hyperthyroidism (elevated thyroxine levels) is definitely indicated to decrease morbidity in both mother and fetus. Thionamide therapy with the judicious use of beta-blockers until thyroid hormone levels are reduced into the high normal range for pregnancy is the preferred treatment because radioiodine readily crosses the placenta and will be concentrated by the fetal thyroid after 10 to 12 weeks of gestation.

34. **Should subclinical hyperthyroidism be treated in pregnancy?**

No. TSH remains suppressed normally in some pregnant women and in a series of more than 400 women with subclinical hyperthyroidism, pregnancy outcomes in untreated women were no different from those of women without a suppressed TSH (Casey 2006). Furthermore, such treatment risks the unnecessary exposure of the fetus to antithyroid drugs. Therefore no matter the etiology (Graves' vs. hCG-mediated vs. warm nodule), a suppressed TSH alone without elevated thyroid hormones should not be treated in pregnancy.

35. **Which is preferable in pregnant and breast-feeding women, PTU or MMI?**
PTU remains the preferred antithyroid medication in the United States because of previous reports that it crosses the placenta less well than MMI and that MMI may be infrequently associated with a scalp deformity in the infant (aplasia cutis) or rarely choanal or esophageal atresia. Both of these concerns about MMI have been recently challenged, however, and it is currently believed that MMI can be used safely if necessary, but it is a second-line agent. Because PTU is more highly protein bound and crosses less efficiently into breast milk than MMI, it is also considered preferable to use PTU in women who breast-feed their infants.

36. **How are PTU and MMI dosed during pregnancy?**
Because both PTU and MMI cross the placenta, the lowest possible dosages should be given with a goal of maintaining the mother's serum free T_4 in the high-normal range or the TT_4 at approximately 1.5 times the nonpregnancy range. The serum TSH level often remains persistently suppressed in women with free T_4 and TT_4 levels in this range and should never be used to titrate the dose of antithyroid drugs during pregnancy. Approximately 1% to 3% of newborns exposed to PTU in utero develop transient neonatal hypothyroidism or a small goiter. However, this is rare when PTU doses are titrated to maintain free T_4 in the upper limits of the normal range but more common if the thyroxine levels fall into the mid- or lower- normal range or if attempts are made to normalize the TSH.

37. **When can doses of PTU and MMI be reduced?**
Fortunately, antithyroid drugs can usually be markedly decreased by the second and especially third trimester because of the decreasing levels of TSI that accompany the natural immunosuppression of pregnancy. In fact, many women require minimal or no drug at term, especially if they have a small goiter, but it is important to ensure that they are not hyperthyroid at delivery to reduce the risk of hyperthyroid complications to the cardiovascular system. The majority of women have a rebound in their hyperthyroidism postpartum, and postpartum thionamide therapy must be increased.

38. **Discuss the role of beta-blockers during pregnancy.**
Beta-blockers are indicated to treat symptomatic hyperadrenergic signs and symptoms until antithyroid drug therapy has rendered the patient euthyroid. However, they should be discontinued when the patient becomes euthyroid because long-term treatment with beta-blockers has been associated with intrauterine growth restriction. No compelling data indicate that one beta-blocker is safer than another; however, metoprolol and propanolol are usually favored over atenolol.

39. **Why is radioactive iodine contraindicated in pregnancy?**
Radioactive iodine is contraindicated in pregnancy because after 12 weeks' gestation the fetal thyroid gland has avidity for iodine that is 20 to 50 times that of the maternal thyroid. Accordingly, any dosage of radioiodine will be more highly concentrated in fetal thyroid tissue and can easily ablate the fetal gland.

40. **Can cold iodine be given during pregnancy?**
Cold iodine (e.g., Lugol's solution or saturated solution of potassium iodide [SSKI]) should also be avoided in pregnancy except in women with thyroid storm. If it must be given after 10 to 12 weeks, the fetus should be monitored for the development of a goiter, and the duration should be limited if possible to 3 days.

41. Does surgery have a role during pregnancy?

Surgery is rarely indicated during pregnancy but may be necessary in women who are unable to take antithyroid drugs (i.e., because of agranulocytosis) or who are refractory to high dosages of antithyroid medications. If necessary, it is best to perform surgery in the second trimester before fetal viability. The rationale for this timing is that there is a significant increase in the risk of miscarriage in the first trimester and of preterm labor when surgery is performed after 24 weeks.

42. Should a woman be counseled to terminate a pregnancy if she inadvertently receives a ^{123}I scan or an ablative dose of ^{131}I?

A woman who receives ^{123}I for a thyroid scan early in pregnancy can be reassured for the most part because the fetus has not developed the ability to concentrate iodine before 10 weeks and the radiation exposure from this test is low with a half-life of only approximately 8 hours. An ablative dose of ^{131}I given early in pregnancy, however, is cause for greater concern because the half-life of ^{131}I is 8 days, and the radiation is more destructive to the thyroid gland. Generally, if the dose is given very early, when the fetal thyroid gland is not yet trapping iodine, the relatively low thyroid and total body irradiation dose is probably not sufficient to justify termination of the pregnancy.

43. How may the risk to the fetus be minimized?

It may be useful to give PTU to block the recycling of ^{131}I in the fetal thyroid gland if it can be given within 1 week of ^{131}I treatment. Fetal hypothyroidism can be diagnosed in utero by percutaneous umbilical sampling, and T_4 treatment may be given through amniotic fluid injections, although such treatment is still experimental. Certainly, all women of childbearing age regardless of contraceptive measures should have a pregnancy test before receiving any dose of ^{123}I or ^{131}I.

44. How should women with Graves' disease be counseled about treatment alternatives before becoming pregnant?

Many experts recommend definitive treatment with ^{131}I (after a negative pregnancy test) in a woman of childbearing age who wishes to become pregnant. In a series of nearly 300 women given radioiodine for cancer therapy, no significant difference in stillbirths, preterm births, low-birth-weight infants, or congenital malformations were reported in subsequent pregnancies. Effective birth control must be established, and then women should optimally wait for at least 6 months after regaining a stable euthyroid status before trying to conceive. Women who are stable on low doses of thionamides should not have a problematic pregnancy, but it is highly likely that thionamide doses will have be adjusted during pregnancy and the postpartum period. Women requiring high doses or who have large goiters should be counseled about the benefits of definitive therapy before becoming pregnant.

45. Describe the natural history of Graves' disease in the postpartum period.

Approximately 70% of women have a postpartum relapse of Graves' disease, usually within the first 3 months after delivery, as the natural immunosuppression of pregnancy disappears. Antithyroid therapy must almost always be increased during this time.

46. What treatment options can be recommended for women who wish to breast-feed?

For the nursing mother, PTU is the preferred antithyroid drug because it is highly protein-bound and crosses less efficiently into breast milk than MMI. Thyroid function in infants appears unaffected by maternal ingestion of therapeutic doses of PTU or MMI, and it is unnecessary to monitor neonatal thyroid function unless dosage requirements are unusually high.

47. Can a nursing mother undergo a diagnostic ^{123}I scan if the cause of the hyperthyroidism is in question?

A diagnostic ^{123}I scan can be performed if the woman is willing to interrupt breast-feeding for 2 to 3 days. Both ^{123}I and ^{99}Tc pertechnetate are excreted into breast milk with an effective half-life of 5 to 8 and 2 to 8 hours, respectively.

48. **Can ablative therapy with ^{131}I be offered to nursing women?**
    Ablative therapy with ^{131}I cannot be offered unless the women is willing to give up nursing altogether, because even a 5-mCi dosage requires discontinuation of breast-feeding for at least 56 days.

49. **Can beta-blockers be used in nursing women?**
    Beta-blockers can be used if necessary in breast-feeding mothers. However, atenolol may produce higher breast milk concentrations than other beta-blockers, and there are rare reports of neonatal bradycardia in infants of mothers who nursed while taking this drug.

50. **When should a nursing woman take antithyroid drugs?**
    It is always best if a mother takes antithyroid drugs immediately after nursing to avoid exposing the infant to peak concentrations of the drug.

51. **Does hypothyroidism pose a risk to the pregnant patient and should all pregnant women be screened?**
    Hypothyroidism occurs in approximately 2.5% of pregnancies, and because of maternal and fetal concerns, a case can be made to screen pregnant women in the first trimester (Vaidya 2007). However, it has not yet been demonstrated that screening all pregnant women and appropriately treating abnormal thyroid functions decreases adverse pregnancy outcomes. Certainly any pregnant woman with risk factors for hypothyroidism, including a positive family history, a history of any type of thyroid disease, presence of a goiter, known thyroid antibodies, symptoms suggestive of thyroid disease, women with autoimmune disorders including type 1 diabetes mellitus, women with a history of head or neck irradiation, or women with a history of preterm delivery should be screened. Untreated hypothyroidism can cause maternal anemia, myopathy, congestive heart failure, preterm delivery, and an increased risk of preeclampsia, low-birth-weight infants, postpartum hemorrhage, and the possibility of neurodevelopmental delay in the infant.

52. **Should pregnant women with recurrent pregnancy loss be screened for TPO antibodies and if found, should thyroid hormone be offered despite a normal TSH?**
    There are both positive and negative studies suggesting that TPO antibodies may be related to pregnancy loss despite a euthyroid state and on balance, there appears to be a positive association. It is not clear whether these women have decreased thyroid reserve as a possible etiology given that women with positive TPO antibodies are more likely to develop subclinical hypothyroidism later in gestation. It is also unknown whether these antibodies could directly cause miscarriage or are simply markers of other autoimmune diseases that could be associated with pregnancy loss. A single randomized controlled trial suggested that treating unselected euthyroid women who were TPO antibody positive with low dosages of thyroid hormone could decrease first trimester loss but not later loss (Negro 2006). Many of the losses occurred so early that initiating treatment before the loss would not have been possible, and it is difficult to understand on a mechanistic basis how only several days of treatment could prevent pregnancy loss. This study also demonstrated that delivery at less than 37 weeks was decreased in the treated group but gestational age of the groups were not reported. Therefore until further studies support or refute this study, it is not recommended that women be checked for TPO antibodies unless there is a suspicion of thyroid disease. Women who are known to be TPO antibody positive clearly have a approximately 15% risk of developing subclinical hypothyroidism later in pregnancy and a 50% chance of postpartum thyroiditis; they should be monitored closely for these developments.

53. **How do thyroid hormone requirements change during pregnancy?**
    Thyroid hormone requirements in treated hypothyroid patients often increase during pregnancy, with up to 75% of pregnant women requiring an increase in thyroxine dosage of up to 50 mcg

over the prepregnancy dose. A recent study confirmed that 85% of pregnant woman required an increase in levothyroxine of 47% by 16 weeks gestation (Alexander 2004), although most of these women were athyreotic. Because requirements increased as early as 5 weeks gestation, women who are athyreotic may need to increase their thyroid hormone dosage by 20% to 25% as soon as pregnancy is confirmed.

KEY POINTS: THYROID DISEASE IN PREGNANCY

1. Approximately 15% of normal pregnant women have a suppressed thyroid-stimulating hormone (TSH), especially in the first trimester.

2. All women at risk for thyroid disease should be screened in the first trimester.

3. TSH norms change in pregnancy and free T_4 assays by analog methods may be inaccurate.

4. Hyperemesis gravidarum can cause overt hyperthyroidism.

5. Graves' disease most often presents in the first trimester with improvement in later pregnancy but commonly exacerbates after delivery.

6. Subclinical hyperthyroidism should not be treated in pregnancy.

7. Thyroid hormone requirements usually increase in pregnancy, beginning in the first trimester.

8. Postpartum thyroiditis occurs in approximately 5% of normal women and approximately 25% of women with type 1 diabetes.

54. **What causes the rapid increase in thyroid hormone requirements?**
The rapid increase in thyroid hormone requirements that occurs in the first trimester may be due to the sudden increase in the estrogen-stimulated TBG pool associated with pregnancy. This can be especially striking in women undergoing assisted reproduction during which hormonal therapy may stimulate very high estrogen levels.

55. **When should serum TSH levels be checked, and at what level of TSH should therapy be directed?**
The serum TSH level should be checked as soon as pregnancy is confirmed, and an appropriate increase in thyroid hormone should be given. A recent study suggests that athyreotic women requiring full replacement dosages should receive a 25% dosage increase as soon as pregnancy is confirmed despite a normal TSH (Alexander 2004). As discussed earlier, the TSH may be mildly suppressed in normal women during the first trimester as a result of the thyrotropic influence of hCG. Therefore unless a woman is symptomatically hyperthyroid or has frankly elevated serum free T_4 levels, the thyroxine dosage should not be reduced in response to the finding of a low first-trimester TSH level. The TSH should be checked 4 to 6 weeks after a dosage change and at least every trimester to maintain a normal serum TSH concentration which is less than 3.0 mU/L in the first trimester and 3.5 mU/L or less in the second and third trimesters. In women who have had a thyroidectomy for thyroid cancer, the goal of maintaining a suppressed serum TSH without rendering the woman thyrotoxic should be adhered to during pregnancy. Thyroid hormone should be reduced almost immediately after delivery to avoid hyperthyroidism postpartum. Prepregnancy dosages may be instituted as soon as the woman has lost the majority of her pregnancy weight gain.

56. When should a pregnant woman take her thyroid hormone?

It is extremely important to advise the pregnant woman to take her thyroid hormone and her prenatal vitamins or iron supplements at different times, because ferrous sulfate can bind to thyroxine and decrease its bioavailability.

57. What is the risk of abnormal fetal and neonatal intellectual development in infants born to mothers who are hypothyroid during the first trimester of pregnancy?

All newborns in the United States are screened for hypothyroidism, because it is well established that infants who have severe congenital hypothyroidism but receive thyroid hormone replacement at birth appear to have fairly normal intellectual growth and development. However, the fetal effects of maternal hypothyroidism during the first trimester, when the fetal brain is dependent on maternal thyroid hormone, is a subject of ongoing debate. Several recent publications suggest that psychomotor and intellectual development might be impaired in infants born to mothers who were hypothyroid during the first trimester of pregnancy, although the differences from control subjects in these studies were small and often became insignificant when the infants were tested later in childhood.

58. What strategies can reduce the risk to the fetus?

It seems prudent to attempt to identify and appropriately treat hypothyroidism in women of childbearing age who wish to become pregnant (preconception), as well as in pregnant women in the first trimester. It must be remembered, however, that serum TSH levels often decline in the first trimester as a result of the influence of hCG. Thus a TSH level greater than 3.5 mU/L in the first trimester may be inappropriately high, whereas a TSH level of 0.1 mU/mL may be appropriately low because of the thyroid-stimulating activity of high levels of hCG.

59. How should a thyroid nodule be evaluated during pregnancy?

The evaluation of a solitary or dominant nodule in a pregnant woman is similar to that in nonpregnant women. Fine-needle aspiration (FNA) should be offered when nodules are greater than 1 to 2 cm, especially if they are detected before 20 weeks or if there are other risk factors for malignancy, such as lymphadenopathy or rapid growth. FNA specimens should be evaluated using the same criteria as established for nonpregnant patients.

60. What is the likelihood that thyroid nodules discovered during pregnancy are malignant?

Data suggest that thyroid nodules discovered during pregnancy may have a higher risk of being malignant. However, this finding is likely due in part to selection or sampling bias, because many young women do not have systematic health examinations until they become pregnant. Depending on the patient population, the incidence of biopsied nodules being benign is greater than 80%, whereas differentiated thyroid cancer has been found in 5% to 40% of cases. The majority of malignant nodules are papillary thyroid carcinoma. FNA cytology is highly accurate in diagnosing papillary carcinoma, whereas cytology showing a follicular or Hürthle cell neoplasm predicts only a 5 to 15% risk of malignancy. When the serum TSH is normal, fewer than 20% of FNA specimens are nondiagnostic. In one series of 61 patients with differentiated thyroid cancer (87% papillary), there were no differences in the rates of recurrence, distant spread, or outcomes related to whether neck surgery was performed during or after pregnancy.

61. How should a thyroid nodule be managed during pregnancy?

If the cytology is suspicious or confirms papillary thyroid cancer, the best time to offer a thyroidectomy is probably in the second trimester, to avoid the risk of miscarriage in the first trimester and preterm labor in the third trimester. If the nodule is less than 2 cm, has not rapidly increased in size, and the patient has no lymphadenopathy, it may be reasonable to postpone thyroidectomy until after pregnancy and place the woman on thyroid suppression therapy in the meantime with careful attention to avoiding elevated thyroxine levels.

62. **How common is postpartum thyroiditis? Who is at risk?**
Postpartum thyroid dysfunction occurs in approximately 5 to 10% of women, with a much higher incidence in certain populations. In one series, 25% of women with type 1 diabetes mellitus developed postpartum thyroid dysfunction; it is therefore recommended that this population should be screened in the postpartum period on a routine basis. In another series of 152 women with TPO antibodies detected at 16 weeks' gestation, postpartum thyroiditis occurred in 50%; of these, 19% had hyperthyroidism alone, 49% had hypothyroidism alone, and the remaining 32% had hyperthyroidism followed by hypothyroidism. Women with a family history of thyroid disease are also at increased risk and may be candidates for screening with TPO antibodies during pregnancy or with thyroid function tests in the postpartum period. Women known to be TPO antibody positive should have a TSH performed at 3 and 6 months postpartum.

63. **Characterize the histopathology of postpartum thyroiditis.**
The disorder is highly associated with circulating TPO antibodies, and the histology is identical to that of Hashimoto's thyroiditis with profuse mononuclear cell infiltration and destruction of thyroid follicles.

64. **Summarize the clinical course of postpartum thyroiditis.**
Classically, the clinical course consists of three phases, but not all women manifest each phase.

65. **Describe phase 1 of postpartum thyroiditis.**
At 1 to 3 months after delivery, affected women often develop hyperthyroidism as a result of immunologically mediated destruction of thyroid follicles, which results in the release of stored thyroid hormone into the circulation. Such women may experience anxiety, irritability, palpitations, fatigue, and insomnia, but commonly this phase does not come to the attention of the clinician. Symptomatic patients are best treated with beta-blockers, which must soon be tapered and discontinued as the thyrotoxic phase spontaneously resolves. Use of PTU or methimazole is not indicated given that these patients have hyperthyroidism due to destruction of their gland, not to increased synthesis of thyroid hormone.

66. **How can phase 1 of postpartum thyroiditis be distinguished from Graves' disease?**
Occasionally there is a question about the cause of the hyperthyroidism, because Graves' disease commonly appears or exacerbates in the first several months postpartum. Distinguishing between the two conditions is facilitated by measurement of a serum thyroglobulin level and TPO antibodies (both are high in postpartum thyroiditis) and TSH receptor-stimulating antibodies (often elevated with Graves' disease). However, the most definitive test is a ^{123}I-uptake test (low in postpartum thyroiditis and high in Graves' disease), if the mother is willing to interrupt nursing for 2 to 3 days.

67. **Describe phase 2 of postpartum thyroiditis.**
More commonly, women present with stage 2 of postpartum thyroiditis, which is characterized by hypothyroidism alone at about 4 to 8 months after delivery. Nonspecific symptoms include fatigue, depression, impaired concentration, poor memory, aches and pains, dry skin, and weight gain, all of which may be overlooked by the clinician. Symptoms may predate the onset of thyroid function abnormalities in women with positive TPO antibodies and may persist for some time after a euthyroid state is achieved.

68. **How is phase 2 of postpartum thyroiditis treated?**
Women with abnormal thyroid function tests and symptoms consistent with hypothyroidism should be treated with thyroxine replacement for approximately 6 to 12 months or at least until

1 year after delivery. At that time, discontinuation of thyroxine therapy can be attempted to identify the 80% of women who will return to the euthyroid state by 12 months after delivery.

69. Describe the natural history of postpartum thyroiditis.

Most women will return to a euthyroid state at 12 to 18 months postpartum. However, thyroid function testing should then be followed at least annually in women who become euthyroid. In one series of 43 patients with postpartum thyroiditis, 23% of the women were hypothyroid at 2 to 4 years, and, in a longer series, 48% of women were hypothyroid 7 to 9 years later. Women with the highest TPO antibody titers and the most severe hypothyroidism appear to be at the highest risk of developing permanent hypothyroidism. If a woman becomes euthyroid within a year postpartum, she has a high likelihood (70%) of developing postpartum thyroiditis after a subsequent pregnancy.

BIBLIOGRAPHY

1. ACOG Practice Bulletin: Thyroid disease in pregnancy. Int J Gynaecol Obstet 79:171–180, 2002.

2. Alexander EK, Marqusee E, Lawrence E, et al: Timing and magnitude of increases in levothyroxine requirements during pregnancy in women with hypothyroidism. N Engl J Med 351:241–249, 2004.

3. Azizi F, Khoshniet M, Bahrainian M, Hedayati M: Thyroid function and intellectual development of infants nursed by mothers taking methimazole. J Clin Endocrinol Metab 85:3233–3238, 2000.

4. Casey BM, Dashe JS, Wells CE, et al: Subclinical hyperthyroidism and pregnancy outcomes. Obstet Gynecol 107:337–341, 2006.

5. Chopra IJ, Baber K: Treatment of primary hypothyroidism during pregnancy: is there an increase in thyroxine dose requirement in pregnancy? Metab Clin Exper 52:122–128, 2003.

6. Endocrine Society Committee: Guidelines for management of thyroid dysfunction during pregnancy and postpartum. J Cl n Endocrinol Metabol 17:1159–1167, 2007.

7. Gerstein HC: Incidence of postpartum thyroid dysfunction in patients with type I diabetes mellitus. Ann Intern Med 118:419–423, 1993.

8. Glinoer D: Management of hypo- and hyperthyroidism during pregnancy. Growth Horm IGF Res 13:45–54, 2003.

9. Glinoer D, Rihai M, Grun JP: Risk of subclinical hypothyroidism in pregnant women with asymptomatic autoimmune thyroid disorders. J Clinc Endocrinol Metab 79:197–204, 1994.

10. Goodwin TM, Hershman JM: Hyperthyroidism due to inappropriate production of human chorionic gonadotropin. Clin Obstet Gynecol 40:32–44, 1997.

11. Hay ID: Nodular thyroid disease diagnosed during pregnancy: how and when to treat. Thyroid 9:667–670, 1999.

12. Kahric-Janic N, Soldin SJ, Soldin OP, et al: Tandem mass spectrometry improves the accuracy of free thyroxine measurements during pregnancy. Thyroid 17:303–311, 2007.

13. Kempers MJE, Van Tijn DA, Van Trotensburg ASP, et al: Central congenital hypothyroidism due to gestational hyperthyroidism: detection where prevention failed. Clin Endocrinol Metab 88:5851–5857, 2003.

14. Lazarus JH: Thyroid disorders associated with pregnancy: etiology, diagnosis, and management. Treat Endocrinol 4:31–41, 2005.

15. Luton D, Le Gac I, Vuillard E, et al: Management of Grave's disease during pregnancy: the key role of fetal thyroid gland monitoring. J Clin Endocrinol Metab 90:6093–6098, 2005.

16. Mandel S, Cooper D: The use of antithyroid drugs in pregnancy and lactation. J Clin Endocrinol Metab 86:2354–2359, 2001.

17. Mandel SJ, Larsen PR, Seely EW, Brent GA: Increased need for thyroxine during pregnancy in women with primary hypothyroidism. N Engl J Med 323:91–96, 1990.

18. Mestman JH, Goodwin TM, Montoro MM: Thyroid disorders of pregnancy. Endocrin Metab Clin N Am 24:41–71, 1995.

19. Momotani N, Yamashita R, Makino F, et al: Thyroid function in wholly breast-feeding infants whose mothers take high doses of propylthiouracil. Clin Endocrinol 53:177–181, 2000.

20. Moosa M, Mazzaferri EL: Outcome of differentiated thyroid cancer diagnosed in pregnant women. J Clin Endocrinol Metab 82:2862–2866, 1997.

21. Nachum Z, Rakover Y, Weiner E, et al: Grave's disease in pregnancy: prospective evaluation of a selective invasive treatment protocol. Am J Obstet Gynecol 189:159–165, 2003.

22. Negro R, Formoso G, Mangieri T, et al: Levothyroxine treatment in euthyroid pregnant women with autoimmune thyroid disease: effects on obstetrical complications. J Clin Endocrinol Metab 91:2587–2591, 2006.

23. Panesar NS, Li CY, Rogers MS: Reference intervals for thyroid hormones in pregnant Chinese women. Ann Clin Biochem 38:329–332, 2001.

24. Pelag D, Cada S, Peleg A, et al: The relationship between maternal serum thyroid-stimulating immunoglobulin and fetal and neonatal thyrotoxicosis. Obstet Gynecol 99:1040–1043, 2002.

25. Pop V, Brouwers EP, Vader HL, et al: Maternal hypothyroxinaemia during early pregnancy and subsequent child development: a 3-year follow-up study. Clin Endocrinol (Oxf) 59:282–288, 2003.

26. Rushworth FH, Backos M, Rai R, et al: Prospective pregnancy outcome in untreated recurrent miscarriers with thyroid autoantibodies. Hum Reprod 15:1637–1639, 2000.

27. Sapin R, D'Herbomez M, Schlienger JL: Free thyroxine measured with equilibrium dialysis and nine immunoassays decreased in late pregnancy. Clin Lab 50:581–584, 2004.

28. Soldin OP, Tractenberg RE, Hollowell, et al: Trimester-specific changes in maternal thyroid hormone, thyrotropin, and thyroglobulin concentrations: trends and associations across trimester in iodine sufficiency. Thryoid 14:1084–1090, 2004.

29. Stagnaro-Green A: Postpartum thyroiditis. Best Pract Res Clin Endocrinol Metab 18:303–316, 2004.

30. Vaidya B, Anthony S, Bilous M: Detection of thyroid dysfunction in early pregnancy: universal screening or target high-risk case finding? J Clin Endocrinol Metab 92:203–207, 2007.

31. Vulsma T, Gons MH, de Vijlder JJ: Maternal-fetal transfer of thyroxine in congenital hypothyroidism due to a total organification defect or thyroid agenesis. N Engl J Med 321:13–16, 1989.

32. Zimmerman D: Fetal and neonatal hyperthyroidism. Thyroid 9:727–733, 1999.

CHAPTER 41

PSYCHIATRIC DISORDERS AND THYROID DISEASE

James V. Hennessey

1. **How well established is the relationship between thyroid disease and psychiatric symptoms?**

   For more than a century, since the publication of the Clinical Society of London's "Report on Myxoedema" in 1888, it has been recognized that thyroid disease may give rise to psychiatric disorders that can be corrected by reestablishment of normal thyroid function. Later, Asher reemphasized the fact that patients with profound hypothyroidism may present with depressive psychosis. As outlined in Table 41-1, the symptoms of hypothyroidism often mimic those of depression, whereas those of hyperthyroidism include anxiety, dysphoria, emotional lability, and intellectual dysfunction, as well as mania or depression, the latter being especially characteristic among the elderly presenting with (so-called) apathetic thyrotoxicosis.

TABLE 41-1. CLINICAL FEATURES COMMON TO BOTH THYROID DISEASES AND MOOD DISORDERS			
	Hypothyroidism	**Mood Disorders**	**Hyperthyroidism**
Depression	Yes	Yes	Yes
Diminished interest	Yes	Yes	Yes
Diminished pleasure	Yes	Yes	No
Decreased libido	Yes	Yes	Sometimes
Weight loss	No	Yes	Yes
Weight gain	Yes	Sometimes	Occasionally
Appetite loss	Yes	Yes	Sometimes
Increased appetite	No	Yes	Yes
Insomnia	No	Yes	Yes
Hypersomnia	Yes	Yes	No
Agitation/anxiety	Occasionally	Yes	Yes
Fatigue	Yes	Yes	Yes
Poor memory	Yes	Yes	Occasionally
Cognitive dysfunction	Yes	Yes	Yes
Impaired concentration	Yes	Yes	Yes
Constipation	Yes	Sometimes	No

(Adapted from Hennessey JV, Jackson IMD: The interface between thyroid hormones and psychiatry. Endocrinologist 6:214–223, 1996.)

2. **What abnormalities of thyroid function are found in psychiatric disorders?**
Because patients with thyroid disease may manifest frank psychiatric disorders that are reversible with endocrine therapy, the thyroid axis has been extensively studied in patients presenting with a wide variety of behavioral disturbances. Various abnormalities of thyroid function have been identified, particularly in depression. In most depressed subjects the basal serum thyroid-stimulating hormone (TSH), thyroxine (T_4) and triiodothyronine (T_3) are within the normal range, though in one report a third of such patients were observed to have suppressed TSH levels.

3. **What abnormalities of TRH stimulation may be observed in the depressed patient?**
Patients with depression have a "blunted" TSH response to thyrotropin-releasing hormone (TRH) administration (as defined by a TSH rise $<5\mu U/mL$) in approximately 25% of such subjects. Blunted TSH response is more likely in unipolar than bipolar depression, but differentiating these disorders with TRH stimulation has been disappointing.
The blunted TSH response is a "state" marker that normalizes upon recovery from the depression.

4. **Describe the mechanism for blunted TSH response in affective disorders.**
The mechanism for the blunted TSH response in affective disorders is not known; however, glucocorticoids, known to inhibit the hypothalamic-pituitary-thyroid axis, are elevated in depression and could be responsible.
The suppressed TSH response to TRH is not specific to depression and may be observed in alcohol withdrawal, starvation, normal aging males, renal failure, acromegaly, Cushing's syndrome, and hypopituitarism. The blunting may also be due to medications such as thyroxine, glucocorticoids, growth hormone, somatostatin, dopamine, and phenytoin, all of which have been reported to diminish this response.

5. **Can abnormalities in the TSH circadian rhythm be identified in depression?**
In normal subjects, TSH begins to rise in the evening before the onset of sleep, reaching a peak between 11:00 p.m. and 4 a.m. In depression, the nocturnal surge of TSH is frequently absent, resulting in a reduction in thyroid hormone secretion, supporting the view that functional central hypothyroidism might occur in some depressed subjects. Sleep deprivation, which has an antidepressant effect, returns TSH circadian rhythm to normal. The mechanism responsible for the impaired nocturnal rise of TSH is unknown.

6. **Is autoimmune thyroid disease frequently present in the depressed patient?**
Although the blunted TSH response is well recognized in depression, it is less clearly appreciated that an enhanced response may occur in up to 15% of depressed subjects with normal baseline thyroid function tests. The majority of such patients have antithyroid antibodies, suggesting that the TSH hyperresponse may indicate latent hypothyroidism caused by autoimmune thyroiditis. When autoimmunity is tested using the antithyroid peroxidase antibody (anti-TPO) rather than the less specific antimicrosomal antibody, the prevalence of autoimmune thyroid disease is even higher. Not all studies, however, have found an increased prevalence of antithyroid antibodies in depressed subjects when compared with matched control groups.

7. **What is the frequency of elevated thyroxine values in the psychiatric patient?**
Approximately 20% of patients admitted to the hospital with acute psychiatric presentations, including schizophrenia and major affective disorders, but rarely dementia or alcoholism, may demonstrate mild elevations in their serum T_4 levels, and less often their T_3 levels. The basal TSH is usually normal but may demonstrate blunted TRH responsiveness in up to 90% of such patients. These findings do not appear to represent thyrotoxicosis, and the abnormalities spontaneously resolve within 2 weeks without specific therapy. Such phenomena may be due to central activation of the hypothalamic-pituitary-thyroid axis resulting in enhanced TSH secretion with consequent elevation in circulating thyroxine levels.

8. **What is the most consistent abnormality of the thyroid axis in hospitalized depressed patients?**
In depressed patients, the most consistent abnormality of the thyroid axis may be an increase in serum total or free T_4 levels, although usually within the conventional normal range. This generally regresses following successful treatment of the depression.

9. **What is the prevalence of hypothyroid dysfunction seen in psychiatric populations?**
Thyroid function test abnormalities are common in older individuals. In otherwise normal female subjects aged over 60 years, the prevalence of elevated TSH values, positive antithyroid antibodies, or both is 10% or more. Subjecting apparently asymptomatic individuals with slight elevations of serum TSH but normal T_4 and T_3 levels to a battery of psychological tests has revealed significant differences from control subjects on scales measuring memory, anxiety, somatic complaints, and depression. It is becoming increasingly recognized that depression is much more common in elderly individuals. Whether borderline hypothyroidism plays a role in these behavioral disturbances requires further investigation. Among alcoholics and those suffering from anorexia nervosa, suppressed T_3 levels with elevations in reverse T_3 and normal TSH values are consistent with the "sick thyroid state." These findings likely result from caloric deprivation.

10. **Which medications affect thyroid function and thyroid function tests?**
Medications commonly used to treat psychiatric illness have been shown to affect thyroid function tests. See Table 41-2.

TABLE 41-2. IMPACT OF PSYCHOTROPIC MEDICATIONS ON THYROID FUNCTION TESTS

Medication	Mechanism	Test Findings
Lithium carbonate	↓ thyroglobulin hydrolysis	TSH ↑ (transiently)
	↓ T4 and T3 release	Hypothyroidism, goiter
Antipsychotics		
Perphenazine	↑ TBG concentration	↑ (T4, nl free T4)
Anticonvulsants		
Phenytoin	↑ Hepatic clearance of T4	↓ T4, ± ↓ free T4, nl TSH
Carbamazepine	↓ T4 binding, ↑ hepatic clearance	↓ T4, ± ↓ free T4, nl TSH
Phenobarbital	↑ hepatic clearance	↓ T4, ± ↓ free T4, nl TSH
Valproic acid	↓ T4 binding (?), ↑ hepatic clearance (?)	↓ T4, ± ↓ free T4, nl TSH
Narcotics		
Heroin	↑ TBG concentration	↑ T4, nl free T4
Methadone	↑ TBG concentration	↑ T4, nl free T4
Miscellaneous		
Amphetamines	↑ TSH secretion (?)	↑ T4, ↑ free T4

T_3, triiodothyronine; T_3RU, T_3 resin uptake; T_4, thyroxine; TBG, thyroxine-binding globulin; TSH, thyroid-stimulating hormone.

(Adapted from Hennessy JV, Jackson IMD: The interface between thyroid hormones and psychiatry. Endocrinologist 6:214–223, 1996.)

11. How does lithium affect the pituitary-thyroidal axis?
Lithium carbonate, used to treat bipolar disorders, interferes with both the release and organification of thyroid hormone. Therapeutic lithium levels diminish both T_3 and T_4 release from the thyroid gland, and at higher (probably toxic) levels, iodine uptake and organification may also be inhibited. Following a 3-week therapeutic course of lithium carbonate, suppression of serum T_4 and T_3 levels and associated elevations of basal serum TSH values and exaggerated TSH responses to TRH administration may be noted; these abnormalities generally return to normal within 3 to 12 months, even if the medication is continued.

12. What is the most common thyroid disorder in lithium-treated patients?
Goiter is the most common thyroid disorder occurring in lithium-treated patients. Hypothyroidism can also occasionally develop, particularly in patients who have thyroid glands that have been compromised by disorders such as Hashimoto's thyroiditis and Graves' disease previously treated with ^{131}I therapy. However, it is uncommon for hypothyroidism to occur if pretreatment thyroid function is completely normal and patients are thyroid antibody-negative. If considered clinically necessary, lithium may be continued and thyroxine added to treat patients who develop goiter or hypothyroidism.

13. How does phenytoin affect laboratory tests and the function of the thyroid?
The effects of phenytoin (Dilantin), occasionally used for bipolar disorder, on thyroid function are complex. Suppressed values of total and, occasionally, free thyroxine are observed in a significant minority of patients who are chronically treated with phenytoin alone and in upward of 75% of those in whom the drug is combined with carbamazepine (Tegretol). The lower total T_4 levels are likely due to displacement of T_4 from thyroxine-binding globulin (TBG), whereas the reduced free T_4 levels result from enhanced clearance of T_4 through phenytoin-induced hepatic microsomal oxidative enzyme activity. Generally, the suppressed T_4 levels are accompanied by normal T_3 and free T_3 levels and normal TSH concentrations. Normal basal TSH values with diminished TSH responses to TRH have been attributed to potential phenytoin agonism at the T_3 receptor. However, other studies have suggested that this may be an assay artifact because free T_4 values have been found to be normal or mildly elevated in analyses using undiluted serum.

14. Describe the effects of carbamazepine on thyroid function.
Carbamazepine (Tegretol) is used increasingly in bipolar disorder. Chronic use with maintenance of therapeutic serum levels may suppress serum T_4 values in more than 50% of patients. This may be because of the enhanced hepatic metabolism of thyroxine. TRH stimulation testing before and after initiation of Tegretol therapy reveals that TSH responsiveness is reduced by the addition of this drug; this has led to speculation that carbamazepine may inhibit thyroid function through effects on the pituitary gland. Displacement of T_4 from TBG, similar to that seen with phenytoin, has additionally been cited as a potential effect.

15. How do phenobarbital, valproic acid, and other psychotropic medications affect thyroid function?
Both phenobarbital and valproic acid are reported to lower serum levels of T_4 in chronically treated patients, the former through enhanced hepatic T_4 clearance and the latter likely because of protein binding changes. Heroin, methadone, and perphenazine commonly increase serum TBG levels and therefore may elevate serum total T_4 levels, although TSH and free thyroxine values remain normal. Amphetamines induce hyperthyroxinemia through enhanced secretion of TSH, an effect that appears to be centrally mediated.

16. How do antidepressant therapies affect thyroid function?
Antidepressants do not generally cause abnormal peripheral thyroid hormone levels but may affect thyroid hormone metabolism in the central nervous system (CNS). However, circulating total T_4 and free T_4, but not T_3, levels often show a modest decline, although still within the

normal range, after treatment with various pharmacological classes of antidepressants, as well as with electroconvulsive therapy (ECT).

17. **Are there caveats of antidepressant usage in individuals with thyroid disease?**
The use of tricyclic antidepressants (TCA) in thyrotoxic patients should be pursued with caution, because cardiac dysrhythmias may be exacerbated or precipitated. Further, the monoamine oxidase inhibitors may cause hypertension in thyrotoxic patients, although they generally do not affect thyroid function or serum thyroid hormone levels.

18. **Has thyroxine been used as sole treatment for depression?**
Asher's report on "myxoedema madness" demonstrated that thyroid hormone deficiency resulted in depression that reversed with thyroid hormone administration. This led to studies of the role of thyroid hormone therapy alone in the treatment of depression and other psychiatric diseases and open studies of high-dosage thyroxine for refractory bipolar and unipolar depression. Euthyroid individuals with typical hypothyroid symptoms, considered depressed on psychological testing, do not improve when treated with thyroxine. In fact, patients presenting with symptoms of hypothyroidism with normal thyroid function tests respond more positively to placebo. Although initial reports of T_3 as single therapy were promising, these studies were methodologically flawed, so that the role of thyroid hormone by itself in the treatment of depression in the absence of abnormalities of thyroid function has not been established.

19. **Are neuropsychiatric abnormalities demonstrable among patients with mild thyroid failure?**
Recent studies have shown that symptomatic patients with subclinical hypothyroidism (elevated serum TSH but normal T_4 and T_3 levels) can have significant impairment of memory-related abilities, health status, mood, anxiety, somatic complaints, and depressive features when compared with euthyroid control subjects (Monzani 1993). Normalization of the serum TSH with L-thyroxine therapy may completely reverse these neuropsychiatric features. Further, when thyroid hormone is withdrawn from subjects with underlying hypothyroidism, gradually increasing cognitive findings, sadness, and anxiety symptoms are observed over the ensuing few weeks. These findings indicate that the patient presenting with depression must be assessed for thyroid dysfunction, because the presence of even subclinical hypothyroidism may provide an opportunity for resolution of the depression with thyroid hormone treatment.

20. **How effective is the combination of L-thyroxine and T_3 in the treatment of neuropsychiatric symptoms of hypothyroidism?**
Since the 1960s, multiple reports have appeared evaluating the effectiveness of combining T_3 with thyroxine to improve outcomes. The report of Bunevicius et al, for example, seemed to indicate that substituting 12.5 μg of T_3 for 50 μg of the individual's usual thyroxine dose resulted in improvement in mood and neuropsychological function. Several double-blind randomized controlled trials designed to correct design flaws of previous trials have subsequently failed to reproduce the positive effects reported by Bunevicius and do not demonstrate improvement in self-rated mood, well-being, or depression scales with the addition of T_3 to T_4 therapy. In addition, these studies fail to demonstrate differences in cognitive function, quality of life, or subjective satisfaction with treatment but do report that anxiety scores were significantly worse in those treated with the T_4/T_3 combination. At this point in time, it would not appear justified to use combined thyroxine and T_3 treatment in hypothyroid patients who complain of depressive symptoms after biochemical euthyroidism is restored.

21. **Can combination thyroid hormone and antidepressant enhance response to depression treatment?**
Adjuvant therapy has been said to be logical when depression fails to resolve after 6 weeks of adequate antidepressant medication. Such resistance occurs in approximately 30% to 45%

of cases. The role of adjuvant thyroid hormone with TCAs, has been investigated in euthyroid patients with depression for more than 25 years. T_3 dosages of 25 to 50 μg daily increase serum T_3 levels and cause suppression of serum TSH and T_4 values. Two separate therapeutic effects of T_3 therapy have been studied: first, its ability to accelerate the onset of the antidepressant response; second, its ability to augment antidepressant responses among those considered pharmacologically resistant.

22. **How effective is thyroid hormone for the acceleration of the antidepressant response?**
    The antidepressant effect of TCAs is known to be delayed, and the role of T_3 in accelerating the therapeutic onset of these drugs has been investigated. Several reports detailing the clinical outcomes of starting T_3 (5–40 μg daily) along with varying doses of TCAs as well as selective serotonin reuptake inhibitors (SSRIs) at the outset of therapy have appeared in the literature. The study populations were inhomogeneous, consisting of patients with various types of depression. Furthermore, there were important methodological limitations, including small sample sizes, inadequate medication doses, lack of serum medication level monitoring, and variable outcomes measures. Because two relatively large, prospective, randomized placebo controlled studies have recently come to opposite conclusions, it still has not been clearly established that T_3 accelerates the antidepressant effect of TCAs.

23. **Can triiodothyronine augment the clinical antidepressant response?**
    An additional hypothesis is that adding small dosages of T_3 to the antidepressant therapy of patients who have little or no or initial response will enhance the clinical effectiveness of the antidepressant. Resistance to antidepressants is defined as inadequate remission after two successive trials of monotherapy with different antidepressants at adequate dosages, each for 4 to 6 weeks, before changing to alternative therapies. However, 8 to 12 weeks of ineffective antidepressant therapy is commonly deemed unacceptable, and strategies designed to augment the response are being sought. Early studies assessing T_3 effectiveness in augmenting the antidepressant response were neither placebo controlled nor focused on patient populations that could be directly compared. The first placebo-controlled, double-blind, randomized study reported results in 16 unipolar depressed outpatients who had experienced no improvement in their clinical outcomes with TCAs alone. The intervention consisted of adding 25 μg of T_3 or placebo daily for 2 weeks before the patients were crossed over to the opposite treatment for an additional 2 weeks. No beneficial effect of T_3 was apparent. The only other placebo-controlled, randomized, double-blind trial investigating this question involved 33 patients with unipolar depression treated with either desipramine or imipramine for 5 weeks before random assignment to placebo or 37.5 μg of T_3 daily. After 2 weeks of observation on T_3, during which TCA levels were monitored, significantly more patients treated with T_3 (10 of 17; 59%) had a positive response than did placebo treated patients (3 of 16; 19%). A subsequent open clinical trial of imipramine-resistant depression, using a prolonged period of TCA treatment preceding the addition of T_3, showed no demonstrable T_3 effect.

24. **What evidence is there that the effect of SSRIs and ECT may be enhanced by the addition of T_3?**
    The SSRI group of substances (including fluoxetine and sertraline) is the preferred antidepressant category in the United States today. Case reports suggest that SSRIs behave similarly to TCAs in this regard. A recent, large, double-blind, placebo-controlled study to determine the role of T_3 as augmentation therapy did not demonstrate an effect of T_3 in augmenting the response of paroxetine (an SSRI) therapy in patients with major depressive disorder but a similar study using sertraline and T_3 seemed to a demonstrate positive response. Responders in the Cooper-Karaz report seemed to have had lower circulating thyroid hormone levels before treatment and to have experienced greater decrease in TSH levels as a result of the intervention. This may indicate that those benefiting from the addition of T_3 may have been

subtly hypothyroid, and the addition of T_3 compensated for this deficiency. Of interest, T_3 has been reported to augment the antidepressant effect of ECT.

25. **Are any psychiatric conditions recognized to respond to pharmacological doses of thyroxine?**

For the 10% to 15% of bipolar disorder patients with four or more episodes of manic-depressive psychosis yearly (rapid cyclers), the prevalence of autoimmune thyroid disease may reach 50% or higher. Therapeutic intervention with standard therapy such as lithium is frequently disappointing. Open-label studies treating such patients with levothyroxine in pharmacological dosages sufficient to suppress serum TSH and elevate T_4 levels to approximately 150% of normal may decrease the manic and depressive phases in both amplitude and frequency and has led to remission in some of the patients. Given these encouraging results, controlled studies on the efficacy of levothyroxine or triiodothyronine seem warranted.

26. **Are mechanisms of thyroid hormone action on the brain known?**

Thyroid hormones play a critical role in the development and function of the central nervous system. Triiodothyronine receptors are widely distributed throughout the brain, and there is much evidence that thyroid hormone regulates brain function through interaction with the catecholaminergic system. Thyroid hormone action in brain tissue is accomplished through the binding of T_3 to its nuclear receptor. The T_3 is derived from T_4 by the action of type II 5′-deiodinase (5′D-11), which is located throughout the CNS.

27. **Should T_4 or T_3 be used in treating the depressed patient?**

Most studies using thyroid hormone as adjuvant therapy have used T_3 rather than T_4, and in those reports in which the advantages of one over the other were assessed, T_3 was considered superior. In a randomized trial combining T_4 or T_3 with antidepressants, only 4 of 21 patients (19%) treated with 150 µg/day of T_4 for 3 weeks responded, whereas 9 of 17 (53%) responded with 37.5 µg/day of T_3. Further studies of open T_4 treatment in antidepressant-resistant patients have appeared, but the lack of control makes outcome interpretation difficult. One of these indicated that responders to levothyroxine had significantly lower pretreatment serum T_4 and reverse T_3 levels, leading the authors to believe that the responders might have been subclinically hypothyroid. Combination therapy with T_4 rather than T_3 may be indicated when subclinical hypothyroidism or rapid-cycling bipolar disease is present. Because T_4 equilibrates in tissues more slowly than T_3, treatment with T_4 for at least 6 to 8 weeks, and preferably longer, would be necessary to determine its efficacy in this situation.

28. **Describe the proposed mechanisms linking thyroid function and depression.**

It has been postulated that 5′D-II activity in the CNS is deficient in depression giving rise to a state of brain hypothyroidism coexisting with systemic euthyroidism. Alternatively, 5co-existing D-II activity may be depressed by the elevated cortisol levels seen in depression and stress resulting in T_4 being converted to reverse T_3 by "inner ring" brain 5 deiodinase (type III deiodinase [5D-III]) activity resulting in decreased brain T_3 and increased rT_3 levels. Of note is the fact that T_3 treatment is feasible as T_3 is not dependant on transport by transthyretin, which is noted to be low in depression, and therefore would ensure adequate T_3 delivery to the brain across the blood-brain barrier.

29. **Do antidepressant medications have a mechanistic connection to the action of thyroid hormone in the brain?**

It has been shown that desipramine, a TCA, and fluoxetine, a SSRI, both enhance type II 5′-deiodinase activity in the CNS, thus presumably increasing the availability of T_3 in the brain. This could conceivably account for the clinical efficacy of these classes of drugs.

30. **What recommendations can be made for the thyroid evaluation in the psychiatric patient?**

It seems prudent to check thyroid function tests in those psychiatric patients who are at increased risk for developing thyroid disease. Women over 45 years of age, patients with known autoimmune diseases, individuals with a family history of thyroid disease, and those receiving lithium or suffering from dementia should be screened for underlying thyroid abnormalities. Patients receiving medications known to influence the interpretation of thyroid function tests should have these considered when interpreting the results of testing.

31. **Who should receive thyroid hormone with the intent of relieving psychiatric symptoms?**

It is recommended that thyroxine therapy be offered to any depressed patient with an elevated serum TSH, especially if accompanied by increased antithyroid antibody titers or low free T_4. Thyroid hormone replacement may alleviate the depression in these individuals. On the other hand, antidepressant therapy, if required, may be ineffective before normalization of thyroid axis parameters. In patients with refractory depression but normal systemic thyroid function, adjuvant T_3 therapy may not be worth considering.

KEY POINTS: PSYCHIATRIC DISORDERS AND THYROID DISEASE

1. The symptoms of hypothyroidism often mimic those of depression, whereas those of hyperthyroidism may be confused with mania or depression.

2. Approximately 20% of patients admitted to the hospital with acute psychiatric presentations, including schizophrenia and major affective disorders, but rarely dementia or alcoholism, may demonstrate mild elevations in their serum thyroxine (T_4) levels, and less often their triiodothyronine (T_3) levels.

3. Normalization of the serum TSH with L-thyroxine therapy may completely reverse the neuropsychiatric features of hypothyroidism.

4. Based upon the results of recent prospective controlled studies, it would not appear justified to use combined thyroxine and T_3 treatment in hypothyroid patients who complain of depressive symptoms after biochemical euthyroidism is restored.

5. A recent, fairly large double-blind, placebo-controlled study to determine the role of T_3 as augmentation therapy did not demonstrate an effect of T_3 in augmenting the response of paroxetine therapy in patients with major depressive disorder.

6. It is recommended that thyroxine therapy be offered to any depressed patient with an elevated serum TSH, especially if accompanied by increased antithyroid antibody titers or low free T_4.

BIBLIOGRAPHY

1. Applehof BC, et al: Triiodothyronine addition to paroxetine in the treatment of major depressive disorder. J Clin Endocrinol Metab 89:6271–6276, 2004.

2. Asher R: Myxedematous madness. Br Med J 22:555–562, 1949.

3. Bauer M, et al: Effects of supraphysiological thyroxine administration in healthy controls and patients with depressive disorders. J Affective Disorders 68:285–294, 2002.

4. Bauer M, Whybrow PC: Thyroid hormones and the central nervous system in affective illness: interactions that may have clinical significance. Integr Psychiatry 6:75–100, 1988.

5. Bocchetta A, Loviselli A: Lithium treatment and thyroid abnormalities. Clin Pract Epidemiol Ment Health 2:23, 2006.

6. Bunevicius R, et al: Effects of thyroxine as compared with thyroxine plus triiodothyronine in patients with hypothyroidism. N Engl J Med 340:424–429, 1999.

7. Chopra IJ, Solomon DH, Huang TS: Serum thyrotropin in hospitalized psychiatric patients: evidence for hyperthyrotropinemia as measured by ultrasensative thyrotropin assay. Metabolism 93:538–543, 1990.

8. Cooper-Karaz R, et al: Combined treatment with sertraline and liothyronine in major depression. Arch Gen Psychiatry 64:679–688, 2007.

9. Fava M, et al: Hypothyroidism and hyperthyroidism in major depression revisited. J Clin Psychiatr 56:186–192, 1995.

10. Fliers E, et al: Efficacy of triiodothyronine (T_3) addition to Paroxetine in major depressive disorder: a randomized clinical trial. In Annual Meeting of the Endocrine Society, The Endocrine Society, 2003, Philadelphia, p. S19–22.

11. Gharib H, et al: Consensus statement: Subclinical thyroid dysfunction: a joint statement on management from the American Association of Clinical Endocrinologists, the American Thyroid Association, and the Endocrine Society. J Clin Endocrinol Metab 90:581–585, 2005.

12. Grozinsky-Glasberg S, et al: Thyroxine-triiodothyronine combination therapy versus thyroxine monotherapy for clinical hypothyroidism: meta-analysis of randomized controlled trials. J Clin Endocrinol Metab 91:2592–2599, 2006.

13. Gulseren S, et al: Depression, anxiety, health-related quality of life, and disability in patients with overt and subclinical thyroid dysfunction. Arch Med Res 37:133–139, 2006.

14. Hein MD, Jackson IMD: Thyroid function in psychiatric illness. Gen Hosp Psych 12:232–244, 1990.

15. Hennessey JV, Jackson IMD: The interface between thyroid hormones and psychiatry. Endocrinologist 6:214–223, 1996.

16. Jackson IMD: The thyroid axis and depression. Thyroid 8:951–956, 1998.

17. Jackson IMD, Whybrow PC: The relationship between psychiatric disorders and thyroid function. Thyroid Update 9:1–7, 1995.

18. Joffe RT: Is the thyroid still important in major depression? J Psychiatry Neurosci 31:367–368, 2006.

19. Monzani F, et al: Subclinical hypothyroidism: Neruo-behavioral features and beneficial effect of L-thyroxine treatment. Clin Invest 71:367–371, 1993.

20. Nelson JC: Augmentation strategies in depression 2000. J Clin Psychiatr 61(Suppl 1):13–19, 2000.

21. Pardridge WM: Carrier medicated transport of thyroid hormones through the rat blood-brain barrier: primary role of albumin bound hormone. Endocrinology 105:605–612, 1979.

22. Pollock MA, et al: Thyroxine treatment in patients with symptoms of hypothyroidism but thyroid function tests within the reference range: randomized double blind placebo controlled crossover trial. Br Med J 323:891–895, 2001.

23. Report on myxoedema. Transactions Clin Soc London, 1888.

24. Samuels MH, et al: Health status, mood, and cognition in experimentally induced subclinical hypothyroidism. J Clin Endocrinol Metab 92:2545–2551, 2007.

25. Saravanan P, et al: Psychological well-being in patients on "adequate" doses of L-thyroxine: results of a large, controlled community-based questionnaire study. Clin Endocrinol 57:577–585, 2002.

26. Sarne D, DeGroot LJ: Effects of the environment, chemicals and drugs on thyroid function. Endocrine Education, Inc., 2002. Available at: http://www.thyroidmanager.org.

27. Sawka AM, et al: Does a combination regimen of thyroxine (T_4) and 3,5,3′-triiodothyronine improve depressive symptoms better than T_4 alone in patients with hypothyroidism? Results of a double-blind, randomized, controlled trial. J Clin Endocrinol Metab 88:4551–4555, 2003.

28. Tremont G, Stern RA: Use of thyroid hormone to diminish the cognitive side effects of psychiatric treatment. Psychopharmacol Bull 33:273–280, 1997.

29. Walsh JP, et al: Combined thyroxine/liothyronine treatment does not improve well-being, quality of life, or cognitive function compared to thyroxine alone: a randomized controlled trial in patients with primary hypothyroidism. J Clin Endocrinol Metab 88:4543–4550, 2003.

30. Whybrow PC: The therapeutic use of triiodothyronine and high dose thyroxine in psychiatric disorders. Acta Med Aust 21:47–52, 1994.

DISORDERS OF SEXUAL DIFFERENTIATION

Craig E. Taplin and Robert H. Slover

CHAPTER 42

1. Describe the first level of sexual differentiation.

The first level of sexual differentiation is the establishment of chromosomal sex. The vast majority of infants are 46XX females or 46XY males. Genetic sex determines gonadal sex. Gonadal structures differentiate from the "bipotential," or primordial, gonadal ridge. The Y chromosome contains an area known as the sex-determining region, or SRY. The SRY gene initiates the differentiation of the bipotential gonad into a testis.

2. What is the next level of sex determination?

The next level of sex determination involves the genital duct structures. The genital duct structures are initially identical in the male and female. In the normal male, testicular Leydig cells produce testosterone, which is necessary to maintain ipsilateral Wolffian duct structures (e.g., vas deferens, epididymis, seminal vesicles). The Sertoli cells of the testis produce Müllerian-inhibiting factor (MIF), which acts ipsilaterally to cause regression of Müllerian duct structures (Fallopian tubes, uterus, upper third of the vagina). In the absence of testosterone and MIF, Müllerian duct structures are preserved and Wolffian duct structures regress.

3. Discuss the development of the external genitalia.

Male and female external genitalia arise from the same embryologic structures. In the absence of androgen stimulation, these structures remain in the female pattern, whereas the presence of androgens causes male differentiation (virilization). For complete virilization, testosterone must be converted to dihydrotestosterone (DHT) by the enzyme 5-alpha reductase, and androgen receptors must be functional. Excessive androgens virilize a female. Inadequate production of androgens, inability to convert testosterone to DHT, or inability to respond to androgens, as in androgen receptor defects, result in undervirilization of a male.

4. How is the decision about sex assignment made?

Exogenous and endogenous hormones are clearly important, as is the appearance of the genitalia. The decision about sex assignment must be carefully made, taking into consideration each "level" of sex determination. That decision requires a multidisciplinary approach including genetics, endocrinology, urology, neonatology, and psychology. It is vital that parents completely understand and support the decision, because ambivalence about sex of rearing may result in gender confusion and psychological trauma.

5. What is testis-determining factor?

The testis-determining factor (TDF) promotes differentiation of the gonad into a testis; SRY was eventually characterized as the TDF. SRY belongs to a family of DNA binding proteins. Specific manipulations have shown that the introduction of SRY results in sex reversal of XX mice, and site-directed mutagenesis of the SRY gene in XY mice yields an XY female. The activation of SRY is influenced by the Wilms tumor suppressor gene, WT1. Other genes that play a role downstream of SRY include SOX9 and GATA4.

6. **Describe the Lyon hypothesis. In which cells are two X chromosomes necessary for normal development?**
   Dr. Mary Lyon addressed the question of the extra X chromosomal material in females. Simply put, if two X chromosomes are necessary in each cell, how can males be developmentally normal? Lyon suggested that in each cell, one of the two X chromosomes is inactive and that in any given cell line, which X is active is randomly determined. In fact, the inactive X may be identified in many cells as a clump of chromatin at the nuclear membrane (Barr body). The important exception is in the ovary, where two functional X chromosomes are necessary for normal sustained ovarian development. Without two X chromosomes per cell (as in 45 XO Turner syndrome), the ovary involutes and leaves only fibrous tissue.

7. **Discuss normal male sexual differentiation.**
   The fetus is sexually bipotential. Figure 42-1 shows schematically how male development is accomplished. The undifferentiated gonad is derived from coelomic epithelium, mesenchyme, and germ cells, which, in the presence of SRY, give rise to Leydig cells, Sertoli cells, seminiferous tubules, and spermatogonia. Testes are formed at 7 weeks. Testicular production of testosterone (Leydig cells) leads to Wolffian duct development, whereas MIF (Sertoli cells) leads to Müllerian duct regression. Masculinization of the external genitalia is mediated by DHT, which is produced from testosterone by the action of the enzyme 5-alpha reductase.

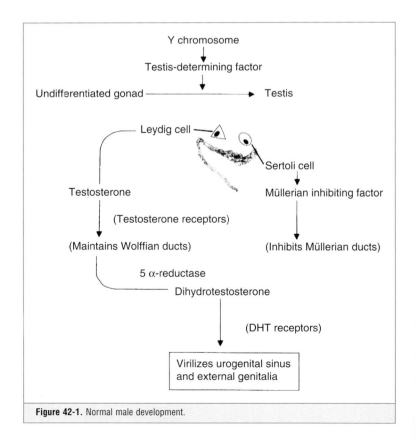

Figure 42-1. Normal male development.

8. Describe normal female sexual differentiation.
In the absence of SRY, the undifferentiated gonad gives rise to follicles, granulosa cells, theca cells, and ova. Ovarian development occurs in the 13th to 16th week of gestation. Lack of testosterone and MIF allows regression of the Wolffian ducts and maintenance of the Müllerian ducts, respectively. Lack of DHT results in the maintenance of female external genitalia.

9. How is external genital development determined?
The external genitalia arise from the urogenital tubercle, urogenital swelling, and urogenital folds. In females, these become the clitoris, labia majora, and labia minora, respectively. In males, under the influence of DHT, the genital tubercle becomes the glans of the penis, the urogenital folds elongate and fuse to form the shaft of the penis, and the genital swellings fuse to form the scrotum. Fusion is completed by 70 days of gestation and penile growth continues to term.

Female differentiation does not require ovaries or hormonal influence, whereas normal development of male genitalia requires normal testosterone synthesis, conversion to DHT by 5-alpha reductase, and normal androgen receptors. See Fig. 42-2.

KEY POINTS: DISORDERS OF SEXUAL DIFFERENTIATION

1. Sexual ambiguity in a newborn must be seen as a medical, social, and psychological emergency requiring a multidisciplinary team approach to assign a sex of rearing. Members of the team include the pediatric endocrinologist, urologist, geneticist, pediatrician, and appropriate counselors.

2. Evaluation of ambiguity must consider the four major categories of children presenting with this problem; namely, virilized 46XX females, undervirilized 46XY males, disorders of gonadal differentiation, and unclassified forms (cryptorchidism, hypospadias, developmental anomalies).

3. The most common cause of sexual ambiguity in newborns is congenital adrenal hyperplasia due to 21-hydroxylase deficiency.

4. As a general rule, gonadal tissue containing Y chromosomal material is at higher risk for development of malignancy. Consideration must be given to surgical removal of such gonads at some point.

10. The differential diagnosis of sexual differentiation disorders is complex but may be simplified by an approach based on an understanding of the process of sexual differentiation. Can you devise such a classification?
There are four large categories of ambiguity (Table 42-1):
1. Virilized 46 XX females
2. Undervirilized 46 XY males
3. Disorders of gonadal differentiation
4. Unclassified forms, including cryptorchidism, hypospadias, and developmental anomalies

11. What is a virilized female?
A virilized female (previously called female pseudohermaphroditism) is characterized by a 46 XX karyotype, ovaries, normal Müllerian duct structures, absent Wolffian duct structures, and virilized genitalia due to exposure to androgens during the first trimester.

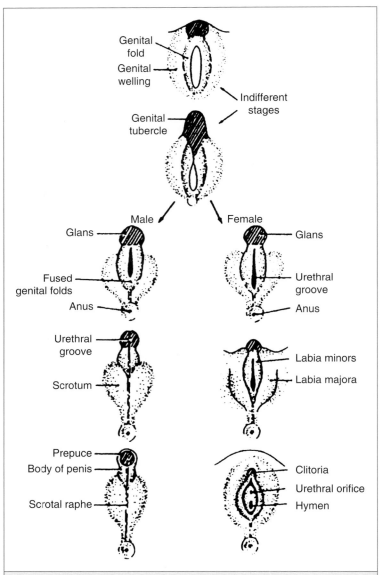

Figure 42-2. Differentiation of the external genitalia of male and female.

12. **What is the most common cause of a virilized female?**

The most common cause is congenital adrenal hyperplasia (CAH) due to 21-hydroxylase deficiency. In fact, this disorder is the single most common cause of sexual ambiguity. In this condition, the gene responsible for encoding the 21-hydroxylase enzyme is inactive. This enzyme blockage occurs along the pathway to cortisol and aldosterone. Because of low or absent levels of cortisol, the feedback mechanism produces increased adrenocorticotropic hormone (ACTH), which drives the pathway further and results in accumulation of precursor

TABLE 42-1. DIFFERENTIAL DIAGNOSIS OF SEXUAL AMBIGUITY

Virilized 46 XX females (female pseudohermaphroditism)
Congenital adrenal hyperplasia

21-hydroxylase deficiency

11-β-hydroxylase deficiency

3-β-hydroxysteroid dehydrogenase deficiency

Maternally derived androgens and synthetic progesterones

Undervirilized 46 XY males (male pseudohermaphroditism)

Testicular unresponsiveness to human chorionic gonadotropin (hCG) and luteinizinghormone (LH) (Leydig cell agenesis or hypoplasia)

Testosterone biosynthesis defects

Congenital lipoid adrenal hyperplasia (Steroidogenic acute regulatory protein/StAR deficiency)

3-β-hydroxysteroid dehydrogenase deficiency

17-α-hydroxylase deficiency

17,20-lyase (desmolase) deficiency

17-β-hydroxysteroid dehydrogenase deficiency

Peripheral unresponsiveness to androgen

Androgen insensitivity syndromes (receptor defects)

5-α-reductase deficiency

Defects in synthesis, secretion or response to Müllerian-inhibiting factor

Maternal estrogen or progesterone ingestion

Disorders of gonadal differentiation

46 XY partial gonadal dysgenesis

45 X/46 XY gonadal dysgenesis

"Vanishing testes" (embryonic testicular regression; 46 XY agonadism; anorchia)

True hermaphroditism

Unclassified

In males

Hypospadias

Cryptorchidism

Ambiguity secondary to congenital anomalies

In females

Absence or anomalous development of vagina, uterus and tubes (Rokitansky syndrome)

hormones, the measurement of which is useful for making a diagnosis. Increased ACTH also drives the production of excess adrenal androgens, which result in virilization. Virilization may also may be caused by maternal ingestion of androgens or synthetic progesterones during the first trimester of pregnancy.

13. **How do virilized female infants present?**

    Of importance, affected infants may present with a wide spectrum of ambiguity, ranging from clitoromegaly alone to complete fusion of the labial swellings to form a scrotum and large phallus. (Beware the infant with bilaterally undescended testes!) Even in the most virilized girls, a penile urethra is rare.

14. **What is an undervirilized male?**

    An undervirilized male (previously called male pseudohermaphroditism) refers to a 46 XY male who has ambiguous or female external genitalia. The abnormality may range from hypospadias to a completely female phenotype. Such disorders result from deficient androgen stimulation of genital development and most often are due to Leydig cell agenesis, testosterone biosynthetic defects, 5-alpha-reductase deficiency, and partial or total androgen resistance (androgen receptor defects).

15. **Which boys with hypospadias should be evaluated for sexual ambiguity?**

    First-degree (coronal or glandular) hypospadias as the sole presenting genital abnormality has no apparent endocrine basis and need not be evaluated. The incidence of this anomaly is between 1 and 8 in 1000 births. In contrast, perineoscrotal hypospadias is a feature of many etiologies of sexual ambiguity, and a child with this finding should be fully evaluated as ambiguous.

16. **What is gonadal dysgenesis?**

    Patients with Y-related chromosomal or genetic disorders that cause maldevelopment of one or both testes are said to have gonadal dysgenesis. They present with ambiguous genitalia and may have hypoplasia of Wolffian duct structures and inadequate virilization. MIF may be absent, allowing Müllerian duct structures to persist. Duct asymmetry is therefore common. The Y-containing dysgenetic testes are at risk for developing gonadoblastomas and must be removed.

17. **An infant is born with ambiguous genitalia, and the sex of the infant is uncertain. How do you approach the parents?**

    Honesty and diplomacy are essential. Explain that the genitalia are not yet fully developed and that further testing is necessary to determine the infant's sex. Reference to more commonly understood birth defects may be useful. Explain that several days may be necessary to complete the testing and that a team will participate to make an accurate diagnosis and a considered recommendation. Completion of the birth certificate should be postponed, and the infant should be admitted to the nursery without a sex assignment. You should encourage the family to delay naming the baby and not to give a name applicable to either sex.

18. **What history is necessary to evaluate the infant?**

    Maternal history is particularly important and should include illnesses, drug ingestion, alcohol intake, and ingestion of hormones during pregnancy. Was progestational therapy used for threatened abortion or androgens for endometriosis? Does the mother have signs of excessive androgen? Explore family history for occurrence of ambiguity, neonatal deaths, consanguinity, or infertility.

19. **How should you direct the physical examination?**

    The diagnosis of the etiology of sexual ambiguity can rarely be made by examination alone, but physical findings can help to direct further evaluation. Look for the following:
    1. Are gonads present? Are they normal in size, consistency, and position? Because gonadal descent is tied to Müllerian duct regression, a palpable gonad implies MIF action on that side.
    2. What is the phallic length? Measure along the dorsum of the phallus from the pubic ramus to the tip of the glans. At term, a stretched phallic length of 2.5 cm is 2.5 SD below the mean. Assess phallic width and development.

3. Note the position of the urethral meatus, and look for evidence of hypospadias and chordee (ventral curvature secondary to shortened urethra).
4. What is the degree of fusion of the labioscrotal folds? The folds may range from normal labia majora to a fully fused scrotum. In subtle cases, the ratio of the distance from the posterior fourchette to the anus is compared with the total distance from the urethral meatus.
5. Is there an apparent vaginal orifice?

20. What other areas should be evaluated?
Certain forms of congenital adrenal hyperplasia may cause areolar or genital hyperpigmentation, dehydration or hypertension. Turner's stigmata may be present, including webbed neck, low hairline, and edema of hands and feet. Other associated congenital anomalies may indicate a complex that includes ambiguity.

21. Explain which radiographic studies are necessary.
Structural studies are needed to address the presence of gonads and Müllerian structures. Pelvic ultrasound by qualified and experienced personnel should be performed as soon as possible to look for a uterus. The presence of gonads, Fallopian tubes, and a vaginal vault may also be determined. If necessary, a genitogram may be performed by inserting contrast material into the urogenital orifice (or vaginal orifice) to define vaginal size, presence of a cervix, and any fistulae.

22. Explain the role of karyotyping.
A karyotype is essential and must be obtained expeditiously. Buccal smears are absolutely contraindicated because they are inaccurate. In many laboratories, a karyotype can be completed within 48 to 72 hours. Some labs can also do rapid fluorescence in situ hybridization analysis for the presence of the SRY gene.

23. What laboratory test is very helpful?
Because 21-hydroxylase deficiency is a common cause of sexual ambiguity, we assess the level of 17-hydroxyprogesterone in all such infants who do not have palpable gonads.

24. How is further evaluation directed?
Further evaluation must be directed by information provided through the history, examination, and initial studies. Determining presence or absence of palpable gonads (presumably testes), presence or absence of a uterus, and karyotype allows classification of the infant as virilized female, undervirilized male, a disorder of gonadal differentiation, or one of the unclassified forms.

25. The infant has no palpable gonads and has fused labioscrotal folds and a prominent phallus. The ultrasound reveals a uterus and tubes with possible ovaries. The karyotype is 46 XX. How do you proceed now?
The infant is a virilized female. If there is no history of maternal androgen ingestion or virilization, the infant has one of three forms of CAH. Of these, 21-hydroxylase deficiency is most common and is confirmed by finding an elevated serum level of 17-hydroxyprogesterone. In 11-beta-hydroxylase deficiency, 11-deoxycortisol is elevated, whereas 17-hydroxypregnenolone and dehydroepiandrosterone (DHEA) are elevated in 3-beta-hydroxysteroid dehydrogenase deficiency. The baseline levels are usually diagnostic but can be confirmed by an ACTH stimulation test. The electrolyte disturbances seen with such disorders do not usually occur until 8 to 14 days of life; however, plasma renin activity will be elevated earlier and should be measured as a marker of salt wasting. Screening of newborns for CAH with measurement of a 17-OHP level is now mandated in all fifty of the United States and in many countries throughout the world.

26. **An undervirilized male represents a more complex diagnostic dilemma. In an infant with palpable gonads, no Müllerian structures and a 46 XY karyotype, how do you proceed?**

Defects in testosterone synthesis include three enzyme blocks common to the adrenal and testicular pathways (StAR defect, 3-beta-hydroxysteroid dehydrogenase deficiency, and 17-α-hydroxylase deficiency). Enzyme blocks are diagnosed with ACTH stimulation testing and measurement of steroid precursors. Those with StAR defects have no measurable precursors but show high levels of ACTH and a low cortisol response. Patients with 17-α-hydroxylase deficiency have elevated levels of progesterone, desoxycorticosterone and corticosterone, with associated hypertension. Infants with 3-beta hydroxysteroid dehydrogenase deficiency have elevated levels of 17-hydroxypregnenolone and DHEA. See Fig. 42-3.

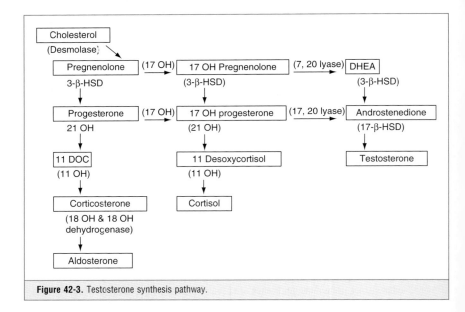

Figure 42-3. Testosterone synthesis pathway.

27. **Discuss the two remaining defects that involve deficiencies of testicular, rather than adrenal, enzymes.**

The two remaining defects in testosterone synthesis involve deficiencies of testicular rather than adrenal enzymes: 17,20-lyase and 17-beta-hydroxysteroid dehydrogenase. Thus they are not associated with elevations of ACTH or electrolyte disturbances. Both deficiencies are diagnosed by measuring the precursor response to administration of human chorionic gonadotropin (hCG). Infants with 17,20-lyase deficiency have elevated levels of 17-hydroxypregnenolone and 17-hydroxyprogesterone, whereas infants with 17-beta-hydroxysteroid dehydrogenase deficiency have elevated levels of DHEA and androstenedione.

28. **What other possibilities should be investigated?**

- Infants with Leydig cell hypoplasia have low levels of testosterone after hCG stimulation but normal adrenal function. Testicular biopsy reveals normal seminiferous tubules but absent or few Leydig cells.
- Stimulation with hCG also allows measurement of the testosterone-to-dihydrotestosterone ratio. If the ratio is elevated, 5-alpha-reductase deficiency should be suspected and may be confirmed by cultures of genital skin fibroblasts.

■ Finally, normal testosterone levels with no abnormalities in ACTH and hCG testing lead to the diagnosis of partial androgen insensitivity (androgen receptor defects). The diagnosis is made by demonstrating abnormal androgen binding in cultures of genital skin fibroblasts in a research laboratory, or molecular analysis.

29. What is complete androgen insensitivity?

The androgen receptor, encoded on the X chromosome, binds testosterone and, more avidly, dihydrotestosterone. Androgen insensitivity results from abnormalities of the androgen receptor. Complete androgen resistance occurs with a frequency of 1 in 20,000 to 1 in 64,000 XY individuals.

30. How do infants with complete androgen insensitivity present?

Complete androgen insensitivity (testicular feminization) rarely presents as ambiguity in the newborn period or early childhood. Unless the testes have descended and are palpable in the labia majora, affected infants appear as phenotypically normal females.

Affected children grow as normal females until puberty. They feminize with normal breast development at puberty because high levels of testosterone are aromatized to estrogen, but they have no pubic or axillary hair and no menses. Because they produce MIF, they lack Müllerian duct structures. Wolffian duct structures are also rudimentary or absent because they lack normal testosterone receptors. Gender identity is usually female. Patients come to medical attention because of primary amenorrhea. The diagnosis is therefore frequently made when patients are in their mid- to late teens.

31. When should intra-abdominal testicular tissue be removed?

The intra-abdominal testes of androgen insensitivity or XY gonadal dysgenesis are at risk for malignancy (up to 20% in some series), particularly after the onset of puberty. Timing of gonadectomy is debated. Because the risk of malignancy is low until puberty, some prefer to leave the gonads intact until spontaneous pubertal development; however, because carcinoma in situ has been found in prepubertal patients, others recommend early removal. If the testes are removed before puberty, estrogen therapy is necessary for normal pubertal progression. Because the upper section of the vagina is Müllerian in origin, affected individuals may have shortened vaginas and require plastic surgical repair.

32. Summarize the physiologic results of 5-alpha-reductase deficiency.

Deficiency of 5-alpha reductase impairs the conversion of testosterone to DHT, leading to incomplete virilization and differentiation of the external genitalia, which is dependent on the action of DHT. The disorder is particularly well documented in large kindreds in the Dominican Republic and Gaza, in whom it is inherited as an autosomal recessive condition.

33. Describe the clinical picture in children with 5-alpha-reductase deficiency.

Male infants with 5-alpha-reductase deficiency are born with sexual ambiguity. External genitalia range from a penis with simple hypospadias to a blind vaginal pouch and clitoris-like phallus. The most common presentation is a urogenital sinus with a blind vaginal pouch. During puberty, affected boys undergo virilization; affected females are normal.

Traditionally, infants with 5-alpha-reductase deficiency were raised as females until puberty, then continued life as males and, in some cases, achieved fertility. Recently, however, the condition has been recognized early in life, and affected males are now raised from infancy as boys.

34. What is a "true hermaphrodite"?

True hermaphroditism, a disorder of gonadal differentiation, refers to individuals with both ovarian and testicular elements. Affected children may have bilateral ovotestes, an ovary or testis on one side with an ovotestis on the other, or an ovary on one side and testis on the other.

Because the effects of MIF and testosterone on duct structures are ipsilateral and localized, internal duct development is often asymmetrical. Thus a Fallopian tube and unicornuate uterus, with absent or vestigial male duct structures, may develop on the side without testicular elements, whereas epididymis, vas deferens and seminal vesicles without Müllerian structures may develop on the side with testicular elements. The genitalia may be male, female, or ambiguous depending on the amount of functioning testicular tissue.

35. **Why is a multidisciplinary team necessary in approaching an infant with sexual ambiguity?**
Sexual ambiguity is a complex issue. Accurate diagnosis is essential and may take some time. Sex of assignment must be based not only on underlying diagnosis and karyotype but also on potential for adult sexual function, fertility, and psychological health. For these reasons, input from several specialties, including endocrinology, genetics, neonatology, psychology, and urology, is important. All members of the team must communicate adequately with each other. Parents must fully understand the medical recommendation for sex assignment and required therapy. They must whole-heartedly agree and support the assigned sex to avoid ambivalence, which can lead to gender confusion and psychological trauma for the child.

36. **After the etiology of sexual ambiguity has been determined in an infant, what factors should be considered in assigning a sex of rearing?**
Arriving at a precise diagnosis provides the treating team an understanding of potential risks and benefits of either sex assignment. For example, in a poorly virilized male, the difference in outcome among children with defects in testosterone synthesis, complete androgen insensitivity, and 5-alpha-reductase deficiency is enormous. A child with defective synthesis of testosterone may be raised male or female, depending on other factors; a child with complete androgen insensitivity should be raised female; and a boy with 5-alpha-reductase deficiency usually is raised male. Yet children affected by any of the three conditions have 46 XY karyotypes.

37. **What other factors must be considered?**
   - What is the potential for unambiguous genital appearance?
   - What is the potential for normal sexual function?
   - Is there a potential for fertility?
   - What was the in utero hormone exposure, with particular reference to exposure of the developing brain to excess androgen?
   - What are the factors likely to affect gender identity and psychological health?
   - Phallic size, urethral position, vaginal anatomy, and presence or absence of Müllerian or Wolffian duct structures, as well as gonadal characteristics and karyotype, must all be considered.

38. **To which gender are virilized females usually assigned?**
Virilized females are usually assigned a female sex. They have normal ovaries as well as Müllerian structures and, with surgical correction and steroid replacement, can have normal sexual function and achieve fertility.

39. **How is sex assignment determined in undervirilized males?**
Undervirilized males are often infertile, and sex assignment has usually been based on phallic size. Because a stretched penile length of 2.5 cm is 2.5 SD below the mean, an infant with a phallus smaller than 2.5 cm may be assigned a female sex of rearing. However, phallic size (penis or clitorus) has been challenged as a major factor in decisions of gender assignment. Adult social and fulfilling sexual function should be the primary goals of gender assignment. If male sex assignment is contemplated, a trial of depot testosterone (50 mg every 3–4 weeks) for 1 to 3 months indicates whether phallic growth is possible.

40. **Summarize the factors that determine sex assignment in patients with gonadal dysgenesis.**

In patients with gonadal dysgenesis and Y chromosomal material, gonadectomy is necessary and fertility is not possible. Internal duct structure is also frequently deranged. Small phallic size usually leads to a female sex assignment.

41. **How is sex assignment determined in true hermaphrodites?**

True hermaphrodites who have a unilateral ovary and Müllerian structures may have spontaneous puberty and normal fertility and may be raised as females. External genital size and structure may allow male assignment, but more commonly, external genitalia are poorly virilized and affected infants are assigned a female sex.

42. **What principles should be kept in mind when sex assignments are made?**

We have much to learn about gender identity and must consider which decisions might be made later than previously thought (such as surgery). Some surgical interventions are cosmetic, and some affected patients have expressed the wish that they should make the decisions in adolescence or adulthood. This field challenges many of our perceptions of sex and gender and our role as physicians. Although the infant with genital ambiguity presents a medical and social emergency, decisions should be made carefully, cautiously, and with all necessary biochemical and anatomical information available. Most important, the multidisciplinary team approach must involve the parents in an open and honest discussion of the options.

BIBLIOGRAPHY

1. Brown J, Warne G: Practical management of the intersex infant. J Pediatr Endocrinol Metab. 18:3–23, 2005.

2. Eugenides J: *Middlesex* [novel]. Picador, 2003, New York.

3. Goodall J: Helping a child to understand her own testicular feminization. Lancet 337:33–35, 1991.

4. Houk CP, Lee PA: Intersexed states: diagnosis and management. Endocr Metab Clin N Am 34:791–810

5. Jasso N, Boussin L, Knebelmann B, et al: Anti-müllerian hormone and intersex states. Trends Endocrinol Metab 2:227–233, 1991.

6. Kaplan S: *Clinical Pediatric Endocrinology.* Philadelphia, W.B. Saunders, 1990.

7. Low Y, Hutson JM: Murdoch Childrens Research Institute Sex Study Group: rules for clinical diagnosis in babies with ambiguous genitalia. J Paediatr Child Health 39:406–413, 2003.

8. McGillivray BC: The newborn with ambiguous genitalia. Semin Perinatol 16:365–368, 1992.

9. Meyers-Seifer CH, Charest NJ: Diagnosis and management of patients with ambiguous genitalia. Semin Perinatol 16:332–339, 1992.

10. Mulaikal RM, Migeon CJ, Rock JA, et al: Fertility rates in female patients with congenital adrenal hyperplasia due to 21-hydroxylase deficiency. N Engl J Med 316:178–182, 1987.

11. Pagona R: Diagnostic approach to the newborn with ambiguous genitalia. Pediatr Clin North Am 34:1019–1031, 1987.

12. Penny R: Ambiguous genitalia. Am J Dis Child 144:753, 1990.

13. Rangecroft L: British association of paediatric surgeons working party on the surgical management of children born with ambiguous genitalia: surgical management of ambiguous genitalia. Arch Dis Child 88:799–801, 2003.

14. Thigpen AE, Davis DL, Gautier T, et al: Brief report: the molecular basis of steroid 5 alpha-reductase deficiency in a large Dominican kindred. N Engl J Med 327:1216–1219, 1992.

15. Warne GL, Kanumakala S: Molecular endocrinology of sex differentiation. Semin Reprod Med 20:169–180, 2002.

16. Zucker KJ, et al: Psychosexual development of women with congenital adrenal hyperplasia. Hormone Behav 30:300–318, 1996.

CHAPTER 43

DISORDERS OF PUBERTY

Christina M. Gerhardt, Sharon H. Travers, and Robert H. Slover

1. **What physiologic events initiate puberty?**

   Maturation of the hypothalamic-pituitary axis initiates puberty. The hypothalamus begins to secrete gonadotropin-releasing hormone (GnRH) in pulses during sleep and eventually during waking hours as well. GnRH pulses stimulate the pituitary gland to secrete pulses of gonadotropins, of which there is a luteinizing hormone (LH) predominance. In response to the increased secretion of gonadotropins, there is increased secretion of gonadal hormones that lead to the progressive development of secondary sexual characteristics and gametogenesis.

2. **Define adrenarche.**

   Adrenarche refers to the time during puberty when the adrenal glands increase their production and secretion of adrenal androgens. Plasma concentrations of dehydroepiandrosterone (DHEA) and DHEA-sulfate(s), the most important adrenal androgens, begin to increase in children by approximately 6 to 8 years. However, the signs of adrenarche, such as pubic and axillary hair development, acne, and body odor, do not typically occur until early to midpuberty. The control of adrenal androgen secretion is not clearly understood, but it appears to be separate from GnRH and the gonadotropins.

3. **What is the normal pattern of puberty in males?**

   The mean age of onset of puberty in boys is 11.5 years with a range of 9 to 14 years. In both sexes, puberty requires maturation of gonadal function and increased secretion of adrenal androgens (adrenarche). The first evidence of puberty in the majority of boys is enlargement of the testes to greater than 4 mL in volume or greater than 2.5 cm in length. It is not until midpuberty, when testosterone levels are rapidly rising, that boys experience voice change, axillary and facial hair, and the peak growth spurt. Spermatogenesis is mature at a mean age of 13.3 years.

4. **Describe the normal pattern of female pubertal development.**

   Girls normally begin puberty between ages 8 and 13 years (mean age: 10.6 years for white girls, 9.8 years for hispanic girls, and 9.5 years for black girls). The initial pubertal event is typically the appearance of breast buds, although in a small percentage of girls, pubic hair development may appear first, and in an even smaller percentage of girls, menstrual cycling may appear first. Initial breast development often occurs asymmetrically and should not be of concern. Breast development is primarily under the control of estrogens secreted by the ovaries, whereas pubic and axillary hair growth result mainly from adrenal androgens. Unlike boys, the pubertal growth spurt in girls occurs at the onset of puberty. Menarche usually occurs 18 to 24 months after the onset of breast development (mean age: 12.8 years). Although most girls have reached about 97.5% of their maximum height potential at menarche, this can vary considerably. Consequently, age of menarche is not necessarily a good predictor of adult height.

5. **What controls the pubertal growth spurt?**

   In both boys and girls, the pubertal growth spurt is primarily controlled by the gonadal steroid, estrogen. In both sexes, gonadal (and adrenal) androgens are aromatized to estrogens. Estrogens augment growth hormone and insulin-like growth factor type 1 secretion. Estrogens also suppress osteoclastic activity and prolong the life span of osteoblasts and osteocytes. Androgens primarily contribute to the pubertal growth spurt by being aromatized to estrogens;

however, they have a small independent role in maintenance of adequate bone mineral density. At the end of puberty, linear growth is nearly complete as a result of the effects of gonadal steroids on skeletal maturation and epiphyseal fusion.

6. **How is pubertal development measured?**
   Sexual maturity is determined by examination and is described by a scale devised by John Tanner in 1969 (Table 43-1). Because of the distinct actions of adrenal androgens and gonadal steroids, it is important to distinguish between breast and pubic hair development in girls and between genital and pubic hair development in boys. In all cases, Tanner stage I is prepubertal and Tanner stage V is complete maturation. In addition to the physical examination, the tools to assess pubertal development may include determination of bone age, growth velocity and pattern, and specific endocrine studies.

TABLE 43-1. TANNER STAGES OF PUBERTAL DEVELOPMENT

Stage	Characteristics	Stage	Characteristics
Girls:	**Breast development**	**Girls:**	**Pubic hair development**
I	Prepubertal; elevation of papilla only	I	Prepubertal; no pubic hair
II	Breast buds are noted or palpable; enlargement of areola	II	Sparse growth of long, straight, or slightly curly, minimally pigmented hair, mainly of labia
III	Further enlargement of breast and areola, with no separation of their contours	III	Considerably darker and coarser hair spreading over mons pubis
IV	Projection of areola and papilla to form secondary mound above level of breast	IV	Thick, adult-type hair that does not yet spread to medial surface of thighs
V	Adult contour breast with projection of papilla only	V	Hair adult in type and distributed in classic inverse triangle
Boys:	**Genital development**	**Boys:**	**Pubic hair development**
I	Prepubertal; testicular length <2.5 cm	I	Prepubertal; no pubic hair
II	Testes >2.5 cm in longest diameter, scrotum thinning and reddening	II	Sparse growth of slightly pigmented, slightly curly pubic hair, mainly at base of penis
III	Growth of penis in width and length and further growth of testes	III	Thicker, curlier hair, spread to mons pubis
IV	Penis further larger, with enlarged; testes darker scrotal skin color	IV	Adult-type hair that does not yet spread to medial surface of thighs
V	Genitalia adult in size and shape	V	Adult-type hair spread to medial thighs

Data from Marshall WE, Tanner JM: Variations in the pattern of pubertal changes in girls. Arch Dis Child 44:291–303, 1969; Variations in the pattern of pubertal changes in boys. Arch Dis Child 45:13–23, 1970.

7. What constitutes sexual precocity in boys and girls?

Precocious puberty is defined as pubertal development occurring below the limits of age set for normal onset of puberty. In girls, this is puberty before 8 years and for boys, before 9 years. Breast development can occur normally as early as 7 years in white girls and 6 years in black girls. Consequently, evaluation and treatment of girls who start puberty between 6 and 8 years should depend on factors such as family history, rapidity of development, presence of central nervous system (CNS) symptoms, and family concern. Girls who are short and start puberty between 6 and 8 years may also benefit from evaluation. In children who present with early pubertal signs, precocious puberty must be distinguished from normal variants of puberty, such as benign premature thelarche and benign premature adrenarche.

8. What clinical findings are associated with precocious puberty?

Precocious puberty, regardless of the cause, is associated with increased linear growth and skeletal maturation secondary to elevated sex steroid levels. Children with precocious puberty are often tall for their age during childhood. However, skeletal maturation may become more advanced than stature, leading to premature fusion of the epiphyseal growth plates and a compromised adult height. In addition to the physical consequences of early puberty, there are social and psychological aspects that the practitioner should consider.

9. In which sex is precocity more prevalent?

Precocious puberty predominantly affects girls. The disparity in overall prevalence of precocity is explained by the large numbers of precocious girls with central idiopathic precocity, a condition that is unusual in boys. At least 80% of all precocious puberty in girls is central idiopathic in nature. The prevalence of organic etiologies of precocious puberty (CNS lesions, gonadal tumors, and specific underlying diseases) is similar in both sexes.

10. Which two common benign conditions in girls are often confused with precocious puberty?

- Premature thelarche is defined as isolated breast development in girls without accompanying signs of adrenarche, such as pubic/axillary hair, body odor, and acne.
- Premature adrenarche, which occurs in both sexes, is defined as the early development of pubic hair with or without axillary hair, body odor, and acne. There are no signs of gonadarche in this condition; thus girls have no breast development and boys show no testicular enlargement.

11. How is benign premature thelarche diagnosed?

Several characteristics of premature thelarche distinguish it from the breast development that occurs in precocious puberty. First of all, premature thelarche is most common in girls who are either under 2 years or between 6 and 8 years of age. Girls with premature thelarche may have a history of slowly progressing breast development or waxing and waning of breast size. Growth rate and bone age are not accelerated on physical examination, and the breast tissue rarely develops beyond Tanner stages II or III. GnRH stimulation may provoke a follicle-stimulating hormone (FSH)-predominant response as opposed to the typical LH-predominant response seen in true central precocity.

12. How is benign premature thelarche treated?

The natural course of benign thelarche is for the breast tissue to regress or fail to progress. Because of its benign nature, treatment is not necessary except for reassurance and follow-up. Follow-up is critical because premature thelarche occasionally is the first sign of what later becomes apparent as central precocious puberty. Measurement of breast tissue diameter during the clinic visit can be helpful for comparison at a later visit.

13. **How is benign premature adrenarche diagnosed?**

Premature adrenarche is caused by early secretion of the adrenal androgens, primarily DHEA and DHEA-S, and is suspected when clinical signs of androgen exposure are present including pubic or axillary hair growth and body odor. A child who has premature adrenarche and Tanner stage II pubic hair development will have adrenal androgen values similar to those normally found in a pubertal child at the same stage of development. As in premature thelarche, growth rate and bone age are not accelerated. If signs of puberty are rapidly progressing or if there is evidence of increased linear growth and advanced bone age, measurement of androgens (DHEA-S, androstenedione, and testosterone) is performed to evaluate for a serious virilizing disorder, such as congenital adrenal hyperplasia (CAH) or an adrenal tumor. A 17-hydroxyprogesterone (17-OHP) level may be drawn as the first screen for late onset or missed nonclassical 21-hydroxylase-deficient CAH.

14. **How is benign premature adrenarche treated?**

The natural course of premature adrenarche is for the signs to progress slowly without having an effect on the timing of true puberty. Because pubic hair development may be the first sign of puberty, especially in girls, follow-up is necessary to evaluate for evidence of gonadarche (i.e., breast development).

15. **How does GnRH-dependent (central) precocious puberty differ from GnRH-independent (peripheral) precocious puberty?**

Central precocious puberty involves activation of the GnRH pulse generator, an increase in gonadotropin secretion, and a resultant increase in the production of sex steroids. Consequently, the sequence of hormonal and physical events in central precocious puberty is identical to the progression of normal puberty. Peripheral precocious puberty occurs independent of gonadotropin secretion. The causes of precocious puberty are listed in Table 43-2.

16. **How is the diagnosis of precocious puberty made?**

The diagnosis of precocious puberty requires the appearance of the physical signs of puberty before the age of 8 years in girls or 9 years in boys. In both boys and girls, a complete history should be taken, with careful consideration of any exposure to exogenous steroids or estrogen receptor agonists (such as lavendar oil or tea tree oil), onset of pubertal signs and rate of progression, presence or history of CNS abnormalities, and pubertal history of other family members. Height measurements should be plotted on a growth chart to determine growth velocity. A physical examination is performed with focus on Tanner staging, presence of café-au-lait spots, and neurologic signs. One of the first steps in evaluating a child with early pubertal development is obtaining a radiograph of the left hand and wrist to determine skeletal maturity (bone age). If the bone age is advanced, further evaluation is typically warranted.

17. **After making the general diagnosis of precocity, how do I proceed to a specific diagnosis?**

It is usually difficult to distinguish GnRH-dependent (central) from GnRH-independent (peripheral) precocity on physical examination, although in boys a lack of testicular enlargement suggests peripheral precocity. Although the possible causes of peripheral precocious puberty are more numerous (see Table 43-2), central precocity accounts for the overwhelming majority of cases. Sex steroid levels, especially in boys, should be measured; testosterone levels above the prepubertal range (>10 ng/dL) confirm pubertal status but do not indicate the cause. Estrogen values in girls are not as helpful because slightly elevated levels may indicate either early puberty or benign thelarche.

18. **What is the single most important test in establishing a specific diagnosis?**

The single most important test is a GnRH stimulation test to determine whether gonadotropin responses are consistent with central or peripheral precocious puberty. The diagnosis of central precocious puberty is made by demonstrating an LH response to GnRH. Measurement of

TABLE 43-2. CAUSES OF PRECOCIOUS PUBERTY

Central (GnRH-Dependent)

Idiopathic true precocious puberty

CNS tumors (hamartomas, hypothalamic tumors)

CNS disorders (meningitis, encephalitis, hydrocephalus, trauma, abscesses, cysts, granulomas, radiation therapy)

Peripheral (GnRH-Independent)

Males

  Human chorionic gonadotropin (hCG)-secreting tumors (CNS, liver)

  CAH (21-hydroxylase, 3-beta-hydroxysteroid dehydrogenase, or 11-hydroxylase deficiency)

  Adrenal tumors

  Leydig cell testicular tumors

  Familial gonadotropin-independent Leydig cell maturation (testotoxicosis)

  McCune-Albright syndrome (polyostotic fibrous dysplasia)

Females

  Follicular cysts

  Ovarian tumors

  Adrenal tumors

  CAH (21-hydroxylase, 3-beta-hydroxysteroid dehydrogenase, or 11-hydroxylase deficiency)

  Exogenous estrogen

  McCune-Albright syndrome (polyostotic fibrous dysplasia)

CAH, congenital adrenal hyperplasia; CNS, central nervous system; GnRH, gonadotropin-releasing hormone; hCG, human chorionic gonadotropin.

random gonadotropins is typically not helpful because of overlap between prepubertal and early pubertal values until at least Tanner stage III. If random gonadotropins are measured, a third-generation assay is recommended because it has better discrimination between prepubertal and pubertal levels.

19. **When is a magnetic resonance imaging study of the brain indicated?**
   In girls younger than 6 years and boys of any age who are diagnosed with central precocious puberty, a magnetic resonance imaging (MRI) study of the brain should be done to evaluate for CNS lesions. It is unlikely that an abnormality will be found in girls between 6 and 8 years, so the need for an MRI in this age group should be individually assessed.

20. **What findings suggest peripheral precocious puberty?**
   A suppressed or prepubertal LH response to GnRH suggests that high sex steroid levels (causing negative feedback) are being produced independently of gonadotropin stimulation, a pattern consistent with peripheral precocious puberty. In girls, pelvic ultrasound and serum estradiol levels are obtained in this scenario to evaluate for an ovarian cyst, tumor, or McCune-Albright syndrome. In boys with suspected peripheral precocious puberty, additional laboratory

studies should include serum hCG, DHEA-S, and androstenedione levels. Elevated adrenal androgens could indicate an adrenal tumor or CAH. To evaluate further for CAH, measurement of baseline or adrenocorticotropic hormone (ACTH)-stimulated steroid intermediates (e.g., 17-OHP, 17-hydroxypregnenolone, 11-deoxycortisol) is recommended. Asymmetric or unilateral enlargement of the testes suggests a Leydig cell tumor.

21. **How is central idiopathic precocious puberty treated?**
Children with central precocious puberty can be treated with GnRH analogs, such as leuprolide. GnRH analogs downregulate pituitary GnRH receptors and thus decrease gonadotropin secretion. With treatment, physical changes of puberty regress or cease to progress, and linear growth slows to a prepubertal rate. Typically, pubic and axillary hair may persist. Projected final heights often increase as a result of slowing of skeletal maturation. Usually, GnRH analogs are given as a monthly depot intramuscular injection, and side effects are rare. After discontinuation of therapy, pubertal progression resumes, and in girls ovulation and pregnancy have been documented. Therapy is considered for both psychosocial and final height considerations. For example, in a girl who is near the normal age of puberty and who has slowly progressing development, treatment would not necessarily be indicated. However, the same aged girl who has already progressed to menarche may benefit psychosocially from treatment. Children on GnRH analogs should be monitored every 4 to 6 months.

22. **What is the association of hypothyroidism with precocity?**
Rare cases of primary hypothyroidism in children may cause breast development in girls and increased testicular size in boys. The mechanism is most likely related to excessive thyroid-stimulating hormone or alpha-subunit secretion, which can activate gonadotropin receptors. These children generally present with growth deceleration rather than acceleration as typically seen in precocious puberty. Bone ages are typically delayed. Thyroid hormone replacement results in regression of pubertal changes and no other therapy is necessary.

23. **What is McCune-Albright syndrome? How is it treated?**
McCune-Albright syndrome is a triad consisting of irregular (coast-of-Maine) café-au-lait lesions, polyostotic fibrous dysplasia, and GnRH-independent precocious puberty. It affects both sexes but is seen infrequently in boys. In girls, breast development and vaginal bleeding occur with sporadic increases in estradiol from autonomously functioning ovarian cysts. Serum gonadotropin levels are low, and GnRH testing elicits a prepubertal response. With time, however, increased estradiol may mature the hypothalamus, thus leading to true central GnRH-dependent precocity. The syndrome is often associated with other endocrine dysfunction, including hyperthyroidism, hyperparathyroidism, adrenal hyperplasia, Cushing's syndrome, and growth hormone excess. In affected tissues, there is an activating mutation in the gene that encodes the alpha-subunit of Gs, the G-protein that stimulates adenylate cylase. Endocrine cells with this mutation have autonomous hyperfunction and secrete excess amounts of their respective hormones.

24. **How is McCune-Albright treated?**
Girls with McCune-Albright syndrome are generally treated with a medication that inhibits the aromatization of testosterone to estrogen such as letrozole. Other trials have been performed using tamoxifen, an estrogen receptor antagonist. In boys, treatment consists of either inhibiting androgen production with ketoconazole or a combination of an aromatase inhibitor that blocks the conversion of androgen to estrogen and an antiandrogen that antagonizes androgen at the receptor.

25. **Describe testotoxicosis. How is it treated?**
Familial testotoxicosis is an autosomal dominant, gonadotropin-independent form of male precocity. Boys with this condition begin to develop true precocity with bilateral testicular and

phallic enlargement and growth acceleration by the age of 4 years. Serum testosterone levels are high, but serum gonadotropins are low and GnRH testing shows a prepubertal response. By midadolescence to adulthood, GnRH stimulation demonstrates a more typical LH-predominant pubertal response. The cause, in some families, has been found to be an activating mutation in the gene encoding the LH receptor. The mutant LH receptors in the testes are constitutively overactive and do not require LH binding for their activity but produce testosterone autonomously. Treatment options are the same as for boys with McCune-Albright syndrome. If central precocious puberty has been induced, GnRH agonists may also be part of the treatment plan.

26. How does 21-hydroxylase-deficient CAH present in boys?
The most common adrenogenital syndrome is 21-hydroxylase deficiency. Girls usually develop virilization in utero, resulting in a degree of sexual ambiguity. They are discovered at birth and should be diagnosed within the first few days of life by the finding of greatly elevated serum 17-OHP levels. Boys have normally formed genitalia and therefore are not picked up on physical examination at birth. In the more common salt-losing form of this disease, boys present with vomiting, shock, and electrolyte disturbances at 7 to 10 days. Fortunately, with neonatal screening for 21-hydroxylase deficiency, boys are being diagnosed before developing life-threatening electrolyte abnormalities. A small subset of affected boys and girls do not waste salt and may present in early or late childhood with signs of adrenarche, such as pubic hair, acne, body odor, acceleration of linear growth, and skeletal maturation.

27. Summarize the treatment of CAH.
Treatment for all forms of CAH is directed at reducing serum androgen levels by replacing glucocorticoids to reduce pituitary secretion of ACTH. Insufficient glucocorticoid replacement will lead to a compromise in final adult height because of advanced skeletal maturation, whereas excessive glucocorticoid replacement will lead to short stature because of direct effects of glucocorticoid on bone. Serum markers, growth curves, and bone age x-rays must be carefully monitored. In salt-wasting CAH, the mineralocorticoid florinef is also required. This is not necessary in the nonsalt-wasting forms.

28. What is adolescent gynecomastia? When and how should it be treated?
Normal boys often have either unilateral or bilateral breast enlargement during puberty. Breast development generally starts during early puberty and resolves within 2 years. The cause of gynecomastia is not clearly understood but may be related to an elevated ratio of estradiol to testosterone levels. Treatment consists primarily of reassurance and support; however, if resolution does not occur or if the breast enlargement is excessive, surgery may be warranted. Surgery should be avoided until puberty is complete to avoid reoccurence of gynecomastia. Pathologic conditions associated with gynecomastia include Klinefelter syndrome and various other testosterone-deficient states. Tea tree oils and lavendar oils have recently been associated with gynecomastia in boys. Some prescription medications cause gynecomastia and galactorrhea. Evidence is mixed regarding the connection of cannibus abuse and gynecomastia.

29. At what age does failure to enter puberty necessitate investigation?
Delayed puberty should be evaluated if there are no pubertal signs by 13 years in girls and by 14 years in boys. An abnormality in the pubertal axis may also present as lack of normal pubertal progression, which is defined as more than 4 years between the first signs of puberty and menarche in girls or more than 5 years for completion of genital growth in boys.

30. What is constitutional growth delay? How does it affect puberty?
Constitutional growth delay is the most common cause of delayed puberty. Children with this growth pattern have a fall-off in their linear growth within the first 2 years of life; after this, growth returns to normal, albeit at a lower growth channel than would be expected for parental heights. Skeletal maturation is also delayed, and the onset of puberty is commensurate with

bone age rather than chronologic age. For example, a 14-year-old boy with a bone age of 11 years will appropriately start puberty when his bone age is closer to 11.5 to 12 years. The delay in puberty postpones the pubertal growth spurt and closure of growth plates, so that the child continues to grow after his or her peers have reached their final height. A key feature of this growth pattern is normal linear growth after 2 years of age. There is often a family history of "late bloomers."

31. When is hypogonadism diagnosed?

Functional or permanent hypogonadism should be considered when there are no signs of puberty and bone age has advanced to beyond the normal ages for puberty to start. An eunuchoid body habitus is often evident in children with abnormally delayed puberty; a decreased upper to lower body ratio and long arm span characterize this habitus. As a rule, serum gonadotropin levels are measured first to determine whether there is hypogonadotropic hypogonadism (gonadotropin deficiency) or hypergonadotropic hypogonadism (primary gonadal failure). If a child's bone age is below the normal age for puberty to start, gonadotropin levels are not a reliable means of making an accurate diagnosis.

32. What causes hypogonadotropic hypogonadism?

Normal or suppressed gonadotropins indicate that there is a failure of the pituitary to stimulate gonadal steroid production. Chronic illnesses, malnutrition, exercise, and anorexia can cause a functional deficiency of gonadotropins that reverses when the underlying condition improves. Hyperprolactinemia can also present as delayed puberty, and only 50% of the time will there be a history of galactorrhea. Other endocrinopathies such as diabetes mellitus, glucocorticoid excess, and hypothyroidism can cause hypogonadotripic hypogonadism when untreated. Permanent gonadotropin deficiency is suspected if these conditions are ruled out and gonadotropin levels are low. Gonadotropin deficiency may be associated with other pituitary deficiencies from conditions such as septo-optic dysplasia, tumors such as craniopharyngioma, trauma, empty sella syndrome, pituitary dysgenesis, Rathke's pouch cysts, or cranial irradiation. Various syndromes, such as Kallmann Syndrome, Laurence-Moon-Bardet-Biedl Syndrome, and Prader-Willi syndrome, are also associated with gonadotropin deficiency. Drug abuse, particularly with heroin or methadone, has been associated with hypogonadotropic hypogonadism. Isolated gonadotropin deficiency (i.e., occurring without another pituitary deficiency) is often difficult to diagnose because hormonal tests do not absolutely distinguish whether a child can produce enough gonadotropins or whether he or she simply has very delayed puberty. If gonadotropin deficiency cannot be clearly distinguished from delayed puberty, a short course of sex steroids can be given. Patients with constitutional delay often enter puberty after such an intervention. If spontaneous puberty does not occur after this treatment or after a second course, the diagnosis of gonadotropin deficiency may be made.

33. What is Kallmann syndrome?

Kallmann syndrome is one of a class of disorders referred to as idiopathic hypogonadotropic hypogonadism or idiopathic hypothalamic hypogonadism. It occurs as frequently as 1:10,000 boys and 1:50,000 girls. The classic form is characterized by hypogonadotropic hypogonadism with hyposmia or anosmia. It is caused by aplasia or hypoplasia of the olfactory bulbs and is associated with hypoplasia or aplasia of other structures of the rhinencephalon (e.g., cleft lip/cleft palate, congenital deafness, and color blindness). Undescended testes and gynecomastia are common.

34. What causes hypergonadotropic hypogonadism?

Elevated gonadotropin levels indicate that there is a failure of the gonads to produce enough sex steroids to suppress the hypothalamic-pituitary axis. These levels are diagnostic for gonadal failure at two periods of time: before 3 years of age, and after the bone age is at or beyond the normal age for puberty to start. Potential etiologies are as follows:

- Variants of ovarian and testicular dysgenesis (Turner syndrome, Klinefelter syndrome, pure XX or XY gonadal dysgenesis)
- Gonadal toxins (chemotherapy, particularly alkylating agents, radiation treatment)
- Androgen enzymatic defects (17-a-hydroxylase deficiency in the genetic male or female; 17-ketosteroid reductase deficiency in the genetic male)
- Complete and partial androgen insensitivity syndrome
- Other miscellaneous disorders (infections, gonadal autoimmunity, vanishing testes, trauma, surgical, torsion)
- Galactosemia (in girls only)

35. **How is gonadal failure with no apparent cause evaluated in boys?**
Boys may have gonadal failure secondary to testicular torsion, radiation, chemotherapy, or the vanishing testis syndrome. Noonan and Klinefelter syndromes (47XXY) are other potential causes of primary testicular insufficiency. Consequently, in a boy with unexplained gonadotropin elevations, a karyotype should be performed.

36. **Describe the evaluation of gonadal failure in girls.**
In girls with gonadal failure (indicated by elevated gonadotropin levels) and no apparent cause, a karyotype evaluation should be performed; Turner syndrome will be the most likely explanation. 46XX gonadal dysgenesis can also occur and may be inherited as an autosomal recessive trait. A karyotype also identifies 46XY gonadal dysgenesis in a phenotypic female who is actually a genetic male. In this condition, there is complete lack of testicular development and consequently, except for the absence of gonads, normal female genital differentiation occurs. If the karyotype is normal, then the evaluation should look for causes of premature ovarian failure as discussed in question 34.

37. **What is Turner syndrome?**
Any consideration of pubertal delay in girls must include the possibility of Turner syndrome. An absent or structurally abnormal second X chromosome characterizes Turner syndrome. The incidence of Turner syndrome is approximately 1:2000 live female births. However, the chromosomal abnormality is actually more common than this; 90% or more of Turner conceptuses do not survive beyond 28 weeks gestation, and the XO karyotype occurs in 1 out of 15 miscarriages. In the absence of a second functional X chromosome, oocyte degeneration is accelerated, leaving fibrotic streaks in place of normal ovaries. Because of primary gonadal failure, serum gonadotropin levels rise and are elevated at birth and again at the normal time of puberty.

38. **What are the clinical findings in patients with Turner syndrome?**
See Table 43-3.

TABLE 43-3. CLINICAL FINDINGS IN PATIENTS WITH TURNER SYNDROME		
Primary Defects	**Secondary Features**	**Incidence (%)**
Physical Features		
Skeletal growth disturbances	Short stature	100
	Short neck	40
	Abnormal upper to lower segment ratio	97
	Cubitus valgus	47

(Continued)

TABLE 43-3. CLINICAL FINDINGS IN PATIENTS WITH TURNER SYNDROME (CONTINUED)

Primary Defects	Secondary Features	Incidence (%)
	Short metacarpals	37
	Madelung deformity	7.5
	Scoliosis	12.5
	Genu valgum	35
	Characteristic facies with micrognathia	60
	High arched palate	36
Lymphatic obstruction	Webbed neck	25
	Low posterior hairline	42
	Rotated ears	Common
	Edema of hands/feet	22
	Severe nail dysplasia	13
	Characteristic dermatoglyphics	35
Unknown factors	Strabismus	17.5
	Ptosis	11
	Multiple pigmented nevi	26
Physiologic Features		
Skeletal growth disturbances	Growth failure	100
	Otitis media	73
Germ cell chromosomal defects	Gonadal failure	96
Infertility		99.9
	Gonadoblastoma	4
Unknown factors—embryogenic	Cardiovascular anomalies	55
	Hypertension	7
	Renal and renovascular anomalies	39
Unknown factors—metabolic	Hashimoto's thyroiditis	34
	Hypothyroidism	10
	Alopecia	2
	Vitiligo	2
	Gastrointestinal disorders	2.5
	Carbohydrate intolerance	40

Data from Hall J, Gilchrist D: Turner syndrome and its variants. Pediatr Clin North Am 37:1421, 1990.

39. **How is Turner syndrome treated?**
    Approximately 10% to 20% of girls with Turner syndrome have some ovarian function at puberty that allows for early breast development. A small percentage of this group also have normal

periods, and an even smaller percentage ($<$1% of all girls with Turner syndrome) are actually fertile. Most girls with Turner syndrome require exogenous gonadal steroid replacement. Low-dose unopposed estradiol, followed by cycling with estrogen and progestin, allows development of secondary sexual characteristics. The timing for initiation of estrogen is critical and should be decided by an endocrinologist through discussions with each patient and her family. The decision includes several factors including final height and psychosocial factors. The short stature of girls with Turner syndrome is treated with growth hormone. Final height in girls with Turner syndrome is related to when growth hormone is initiated, with better outcomes in girls who are started at a young age. Consequently, early diagnosis of Turner syndrome is essential.

40. **Why do boys with Klinefelter syndrome have pubertal delay?**
    Klinefelter Syndrome is the most common cause of testicular failure. Leydig cell function (testosterone production) is variable however seminiferous tubular function is almost always abnormal. Although some boys with Klinefelter Syndrome do have reproductive ability this is very rare. Many boys have spontaneous onset of pubic hair growth however with inappropriately small testes. Even these boys may fail to continue to progress through appropriate patterns of pubic hair growth. Testosterone supplementation is indicated in many boys over time and in some it is required to initiate puberty.

41. **What features help to diagnose Klinefelter syndrome?**
    Klinefelter syndrome results from at least one extra X chromosome; thus the most common karyotype is 47XXY. The incidence is 1:1000 male births. Eunuchoid proportions are present from early childhood. Associated features include gynecomastia, tall stature, small testes, and elevated serum gonadotropins. Learning disabilities and behavioral problems may also be present.

42. **Describe the appropriate history for an adolescent with pubertal delay.**
    The history should include questions regarding the presence of chronic illnesses, autoimmune disorders, nutritional disorders, exercise history, galactorrhea, family history of infertility, and timing of puberty in parents and siblings. Weight gain or loss should also be noted.

43. **Describe the physical examination of an adolescent with pubertal delay.**
    Physical examination should include measurement of arm span and upper-to-lower segment ratio. Eunuchoid proportions occur early in patients with Klinefelter syndrome and late in those with other forms of hypogonadism. Signs of any chronic illness, malnutrition, anorexia, hypothyroidism, glucocorticoid excess, and features of Turner syndrome (girls) and Klinefelter syndrome (boys) should be noted. A careful search should be made for any signs of puberty, such as pubic hair and axillary hair, acne, testicular size and penile length (boys), and breast development (girls). Pubic hair may represent only adrenal androgen production. Testicular volume of greater than 4 mL (length of greater than 2.5 cm) indicates gonadotropin stimulation. Estrogen effect is evaluated by breast development and vaginal maturity. In addition, visual field and olfaction should be evaluated (80% of boys with Kallmann syndrome have reduced, or absent, sense of smell). The growth chart should be analyzed to determine if there is short stature and if linear growth has been normal.

44. **How are radiographic studies and gonadotropin levels helpful in the diagnosis of pubertal delay?**
    Assessment of bone age is critical in determining biological age and the time of expected pubertal development. If linear growth is normal and the bone age is less than the normal age for pubertal onset, the diagnosis is likely to be constitutional growth delay. If linear growth is subnormal with bone age delay, it may be necessary to investigate the poor growth with evaluation of growth hormone or thyroid status. If bone age has advanced to beyond the age for normal puberty, gonadotropin levels are helpful to distinguish between gonadotropin deficiency and primary gonadal failure.

45. What other lab tests may be needed?

Additional laboratory studies may include chemistry panels including electrolytes, thyroid function tests, estradiol (girls), testosterone (boys), and prolactin levels. If gonadotropins are elevated, chromosome analysis is indicated for both genders to evaluate for Turner syndrome in girls and Klinefelter syndrome in boys. In the case of low serum gonadotropins, olfactory testing and cranial MRI are recommended.

46. How is delayed puberty managed?

The treatment of delayed puberty depends on the underlying cause. If the delayed pubertal development is secondary to anorexia, hypothyroidism, or illness, treatment of these underlying conditions results in spontaneous onset of puberty. Puberty also begins spontaneously, albeit late, in constitutional growth delay so that reassurance alone to the patient and family may be sufficient. In some patients with constitutional delay, initiation of puberty may be appropriate. For boys, a 4- to 6-month course of low-dose depot testosterone (50–100 mg intramuscularly every 4 weeks) can be offered if the bone age is at least 11 to 12 years. This treatment results in some early virilization without adversely affecting final height. Spontaneous puberty usually begins, as evident by testicular enlargement, 3 to 6 months after the end of the testosterone course. For girls, a 3-month course of low-dose estradiol (0.25–0.5 mg orally every day) can be offered if the bone age is at least 10 to 11 years. Therapy is then stopped, and physical changes are evaluated. Withdrawal bleeding is unusual after one course of estrogen therapy but may occur with subsequent courses.

47. Describe the treatment of boys with hypogonadism.

In boys with hypogonadotropic hypogonadism for whom fertility is not an immediate issue and in all boys with primary hypogonadism, long-term testosterone therapy is required. While the patient is growing, careful attention must be paid to growth velocity and bone age. Most commonly, depot testosterone esters (enanthate or cypionate) are used in 25- to 50-mg doses every 3 to 4 weeks for the first 1 to 2 years of therapy. By the second or third year, the dosage is raised to 50 to 100 mg intramuscularly every 3 to 4 weeks. The adult maintenance level is 200 to 300 mg intramuscularly every 3 to 4 weeks. Alternatively, the cutaneous testosterone patch or gel may be used.

48. How is estrogen treatment given for girls with hypogonadism?

Replacement therapy in hypogonadal girls is begun with very low-dose unopposed estrogen treatment for 12 to 18 months. The dosages used vary on the basis of height projections and individual response. Following this period of unopposed estrogen, progesterone is added for 10 to 12 days of each month, or a birth control pill may be prescribed. Progesterone therapy is necessary to counteract the effects of estrogen on the uterus; unopposed estrogen can cause endometrial hyperplasia and carcinoma. Replacement of gonadal steroids in both sexes is also necessary for normal bone mineralization and to prevent osteoporosis.

49. How do body habitus and lifestyle influence the timing of puberty?

There is a high incidence of primary amenorrhea and delay of puberty in girls with anorexia nervosa and in girls who are highly competitive athletes. These girls have hypogonadotropic hypogonadism which appears to be directly related to their low fat-lean ratios. The girls with the lowest body mass index (BMI) also have the lowest circulating leptin and estrogen levels and are the most affected by pubertal delay or menstrual dysfunction. Leptin is a hormone produced by adipocytes and is important in hypothalamic-pituitary-gonadal feedback signaling. Deficiency has been associated with both anorexia and obesity with hypogonadotropic hypogonadism present in both phenotypes. There appears to be a minimum leptin level that is permissive for pubertal development. When severely underweight girls improve their BMI, puberty quickly ensues and progresses to menarche.

50. Define amenorrhea.

A girl who has not had menarche by 16 years of age or within 4 years after the onset of puberty is considered to have primary amenorrhea. Secondary amenorrhea is diagnosed if more than 6 months has elapsed since the last menstrual period or if more than the length of three previous cycles has elapsed with no menstrual bleeding.

51. How do you begin to evaluate a girl with amenorrhea?

To sort out the many causes of amenorrhea, it is helpful to distinguish girls who produce sufficient estrogen from those who do not by performing a progesterone challenge. Girls who are producing estrogen have a withdrawal bleed after 5 to 10 days of oral progesterone, whereas those who are estrogen-deficient have no or very little bleeding. There are two situations in which girls have sufficient estrogen but do not have a withdrawal bleed: obstruction of the cervix or absence of the cervix or uterus. In Rokitansky's syndrome, maldevelopment of the Müllerian structures leads to an absent or hypoplastic uterus or cervix (or both). Complete androgen insensitivity syndrome (testicular feminization) in a genetic male results in a phenotypic female who has normal breast development secondary to the aromatization of testosterone to estrogen The production of Müllerian-inhibiting factor in patients with androgen insensitivity syndrome leads to regression of the Müllerian structures and thus the absence of a uterus. The absence of a cervix is a diagnostic finding in both Rokitansky's syndrome and complete androgen insensitivity syndrome; consequently, a pelvic examination should be considered in all girls who present with amenorrhea, especially primary amenorrhea. The causes of amenorrhea associated with estrogen insufficiency include hypogonadism, which is described in the previous section about delayed puberty.

52. What causes amenorrhea in girls who are producing estrogen and do not have an outflow tract obstruction?

Amenorrhea in girls who are producing normal or even elevated amounts of estrogen is a manifestation of anovulatory cycles. Irregular menses may also be a sign of chronic anovulation; estrogen production, unopposed by progesterone, leads to endometrial hyperplasia and intermittent shedding. Because menarche is normally followed be a period of anovulatory cycles and irregular menses, many adolescents with a pathologic etiology may be missed. Consequently, it is important to evaluate all girls who do not have regular menses by 3 years after menarche. The most common cause of chronic anovulation is polycystic ovarian syndrome (PCOS), a disorder characterized by increased ovarian androgen production. The clinical presentation varies and may include amenorrhea, oligomenorrhea, dysfunctional uterine bleeding, hirsutism, acne, and obesity. PCOS is further discussed in a separate chapter.

KEY POINTS: DISORDERS OF PUBERTY

1. Central precocious puberty occurs more frequently in girls than boys. Boys with central precocity, however, have a much higher incidence of underlying central nervous system pathology.

2. Precocious puberty must be distinguished from normal variants of early development, that is, benign premature thelarche and adrenarche.

3. The most useful diagnostic test to evaluate precocious puberty is a gonadotropin-releasing hormone stimulation test.

4. Children with delayed puberty and normal linear growth will most likely have constitutional growth delay.

5. Bone age assessment is the first step in evaluating a child with delayed puberty.

6. After it has been determined that a child has abnormally delayed puberty, gonadotropins should be obtained. If gonadotropins are elevated, obtaining chromosomes is generally the next step.

BIBLIOGRAPHY

1. Comite F, Shawker TH, Pescovitz OH, et al: Cyclical ovarian function resistant to treatment with an analogue of luteinizing hormone-releasing hormone in McCune-Albright syndrome. N Engl J Med 311:1032, 1984.

2. Evans SJ: The athletic adolescent with amenorrhea. Pediatr Ann 13:605, 1984.

3. Frisch R, Wyshak G, Vincent L: Delayed menarche and amenorrhea in ballet dancers. N Engl J Med 303:17, 1980.

4. Ghai K, Cara JF, Rosenfeld RL: Gonadotropin releasing hormone agonist (Nafarelin) test to differentiate gonadotropin deficiency from constitutionally delayed puberty in teen-age boys—a clinical research center study. J Clin Endocrinol Metab 80:2980, 1995.

5. Grumbach MM, Styne DM: Puberty: ontogeny, neuroendocrinology, physiology, and disorders. In Wilson JD, Foster DW, Kronenberg HM, Larsen PR, editors, Williams textbook of endocrinology, ed 9, Philadelphia, 1998, W.B. Saunders, pp. 1509–1625.

6. Grumbach MM: The neuroendocrinology of human puberty revisited. Horm Res 57(suppl 2):2–14, 2002.

7. Hall J, Gilchrist D: Turner syndrome and its variants. Pediatr Clin North Am 37:1421, 1990.

8. Herman-Giddens ME, Slora EJ, Wasserman RC, et al: Secondary sexual characteristics and menses in young girls seen in office practice: a study from the Pediatric Research in Office Setting network. Pediatrics 99:505–512, 1997.

9. Ibanez L, Virdis R, Potau N, et al: Natural history of premature pubarche and auxological study. J Clin Endocrinol Metab 74:254, 1992.

10. Kaplan S, editor: Clinical pediatric endocrinology. Philadelphia, 1990, W.B. Saunders.

11. Kaplan S, Grumbach M: Pathophysiology and treatment of sexual precocity. J Clin Endocrinol Metab 71:785, 1990.

12. Kappy MS, Ganong CS: Advances in the treatment of precocious puberty. Adv Pediatr 41:223, 1994.

13. Kulin H, Rester E: Managing the patient with a delay in pubertal development. Endocrinologist 2:231, 1992.

14. Levine M: The McCune-Albright syndrome: the whys and wherefores of abnormal signal transduction. N Engl J Med 325:1738, 1991.

15. Matejek N, Weimann E, Witzel C, et al: Hypoleptinaemia in patients with anorexia nervosa and in elite gymnasts with anorexia athletica. Int J Sports Med 20:451–456, 1999.

16. Pescovitz O: Precocious puberty. Pediatr Res 11:229, 1990.

17. Root AW: Precocious puberty. Pediatr Rev 21:10–19, 2000.

18. Root AW, Diamond FB Jr: Calcium metabolism, normal homeostasis. In Sperling MA, editor, Pediatric endocrinology, Philadelphia, 2002, W.B. Saunders, pp. 88–89.

19. Rosenfeld R: Diagnosis and management of delayed puberty. J Clin Endocrinol Metab 70:559, 1990.

20. Rosenfield RL: The ovary and female sexual maturation. In Sperling MA, editor, Pediatric endocrinology Philadelphia, 1996, W.B. Saunders, pp. 75–86.

21. Styne DM: The testes: disorders of sexual differentiation and puberty. In Sperling MA, editor, Pediatric endocrinology, Philadelphia, 1996, W.B. Saunders, pp. 423–476.

22. Theinz G, Howald H, Weiss U, Sizonenko PC: Evidence for a reduction of growth potential in adolescent female gymnasts. J Pediatr 122:306, 1993.

23. Wheeler M, Styne DM: Diagnosis and management of precocious puberty. Pediatr Clin North Am 37:1255, 1990.

24. Wu T, Mendola P, Buck GM: Ethnic differences in the presence of secondary sex characteristics and menarche among US girls: the Third National Health and Nutrition Examination Survey, 1988–1994. Pediatrics 110:752–757, 2002.

25. Zachman M: Therapeutic indications for delayed puberty and hypogonadism in adolescent boys. Horm Res 35:141, 1991.

CHAPTER 44

MALE HYPOGONADISM

Derek J. Stocker and Robert A. Vigersky

1. **Define male hypogonadism.**
   Male hypogonadism refers to the clinical or laboratory syndrome that results from a failure of the testis to work properly. The normal testis has two functions: synthesis and secretion of testosterone (from the Leydig cells) and production of sperm (from the seminiferous tubules). Deficiency of one or both functions is termed male hypogonadism. This can be due to a disruption at one or more levels of the hypothalamic-pituitary-gonadal axis. Depending on the stage of development, hypogonadism may have varied manifestations.

2. **What are the manifestations of in utero hypogonadism?**
   In utero androgen deficiency leads to a female phenotype or ambiguous genitalia (male pseudohermaphroditism), most commonly caused by a block in the production of testosterone due to congenital testosterone biosynthetic enzyme defects. Rarely, peripheral tissues cannot respond normally to testosterone, resulting in the androgen-insensitivity syndromes of testicular feminization (complete) and Reifenstein's syndrome (incomplete). Other manifestations include micropenis, hypospadias, and cryptorchidism.

3. **Describe the manifestations of peripubertal hypogonadism.**
   Childhood androgen deficiency results in delayed, incomplete, or absent pubertal development. Common manifestations include:
   - Eunuchoid proportions (ratio of pubis-to-vertex/pubis-to-floor is less than 0.9; arm span is greater than 5 cm more than height (due to the delayed closure of the epiphyses)
   - Small testes ($<$20 mL or $< 4.5 \times 3.0$ cm)
   - Decreased body hair
   - Gynecomastia
   - Reduced peak bone mass
   - Reduced male musculature
   - Persistently higher-pitched voice

4. **Summarize the manifestations of hypogonadism in early adulthood.**
   In early adulthood, a decrease in sperm output (azoospermia/oligospermia) without deficient production of testosterone is common and results in male infertility; thus infertility is a form of male hypogonadism. A decrease in production of testosterone in adulthood is usually accompanied by a decline in production of sperm. When it is not, the term "fertile eunuch" (eunuchoid proportions, low levels of luteinizing hormone [LH], low levels of testosterone, normal levels of follicle-stimulating hormone [FSH], and spermatogenesis) is appropriately applied. Libido and potency may be diminished.

5. **What are the manifestations of hypogonadism in mid-to-late adulthood?**
   The most frequent circumstance in which adult hypogonadism occurs is in the middle-aged or senescent man complaining of decreased libido or potency. Semen analysis is rarely performed in these men because they are usually not concerned with fertility. Other findings may include osteoporosis, diminished androgen production, and small prostate. If the onset of hypogonadism is acute, the patient may experience hot flashes and sweats.

6. **How is production of testosterone normally regulated?**

LH is episodically secreted from the anterior pituitary in response to pulses of gonadotropin-releasing hormone (GnRH), thus stimulating production of testosterone by Leydig cells. After testosterone is secreted into the bloodstream, it is bound by sex hormone–binding globulin (SHBG). The non-SHBG-bound (or "free") testosterone provides negative feedback to the hypothalamic-pituitary unit and thus inhibits output of LH. This classic endocrine feedback loop serves to maintain serum testosterone at a predetermined level; if serum testosterone falls below the set point, the pituitary is stimulated to secrete LH, which in turn stimulates testicular output of testosterone until serum levels return to the set point. Conversely, if serum testosterone rises above the set point, decreased output of LH results in decreased testicular output of testosterone until serum levels have declined to the set point. Although most automated total testosterone assays are reliable and generally able to distinguish hypogonadal from eugonadal men, abnormalities in the SHBG level may give falsely low or high total testosterone levels. Equilibrium dialysis is the gold standard for measuring the free testosterone but is not commonly available and should only be performed in a reliable reference laboratory. Analog methods for determining free testosterone are more widely available but are not accurate in the low ranges.

7. **What are some conditions associated with decreased or increased serum SHBG levels?**

Moderate obesity, nephrotic syndrome, hypothyroidism, and the use of certain medications (notably glucocorticoids and androgenic steroids) will decrease SHBG levels, giving a low total serum testosterone level, whereas anticonvulsant use, estrogen use, hepatic cirrhosis, HIV infection, and hyperthyroidism may all increase SHBG, causing a high level of total testosterone.

8. **Describe how production of sperm is normally regulated.**

The regulation of sperm production is complex and less clearly understood than regulation of testosterone production. Both hormonal and nonhormonal factors are important. The Sertoli cells within the seminiferous tubules seem to play an important coordinating role. Sertoli cells respond to FSH by producing inhibin (secreted into the blood) and androgen-binding protein, transferrin, and other proteins (secreted into the seminiferous tubular lumen). Inhibin appears to inhibit the output of FSH from the pituitary gland, thus completing a feedback loop. In theory, if spermatogenesis declines, production of inhibin also should decline; thus the negative feedback effect on the pituitary would be reduced, leading to an increased output of FSH, which then presumably stimulates spermatogenesis. However, not all aspects of this feedback loop (FSH-inhibin-spermatogenesis) have been verified experimentally. Moreover, spermatogenesis depends on intratesticular production of testosterone mediated by androgen receptors within Sertoli cells. Initiation of spermatogenesis during puberty requires both LH and FSH. However, reinitiation of the process if it is disrupted by exogenous factors (see the following), requires only LH (or human chorionic gonadotropin [hCG]), although FSH may be necessary to produce a normal number of sperm.

9. **Define primary hypogonadism and secondary hypogonadism.**

Failure of testicular function may result from a defect either in the testis or at the hypothalamic-pituitary level. Testicular disorders leading to hypogonadism are termed primary hypogonadism (Fig. 44-1), whereas disorders of hypothalamic-pituitary function leading to hypogonadism are termed secondary hypogonadism (Fig. 44-2). This distinction has therapeutic implications. In men with secondary hypogonadism, fertility can generally be restored with appropriate hormonal treatment. Men with primary hypogonadism have fewer options and more limited success with improvement in fertility. In addition, the evaluation of secondary hypogonadism can reveal a pituitary mass or systemic illness as the underlying cause.

Figure 44-1. Primary hypogonadism.

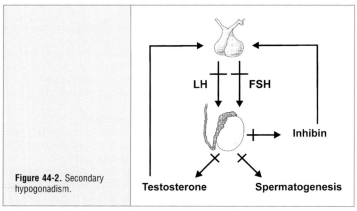

Figure 44-2. Secondary hypogonadism.

10. **List the congenital causes of primary hypogonadism.**
   - Klinefelter's syndrome (47XXY and mosaics)
   - Microdeletions of azoospermia factor (AZF) regions of Yp telomere (15% of men with nonobstructive azoospermia; 5%–10% of those with oligospermia)
   - Cryptorchidism
   - Myotonic dystrophy
   - Congenital adrenal hyperplasia (3-b-hydroxysteroid dehydrogenase, 17-a-hydroxylase, or 17-b-hydroxysteroid dehydrogenase deficiency)
   - Androgen receptor gene mutations (qualitative or quantitative)
   - LH receptor mutations (male phenotype, if mild; female phenotype, if severe)

11. **List the acquired causes of primary hypogonadism**
   - Cancer therapy: chemotherapy (alkylating agents > cisplatin and carboplatin) and radiation therapy (may be permanent with external radiation; usually transient with radioactive iodine)
   - Drugs (e.g., ketoconazole)
   - Testicular injury
   - Hyperthyroidism
   - Infiltrative disease (e.g., hemochromatosis)
   - Infections (e.g., HIV [may be multifactorial], mumps orchitis)
   - Systemic illness (e.g., uremia, cirrhosis): may be multifactorial
   - 5-alpha reductase inhibitors (finasteride and dutasteride) reduce sperm counts

12. **Is normal aging associated with primary hypogonadism?**

Symptomatic hypogonadism is present in about 5% of the adult male population, but in those men aged over 70 years, it is about 18%. Not all hypogonadism is symptomatic. Nevertheless, a number of cross-sectional studies have noted that older men seem to have mildly reduced levels of total serum testosterone but significantly reduced levels of free testosterone (due to a rise in SHBG with age) compared with younger men. This decline is associated with a rise in LH and FSH, suggesting that it is due to a primary gonadal cause. Studies have demonstrated an average 1% to 2% decline in serum testosterone per year associated with normal aging. Further complicating the situation is the controversial observation that there has been a population-level decrease in serum testosterone levels in American men since the mid-1950's.

13. **Discuss the causes of secondary hypogonadism.**

Any disease that affects the hypothalamic-pituitary axis can cause secondary hypogonadism. Involvement of the hypothalamus or pituitary stalk interferes with the secretion of GnRH or the ability of GnRH to communicate with the pituitary. Various anatomical lesions of the pituitary cause secondary hypogonadism by interfering with the release of LH and FSH. Such lesions include benign tumors and cysts, malignant tumors (both primary central nervous system tumors and metastatic tumors from distant sources), vascular aneurysms, infiltrative diseases (e.g., hemochromatosis), pituitary hemorrhage, and pituitary trauma. Certain inflammatory diseases (such as sarcoidosis and histiocytosis) can also affect the hypothalamus and pituitary and decrease testosterone production. Congenital disorders, in which output of LH and FSH is impaired, such as Kallmann's syndrome, also lead to secondary hypogonadism. Both obesity and HIV/AIDS are associated with secondary hypogonadism as well. Others include the use of narcotic analgesics or the abuse of anabolic steroids by athletes.

14. **What is the most common pituitary tumor in adults?**

The most common pituitary tumor found in adults is a prolactin-secreting adenoma. These tumors primarily cause hypogonadism as a result of local destruction and compression, inhibiting the production and release of LH and FSH. Elevated prolactin levels can also interrupt secretion of GnRH, although this is usually of much less significance in men than the mass effect.

15. **How do other pituitary adenomas cause hypogonadism?**

Pituitary adenomas that produce growth hormone (acromegaly) or adrenocorticotropic hormone (Cushing's disease) and nonfunctioning pituitary tumors may similarly cause secondary hypogonadism by their mass effects.

16. **What clinical symptoms are seen in male hypogonadism?**

Loss of the sperm-producing function of the testis leads to infertility, usually defined as failure of a normal female partner to conceive after 12 months of unprotected intercourse. Loss of the testosterone-producing function of the testis may lead to loss of libido and erectile dysfunction, as well as diminution of secondary sexual characteristics, such as facial and pubic hair, and decrease in testicular volume to < 20 ml or 3 cm × 5 cm. Decreased production of testosterone may also cause more generalized symptoms, such as decreased muscle mass and strength, malaise, and fatigue. In boys who develop hypogonadism before sexual maturation, delay or absence of the onset of puberty is typical. Tender gynecomastia is frequently seen in hypogonadism. A number of nonspecific features are also commonly associated with hypogonadism, such as a normochromic, normocytic anemia, poor concentration, depressed mood, and increased body fat and body mass index.

17. **How does hypogonadism affect bone architecture?**

Osteoporosis is now a well-recognized result of both primary and secondary hypogonadism. Trabecular architecture (and bone strength) is even more severely disturbed than bone density in men with hypogonadism. Thus it is not surprising that hypogonadism is found in up to 30% of men with vertebral fractures. Estradiol that is aromatized from testosterone may be the most important factor in preserving bone architecture and density in both men and women. However, androgen receptors are also found in bone and may explain the sexual dimorphism of bone density.

18. **What laboratory tests help to confirm a suspected diagnosis of male hypogonadism?**

The main functions of the testis, production of sperm and production of testosterone, are readily assessed by semen analysis and measurement of serum testosterone, respectively. Normal semen analysis values in men following 2 to 3 days of abstinence are 20 million sperm/mL and greater than 60% motility of the sperm. Because sperm density is highly variable from day to day in all men, accurate assessment usually involves several semen analyses performed with the same abstinence period each time. The best initial test for testosterone production is measurement of the nonfasting early (by 0800 hours) morning serum total testosterone level. Serum testosterone also varies considerably from moment to moment and from morning to night in response to LH secretion; again, several samples may be necessary to establish an accurate measurement. In addition, most testosterone in serum is bound to plasma proteins, particularly SHBG; thus in patients who have increased and decreased SHBG levels (discussed earlier) and in those men in whom plasma protein levels may be disrupted, measurement of the physiologically active "free" testosterone may prove informative. Bone density measurement using a Dual Energy X-ray Absorpiometry (DXA) scan may provide helpful baseline information and assist in deciding whether to provide androgen replacement therapy.

KEY POINTS: MALE HYPOGONADISM

1. The manifestations of hypogonadism vary depending on the stage of development of the patient when the hypogonadism occurs.

2. A reduction in testicular volume (below 20 mL 3 cm × 5 cm) is the most common manifestation of hypogonadism and is seen in nearly all cases of long-standing hypogonadism.

3. The diagnosis of hypogonadism is readily confirmed with a correctly obtained total serum testosterone measurement or semen analysis.

4. Hypogonadism should be characterized as primary (a disorder at the level of the testes) or secondary (a disorder at the level of the hypothalamic-pituitary unit) based on the LH and FSH levels.

5. Hypogonadism should be corrected to the mid-normal range with testosterone given in one of the following ways: injection, scrotal or dermal patch, topical gel, or buccal tablet.

6. Patients on testosterone replacement should be monitored for gynecomastia, prostate size and symptoms, increases in prostate-specific antigen, polycythemia, sleep apnea, and psychological difficulties.

19. **Can laboratory tests help to distinguish primary from secondary hypogonadism?**

Primary hypogonadism resulting from a testicular disorder leads to a decline in production of testosterone and sperm, a consequent decrease in the negative feedback effects on the pituitary and a corresponding increase in serum levels of LH and FSH. Conversely, in secondary hypogonadism due to a hypothalamic-pituitary disorder, serum LH and FSH may be subnormal or "inappropriately" normal (explainable, in part, by decreased bioactivity) despite a low testosterone. A subnormal sperm count and normal testosterone level with a normal LH and elevated FSH suggests primary hypogonadism with a dysfunction of the seminiferous tubules and sperm production but intact Leydig cell function.

20. **What other diagnostic tests are useful in defining the cause of male hypogonadism?**
Additional diagnostic testing should be based on clinical suspicion and the results of preliminary testing. For example, in cases of secondary hypogonadism, measurement of serum prolactin and pituitary radiography, preferably magnetic resonance imaging (MRI) with gadolinium, should be performed. Computed tomography of the sella usually detects macroadenomas (>1.0 cm) but will miss many clinically significant microadenomas and therefore MRI is preferred. Plain skull or sella turcica films are not adequate for diagnosis. Measurement of other pituitary hormones also may be appropriate to assess either possible tumoral hypersecretion (e.g., Cushing's disease, acromegaly) or tumor-related hypopituitarism. Visual field testing is indicated if a macroadenoma is present or there is suprasellar extension. Likewise, the initial findings in primary hypogonadism may suggest additional tests. For example, small firm testes, gynecomastia, azoospermia, modestly reduced serum testosterone, and high levels of serum LH and FSH in a young man may lead to chromosome analysis to confirm a presumptive diagnosis of Klinefelter's syndrome. Measurement of serum estradiol levels may be helpful when feminization is prominent clinically, as with secondary hypogonadism related to production of estrogen by testicular or adrenal tumors. If infertility is the primary issue and no hormonal abnormality is found, genetic causes should be investigated. This includes testing for Y chromosome microdeletion syndromes. Testis biopsy rarely provides information that is useful in establishing a specific diagnosis, prognosis, or treatment.

21. **Define hermaphrodite.**
The term hermaphrodite refers to individuals who have both ovarian and testicular elements in their body. They usually have a 46XX or 46XX/46XY karyotype. Such individuals may have an ovary and a testis or an ovotestis. They most often have ambiguous genitalia.

22. **Define pseudohermaphrodite.**
Pseudohermaphrodite refers to someone whose external genitalia are not consistent with his or her gonadal sex. A male pseudohermaphrodite, for example, has a 46XY karyotype and testes but has either ambiguous genitalia or a complete female phenotype. Most often this results from genetic disorders of testosterone biosynthetic enzymes, the androgen receptor or the 5-a-reductase enzyme; the severity of the phenotype depends on the severity of the genetic defect. A female pseudohermaphrodite, in contrast, has a 46XX karyotype and ovaries but has ambiguous external genitalia. The most common cause of this is congenital adrenal hyperplasia, which results in virilization of the female fetus in utero.

23. **How is hypogonadism treated?**
Deficiency of testosterone is easily treated with testosterone replacement therapy (TRT) (see Table 45-2). In general, the treatment goal for all TRT is normalization of the serum LH in primary hypogonadism and a serum total testosterone level in the mid-normal range for secondary hypogonadism. However, in elderly men, the goal of therapy should be to raise serum testosterone levels to the mid-normal range. There is currently considerable controversy over whether men with age-associated hypogonadism should be treated with testosterone replacement. Although some short-term studies have demonstrated treatment benefits, long-term large studies are lacking and are necessary to clarify the criteria for treatment, as well as the risks and benefits associated with testosterone replacement in this population. Furthermore, some older men with testosterone deficiency are unconcerned about sexual function and may not desire testosterone replacement. However, in testosterone-deficient men of any age, low

bone density or reduced hematopoiesis may be indications for TRT even in the absence of decreased libido or erectile dysfunction. Testosterone preparations are currently designated as schedule III drugs by the Anabolic Steroid Control Act because of their potential for abuse by athletes and others.

24. **What are the potential adverse effects of testosterone treatment?**

Gynecomastia and acne are rare symptoms that may occur in the first few months after initiating testosterone treatment; these side effects may resolve with continued treatment, although temporary dose reduction may be helpful. Abnormalities in liver function are uncommon with currently used injectable and transdermal preparations but can be seen in seldom-used oral preparations. A testosterone-induced increase in hematocrit is common, especially when testosterone injections are used, although clinically significant polycythemia is rare unless the drug is being abused. Testosterone treatment may also precipitate or worsen sleep apnea; marked increases in hematocrit may be a clue to this side effect. Skin reactions are commonly seen in patients using the transdermal patch and are occasionally, but much less frequently, seen with the use of the gel. In boys who have not yet gone through puberty, the rapid increase in serum testosterone after initial treatment may lead to considerable psychological difficulties and physically aggressive behavior; initiating treatment with smaller doses may be helpful. TRT has no adverse effect on lipid profiles compared with eugonadal men, but overtreatment can lead to several lipid abnormalities, including decreases in the high-density lipoprotein cholesterol level. There does not appear to be a significant increase in cardiovascular disease associated with physiologic testosterone replacement, and some studies have even suggested a treatment benefit. However, patients with class III or IV heart failure should be given testosterone replacement cautiously.

25. **Does testosterone replacement affect the prostate in older men?**

In older men, effects of testosterone on the prostate must be considered, including the possibility of precipitating urinary retention due to testosterone-induced enlargement of the prostate. Short-term studies have not shown any histologic or gene expression effects of testosterone replacement. However, prostate volume increases with long-term testosterone therapy to a level comparable to eugonadal men, without any significant associated increase in symptoms, urine flow rates, or residual volumes. Individual men may experience voiding symptoms associated with this enlargement, which they should be told to monitor. Testosterone therapy with a scrotal patch or gel (but not a nonscrotal patch) increases dihydrotestosterone more than testosterone, and it is the former that stimulates the prostate. It is advisable to perform a digital rectal examination (DRE) of the prostate and monitor prostate-specific antigen (PSA) in middle-age and older men before initiating therapy and annually thereafter while they are receiving any testosterone replacement. Although no compelling evidence indicates that testosterone treatment causes prostate carcinoma, the potential for testosterone stimulation of occult prostate carcinoma exists. Men with an elevated PSA level or an abnormal DRE should be evaluated further, potentially including a prostate biopsy, before initiation of testosterone therapy.

26. **How does one treat the deficiency of sperm production in primary hypogonadism?**

In men with primary hypogonadism, as manifested by elevated levels of serum FSH, there seems to be no effective pharmacological treatment for increasing the sperm count. Anatomical lesions, such as varicocele and ejaculatory duct obstructions, can be corrected surgically, but improvement in spermatogenesis may not result. If one plans to use a medication that is known to cause hypogonadism (e.g., cancer chemotherapeutic agents), it may be desirable to cryopreserve semen specimens before treatment, provided that treatment is not unduly delayed.

27. **How does one treat deficient sperm production in secondary hypogonadism?**
    The outlook is much less pessimistic with secondary hypogonadism, particularly if the condition developed after puberty. Treatment with gonadotropins (human chorionic gonadotropin with or without added FSH) may be successful in restoring production of sperm, as well as testosterone. The pretreatment size of the testis is often a clue to prognosis; larger testis size is associated with a better outcome. Production of testosterone and sperm in men with secondary hypogonadism may also be enhanced with pulsatile administration of GnRH through a portable infusion pump, provided that the pituitary retains the capability to make gonadotropins. Treatment with gonadotropins or GnRH tends to be both costly and prolonged.

28. **What reproductive alternative is available to men with hypogonadism who do not respond to therapy?**
    In men with primary or secondary hypogonadism who have not responded to specific therapy when appropriate and who have preservation of some germ cells in either ejaculate or testis, intracytoplasmic sperm injection (ICSI) may offer some hope, although at a high financial cost. The prognosis for successful ICSI is dependent on the site and extent of microdeletions on the Y chromosome. If microdeletions are found, the patient should be counseled about the possibility of transmitting this to his male child. Other fertility options that should be discussed include donor sperm and adoption.

WEBSITES

1. http://www.endosociety.org/publications/guidelines/final/upload/
   AndrogensMenGuideline053006.pdf

2. http://www.aace.com/pub/pdf/guidelines/hypogonadism.pdf

3. http://www.nlm.nih.gov/medlineplus/ency/article/000390.htm

4. http://www.hormone.org/public/other.cfm

5. http://www.mayoclinic.com/health/male-hypogonadism/DS00300

BIBLIOGRAPHY

1. Adamopoulos DA, Lawrence DM, Vassilopoulos P, et al: Pituitary-testicular relationships in mumps orchitis and other viral infections. BMJ 1:1177–1180, 1978.

2. Araujo, AB, Esche GR, Kupelian V, et al: Prevalence of symptomatic androgen deficiency in men. J Clin Endo Metab 92:4241–4247, 2007.

3. Amory JK, Wang, C, Swerdloff RS, et al: The effect of 5 reductase inhibition with dutasteride and finasteride on semen parameters and serum hormones in healthy men. J Clin Endo Metab 92:1659–1665, 2007.

4. Bagatell CJ, Bremner WJ: Androgens in men—uses and abuses. N Engl J Med 334:707–714, 1996.

5. Baker HWG, Burger HF, DeKretser DM, et al: Changes in the pituitary-testicular system with age. Clin Endocrinol 5:349–372, 1976.

6. Bannister P, Handley T, Chapman C, Losowsky MS: Hypogonadism in chronic liver disease: impaired release of luteinising hormone. BMJ 293:1191–1193, 1986.

7. Bhasin S: Approach to the infertile man. J Clin Endo Metab 92:1995–2004, 2007.

8. Bhasin S, Cunningham GR, Hayes FJ, et al: Testosterone therapy in adult men with androgen deficiency syndromes: an Endocrine Society Clinical Practice Guideline. J Clin Endo Metab 91:1995–2010, 2006.

9. Byrne M, Nieschlag E: Testosterone replacement therapy in male hypogonadism. J Endocrinol Invest 26:481–489, 2003.

10. Castro-Magana M, Bronsther B, Angulo MA: Genetic forms of male hypogonadism. Urology 35:195–204, 1990.

11. Dada R, Gupta NP, Kucheria K: Molecular screening for Yq microdeletion in men with idiopathic oligospermia and azoospermia. J Biosci 28:163–168, 2003.

12. Gambineri A, Pelusi C, Vicennati V, et al: Testosterone in ageing men. Expert Opin Investig Drugs 10:477–492, 2001.

13. Griffin JE, Wilson JD: The syndromes of androgen resistance. N Engl J Med 302:198–209, 1980.

14. Gromoll J, Eiholzer U, Nieschlag E, Simoni M: Male hypogonadism caused by homozygous deletion of exon 10 of the luteinizing hormone (LH) receptor: differential action of human chorionic gonadotropin. J Clin Endocrinol Metab 85:2281–2286, 2000.

15. Guo CY, Jones TH, Eastell R: Treatment of isolated hypogonadotropic hypogonadism effect on bone mineral density and bone turnover. J Clin Endocrinol Metab 82:658–665, 1997.

16. Harman SM, Metter EJ, Tobin JD, et al: Longitudinal effects of aging on serum total and free testosterone levels in healthy men. Baltimore Longitudinal Study of Aging. J Clin Endocrinol Metab 86:724–731, 2001.

17. Hayes FJ, Seminara SB, Crowley WF: Hypogonadotropic hypogonadism. Endocrinol Metab Clin North Am 27:739–763, 1998.

18. Hopps CV, Mielnik A. Goldstein M, et al: Detection of sperm in men with Y chromosome microdeletions on the AZFa, AZFb and AZFc regions. Hum Reprod 18:1660–1665, 2003.

19. Hsueh WA, Hsu TH, Federman DD: Endocrine features of Klinefelter's syndrome. Medicine 57:447–461, 1978.

20. Kalyani RR, Gavini S, Dobs AS: Male hypogonadism in systemic disease. Endocrinol Metab Clin North Am 36:333–348, 2007.

21. Kidd GS, Glass AR, Vigersky RA: The hypothalamic-pituitary-testicular axis in thyrotoxicosis. J Clin Endo Metab 48:798–802, 1979.

22. Layman LC: Hypogonadotropic hypogonadism. Endocrinol Metab Clin North Am 36:283–296, 2007.

23. Lee PA, O'Dea LS: Primary and secondary testicular insufficiency. Pediatr Clin North Am 37:1359–1387, 1990.

24. Lieblich JM, Rogol AD, White BJ, Rosen SW: Syndrome of anosmia with hypogonadotropic hypogonadism (Kallman syndrome): clinical and laboratory studies in 23 cases. Am J Med 73:506–519, 1982.

25. Marks LS, Mazer NA, Mostaghel E, et al: Effect of testosterone replacement therapy on prostate tissue in men with late-onset hypogonadism. JAMA 296:2351–2361, 2006.

26. Matsumoto AM, Bremner WJ: Endocrinology of the hypothalamic-pituitary-testicular axis with particular reference to the hormonal control of spermatogenesis. Baillieres Clin Endocrinol Metab 1:71–87, 1987.

27. Rhoden EL, Morgentaler A: Risks of testosterone-replacement therapy and recommendations for monitoring. N Engl J Med 29;350:482–92, 2004.

28. Schwartz ID, Root AW: The Klinefelter syndrome of testicular dysgenesis. Endocrinol Metab Clin North Am 20:153–163, 1991.

29. Seminara SB, Hayes FJ, Crowley WF, Jr: Gonadotropin-releasing hormone deficiency in the human (idiopathic hypogonadotropic hypogonadism and Kallmann's syndrome): pathophysiological and genetic considerations Endocrine Rev 19:521–539, 1998.

30. Silveira LF, MacColl GS, Bouloux PM. Hypogonadotropic hypogonadism. Semin Reprod Med 20:327–338, 2002.

31. Snyder PJ, Peachy H, Berlin JA, et al: Effects of testosterone replacement in hypogonadal men. J Clin Endocrinol Metab 85:2670–2677, 2000.

32. Swerdloff RS, Wang C, Cunningham G, et al: Long-term pharmacokinetics of transdermal testosterone gel in hypogonadal men. J Clin Endocrinol Metab 85:4500–4510, 2000.

33. Szulc P, Munoz F, Claustrat B, et al: Bioavailable estradiol may be an important determinant of osteoporosis in men: the MINOS study. J Clin Endocrinol Metab 86:192–199, 2001.

34. Tenover JL: Male hormone replacement therapy including "andropause." Endocrinol Metab Clin North Am 27:969–987, 1998.

35. Whitcomb RW, Crowley WF: Male hypogonadotropic hypogonadism. Endocrinol Metab Clin North Am 22:125–133, 1993.

CHAPTER 45

IMPOTENCE

Robert A. Vigersky

1. **What is impotence?**

   Classically, impotence has been defined as the inability to attain and maintain an erection of sufficient rigidity for sexual intercourse in 50% or more attempts. A more descriptive term for impotence is erectile dysfunction.

2. **Do men with erectile dysfunction have disturbances in other sexual functions?**

   Most men with erectile dysfunction are able to ejaculate. Premature ejaculation may precede the development of impotence and is sometimes associated with drug therapy. Sexual desire (libido) is also usually preserved; loss of libido is suggestive of hypogonadism or severe systemic or psychiatric illness.

3. **Is impotence common?**

   At least 10 million American men and perhaps as many as 20 million are impotent. Another 10 million may suffer from partial erectile dysfunction. The prevalence of impotence increases with age; about 2% of 40–year–old, 20% of 55–year–old, and 50% to 75% of 80–year–old men are impotent. Of interest, there is a libido–potency gap in that many elderly men continue to have active libidos, but only 15% of them engage in sexual activity.

4. **How does a normal erection occur?**

   Erection is primarily a vascular event that results from the complex interplay of the hormonal, vascular, peripheral nerve, and central nervous system.

5. **Explain the role of the nervous system in achieving erection.**

   Erection is usually initiated by various psychological and/or physiologic stimuli in the cerebral cortex. The stimuli are modulated in the limbic system and other areas of the brain, integrated in the hypothalamus, transmitted down the spinal cord, and carried to the penis via both autonomic and sacral spinal nerves. (For Latin scholars, these are the nervi erigentes derived from the verb *erigo, erigere, erexi, erectus*.) Sensory nerves from the glans of the penis enhance the message and help to maintain erection during sexual activity through a reflex arc.

6. **Explain the hormonal aspects of erection.**

   Nervous system stimuli release neurotransmitters that reverse the tonic smooth muscle constriction maintained by norepinephrine, endothelin, and other vasoconstrictive factors. The most important of these are the potent vasodilators, nitric oxide (NO), and prostaglandin E1 (PGE1). In addition to neural sources, NO is derived from endothelial cells, which may explain why endothelial integrity may be necessary for maintenance of an erection. NO works by increasing cyclic guanosine monophosphate (cGMP) and causing a decrease in intracellular calcium. This results in relaxation of vascular smooth muscle cells due to dissociation of actin–myosin.

7. **What vascular changes in the penis result in erection?**
Within the two spongy corpora cavernosa of the penis are millions of tiny spaces called lacunae, each lined by a wall of trabecular smooth muscle. As neurotransmitters dilatate cavernosal and helicine arteries to the penis and relax the trabecular smooth muscle, the lacunar spaces in the penis become engorged with blood. This results in entrapment of outflow vessels between the expanding trabecular walls and the rigid tunica albuginea that surrounds the corpora cavernosa, thereby greatly reducing venous outflow from the penis. This veno–occlusive mechanism accounts for both rigidity and tumescence. Failure of venous occlusion (venous leak) is one of the intractable causes of impotence.

8. **What types of nerves and neurotransmitters play a role in penile erection?**
At least three neuroeffector systems play a role in penile erection. Adrenergic nerves generally inhibit erection; cholinergic nerves and nonadrenergic, noncholinergic (NANC) substances enhance erection as follows:
   ■ Sympathetic nerves (via beta–adrenergic receptors): constrict cavernosal and helicine arteries, contract trabecular smooth muscle
   ■ Parasympathetic nerves (via cholinergic receptors): inhibit adrenergic fibers, stimulate NANC fibers
   ■ NANC messengers (NO, vasoactive intestinal polypeptide, and PGs or other endothelium–derived factors): dilatate cavernosal and helicine arteries, relax trabecular smooth muscle

9. **How does detumescence occur?**
Phosphodiesterase 5 (PD5), by causing a decrease in cGMP, allows for reversal of the process; that is, detumescence, making PD5 inhibitors, such as sildenafil, vardenafil, and tadalafil, important therapeutic agents for the treatment of impotence (see the following).

10. **What are the common causes of impotence?**
The frequency of the various causes of impotence is difficult to assess because of the large number of patients who do not report the problem, confusion regarding the diagnosis, and variability in the sophistication of the initial evaluation. Primary causes of impotence in men presenting to a medical outpatient clinic are approximated as follows:
   ■ Endocrine factors (including hyper– and hypothyroidism): 30%
   ■ Diabetes mellitus and metabolic syndrome: 15%
   ■ Medications: 20%
   ■ Systemic disease and alcoholism: 10%
   ■ Primary vascular causes: 5% (Alterations of blood flow are thought to play a role in many causes of impotence, but specific lesions amenable to therapy are relatively rare.)
   ■ Primary neurologic causes: 5%
   ■ Psychogenic or unknown causes: 15%

11. **What lifestyles are associated with impotence?**
   ■ Low levels of physical activity
   ■ Overeating/obesity
   ■ Smoking
   ■ Excessive TV viewing
   ■ Alcohol consumption

12. **Besides diabetes mellitus, what are the three most common endocrine causes of impotence?**
   ■ Primary (hypergonadotropic) hypogonadism (increased luteinizing hormone [LH] and decreased testosterone)
   ■ Secondary (hypogonadotropic) hypogonadism (decreased LH and decreased testosterone)
   ■ Hyperprolactinemia

Less common causes include hyperthyroidism, hypothyroidism, adrenal insufficiency, and Cushing's syndrome.

13. **Describe the most common drugs known to induce impotence.**
Nonprescription drugs, such as alcohol (as the porter says to Macduff in Act II, Scene 3, of *Macbeth*, "It provokes the desire but takes away the performance"), and illicit drugs, such as cocaine, methadone, and heroin, can cause impotence. The prescription drugs most commonly associated with impotence include the following:
- Antihypertensive agents, especially methyldopa, clonidine, beta–blockers, vasodilators (e.g., hydralazine), thiazide diuretics, and spironolactone
- Antipsychotic medications
- Antidepressants and tranquilizers
- Others (especially cimetidine, digoxin, phenytoin, carbamazepine, ketoconazole, metoclopramide, and megestrol)

14. **Which antihypertensive agents should be used in patients with impotence?**
Virtually every blood pressure medication has been associated with impotence. Although there is little overall difference in the rate of erectile problems among the commonly prescribed antihypertensive agents, angiotensin–converting enzyme inhibitors, angiotensin–receptor blockers, and calcium channel blockers are the agents least likely to affect erectile ability. When beta blockade is required, selective beta antagonists, such as atenolol or acebutolol, are preferred as they have minimal impact on sexual function.

15. **What is "stuttering" impotence? What is its significance?**
Impotence alternating with periods of entirely normal sexual function is termed stuttering impotence. Multiple sclerosis (MS) is the most significant organic cause of stuttering impotence. It may be the initial manifestation of MS and may be present in up to 50% of men with the disease.

16. **What historical information helps to separate organic from psychogenic impotence?**
True psychogenic impotence is uncommon and should be a diagnosis of exclusion. Questions that may help to separate psychogenic from organic impotence are listed in Table 45-1.

TABLE 45-1. ORGANIC VERSUS PSYCHOGENIC IMPOTENCE		
	Organic	Psychogenic
Was onset abrupt?	No	Yes
Is impotence stress dependent?	No	Yes
Is libido preserved?*	Yes	No
Do you have morning erections?	No	Yes
Do you have orgasms?	Yes	No
Can you masturbate?	No	Yes
Does impotence occur with all partners?	Yes	No

*There is a general relationship of libido to hypogondal levels of testosterone in populations but on an individual basis, libido may not be a reliable discriminator.

17. **Name the essential components of a physical examination in a man complaining of impotence.**
    - Secondary sexual characteristics, such as muscle development, hair pattern, and presence of breast tissue
    - Vascular examination, especially of the femoral and lower extremity pulses and the presence of bruits
    - Focused neurological examination, including assessing the presence of peripheral neuropathy with vibratory and light touch sensation and of autonomic neuropathy using the cremasteric reflex, anal sphincter tone or the bulbocavernosus reflex, evaluation of standing and supine blood pressure, and measurement of the heart rate response to deep breathing and Valsalva (Diabetics rarely have autonomic neuropathy as a cause of impotence in the absence of peripheral neuropathy.)
    - Examination of the genitalia to determine penile size, shape, presence of plaque or fibrous tissue (Peyronie's disease); size and consistency of the testes; prostate examination
    - Thyroid–relevant examination including size, the presence of nodularity, and abnormal reflexes

18. **What is the appropriate laboratory assessment for men with impotence?**
    Laboratory assessment should be based on history and physical examination findings. It can discover previously unknown disease in 6% of men. Generally, it should include the following:
    - Complete blood count
    - Urinalysis
    - Fasting plasma glucose and (in known diabetics) hemoglobin A_{1C} (HbA1C)
    - Fasting serum lipid profile
    - Serum creatinine
    - Serum free thyroxine and thyrotropin
    - Serum testosterone, LH, and FSH

19. **Should prolactin levels be measured in all impotent men?**
    Whether serum prolactin should be measured in all men with impotence is somewhat controversial. In general, patients with normal levels of testosterone and LH and a normal neurological examination do not require measurement of prolactin. However, if testosterone is low and associated with low or low–normal LH or if history or examination suggests a pituitary lesion, prolactin should be measured. Because prolactin interferes with the action of testosterone, prolactin status should be assessed in hypogonadal men unresponsive to testosterone replacement therapy. Hypothyroidism and renal failure also may elevate prolactin.

20. **What is a penile brachial index?**
    Comparison of the penile and brachial systolic blood pressure allows a general assessment of the vascular integrity of the penis. This technique is not highly sensitive, but it is noninvasive and easy to perform and may help to identify men who require more extensive vascular studies. Penile systolic blood pressure obtained with Doppler ultrasound should be the same as brachial systolic pressure (i.e., ratio approximately = 1.0). An index less than 0.7 is highly suggestive of vasculogenic impotence. Diagnostic yield is increased if the penile brachial index is repeated after exercising the lower extremities for several minutes. This maneuver may uncover a pelvic steal syndrome (loss of erection due to pelvic thrusting) that is characterized by a difference of greater than 0.15 between the resting and exercise ratios.

21. **What is nocturnal penile tumescence monitoring?**
    Most men experience 3 to 6 erections during the night that are entrained to rapid eye movement sleep. By monitoring such events, one can assess the frequency, duration, and, with some instruments, even the rigidity of erection. This procedure helps to distinguish organic from psychogenic impotence. This can be done at home either semiquantitatively (using a Snap–Gauge [Dianon Corporation, Stratford, Connecticut]) or more quantitatively (using the RigiScan [Timm Medical Technologies, Inc., Eden Prairie, Minnesota]).

22. What are the therapeutic options in the treatment of impotence?
After drugs with a high likelihood of causing impotence are discontinued or other underlying conditions are aggressively treated (e.g., diabetes mellitus, hypercholesterolemia), the broad categories of available therapy are as follows:
- Medical treatment including lifestyle modifications and weight reduction
- Intracavernosal injection
- Transurethral delivery of alprostadil (PGE1)
- External mechanical aids and vacuum/suction devices
- Surgical treatments
- Psychological therapy (especially in the absence of an obvious organic cause)

23. What options are available for medical treatment?
- Testosterone replacement in hypogonadal men with a goal of achieving a mid–normal level of serum testosterone
- Dopamine agonists (bromocriptine or cabergoline) to reduce hyperprolactinemia in men with normal testosterone unresponsive to testosterone treatment
- PD5 inhibitors, such as sildenafil citrate (Viagra), vardenafil (Levitra), or tadalafil (Cialis)
- Adrenergic receptor blockers (e.g., yohimbine, 5.4 mg t.i.d.)
- Herbal remedies (e.g., Korean red ginseng, 900 mg t.i.d.)
- Selective serotonin reuptake inhibitor for premature ejaculation

24. Summarize the role of intracavernosal injections.
Intracavernosal injection of vasoactive substances (PGE, papaverine, and phentolamine) individually or in combination (Trimix) may be effective for men in whom PD5 inhibitors have failed or are contraindicated.

25. List the surgical procedures used to treat impotence.
- Revascularization procedures
- Obliteration of venous shunts
- Surgical penile implants

26. What are the advantages and disadvantages of the various forms of androgen replacement therapy?
Oral forms of testosterone, such as oxandrolone and methyltestosterone, should not be used for long–term therapy because of their propensity to cause hepatotoxicity and hepatic tumors. Fluoxymesterone (Halotestin) cannot be aromatized to estrogens and therefore may not provide protection against osteoporosis. Contact dermatitis is common with testosterone patches and may preclude their use. Mood changes with intramuscular forms of testosterone and gingival irritation with the buccal delivery system are not uncommon. The recommended forms of testosterone with their relative advantages and disadvantages are listed in Table 45-2.

27. What parameters should be monitored in men on testosterone therapy?
The following should be determined at baseline, at 3 months after initiation of therapy, and then followed at least yearly, after the patient is stabilized:
- Hematocrit and hemoglobin
- Prostate size by digital rectal examination
- Serum prostatic–specific antigen (PSA)
- Liver function tests
- Development of gynecomastia, acne, or edema
- Serum testosterone levels in all forms of treatment
- Serum dihydrotestosterone levels in those receiving scrotal patches or gel
- Development of or worsening of sleep apnea
- Bone mineral density at baseline and at 1 to 2–yearly intervals

TABLE 45-2. RECOMMENDED FORMS OF TESTOSTERONE ADMINISTRATION

	Intramuscular	Scrotal Patch	Dermal Patch	Gel	Buccal
Brand name	Delatestryl/Depo Testosterone	Testoderm	Androderm/ Testoderm TTS	AndroGel/ Testim	Striant
Dose	50–100 mg weekly or 100–200 mg biweekly	4–6 mg q.d.	2.5–5 mg q.d.	50 mg q.d.	30 mg b.i.d.
Reliable delivery/ compliance	4	2	3	3	?
Flexible dosing	4	2	2	2	2
Stable serum levels	1	4	4	4	?
Convenience	1	2	3	3	2
Side effects	2	2	3	1*	?
Cost	1	2	3	3	4

?, data not available; 1, lowest; 4, highest.
*15 minutes of vigorous skin-to-skin contact can transfer significant amounts of testosterone to a female partner.

28. **In what conditions is testosterone therapy absolutely or relatively contraindicated?**
    Absolute contraindication:
    - Carcinoma of the prostate
    - Obstructive sleep apnea
    - Polycythemia vera
    - Symptomatic or severe benign prostatic hypertrophy
    - Breast carcinoma

    Relative contraindication:
    - Prostate nodule that has not been biopsied
    - Elevated serum PSA level
    - Class III or IV congestive heart failure

29. **How effective are PD5 inhibitors?**
    The introduction of the selective PD5 inhibitors (sildenafil citrate [Viagra], vardenafil [Levitra], and tadalafil [Cialis]) has produced a paradigm shift in the approach to the treatment of impotence by reducing the relevance of finding a specific cause of the problem. There appears to be no tachyphylaxis to their effect for at least 5 years. Given 1 hour before anticipated sexual activity (and for Viagra avoiding a fatty meal, which inhibits its absorption by one third), they are successful in up to 80% of men with organic impotence (although only approximately 50% to 70% of diabetic men and 50% of elderly men). There may be a place for testosterone "rescue" in patients who do not respond to PD5 inhibitors and who also have low testosterone levels. Switching from one PD5 inhibitor to another is also sometimes beneficial.

30. Discuss the side effects of PD5 inhibitors.

The few side effects associated with PD5 inhibitors (headache, flushing, dyspepsia, and a blue haze in vision) rarely cause discontinuation of their use. Because they cause vasodilatation similar to that of nitrates, they are contraindicated in men taking any form of nitrates. The long half–life of tadalafil (the so–called "weekend pill") may prove to be particularly troublesome if a patient develops angina within 72 to 96 hours of taking it. In addition, PD5 inhibitors should be given with care in men with a recent myocardial infarction or stroke, resting hypotension, class III or class IV congestive heart failure, and unstable angina.

KEY POINTS: IMPOTENCE

1. Erections are mediated by neural and endothelial NO release, which induce vasodilation.

2. The specific cause of impotence can be diagnosed in 85% of men.

3. The antihypertensives that are least likely to cause impotence are angiotensin–converting enzyme inhibitors, angiotensin–receptor blockers, and calcium channel blockers.

4. PD5 inhibitors (sildenafil, vardenafil, and tadalafil) are the most effective drugs in treating nonhormonal impotence.

5. Men treated with testosterone replacement therapy should be monitored yearly by a digital rectal examination and blood tests for hemoglobin, prostate–specific antigen, hepatic function, and testosterone.

31. What drug interactions are associated with PD5 inhibitors?

Because PD5 inhibitors are metabolized through CYP3A4, any drugs that block that enzyme (e.g., erythromycin and other macrolide antibiotics; ketoconazole and other antifungal drugs; HIV protease inhibitors, such as saquinavir and ritonavir; cimetidine) increase the plasma concentrations of PD5 inhibitors. In such cases, PD5 inhibitors should be started at one fourth to one half of the usual dose. Because PD5 inhibitors may potentiate the hypotensive effect of beta–adrenergic blocking agents, they should be given in lower doses (Viagra) or not at all (Levitra) in men on alpha blockers for control of blood pressure or for benign prostatic hypertrophy.

32. When are intracavernosal or intraurethral injections recommended?

Injection of vasodilatatory substances directly into the corpora cavernosa of the penis should be reserved for men in whom PD5 inhibitors are ineffective, contraindicated, or have produced intolerable adverse effects. Such "PD5 salvage" therapy results in erection satisfactory for intercourse in some men with impotence. PGE1 (Caverject), papaverine, and phentolamine may be used alone or in combination (Trimix).

33. Discuss the side effects of intracavernosal and intraurethral injections.

Side effects, which depend on the type and quantity of substances injected, include hypotension, elevation of liver enzymes, and headache. Local complications include hematoma, swelling, inadvertent injection into the urethra, and local fibrosis with long–term use. The most serious local complication is priapism (a sustained erection) for more than 4 hours, which may necessitate injection of beta–adrenergic agonists or corpora cavernosal aspiration. PGE1 is also available as an intraurethral suppository (medicated urethral system for erection [MUSE]), and because it is less invasive and easier to use, it may be a more appropriate second–line agent than intracavernosal injection. No controlled studies have evaluated the success of either approach in PD5 inhibitor failures.

34. Does the onset of impotence have other health implications?

The development of impotence is associated with a 45% increased risk of cardiovascular events. This is in the same range of other well-known risk factors such as current smoking and a family history of a myocardial infarction.

35. What future treatments may be forthcoming?

There are newer PD5 inhibitors that are in trials. These have shorter onset of actions or intermediate duration of actions. Gene therapy that targets the potassium channels in the penile smooth muscle is being evaluated in safety and efficacy trials.

36. What other modalities are available to treat impotent men?

Vacuum erection devices provide a noninvasive, mechanical solution for impotence. They are somewhat cumbersome to use and require the placement of an occlusive ring at the base of the penis to prevent venous outflow. They may be particularly effective in those men who have a "venous leak" as the etiology of their impotence. The constrictive ring prevents antegrade ejaculation because of the urethral constriction. Surgical revascularization has a limited place in the treatment of impotent men because of its invasiveness and limited success rate. Similarly, penile prosthesis insertion is rarely performed because of the availability of several effective and noninvasive alternatives. In men in whom premature ejaculation is the major problem, intermittent use of selective serotonin reuptake inhibitors has been efficacious in delaying time to ejaculation.

WEBSITES

1. http://www.endosociety.org/publications/guidelines/final/upload/AndrogensMenGuideline053006.pdf

2. http://www.impotence.org/

3. http://kidney.niddk.nih.gov/kudiseases/pubs/impotence/index.htm

4. http://www.hormone.org/public/other.cfm

BIBLIOGRAPHY

1. Adams MA, Banting BD, Maurice DH, et al: Vascular control mechanism in penile erection: phylogeny and the inevitability of multiple overlapping systems. Int J Impotence Res 9:85–95, 1997.

2. Andersson KE: Erectile physiological and pathophysiological pathways involved in erectile dysfunction. J Urol 170:S6–S14, 2003.

3. Bagatell CJ, Bremner WJ: Androgens in men—use and abuses. N Engl J Med 334:707–714, 1997.

4. Bhasin S, Cunningham GR, Hayes FJ, et al: Testosterone therapy in adult men with androgen deficiency syndromes: an Endocrine Society Clinical Practice Guideline. J Clin Endo Metab 91:1995–2010, 2006.

5. Cohan P, Korenman SG: Erectile dysfunction. J Clin Endo Metab 86:2391–2394.

6. Cookson MS, Nadig PW: Long-term results with vacuum constriction device. J Urol 149:290–294, 1993.

7. Esposito K, Giugliano F, Di Palo C, et al: Effect of lifestyle changes on erectile dysfunction in obese men: a randomized controlled trial. J Am Med Assoc 291:2978–2984, 2004.

8. Esposito K, Giugliano F, Martedi E, et al: High proportions of erectile dysfunction in men with the metabolic syndrome. Diabetes Care 28:1201–1203, 2005.

9. Feldman HA, Goldstein I, Hatzichristou DJ, et al: Impotence and its medical and psychosocial correlates: results of the Massachusetts male aging study. J Urol 151:54–61, 1994.

10. Goldstein I, Lue TF, Padma–Nathan H, et al: Oral sildenafil in the treatment of erectile dysfunction. N Engl J Med 338:1397–1404, 1998.

11. Goldstein I, Young JM, Fischer J, et al Vardenafil, a new phosphodiesterase type 5 inhibitor, in the treatment of erectile dysfunction in men with diabetes: a multicenter double–blind placebo–controlled fixed–dose study. Diabetes Care 26:777–783, 2003.

12. Grimm RH Jr, Grandits GA, Prineas RJ, et al (for the TOHMS Research Group): Long–term effects on sexual function of five antihypertensive drugs and nutritional hygienic treatment in hypertensive men and women. Treatment of Mild Hypertension Study (TOHMS). Hypertension 29:8–14, 1997.

13. Hanash KA: Comparative results of goal oriented therapy for erectile dysfunction. J Urol 157: 2135–2139, 1997.

14. Herrmann HC, Chang G, Klugherz BD, Mahoney PD: Hemodynamic effects of sildenafil in men with severe coronary artery disease. N Engl J Med 342:1622–1626, 2000.

15. Hong G, Ji YH, Hong JH, et al: A double–blind crossover study evaluating the efficacy of Korean red ginseng in patients with erectile dysfunction: a preliminary report. J Urol 168:2070–2073, 2002.

16. Krane RJ, Goldstein I, DeTejada JS: Impotence. N Engl J Med 321:1648–1659, 1989.

17. Krassas GE, Tziomalos K, Papadopoulou F, et al: Erectile dysfunction in patients with hyper– and hypothyroidism: how common and should we treat? J Clin Endo Metab 93:1815–1819, 2008.

18. Lerner SF, Melman A, Christ GJ: A review of erectile dysfunction: new insights and more questions. J Urol 149:1246–1252, 1993.

19. Linet OI, Ogring FG, and the Alprostadil Study Group: Efficacy and safety of intracavernosal prostaglandin in men with erectile dysfunction. N Engl J Med 334:873–878, 1996.

20. Melman A: Gene therapy for male erectile dysfunction. Urol Clin N Am 34: 619–630, 2007.

21. McMahon CG, Touma K: Treatment of premature ejaculation with paroxetine hydrochloride as needed: two single–blind placebo controlled crossover studies. J Urol 161:1826–1830, 1999.

22. Morley JE, Kaiser FE: Impotence: the internists' approach to diagnosis and treatment. Adv Intern Med 38:151–168, 1993.

23. Neisler AW, Carey NP: A critical reevaluation of nocturnal penile tumescence monitoring in a diagnosis of erectile dysfunction. J Nerv Ment Dis 178:78–79, 1990.

24. NIH Consensus Conference: Impotence. JAMA 270:83–90, 1993.

25. Padma–Nathan H, Hellstrom WSG, Kaiser FE, et al: (for the Medicated Urethral System for Erection (MUSE) Study Group): Treatment of men with erectile dysfunction with transurethral alprostadil. N Engl J Med 336:1–7, 1997.

26. Park K, Ku JH, Kim SW, Paick JS: Risk factors in predicting a poor response to sildenafil citrate in elderly men with erectile dysfunction. BJU International 95:366–370, 2005.

27. Porst H, Padma–Nathan H, Giuliano F, et al: Efficacy of tadalafil for the treatment of erectile dysfunction at 24 and 36 hours after dosing: a randomized controlled trial. Urology 62:121–125, 2003.

28. Rajfer J, Aronson WJ, Bush PA, et al: Nitric oxide as a mediator of relaxation of the corpus cavernosum in response to nonadrenergic, noncholinergic neurotransmission. N Engl J Med 326:90–94, 1992.

29. Rendell MS, Rajfer J, Wicker PA, et al: Sildenafil for treatment of erectile dysfunction in men with diabetes. A randomized controlled trial. JAMA 281:421–426, 1999.

30. Rosenthal BD, May NR, Metro MJ, et al: Adjunctive use of Androgel (testosterone gel) with sildenafil to treat erectile dysfunction in men with acquired androgen deficiency syndrome after failure using sildenafil alone. Urology 67:571–574, 2006.

31. Sidi AA: Vasoactive intracavernous pharmacotherapy. Urol Clin N Am 15:95–101, 1988.

32. Thompason IM, Tangen CM, Goodman PJ, et al: Erectile dysfunction and subsequent cardiovascular disease. J Am Med Assoc 294:2996–3002, 2005.

33. Witherington R: Mechanical aids for treatment of impotence. Clin Diabetes 7:1–22, 1989.

CHAPTER 46

GYNECOMASTIA

Brenda K. Bell and Micol S. Rothman

1. **Define gynecomastia.**
   Gynecomastia is defined as the presence of palpable breast tissue in a male.

2. **How does gynecomastia present clinically?**
   Gynecomastia usually presents as a palpable discrete button of tissue radiating from beneath the nipple and areolar region. Gynecomastia will feel "gritty" when the breast is pinched between the thumb and forefinger. Fatty tissue, unlike gynecomastia, will not cause resistance until the nipple is reached. If doubt remains, soap and water on the breast can facilitate the examination by decreasing the skin friction.

3. **What is the significance of painful gynecomastia?**
   Gynecomastia is frequently asymptomatic and incidentally discovered. Pain or tenderness implies recent, rapid growth of breast tissue. This may indicate a pathological cause for the gynecomastia and should prompt further evaluation.

4. **Is gynecomastia always bilateral?**
   The involvement tends to be bilateral, but asymmetry is common. Unilateral enlargement is present in 5% to 25% of patients and may be a preliminary stage in the development of bilateral disease. In autopsy studies, unilateral enlargement is often found to be bilateral gynecomastia histologically.

5. **Summarize the pathophysiology of gynecomastia.**
   Gynecomastia results from an imbalance between the stimulatory effect of estrogen on ductal proliferation and the inhibitory effect of androgen on breast development. The imbalance is most commonly caused by increased production of estrogens, decreased production of testosterone, or increased conversion of androgens to estrogens in peripheral tissue. Problems with sex hormone binding globulin and problems with androgen receptor binding and function can also result in gynecomastia.

6. **Where are estrogens produced in the male?**
   Direct testicular production of estrogens accounts for less than 15% of male estrogen production. The majority of estrogens come from the conversion of adrenal and testicular androgens to estrogens in peripheral tissues, particularly adipose tissue and the liver.

7. **What is the most common cause of gynecomastia?**
   Asymptomatic palpable breast tissue is common in normal males, particularly in the neonate (60%–90%), at puberty (60%–70% between the ages of 12 and 15 years), and with increasing age (20%–65% over age 50 years). Because of this high prevalence, gynecomastia is considered a relatively normal finding during these periods of life. Gynecomastia at these ages is often called physiologic or idiopathic.

8. **Why does gynecomastia occur so commonly during these stages of life?**
   Neonatal gynecomastia is due to placental transfer of estrogens. During early puberty, production of estrogens begins sooner than production of testosterone, causing an imbalance in

the ratio of estrogens to androgens. With aging, production of testosterone decreases, and peripheral conversion of androgens to estrogens often increases because of an age-associated increase in adipose tissue.

9. **What are the other causes of gynecomastia?**
   Idiopathic and pubertal gynecomastia makes up the majority of cases. Drugs account for 10% to 20% of cases and primary hypogonadism for another 10%. Adrenal or testicular tumors account for less than 3% of cases—gynecomastia may precede the development of the testicular tumor. Other causes combined account for less than 10% of cases and include secondary hypogonadism, androgen-resistant disorders, malnutrition, cirrhosis, alcohol abuse, renal disease, congenital adrenal hyperplasia, extragonadal tumors, refeeding gynecomastia, and hyperthyroidism.

10. **What drugs cause gynecomastia?**
    Many drugs have been implicated, some with known steroid effects, others with no clear mechanism:

Anabolic steroids	Methyldopa	Nifedipine	Protease inhibitors
Androgens	Reserpine	Verapamil	Amiodarone
Estrogen creams	Marijuana	Amlodipine	Risperidone
Spironolactone	Heroin	Diltiazem	Amphetamines
Flutamide	Methadone	Captopril	Minocycline
Finasteride	Phenytoin	Enalapril	Ethionamide
Cyproterone acetate	Diazepam	Thalidomide	Isoniazid
Ranitidine	Metronidazole	Fluoxetine	Tricyclic antidepressants
Cimetidine	Ketoconazole	Phenothiazines	Growth hormone
Omeprazole	Chemotherapy	Methotrexate	Theophylline
Digitoxin	Pravastatin	Haloperidol	Auranofin
Domperidone	Atorvastatin	Etretinate	Sulindac
Diethylpropion	Gabapentin	Penicillamine	Dong Quai
Metoclopramide	Alcohol	Melatonin	Lavender
Tea tree oil	Antiandrogen treatment for prostate cancer		

11. **How do testicular tumors cause gynecomastia?**
    Germ cell tumors can produce human chorionic gonadotropin (hCG). Like luteinizing hormone (LH), hCG increases testicular production of estradiol. Leydig cell tumors may directly secrete estradiol.

12. **What extragonadal tumors cause gynecomastia?**
    Pancreatic, gastric, and pulmonary tumors, transitional cell carcinoma of the bladder and renal cell carcinoma have been associated with production of hCG. Hepatomas may have increased aromatase activity that results in excess conversion of androgens to estrogens.

13. **Who should undergo evaluation for gynecomastia?**
History and physical examination are indicated in all cases and will determine the cause in 30% to 40% of patients. Gynecomastia is so common, however, that many experts are cautious about attaching importance to the detection of a small amount of breast tissue in an otherwise asymptomatic man. In adolescents, there is no reason to consider endocrine testing unless the enlargement is massive or the gynecomastia persists longer than 2 years. Acute development of enlargement and tenderness in males older than age 20 warrants additional evaluation, as do eccentric, hard masses and lesions greater than 4 cm in size.

14. **What information is significant in the history?**

Age	Other illnesses
	Congenital abnormalities
Thyroid symptoms	Nutritional status and recent changes in weight
Duration of enlargement	Pubertal progression
Drugs	Impotence and libido
Breast symptoms (tenderness, discharge)	
Alcohol use	

15. **What should be noted on the physical examination?**
The most important features include characteristics of the breast tissue (irregular, firm, eccentric, nipple discharge), testes (size, asymmetry), abdomen (liver enlargement, ascites, spider angioma), secondary sexual characteristics, thyroid status (goiter, tremor, reflexes), and any signs of excessive cortisol (buffalo hump, central obesity, hypertension, purple striae, moon facies).

KEY POINTS: GENERAL APPROACH TO GYNECOMASTIA

1. The most important differentiation is between gynecomastia and breast cancer. If doubt remains after physical examination, obtain a mammogram.

2. Most cases are bilateral, asymptomatic, and incidentally discovered. History, physical examination, and reevaluation in 3 to 6 months are appropriate for such men.

3. Rapid enlargement, growth greater than 4 cm, pain, and age less than 10 years or between 20 and 50 years correlate with a systemic illness/pathological cause for the gynecomastia. Such men should be evaluated thoroughly if the cause is not apparent after history and physical examination.

4. Malignant tumors can cause gynecomastia, although rarely. Consider testicular, pulmonary and abdominal tumors (pancreatic, adrenal, gastric, renal/bladder).

16. **Should laboratory tests be ordered?**
Some believe that hormonal testing is not cost-effective and favor checking testicular ultrasound alone to rule out the 3% incidence of feminizing tumors. Most, however, favor measuring liver enzymes, blood urea nitrogen, creatinine, thyrotropin (TSH), and testosterone (total and free). Estradiol, hCG, LH, and follicle-stimulating hormone (FSH) may follow the initial screen. If the

hCG or estradiol level is elevated, a testicular ultrasound is indicated. If this is negative, chest radiograph and abdominal computed tomographic (CT) scan should follow. For prepubertal patients, an adrenal CT scan would precede the testicular ultrasound.

17. **What findings raise the suspicion of breast cancer?**
Breast cancer is rare in men (0.2%). The risk is increased in Klinefelter's syndrome (3%–6%) and in male relatives of young women with breast cancer. Carcinoma is usually unilateral, painless, and nontender. Bloody discharge, ulceration, firmness, fixation to the underlying tissue, eccentric location, and adenopathy are suspicious findings. If doubt remains, mammogram or biopsy should be considered. The sensitivity and specificity of mammogram for the diagnosis of male breast cancer approaches 90%. The diagnostic accuracy of fine-needle aspiration cytology is greater than 90%. Excisional biopsy or mastectomy would be recommended for malignant or suspicious cytology or mammogram appearance.

18. **Will gynecomastia spontaneously regress?**
Gynecomastia of recent onset, less than 3 cm in size, will regress in 85% of patients. It may take 18 to 36 months for gynecomastia to resolve during puberty but resolution will occur in greater than 90% of pubertal boys. Persistence is uncommon after age 17. Gynecomastia due to a medication or underlying disease should also resolve after discontinuing the inciting agent or treating the underlying disease. Persistent tissue becomes more fibrous with time, however, and is less likely to remit spontaneously if it has been present for greater than 12 months. More highly developed breast tissue (Tanner stages III, IV, and V) is also less likely to regress.

19. **What is the treatment when gynecomastia does not regress?**
Hormonal therapy can be attempted. Tamoxifen, clomiphene, danazol, dihydrotestosterone, testolactone, and anastrozole have all been used. Tamoxifen has the fewest side effects and the highest response rate for both improvement in tenderness and decrease in size. Although it is not an improved treatment, partial regression can be seen in approximately 80% of patients and complete regression in about 60%. Medication is more likely to work if gynecomastia has been present less than 4 months and the size of the tissue is less than 3 cm. Tamoxifen is given at a dosage of 10 mg twice daily with follow-up in 3 months to assess response. For recurrent or persistent gynecomastia greater than 3 cm, surgery is the recommended therapy. Liposuction/ultrasound guided liposuction, excision or both may be used. Low-dose bilateral breast irradiation and tamoxifen have also been studied in trials as prophylaxis to prevent the development of gynecomastia caused by estrogens and antiandrogens used in the treatment of prostate cancer.

KEY POINTS: TREATMENT OF GYNECOMASTIA

1. Most cases resolve spontaneously or after removal of the offending medication or treatment of the underlying disease.
2. Medical management with tamoxifen can be attempted for 3 to 6 months if desired.
3. The longer the tissue has been present and the larger the amount of tissue, the less likely the response to tamoxifen. Surgery is indicated for these cases.

BIBLIOGRAPHY

1. Braunstein G: Gynecomastia. N Engl J Med 357:1229–1237, 2007
2. Braunstein G: Pathogenesis and diagnosis of gynecomastia. Up to Date in Endocrinology and Diabetes 11(2): 1–11, 2003.
3. Braunstein G: Prevention and treatment of gynecomastia. Up to Date in Endocrinology and Diabetes 11(3):1–9, 2003.
4. Bowers S, Pearlman N, McIntyre R, et al: Cost-effective management of gynecomastia. Am J Surg 176:638–641, 1998.
5. Ersoz H, Onde M, Terekeci H, et al: Causes of gynecomastia in young adult males and factors associated with idiopathic gynecomastia. Int J Androl 25:312–316, 2002.
6. Evans G, Anthony T, Appelbaum A, et al: The diagnostic accuracy of mammography in the evaluation of male breast disease. Am J Surg 181:96–100, 2001.
7. Fruhstorfer B, Malata C: A systematic approach to the surgical treatment of gynecomastia. Br J Plast Surg 56:237–246, 2003.
8. Gruntmanis U, Braunstein G: Treatment of gynecomastia. Curr Opin Investig Drugs 2:643–649, 2001.
9. Henley DV, Lipson N, Korach KS, et al: Prepubertal gynecomastia linked to lavender and tea tree oils. N Engl J Med 356:479–485, 2007.
10. Ismail A, Barth J: Endocrinology of gynaecomastia. Ann Clin Biochem 38:596–607, 2001.
11. Khan H, Blarney R: Endocrine treatment of physiological gynecomastia. BMJ 327:301–302, 2003.
12. Narula HS, Carlson HE: Gynecomastia. Endocrinol Metab Clin N Am 36:497–519, 2007.
13. Widmark A, Fossa S, Lundmo P, et al: Does prophylactic breast irradiation prevent antiandrogen induced gynecomastia? Urology 61:145–151, 2003.
14. Yaturu S, Harrara E, Nopajaroonsri C, et al: Gynecomastia attributable to HCG secreting giant cell carcinoma of the lung. Endocr Pract 9:233–235, 2003.

CHAPTER 47

AMENORRHEA

Margaret E. Wierman and Micol S. Rothman

1. **Define amenorrhea.**
   Amenorrhea is the absence of menstrual periods. Oligomenorrhea refers to lighter, irregular menses. Primary amenorrhea is the failure to ever begin menses, whereas secondary amenorrhea refers to cessation of menstrual periods after cyclic menses have been established.

2. **Describe the normal timing of puberty.**
   In girls, puberty usually begins after age 8 years and is heralded by the initiation of breast development. The average age for girls in the United States to begin menses is 12 years. This event generally signals the end of the pubertal process, occurring after the growth spurt and most somatic changes are completed.

3. **Summarize the underlying process of pubertal development.**
   The process is triggered by gonadotropin-releasing hormone (GnRH)-induced episodic secretion of luteinizing hormone (LH) and follicle-stimulating hormone (FSH) from the pituitary gland. The pulsatile release of gonadotropins activates the ovaries, causing maturation of follicles and production of estrogen and, later, progesterone. These gonadal steroids give feedback at the level of the hypothalamus and pituitary to regulate GnRH and gonadotropin secretion. A final maturation event is the development of positive feedback by estradiol to induce the midcycle LH surge that stimulates ovulation. In many adolescents, menstrual cycles are anovulatory and thus irregular for the first 12 to 18 months. As the hypothalamic-pituitary-gonadal (HPG) axis matures, ovulatory cycles become more frequent. In normal adult women, all but one or two cycles per year are ovulatory.

4. **What types of disorders cause primary amenorrhea?**
   Primary amenorrhea is defined as lack of menses by age 16 or lack of secondary sexual characteristics by age 14. It usually results from abnormal anatomical development of the female reproductive organs or from a hormonal disorder involving the hypothalamus, pituitary gland, or ovaries (Table 47-1). The presence of normal secondary sexual characteristics in such patients suggests an anatomical problem, such as obstruction or failure of development of the uterus or vagina. In contrast, a lack of secondary sexual characteristics indicates a probable hormonal cause.

5. **What are hypothalamic and pituitary causes of primary amenorrhea?**
   Idiopathic hypogonadotropic hypogonadism (IHH) be due to maturational arrest of GnRH-producing neurons during embryonic development (also called Kallmann syndrome when associated with anosmia). In addition, the kisspeptin/GPR54 system has recently been shown to regulate GnRH secretion at puberty. Mutations in this pathway as well as the GnRH receptor in the pituitary may also cause primary amenorrhea. The pituitary gland may also be compressed by pituitary tumors, craniopharyngiomas, and Rathke's pouch cysts, causing impaired LH and FSH secretion in adolescence disrupting sexual maturation.

TABLE 47-1. CAUSES OF PRIMARY AMENORRHEA
Anatomic
Congenital absence of ovaries, uterus, or vagina
Cervical stenosis
Imperforate hymen
Hormonal
Hypothalamic
GnRH deficiency
Hypothalamic tumor (craniopharyngioma)
Pituitary
Prolactinoma
Rathke's cleft cyst
Panhypopituitarism from a genetic mutation
Ovarian
Gonadal dysgenesis (XO)
Chemotherapy or radiation damage of the ovaries
Androgen resistance syndromes (XY)
Other: congenital adrenal hyperplasia

6. **Summarize the ovarian causes of primary amenorrhea.**

   The ovaries may impaired because of gonadal dysgenesis due to Turner's syndrome (45XO karyotype) or destruction by chemotherapy or radiation before the completion of sexual maturation. The presence of ambiguous genitalia or palpable gonads in the labia or inguinal area may indicate a disorder of sexual differentiation, such as congenital adrenal hyperplasia (CAH) (21-hydroxylase deficiency) or an androgen resistance syndrome (testicular feminization) due to mutations in the androgen receptor.

7. **What disorders cause secondary amenorrhea?**

   Secondary amenorrhea, which is much more common than primary amenorrhea, occurs postpubertally. The causes are outlined in Table 47-2. Pregnancy should be excluded in all amenorrheic women. Onset of irregular menses after having regular menses and association with hot flashes should suggest premature ovarian failure (i.e., premature menopause). Hypothalamic amenorrhea occurs in 3% to 5% of women and is caused by abnormal GnRH- induced gonadotropin secretion often due to stress or eating disorders but is a diagnosis of exclusion. Hyperprolactinemia is an underlying cause in 10% of women. Pituitary tumors can result in secondary amenorrhea. Hyperandrogenic anovulatory disorders present with oligomenorrhea or amenorrhea and signs and symptoms of excess androgens, such as hirsutism and acne.

8. **How do you evaluate a patient with amenorrhea?**

   One must determine whether the disorder is anatomical or hormonal, congenital or acquired, and where the defect is located. A complete history and physical examination provide the first essential clues. Timed measurement of serum gonadotropin levels (LH and FSH) within the first 5 days after the onset of a spontaneous or timed menses separates patients into one of two categories. Patients with low or normal levels of LH and FSH (hypogonadotropic hypogonadism) have a disorder at the level of the hypothalamus or pituitary gland. However, patients with high LH and FSH levels (hypergonadotropic hypogonadism) may have a defect at the level of either

TABLE 47-2. CAUSES OF SECONDARY AMENORRHEA
Pregnancy
Hypogonadotropic hypogonadism
Hyperprolactinemia (from drugs or prolactinoma)
Pituitary tumor inhibiting gonadotropin production
Hypothalamic amenorrhea
Hypergonadotropic hypogonadism
Premature ovarian failure (surgical or autoimmune)
Gonadotropin producing pituitary tumors
Hyperandrogenic anovulation

the ovary or hypothalamic-pituitary unit (e.g., polycystic ovary syndrome [PCOS], in which the hypothalamic GnRH pulse generator is abnormally accelerated or a gonadotrope pituitary tumor that secretes FSH, LH, or both).

9. **Discuss the major congenital causes of hypogonadotropic hypogonadism.**
   Idiopathic hypogonadotropic hypogonadism is due to GnRH deficiency. Female patients present with primary amenorrhea and lack of secondary sex characteristics. When associated with anosmia, the disorder is termed Kallmann syndrome. GnRH deficiency occurs in 1/8000 males and 1/80,000 females and may be X-linked, autosomal dominant, autosomal recessive, or sporadic. The X-linked form is associated with a mutation in the KAL-1 gene that encodes anosmin, a neural cell adhesion protein thought to be important in providing the scaffolding for GnRH neurons in their migration from the olfactory placode to the hypothalamus during embryonic development. Similarly, mutations in FGFR1 also disrupt neuronal migration. Thus GnRH neurons fail to reach their target in the hypothalamus. All other hypothalamic-pituitary function is normal. Recently investigators have found that mutations in the kisspeptin/GPR54 system that is important in GnRH secretion can also cause IHH. Estrogen administration is used to initiate the development of secondary sexual characteristics in these patients, and fertility can be attained using pulsatile GnRH or gonadotropin therapy.

10. **What are the most frequent acquired forms of amenorrhea due to hypogonadotropic hypogonadism?**
    - Hyperprolactinemia
    - Hypothalamic amenorrhea

11. **How does hyperprolactinemia cause amenorrhea?**
    Elevated prolactin levels may be due to prolactinomas, hypothyroidism, medications (usually psychotropic drugs), and pregnancy. Hyperprolactinemia impairs function of the HPG axis at all levels, but the major site of inhibition is the hypothalamic GnRH pulse generator. As prolactin levels rise, luteal phase defects develop, ovulation ceases, and menstrual cycles become shorter and irregular. Higher elevation in prolactin levels are associated with amenorrhea. Treatment of the underlying cause of the elevated prolactin level usually normalizes menstrual cycles.

12. **What is hypothalamic amenorrhea?**
    Hypothalamic amenorrhea refers to amenorrhea resulting from acquired disorders of the GnRH pulse generator. Excessive stress, exercise, and weight loss have been shown to act centrally to disrupt the GnRH-induced pulsatile gonadotropin secretory pattern. In men, GnRH-induced LH pulses normally occur every 2 hours. In contrast, the LH pulse pattern in women must

change across the menstrual cycle, accelerating from every 90 minutes in the early follicular phase to every 30 minutes at ovulation and then slowing from every hour to every 8 hours across the luteal phase. Disruption of this precisely timed pattern results in anovulation, irregular menses, and, eventually, amenorrhea.

13. **What types of GnRH pulse generator defects cause hypothalamic amenorrhea?**
Hypothalamic amenorrhea may result from several types of gonadotropin secretory disorders. Some women with anorexia nervosa have absent LH pulsations (prepubertal pattern), some have pulsations only at night (early pubertal pattern), and still others have LH pulses throughout the 24-hour period but they are significantly reduced in amplitude or frequency.

14. **How do you make a diagnosis of hypothalamic amenorrhea?**
The diagnosis depends on excluding other causes of amenorrhea and then relies heavily on a history of weight loss, high levels of exercise or stress, or a combination of these. Supportive findings on physical examination include evidence of decreased estrogen effects and absence of other major illnesses. Laboratory testing usually reveals low serum estradiol and low or low-normal serum LH and FSH levels; the test for βb-hCG is negative, and the prolactin level is normal. Elevated FSH levels with low estradiol levels, in contrast, indicate probable premature ovarian failure.

15. **What are the consequences of estrogen deficiency?**
Short-term consequences of estrogen deficiency may include painful intercourse, hot flashes, and sleep disturbances. Among the more important long-term consequences are osteoporosis and premature coronary artery disease.

16. **What treatment options are available for hypothalamic amenorrhea?**
Interventions to increase body weight and to reduce stress or exercise should be attempted initially. If these interventions are unsuccessful, estrogen replacement therapy (usually with oral contraceptives) are instituted. Fertility, if desired, may be achieved by ovulation induction with clomiphene in mild cases or with human menopausal gonadotropins or pulsatile GnRH administration if the disorder is more severe.

17. **What disorders cause amenorrhea with hypergonadotropic hypogonadism?**
   - Premature ovarian failure (high FSH, later high LH)
   - PCOS (low FSH, high LH)
   - Gonadotropin-secreting pituitary tumors (high FSH and/or LH)

18. **How do you make a diagnosis of premature ovarian failure?**
Premature ovarian failure, which is defined as menopause before age 40, may be due to surgical removal or autoimmune destruction of the ovaries. Autoimmune destruction of the ovaries is characterized by a history of normal puberty and regular menses followed by the early onset of hot flashes, irregular menses, and eventual amenorrhea. Elevated serum FSH levels are the laboratory hallmark of gonadal failure. To avoid misdiagnosis, blood for FSH measurements, together with estradiol measurement, must be drawn in the early follicular phase (day 1–5 after onset of a spontaneous or induced menses), because FSH levels rise along with LH at midcycle in normally ovulating women. Turner's syndrome mosaics (XO/XX) may have several menses before they undergo menopause; therefore a karyotype may be helpful if ovarian failure occurs in adolescence or the early 20s.

19. **What other disorders may coexist with premature ovarian failure?**
Both patients and family members are at risk for other autoimmune disorders, including primary adrenal insufficiency (Addison's disease), autoimmune thyroid disorders (Graves' disease,

Hashimoto's disease), type 1 diabetes mellitus, pernicious anemia (vitamin B12 deficiency), celiac sprue, and rheumatologic disorders.

20. What are the treatment options for women with premature ovarian failure?
Estrogen replacement therapy, usually in combination with progesterone, is critical to decrease postmenopausal bone loss and premature coronary artery disease. New options for fertility in women with premature ovarian failure include incubation of donor eggs with the partner's sperm in in vitro fertilization protocols, along with hormonal preparation of the patient to enable her to carry the fetus in her uterus.

21. What is hyperandrogenic anovulation?
Hyperandrogenic anovulation refers to the cluster of disorders that present with irregular menses or amenorrhea and signs of androgen excess, such as hirsutism and acne. The disorders in this group include PCOS, androgen-secreting tumors of the ovaries or adrenal glands, Cushing's syndrome, CAH (classic or attenuated form), and obesity-induced amenorrhea.

KEY POINTS: AMENORRHEA

1. Amenorrhea with estrogen deficiency can result in osteoporosis and premature cardiovascular disease.

2. Hyperprolactinemia and hypothalamic amenorrhea are the most common causes of amenorrhea with low estrogen and low follicle-stimulating hormone (FSH) levels.

3. Premature menopause (high FSH, low E) is an autoimmune disease, and patients are at risk for other autoimmune disorders, such as autoimmune thyroid disease, pernicious anemia, celiac sprue, and rheumatologic disorders.

4. Hyperandrogenic anovulation refers to amenorrhea with hirsutism and acne.

5. Polycystic ovarian disease is common, associated with risks of infertility, endometrial cancer, the metabolic syndrome, and type 2 diabetes.

22. How do tumors cause hyperandrogenic anovulation?
Tumors are suggested by rapid progression of hirsutism and virilization (temporal hair recession, clitoris enlargement, breast atrophy) and by high serum androgen levels; they may be excluded by a serum testosterone level less than 200 ng/dL or dehydroepiandrosterone sulfate (DHEAS) levels less than 1000 ng/mL.

23. What clinical and biochemical features suggest a patient with hirsutism has CAH?
CAH (most commonly due to 21-hydroxylase deficiency) presents in infancy with ambiguous genitalia in girls occasionally with salt wasting syndromes. In adolescence, it is detected with early pubarche and irregular menses. Family history and ethnicity (Ashkenazi Jews, Italians, Hispanics) increase the suspicion of CAH. CAH is diagnosed by high basal (>2–3 ng/mL) or adrenocorticotropic hormone (ACTH)-stimulated (>10 ng/mL) levels of 17-hydroxyprogesterone.

24. When should you suspect obesity-induced amenorrhea?
Obesity-induced amenorrhea is suggested by a history of normal puberty and menses until progressive weight gain triggers the development of hirsutism, acne, oligomenorrhea, and, later,

amenorrhea. Affected women have low serum levels of FSH and LH in the follicular phase in contrast to women with PCOS (see subsequent discussion).

25. **Describe the pathophysiology of obesity-induced amenorrhea.**
    Fat tissue contains aromatase and 5-alpha-a-reductase enzymes. Aromatase converts androgens to estrogens; when aromatase is present in increased amounts, as in obesity, constant elevated (rather than normally fluctuating) serum estrogen levels are produced, inhibiting LH and FSH secretion and thereby impairing normal ovulation. Increased activity of 5-alpha-a reductase, which converts testosterone to dihydrotestosterone (DHT), results in excessive DHT production, promoting the development of hirsutism and acne. Primary treatment with weight loss often results in restoration of normal reproductive function.

26. **How does the patient with PCOS present clinically?**
    Most patients with PCOS present in adolescence with a history of early menarche (<12 years) and persistently irregular menses. Hirsutism and acne beginning in the teenage years are other common features of the disorder. Approximately 60% of patients become overweight in their 20s and 30s. Patients also frequently have signs of insulin resistance, including acanthosis nigricans, a velvety, hyperpigmented cutaneous lesion on the neck and in the axillae. Irregular, anovulatory menses lead to infertility, and the resultant unopposed estrogen exposure increases the risk of endometrial hyperplasia and carcinoma.

27. **Describe the pathogenesis of PCOS.**
    Experts disagree as to whether PCOS is a primary disorder of the central nervous system, the adrenal glands, or the ovaries. Existing data support the presence of an abnormal hypothalamic GnRH pulse generator that, in contrast to hypothalamic amenorrhea, which is too slow, is set too fast in PCOS. The pituitary gonadotropin response to GnRH is rate dependent; rapid GnRH pulses stimulate LH secretion but inhibit FSH production. The increased LH/FSH secretory ratio results in multiple ovarian follicle recruitment but no dominant follicle and inability to trigger a GnRH-induced LH surge causing anovulation and the appearance of multiple subcapsular cysts. The GnRH pattern triggers constant estrogen and enhanced androgen production by the ovaries. Some have suggested a primary ovarian defect triggers the abnormal GnRH-induced LH pulse pattern. The ovarian prohormones (dehydroepiandrosterone [DHEA] and androstenedione) and testosterone may be elevated; for unclear reasons, the adrenal androgens, DHEA and DHEAS, may be increased as well. High levels of circulating androgens decrease hepatic production of sex hormone–binding globulin (SHBG), allowing more free androgen to target the skin and hair follicles, inducing the development of acne and hirsutism. Insulin resistance also plays a role in the ultimate picture because hyperinsulinemia augments ovarian androgen production and further reduces SHBG levels.

28. **What are the criteria for diagnosis of PCOS?**
    The 1990 National Institutes of Health criteria were modified by the Rotterdam criteria in 2003. The Rotterdam criteria include two of the three following: oligo-ovulation or anovulation, clinical or biochemical signs of hyperandrogenism and polycystic ovaries. Other etiologies such as Cushing's syndrome, CAH, and androgen-secreting tumor should be excluded.

29. **What are the treatment options for patients with PCOS?**
    The initial goals are to suppress androgen production and action and to ensure regular shedding of the endometrium to decrease the risk of developing endometrial hyperplasia. Birth control pills are the treatment of choice; an antiandrogen, such as spironolactone, may be added if hirsutism is a major problem. Intermittent cycling with medroxyprogesterone (Provera) is an alternative for endometrial protection but does not suppress the elevated androgens and their ultimate impact on ovarian morphology and function. Fertility may be achieved with clomiphene citrate or human menopausal gonadotropinst. A recent trial has shown that clomiphene citrate is

more efficacious than metformin, an insulin sensitizer, for induction of ovulation and increased live births. There was a higher incidence of multiple births in the clomiphene group (5% vs 0) than the metformin group. This trial was in contrast with other previous smaller trials which found similar rates in ovulation between the two medications, but did not report live birth rate. The patients in this trial were also heavier, with an average BMI of 36.0 and 35.6 in the clomiphene and metformin groups respectively, although the results were not different when they looked at the sub group of patients with BMI<30.

30. **Is there a role for insulin sensitizers in the treatment of women with PCOS?**
Studies have shown that reducing insulin resistance and serum insulin levels with metformin results in modest decreases in serum androgen levels, decreased BP, improved lipids, with some improvement in menstrual regularity, and improved ovulation in response to clomiphene citrate. The thiazolidinedione class of insulin sensitizers has shown promise, but recent cardiovascular concerns have limited their use. Data on combination therapy with birth control pills, antiandrogens, and insulin sensitizers are not yet available. Predictors of responders to metformin may include patients with a family history of type 2 diabetes, history of rapid weight gain, and lack of severe obesity. Oral glucose tolerance testing should be considered in patients with PCOS.

31. **What are the long-term consequences of PCOS?**
Long-term consequences include infertility, obesity, metabolic syndrome with hypertension, central adiposity, dyslipidemia and increased risk of glucose intolerance, and type 2 diabetes. Epidemiological studies have not yet defined a clear-cut increase in cardiovascular events, but long-term studies are underway.

BIBLIOGRAPHY

1. Berga SL: Functional hypothalamic chronic anovulation. In Adashi WY, Rock JA, Rosenwaks Z, editors, *Reproductive endocrinology, surgery, and technology*, Philadelphia, 1996, Lippincott-Raven, pp. 1061–1075.

2. Cumming DC: Exercise-associated amenorrhea, low bone density, and estrogen replacement therapy. Arch Intern Med 156:2193–2195, 1996.

3. Kiningham RB, Apgar BS, Schwenk TL: Evaluation of amenorrhea. Am Fam Physician 53:1185–1194, 1996.

4. Legro RS: A 27-year-old woman with a diagnosis of polycystic ovary syndrome. JAMA 297:509–519, 2007.

5. Legro RS, Barnhart HX, Schlaff WD, et al: Clomiphene, metformin, or both for infertility in the polycystic ovary syndrome. N Engl J Med 356:551–566, 2007.

6. Norman RJ, Dewailly D, Legro RS, et al: Polycystic ovary syndrome. Lancet 370:685–597, 2007.

7. Pralong FP, Crowley WF Jr: Gonadotropins: normal physiology. In Wierman ME, editor, *Diseases of the pituitary: diagnosis and treatment*, Totowa, 1997, Humana Press, pp. 203–219.

8. Schlechte JA: Differential diagnosis and management of hyperprolactinemia. In Wierman ME, editor, *Diseases of the pituitary: diagnosis and treatment*, Totowa, 1997, Humana Press, pp. 71–77.

9. Taylor AE, Adams JM. Mulder JE, et al: A randomized, controlled trial of estradiol replacement therapy in women with hypergonadotropic amenorrhea. J Clin Endocrinol Metab 81:3615–3621, 1996.

10. Warren MP: Anorexia, bulimia, and exercise-induced amenorrhea: medical approach. Curr Ther Endocrinol Metab 6:13–17, 1997.

11. Welt CK, Hall JE: Gonadotropin deficiency: differential diagnosis and treatment. In Wierman ME, editor, *Diseases of the pituitary: diagnosis and treatment*, Totowa, 1997. Humana Press, pp. 221–246.

12. Wierman ME: Gonadotropin releasing hormone. In Adashi WY, Rock JA, Rosenwaks Z, editors, *Reproductive endocrinology, surgery, and technology*, Philadelphia, 1996, Lippincott-Raven, pp. 665–681.

CHAPTER 48

GALACTORRHEA

William J. Georgitis

1. **Define galactorrhea.**
   Galactorrhea is discharge of breast milk not associated with breast-feeding. It may also be defined as a milk-like discharge from the breast of a nongravid woman. Milk production persisting for 6 months after weaning should also be considered galactorrhea and properly investigated for a pathologic cause.

2. **Which hormones affect lactation?**
   Estrogen and prolactin are necessary for milk production. Estrogens promote cellular proliferation and ductular development. Prolactin rises dramatically during pregnancy stimulating further differentiation of acini to prepare the breast for production of milk protein. Paradoxically, high levels of estrogen inhibit milk production during pregnancy. Shortly after delivery, estrogen levels decline and lactation begins. As demonstrated by studies with tissue cultures, growth hormone, insulin, and cortisol are necessary permissive factors for mammory cells to grow. Androgens inhibit breast growth and differentiation. Galactorrhea rarely occurs in men but can occur in the presence of prolactin excess and an alteration in the normal ratio of androgen and estrogen (Fig. 48-1).

3. **How common is galactorrhea?**
   Quite common. The lifelong cumulative frequency of galactorrhea ranges from 2% to 20%. Galactorrhea should not occur in nulligravidas, postmenopausal women, or men.

4. **Does galactorrhea have the appearance of milk?**
   Not always. Small amounts of serous fluid can be expressed from the breasts of a majority of normal nulliparous women, making the determination that a nipple discharge is really milk important before ordering additional tests. Breast milk is an emulsion of fat and water with proteins including over 100 known constituents. The fat content of milk varies and the gross appearance may range from milky to opalescent to clear. Microscopic examination can be used to confirm that a breast secretion is galactorrhea by revealing fat globules. Special testing with staining for fat and chemical analysis for lactate or specific milk proteins are rarely necessary to be confident that a breast discharge is milk.

5. **Is galactorrhea always expressed from both breasts?**
   No. Galactorrhea may be unilateral or bilateral. Although patients often are the first to observe galactorrhea due to nipple discharge or stained garments, some may not notice the galactorrhea. Galactorrhea elicited by nipple compression is referred to as expressible galactorrhea in distinction to spontaneous galactorrhea.

6. **List a differential diagnosis for galactorrhea?**
   The differential diagnosis for galactorrhea can be both lengthy and complex. Causes for nonpuerperal galactorrhea are not easily arranged in a logical sequence. Some lists categorize diagnoses by anatomic location, some by causality, and some by symptoms or signs. Most attempts at a structured approach to the differential become less structured as the list progresses. A shift in gender often complicates matters. Table 48-1 lists potential causes for galactorrhea. For clarity, selected examples are given in parentheses.

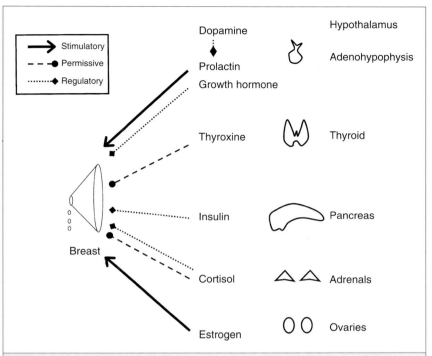

Figure 48-1. Hormones essential for lactation. Bold arrows indicate major stimulatory hormones, dashed arrows indicate permissive hormones, and dotted arrows indicate hormones that play predominantly regulatory roles.

TABLE 48-1. CAUSES OF NONPUERPERAL GALACTORRHEA

Idiopathic	Endocrinopathies
Pituitary tumors	Primary hypothyroidism
Prolactinoma	Hyperthyroidism
Somatotropinoma	Primary adrenal insufficiency
Hypothalamic disorders	Endogenous estrogens
Tumor (craniopharyngioma)	Adrenocortical carcinoma
Infiltrative disease (sarcoid)	Reflex arc activation
Infundibular disruption (trauma)	Nipple stimulation
Medications	Thoracic nerve irritation (shingles)
Psychotropic (risperidone)	Miscellaneous associations
Antihypertensive (methyldopa)	Stress
Cannabinoid (morphine)	Empty sella syndrome
Estrogens (oral contraceptives)	Renal or hepatic failure
Antiemetics (metoclopramide)	Polycystic ovary syndrome

7. **Which medications cause galactorrhea?**
Psychotropic medications are the leading culprits. The most common are phenothiazines, tricyclic antidepressants, haloperidol, benzodiazepines, butyrophenones, amphetamines, and monoamine oxidase (MAO) inhibitors. Other commonly prescribed drugs implicated as causes include cimetidine, metoclopramide, verapamil, and estrogens in numerous formulations. Prolactin levels can rise 10 to 20 times above the upper limit of normal with some antipsychotic medications with 17% to 78% of women experiencing amenorrhea with or without galactorrhea. The pituitary-gonadal axis in men is less affected by psychotropic medications. Risperidone is a particularly noteworthy drug, causing prolactin levels as high as 400 ng/mL.

8. **How often should one obtain a menstrual history from a woman with galactorrhea?**
Always. It is imperative to obtain a comprehensive menstrual history from any woman with galactorrhea. The most common physiological cause for amenorrhea-galactorrhea is pregnancy. This diagnosis should be considered first. A galactorrheic woman without amenorrhea has only a 20% chance of harboring a pituitary tumor. The prevalence of a pituitary tumor increases to 34% when amenorrhea accompanies galactorrhea.

9. **What percentage of women with hyperprolactinemia have galactorrhea?**
Not all women with hyperprolactinemia have galactorrhea. Women with elevated prolactin levels have a prevalence of galactorrhea ranging from 50% to 80%. Also, the degree of prolactin elevation correlates poorly with the amount of lactation. However, the degree of prolactin elevation does provide important clues to etiology as discussed in the following questions.

10. **Discuss the physiological variations in prolactin levels.**
Prolactin is a dynamic, not a static, hormone. It rises after meals and in response to hypoglycemia, seizures, intercourse, and vigorous nipple stimulation. Normal levels range as high as 20 ng/mL and show a diurnal variation. Many laboratories now report sex-specific normal ranges that range higher for women than men.

11. **How does the degree of prolactin elevation help determine the cause for galactorrhea?**
Drug-induced galactorrhea is usually accompanied by moderately elevated serum prolactin levels. Most medications cause galactorrhea by competitively blocking dopamine receptors. Mild hyperprolactinemia may also result from pituitary, hypothalamic, or parasellar processes. Mass lesions compressing or disrupting normal hypothalamic-pituitary portal connections permit prolactin levels to rise from the loss of the normal restraining influence of dopamine. Both drug-induced and non-prolactin-secreting pituitary region tumors are associated with prolactin levels ranging from 20 to 100 ng/mL. Prolactin levels above 100 ng/mL are most often due to pregnancy or prolactinomas. In a nonpregnant individual, the odds of finding a prolactinoma are proportionate to the degree of hyperprolactinemia. Levels above 300 ng/mL usually indicate the presence of a prolactinoma readily demonstratable with current pituitary imaging methods. Patients with levels ranging from 100 to 300 ng/mL should also have pituitary imaging. If a tumor is not found and treatment is not recommended, continued surveillance is necessary; the majority do have microprolactinomas that are not detected because their size is below the resolving power of current imaging modality slice protocols.

12. **What other lab tests should be included in the evaluation of galactorrhea?**
In addition to the mandatory pregnancy test for every potentially fertile woman, a thyroid-stimulating hormone (TSH) should be measured in every patient. Primary hypothyroidism can present as the amenorrhea-galactorrhea syndrome. The accompanying lactotroph hyperplasia in the pituitary may mimic a pituitary adenoma. Massive hyperplasia can even cause bitemporal hemianopsia from optic chiasmal compression as seen with suprasellar extension

of pituitary tumors. Signs of hypothyroidism may be subtle in young women. Therefore it is crucial that a TSH be measured in every case. It would be a serious disservice to the patient to miss primary hypothyroidism as the cause for amenorrhea-galactorrhea for many reasons. Both the pituitary hyperplasia and the amenorrhea-galactorrhea gradually resolve with thyroxine therapy. Treatment with dopamine agonists such as bromocriptine and cabergoline is more expensive than thyroxine therapy for hypothyroidism. Recent concerns about changes in heart valves with these agents used at higher doses for Parkinson's disease led to the withdrawal of pergolide and highlights the importance of using these agents judiciously. Dopamine agonists commonly cause side effects including nausea, although cabergoline is better tolerated than other agents. Finally, treatment of hypothyroidism even in the patient who appears asymptomatic often has benefits recognized by both the physician and the patient in retrospect.

13. **It seems odd that hyperthyroidism is listed just below hypothyroidism as a cause for galactorrhea. How did that come about?**
A single article reported a high prevalence of galactorrhea expressed with breast and nipple compression in hyperthyroid patients. Prolactin levels were normal, and the mechanism for the galactorrhea is obscure. Because these patients did not present with symptomatic galactorrhea with subsequent hyperthyroidism defined as the etiology, and it has not been shown that expressible galactorrhea resolves after treatment of the hyperthyroidism, the relevance of this observation to clinical practice is of questionable significance. Perhaps hyperthyroidism should be dropped from the list of disorders included in the differential diagnosis of galactorrhea.

14. **Describe the proposed mechanism for galactorrhea following thoracic surgery or associated with painful chest wall lesions.**
Galactorrhea sometimes appears after major surgery involving both the thorax and the abdomen. In the postoperative period, a woman's prolactin levels may rise while estrogen levels fall—a relationship that favors lactation. There is not a greater frequency of galactorrhea following chest wall surgery compared with other major surgical procedures. Postoperative hyperprolactinemia is not sustained. Galactorrhea also occurs with *Herpes zoster* involving nerves supplying dermatomes in the pectoral region. Prolactin levels are similar to drug-induced hyperprolactinemia ranging up to about 100 ng/mL. The increased prolactin secretion results from stimulation of a neural reflex arc between the breast and the pituitary-hypothalamic unit.

15. **Galactorrhea in renal failure seems odd. What is the connection?**
Hyperprolactinemia in renal failure is modest in degree. It results from decreased metabolic clearance of prolactin, but medications with dopamine inhibitory actions may also contribute to the elevation in prolactin. Most renal insufficiency patients with elevated prolactin levels do not have galactorrhea.

16. **Can galactorrhea occur in the absence of prolactin excess?**
Yes. One third of women with acromegaly have galactorrhea. Galactorrhea results most often from one of two mechanisms but there is a third mechanism. The first is prolactin secretion by the pituitary tumor itself. The second common mechanism is prolactin release due to pituitary stalk disruption and loss of the constant tonic restraint of dopamine inhibition on lactotroph prolactin secretion.

The third mechanism is seen in the rare acromegalic patient with galactorrhea who has normal, not elevated levels of prolactin. The 191-amino-acid human growth hormone molecule has 16% structural homology with the 198-amino-acid human prolactin. Twenty-four percent of the first 50 amino acids are similar. In normoprolactinemic acromegalic patients with galactorrhea, the galactorrhea probably results from cross-activation of breast prolactin receptors by very high levels of growth hormone.

17. **Is galactorrhea associated with an increased risk of breast cancer?**

    No. When a breast discharge occurs in breast cancer, a palpable mass is usually present. It is not a common presenting feature of breast cancer. Even bloody galactorrhea more often results from benign conditions, including mastitis. Some evidence suggests the risk of breast cancer is reduced in premenopausal women who have lactated.

18. **Are medications used for postpartum galactorrhea?**

    Not any more. Although the dopamine agonists bromocriptine and cabergoline are the drugs of choice for patients with prolactinomas, they are also effective for other causes of galactorrhea including postpartum galactorreha. However, in 1994, the manufacturer of bromocriptine withdrew postpartum lactation as a treatment indication following case reports of vascular side effects attributed to bromocriptine, including stroke and myocardial ischemia. Women who choose not to nurse can use other measures to manage galactorrhea postpartum. Measures to relieve the discomfort of postpartum breast engorgement include garments providing firm breast support, analgesics, and ice packs.

19. **What about galactorrhea in men?**

    Men rarely present for evaluation of galactorrhea as a primary presenting complaint despite the prevalence of 5% men in some series of patients evaluated for galactorrhea. Galactorrhea is uncommon even in hyperprolactinemic men due to the lack of estrogen priming necessary to prepare the breast for milk production. Despite the infrequency of galactorrhea in men, any man with galactorrhea should be examined for feminizing syndromes and a prolactin-producing pituitary tumor.

20. **Does galactorrhea always require treatment?**

    Not always. Generally, galactorrhea unaccompanied by amenorrhea, infertility, low bone mass or fragility fractures, or a pituitary tumor does not have serious long-term consequences if left untreated. Treatment is indicated to restore fertility and may be indicated when a pituitary tumor is present if the tumor is large or causing symptoms.

21. **Do microadenomas require treatment?**

    Microadenomas, which by definition are less than 1 cm in diameter, rarely seem to grow to macroadenomas. Spontaneous improvement with falling prolactin levels and return of menstruation can occur. However, if infertility or estrogen deficiency and low bone mass are present, even microprolactinomas may require treatment. Because macroadenomas do exist, continued observation is necessary in all patients with microprolactinomas.

22. **Why should macroadenomas be treated?**

    Macroadenomas associated with galactorrhea may require treatment to preserve vision threatened by expansion of the tumor towards the optic chiasma. Treatment may be necessary to control the excess cosecretion of another pituitary hormone causing a morbid condition. Cosecretion of growth hormone can cause acromegaly, and thyrotropin excess can result in goiter and hyperthyroidism. Despite the issue of potential secretion of multiple hormones, the fact remains that the most common tumors presenting with galactorrhea are prolactinomas.

23. **How are macroadenomas treated?**

    Transsphenoidal surgery for small prolactinomas initially showed postoperative success in about 80% of cases compared with the lower success rate of 50% for macroprolactinomas. Transsphenoidal surgery as the initial treatment of choice for microprolactinomas fell into disfavor when recurrence rates assessed several years postoperatively ranged from 17% to 91%. Now medical therapy with dopamine agonists is first-line therapy for all size categories of prolactinomas.

24. How do dopamine agonists work in the treatment of macroadenomas?

The dopamine agonists bromocriptine and cabergoline lower prolactin levels, shrink tumors, and can restore cyclic menstrual function in premenopausal women with prolactinomas. Serum prolactin levels must be reduced near or into the normal range to restore menses and control galactorrhea. Galactorrhea can decrease hours after treatment begins. Some reduction in tumor size occurs in 9 out of 10 patients. A 25% reduction in size occurs in nearly 8 out of 10. Surgery and radiation therapy are effective for tumors failing to respond to medications and for the occassional drug-intolerant patient. Radiation therapy stops tumor growth and causes a gradual decline in prolactin levels over many years. This slow decline in prolactin is accompanied by a progressive increase in the prevalence of radiation-induced hypopituitarism. Surgery and radiation should now be viewed as adjuncts to medical treatment rather than primary treatment for most prolactinoma patients.

25. What is macroprolactinemia?

Rarely, hyperprolactinemia results from the formation of prolactin multimers in the serum of patients without any sign of reproductive dysfunction or pituitary tumor. This has been called macroprolactinemia. Laboratories can investigate this by several techniques, including adding polyethylene glycol to the assay and serial dilution studies. Proceeding to pituitary imaging in such cases can be misleading because of the high frequency of unrelated pituitary abnormalities and incidentalomas.

26. What is the syndrome signaled by failure to lactate postpartum?

Sheehan syndrome, which is pituitary necrosis associated with childbirth, can lead to the failure to lactate and menstruate postpartum. Loss of pubic and axillary hair can also occur if deficiencies of prolactin and gonadotropins are accompanied by loss of corticotropin-dependent adrenal androgen secretion. Pituitary necrosis occurs after deliveries complicated by hypotension from sepsis or hemorrhage. In the United States, pituitary insufficiency from Sheehan syndrome is usually limited to deficient anterior pituitary functions. In some areas of the world with less readily available obstetric care, posterior pituitary necrosis can be more extensive, resulting in vasopressin deficiency and neurogenic diabetes insipidus. The mechanism for this is felt to be more prolonged and severe hypotension, leading to extension of the pituitary infarction to involve the neurohypophysis as well as the adenohypophysis.

27. Did Hippocrates speak of amenorrhea or galactorrhea?

His aphorisms show he did: "If a woman who is neither pregnant nor has given birth produces milk, her menstruation has stopped" (Aphorisms, Section V, No. 39).

In current times, it is conceivable that a woman with galactorrhea and amenorrhea after Googling the Internet for medical advice could seek treatment and pituitary imaging having already ruled out pregnancy with a home testing kit, hypothyroidism with a TSH from a self-serve reference laboratory, and confirmation of hyperprolactinemia with results from the same self-directed lab testing.

Hippocrates also spoke of early pregnancy and morning sickness: "If the catamenia are suppressed, without being followed by rigor or fever, but by disinclination for food, pregnancy may be suspected" (Aphorisms, Section V, No. 61). This aphorism reminds us that amenorrhea in women of reproductive age should always make pregnancy a prime consideration.

KEY POINTS: GALACTORRHEA

1. Many medications can cause galactorrhea.

2. Estrogen and prolactin are both necessary for milk production.

3. High levels of estrogen can inhibit lactation.

4. Not all nipple discharges are galactorrhea but if fat globules are present in the fluid the discharge is milk and galactorrhea is present.

5. Hyperprolactinemia can inhibit menstruation.

TOP SECRETS

1. Prolactin levels rise during pregnancy overlapping with the range of elevation found with prolactinomas.

2. Primary hypothyroidism can cause amenorrhea, galactorrhea, and pituitary enlargement and thus mimic a prolactinoma.

3. The absence of lactation postpartum can signify pituitary necrosis (Sheehan syndrome).

4. Painful lesions of the thoracic wall can induce galactorrhea.

5. When prolactin is elevated without disruption in menstrual function or galactorrhea, macroprolactinemia caused by circulating multimers of prolactin is a possible diagnosis.

WEBSITES

Family Practice Notebook. Available at: http://www.fpnotebook.com

BIBLIOGRAPHY

1. Bevan JS, Webster J, Burke CW, Scanlon MF: Dopamine agonists and pituitary tumor shrinkage. Endocr Rev 13:220–240, 1992.

2. Biller BM: Diagnostic evaluation of hyperprolactinemia. J Reprod Med 44(12 Suppl):1095–1099, 1999.

3. Dalkin AC, Marshall JC: Medical therapy of hyperprolactinemia. Endocrinol Metab Clin North Am 18:259–276, 1989.

4. Falkenberry SS: Nipple discharge. Obstet Gynecol Clin North Am. 29:21–29, 2002.

5. Fiorica JV: Nipple discharge. Obstet Gynecol Clin North Am 21:453–460, 1994.

6. Fradkin JE, Eastman RC, Lesniak MA, et al: Specificity spillover at the hormone receptor—exploring its role in human disease. N Engl J Med 320:640–645, 1989.

7. Kapcala LP: Galactorrhea and thyrotoxicosis. Arch Intern Med 144:2349–2350, 1984.

8. Kleinberg DL, Noel GL, Frantz AA: Galactorrhea: a study of 235 cases, including 48 pituitary tumors. N Engl J Med 296:589–600, 1977.

9. Klibanski A, Biller BMK, Rosenthal DI, et al: Effects of prolactin and estrogen deficiency in amenorrheic bone loss. J Clin Endocrinol Metab 67:124–130, 1988.

10. Larsen PR: Physiology and disorders of pituitary hormone axes, prolactin. Disorders of the female reproductive system. In *Williams textbook of endocrinology*, 10th ed, Philadelphia, 2003, Elsevier, pp. 207–208, 614–620.

11. Luciano AA: Clinical presentation of hyperprolactinemia. J Reprod Med 44(12 Suppl):1085–1090, 1999.

12. Mah PM, Webster J: Hyperprolactinemia: etiology, diagnosis, and management. Semin Reprod Med. 20:365–374, 2002.

13. Mehta AE, Reyes FI, Faiman C: Primary radiotherapy of prolactinomas: eight- to 15-year follow-up. Am J Med 83:49–58, 1987.

14. Molitch ME, Elton RL, Blackwell RE, et al: Bromocriptine as primary therapy for prolactin-secreting macroadenomas: results of a prospective multicenter study. J Clin Endocrinol Metab 60:698–705, 1985.

15. Pena KS, Rosenfeld JA. Evaluation and treatment of galactorrhea. Am Fam Physician 63:1763–1770, 2001.

16. Poretsky L, Garber J, Kleefield J: Primary amenorrhea and pseudoprolactinoma in a patient with primary hypothyroidism: reversal of clinical, biochemical and radiologic abnormalities with levothyroxine. Am J Med 81:180–182, 1986.

17. Rayburn WF: Clinical commentary: the bromocriptine (Parlodel) controversy and recommendations for lactation suppression. Am J Perinatol 13:69–71, 1996.

18. Schlechte JA: Prolactinoma. N Engl J Med 349:2035–2041, 2003.

19. Thomson JA, Davies DL, McLaren EH, et al: Ten-year follow-up of microprolactinoma treated by transsphenoidal surgery. BMJ 309:1409–1410, 1994.

20. Wieck A, Haddad PM. Anti-psychotic-induced hyperprolactinemia in women: pathophysiology, severity and consequences. Selective literature review. Br J Psychol 182:199–204, 2003.

CHAPTER 49

HIRSUTISM AND VIRILIZATION

Tamis M. Bright and Raul E. Storey

1. **Define hirsutism.**

   Hirsutism is the excessive growth of terminal hair in androgen-dependent areas: upper lip, chin, side burns, earlobes, tip of the nose, back, chest, areolae, axillae, lower abdomen, pubic triangle, and anterior thighs. Hirsutism is frequently associated with irregular menses and acne. Hirsutism should be distinguished from hypertrichosis, which is a nonandrogen-dependent increase in vellus hair. Hirsutism affects 5% to 10% of females.

2. **Define virilization.**

   Virilization consists of hirsutism, acne, and irregular menses along with signs of masculinization: deepening of the voice, increased muscle mass, temporal balding, clitoromegaly, and increased libido. Virilization results from high circulating levels of androgens, close to or in the male range, and is usually due to an androgen-secreting tumor.

3. **Where are androgens produced?**

   Twenty-five percent of testosterone comes from the ovaries, 25% from the adrenal glands, and 50% from peripheral conversion of androstenedione, which is produced by both the ovaries and adrenals. Testosterone is converted into dihydrotestosterone (DHT) by the enzyme 5-alpha reductase, which is present in hair follicles, or to estradiol by the aromatase enzyme present in adipose tissue (Fig. 49-1). DHT is responsible for the transformation of vellus into terminal hair. Hair follicles also contain the enzymes that convert dehydroepiandrosterone (DHEA), which is produced by the adrenals, and androstenedione into testosterone.

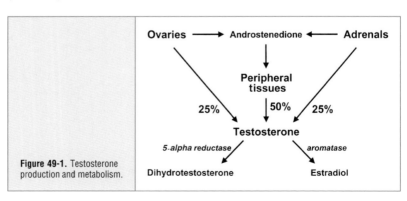

Figure 49-1. Testosterone production and metabolism.

4. **What causes hirsutism?**

   Hirsutism is caused by hyperandrogenism. Androgens transform the fine, downy, minimally pigmented vellus hair in androgen-sensitive areas into coarse, pigmented, terminal hair. An increase in any of the androgenic steroids may cause high levels of DHT in the hair follicle and result in hirsutism.

Low levels of sex hormone–binding globulin (SHBG), which is produced by the liver, may promote hirsutism. Eighty percent of circulating testosterone is bound to SHBG, 19% is bound to albumin, and 1% is free. Decreases in SHBG increase the free fraction of hormone available to androgen-sensitive hair.

Increased activity of 5-alpha reductase, even with normal circulating androgen levels, also may cause hirsutism by the excessive conversion of testosterone into DHT.

5. **List the conditions that result in hirsutism.**
   - Polycystic ovarian syndrome (PCOS)
   - Prolactinoma
   - Congenital adrenal hyperplasia (CAH)
   - Hypothyroidism
   - Idiopathic/familial hirsutism
   - Ovarian hyperthecosis
   - Cushing's syndrome
   - Medications

6. **Describe the pathophysiology of PCOS.**
   The exact cause of PCOS is unknown, but affected patients have been shown to have an accelerated rate of pulsatile gonadotropin-releasing hormone (GnRH) secretion from the hypothalamus. The gonadotropin secretory profile is highly dependent on the rate of GnRH pulsatility. Rapid GnRH pulses stimulate the secretion of luteinizing hormone (LH), but not follicle-stimulating hormone (FSH), from the pituitary gland. The increased LH/FSH secretory ratio results in arrested ovarian follicle development with cyst formation and hypertrophy of theca cells, leading to constant estrogen and increased androgen production with chronic anovulation.

7. **How does PCOS present?**
   PCOS affects 5% to 10% of premenopausal women and is a common cause of hirsutism and oligomenorrhea. The hirsutism is gradually progressive, usually beginning at puberty, and most patients have irregular menses from the onset of menarche. However, in a study of hirsute patients with regular menses, 50% had polycystic ovaries. PCOS patients also frequently have insulin resistance and hyperinsulinemia. Because insulin decreases SHBG and increases the ovarian androgen response to LH stimulation, the hyperinsulinemia contributes to the elevated free androgen levels in PCOS. Thus PCOS presents as a spectrum: some patients have minimal findings, whereas others have the entire constellation of hirsutism, acne, obesity, infertility, amenorrhea or oligomenorrhea, male pattern alopecia, acanthosis nigricans, hyperinsulinemia, and hyperlipidemia.

8. **Describe the pathophysiology of the hyperandrogenism in CAH.**
   CAH results from a deficiency of one of the key enzymes in the cortisol biosynthesis pathway; it often presents with precocious puberty and childhood hirsutism. Partial or late-onset CAH, owing to milder deficiencies of the same enzymes, may cause postpubertal hirsutism. Ninety percent of CAH is due to 21-hydroxylase deficiency, which causes a defect in the conversion of 17-hydroxyprogesterone (17-OHP) to 11-deoxycortisol and of progesterone to desoxycorticosterone (DOC). The resulting low cortisol production rate leads to hypersecretion of pituitary adrenocorticotropic hormone (ACTH), which stimulates overproduction of 17-OHP and progesterone, as well as adrenal androgens, particularly androstenedione (Fig. 49-2). Hirsutism results from the androgen excess.

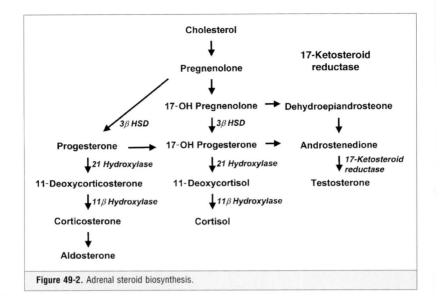

Figure 49-2. Adrenal steroid biosynthesis.

9. **Do any other causes of CAH result in hirsutism?**
   Deficiency of 11-beta-hydroxylase decreases the conversion of 11-deoxycortisol to cortisol and of DOC to corticosterone. This stimulates hypersecretion of ACTH, with consequent overproduction of 11-deoxycortisol, DOC, and androstenedione. Patients also frequently develop hypertension from the mineralocorticoid, DOC. Deficiency of 3-beta-hydroxysteroid dehydrogenase (3β HSD) decreases the conversion of pregnenolone to progesterone and 17-hydroxy-pregnenolone to 17-OHP. This defect increases pregnenolone, 17-hydroxypregnenolone, and the androgens DHEA, dehydroepiandrosterone sulfate (DHEAS), and androstenediol, which promote the development of hirsutism. Deficiency of 17-ketosteroid reductase decreases the conversion of androstenedione to testosterone, DHEA to androstenediol, and estrone to estradiol. Affected patients have elevated basal levels of androstenedione, DHEA, and estrone (see Fig. 49-2).

10. **Describe the pathophysiology of idiopathic and familial hirsutism.**
    Idiopathic hirsutism is believed to be caused by increased cutaneous activity of 5-alpha-reductase or enhanced skin sensitivity to androgens. Familial hirsutism is an ethnic tendency to have a higher density of hair follicles per unit area of skin. Mediterraneans and Hispanics have increased hair density, whereas Asians have lower density. Patients with idiopathic or familial hirsutism usually have the onset of hirsutism shortly after puberty with a slow subsequent progression. They have normal menses and fertility, as well as a normal hormonal profile.

11. **How do Cushing's syndrome, prolactinomas, and hypothyroidism cause hirsutism?**
    All causes of Cushing's syndrome may result in hypertrichosis because of increased vellus hair on the face, forehead, limbs, and trunk owing to cortisol hypersecretion. Cushing's syndrome due to an adrenal tumor also may produce hirsutism and virilization from increased secretion of androgens with cortisol.
    Hyperprolactinemia suppresses GnRH activity, which diminishes pulsatile LH secretion from the pituitary gland, resulting in decreased ovarian estrogen production and amenorrhea. Prolactin also increases the adrenal androgens, DHEA and DHEAS. Hypothyroidism decreases SHBG, leading to an increase in free testosterone.

12. **What is the pathophysiology of the hyperandrogenism in ovarian hyperthecosis?**
    Ovarian hyperthecosis is a nonneoplastic condition of the ovaries with proliferating islands of luteinized thecal cells in the ovarian stroma. Hyperthecosis causes overproduction of testosterone, androstenedione, and DHT to an even higher level than is usually seen in PCOS. LH and FSH are either normal or low, and the degree of insulin resistance and hyperinsulinemia is greater than in PCOS.

13. **Which medications can cause hirsutism?**
    Danazol, testosterone, glucocorticoids, metyrapone, phenothiazines, anabolic steroids, and oral contraceptives containing norgestrel and norethindrone can cause hirsutism. Phenytoin, cyclosporin, diazoxide, minoxidil, glucocorticoids, streptomycin, penicillamine, and psoralens can cause hypertrichosis.

14. **What conditions cause virilization?**

Ovarian Tumors	Adrenal Disorders
Thecoma	CAH
Fibrothecoma	Adenoma
Granulosa and granulosa-theca cell tumors	Carcinoma
Arrhenoblastoma (Sertoli-Leydig cell tumors)	
Hilus cell tumors	
Adrenal rest tumors of the ovary	
Luteoma of pregnancy	

KEY POINTS: PATHOGENESIS OF HIRSUTISM AND VIRILIZATION

1. Hirsutism is the excessive growth of terminal hair and is frequently associated with irregular menses.
2. Virilization consists of hirsutism and irregular menses associated with signs of masculinization.
3. Hirsutism and virilization usually result from excess androgens.
4. The common causes of hirsutism are polycystic ovarian syndrome, congenital adrenal hyperplasia (CAH), idiopathic/familial hirsutism, and medications.
5. The common causes of virilization are ovarian tumors, adrenal tumors, and CAH.

15. **When should a patient be evaluated for hirsutism?**
    Any patient with rapid development of hirsutism or coexistence of amenorrhea, irregular menses, or virilization should be evaluated. A patient with regular menses who shows significant concern about hirsutism also may warrant a workup.

16. **What information is important in the history?**
    - Age of onset, progression, and extent of hair growth
    - Current measures of hair removal and frequency of use
    - Age at menarche, regularity of menses, and fertility
    - Family history of hirsutism
    - Change in libido or change in voice
    - Symptoms of Cushing's disease, prolactinoma, or hypothyroidism
    - Medications

17. **What findings are important on physical examination?**
    - Distribution and degree of hirsutism
    - Increased muscle mass, temporal balding, clitoromegaly, or acne
    - Obesity
    - Acanthosis nigricans
    - Visual field defects
    - Moon facies, plethora, buffalo hump, supraclavicular fat pads, striae, or thin skin
    - Galactorrhea
    - Goiter, loss of lateral eyebrows, periorbital edema, dry skin, or delayed reflexes
    - Abdominal or pelvic masses

18. **What laboratory tests should be ordered for a patient with hirsutism?**
    Laboratory testing should be guided by the results of the history and physical examination. Many authors advocate against testing in patients with regular menses and only gradual progression of hirsutism. However, serum levels of total testosterone, DHEAS, 17-OHP, LH, and FSH can be useful tests, depending on the individual patient. Patients with signs or symptoms of hypothyroidism, hyperprolactinemia, or Cushing's syndrome also should be evaluated with serum TSH, prolactin, or 24-hour urine cortisol testing, respectively. Otherwise, these tests need not be obtained for every patient.

19. **How are the results of these laboratory tests interpreted?**
    For a patient without signs of virilization, it is important to differentiate idiopathic hirsutism, PCOS, and CAH because each is treated differently. Total testosterone, DHEAS, and 17-OHP help in the differentiation. Idiopathic hirsutism has normal levels on all three tests. PCOS has mildly increased testosterone, normal or slightly increased DHEAS, and normal 17-OHP. CAH has elevated testosterone and DHEAS and mild-to-marked elevation of 17-OHP. An early morning follicular phase level of 17-OHP greater than 500 ng/dL (normal $\leq$200 ng/dL) is diagnostic. In most patients with PCOS, LH is elevated, FSH is normal or low, and the ratio of LH to FSH should be greater than 2. However, not all patients with PCOS have an elevated LH, particularly those with obesity; thus LH and FSH are helpful in confirming but not excluding the diagnosis of PCOS.

20. **What do you do if a patient has borderline (200–500 ng/dL) elevations of 17-OHP?**
    A borderline elevated level requires an ACTH stimulation test with assessment of 17-OHP levels at baseline and 60 minutes after stimulation with ACTH. The levels are then plotted on a nomogram to determine normals, heterozygous carriers of the 21-OH gene, and patients with late-onset 21-OH deficiency. Some patients with late-onset 21-OH deficiency have normal baseline 17-OHP levels; however, the ACTH-stimulated levels are usually diagnostic.

21. **What laboratory tests should be ordered in a patient with virilization?**
    A patient with virilization should be evaluated to determine whether she has an ovarian tumor, an adrenal tumor, or CAH. As in patients without virilization, tests should include serum total testosterone, DHEAS, and 17-OHP. A markedly increased testosterone level (>200 ng/dL) with normal values on the other tests points to an ovarian tumor. High levels of DHEAS with or

without high testosterone levels suggest an adrenal tumor. Increased levels of 17-OHP with modest elevations of DHEAS and testosterone are more consistent with CAH. Laboratory values suggesting tumors should be followed with a transvaginal ultrasound of the ovaries or computed tomography (CT) of the adrenals or ovaries. If no mass is found, iodocholesterol scanning of the adrenals or venous sampling of the ovaries or adrenals can be performed for localization before surgical removal.

22. **How is PCOS treated in a patient desiring pregnancy?**
   If the patient's primary concern is fertility, clomiphene is the usual drug of choice. If clomiphene fails to induce ovulation, cyclic gonadotropin administration is often useful. Pulsatile GnRH also has been used with some success. In obese patients, weight reduction alone has been shown to increase the spontaneous ovulation rate. If a component of adrenal androgen (DHEAS) hypersecretion appears to be present, low-dose dexamethasone can be added in doses of 0.125 to 0.375 mg at night. This regimen may improve the ovulation rate, as well as decrease hirsutism. In patients resistant to medical management, surgical destruction of small sections of the ovaries induces ovulation in some patients. Wedge resection of the ovaries has been replaced by laparoscopic ovarian diathermy, in which laser or electrocautery is used to destroy portions of the ovaries.

23. **How is PCOS treated in a patient not desiring pregnancy?**
   If fertility is not the issue, oral contraceptives or cyclic progestins are used to induce regular menses and thereby decrease the risk of endometrial cancer. Preparations containing androgenic progestins, such as norgestrel and norethindrone, should be avoided. Weight reduction should be encouraged. As noted earlier, dexamethasone may be added in patients with an elevated DHEAS; however, this may increase glucose in an already glucose-intolerant patient. If hirsutism does not improve with these measures, the agents listed in questions 24 and 27 through 30 may be necessary.

24. **What can be done about the hyperinsulinemia of PCOS?**
   PCOS patients should be evaluated with a fasting blood glucose or an oral glucose tolerance test and a lipid profile because of the high prevalence of glucose intolerance, diabetes, and hyperlipidemia in this disorder. These problems should be addressed separately because they are not resolved by treating the hyperandrogenism alone. The insulin sensitizers metformin and thiazolidinediones have been used in PCOS patients with and without increased glucose levels. Treatment with troglitazone, the first thiazolidinedione, decreased androgens and increased SHBG but was withdrawn from the market because of liver toxicity. The newer thiazolidinediones rosiglitazone and pioglitazone, as well as metformin, improve insulin resistance, decrease androgens, increase SHBG, improve regularity of menses, and increase fertility. In patients not controlled on metformin alone, there is some added benefit in combination with pioglitazone resulting in further increases in SHBG, insulin sensitivity, and improved menstrual regularity. The hypothalamic peptide somatostatin mainly decreases growth hormone secretion but also decreases the LH response to GnRH and inhibits pancreatic insulin release. Therefore octreotide, a somatostatin analog, and the long-acting release formulation, octreotide-LAR, have been investigated in PCOS treatment. Octreotide-LAR decreases insulin, improves insulin sensitivity, decreases androgens, improves hirsuitism, and increases ovulation. Although the standard octreotide shows similar results, its multiple daily subcutaneously injections make it a poor choice compared to the octreotide-LAR dosing of one intramuscular injection every 28 days.

25. **What is the treatment for CAH?**
   Glucocorticoid replacement decreases ACTH secretion and thereby reduces excessive adrenal androgen production. Mineralocorticoid replacement is also required in some causes of CAH. Treatment with the regimens listed in questions 26 through 30 can hasten improvement of the hirsutism.

26. **Describe how oral contraceptive pills are used for the treatment of hirsutism.**
Oral contraceptive pills (OCPs) are the most commonly used therapy. They increase serum estrogens and SHBG, which decreases free testosterone levels. Monophasic and triphasic preparations work equally well. Preparations containing the progestins desogestrel, norgestimate, drospirenone, and gestodene are believed to be the best because they are the least androgenic. Potential side effects include weight gain, bloating, nausea, emotional lability, breast pain, and deep venous thrombosis.

27. **Describe how antiandrogens are used for the treatment of hirsutism.**
Spironolactone is an androgen receptor blocker and a weak inhibitor of testosterone production. Side effects include diuresis, fatigue, and dysfunctional uterine bleeding. Initial doses are 25 to 100 mg twice daily, tapered to 25 to 50 mg/day after an effect has been seen. Flutamide, another androgen receptor blocker, is dosed at 62.5 to 250 mg once or twice daily. Side effects include increased liver function tests (LFTs) and rare fatal hepatotoxicity. Finasteride, a 5-alpha-reductase inhibitor, effectively decreases hirsutism. Side effects include headache and depression. Dosage is 2.5 to 7.5 mg/day. The antiandrogens are usually used in combination with OCPs for additive effects and to give adequate birth control because antiandrogens can feminize a male fetus.

28. **Describe how GnRH agonists are used for the treatment of hirsutism.**
By providing constant rather than pulsatile GnRH levels to the pituitary, GnRH agonists reduce gonadotropin secretion and thereby decrease ovarian production of both estrogen and androgen. Estrogen replacement must be given to avoid hot flashes, vaginal dryness, and bone density loss. Leuprolide (3.75 mg/month intramuscularly), buserelin or nafarelin nasal spray (3 times/day), and goserelin subcutaneous implants effectively reduce hirsutism. Some studies demonstrate an increased effect over OCPs alone, whereas others show similar effects. The preparations are expensive and thus are usually reserved for severe PCOS.

KEY POINTS: DIAGNOSIS AND TREATMENT OF HIRSUTISM AND VIRILIZATION

1. Appropriate laboratory testing includes at least total testosterone, dehydroepiandrosterone sulfate, and 17-hydroxyprogesterone.

2. Treatment of hirsutism is usually with the combination of oral contraceptive pills, spironolactone, eflornithine, and cosmetic measures; however, gonadotropin-releasing hormone agonists and antiandrogens can be used.

3. Polycystic ovarian syndrome patients may have improvement of symptoms if treated with insulin sensitizers.

4. Treatment of virilization is surgical removal of the tumor or steroid treatment for CAH.

29. **What topical agent is approved for the treatment of hirsutism?**
Eflornithine HCl 13.9% cream is the newest agent for the treatment of facial hirsutism. Eflornithine HCl irreversibly inhibits ornithine decarboxylase, an enzyme necessary for hair follicle cell division. Inhibition of ornithine decarboxylase results in a decreased rate of hair growth. In clinical trials, 58% of patients had marked improvement or some improvement as compared with 34% of controls after 24 weeks of treatment. The most common side effects encountered were acne, pseudofolliculitis barbae, burning, tingling, erythema, or rash over the applied area. Generally, side effects resolved without treatment and rarely required

discontinuation of the medication. The cream is applied to the face twice daily. The patients' hirsutism returned to baseline by 8 weeks following discontinuation of the medication.

30. **What cosmetic measures can be used for the treatment of hirsutism?**
Bleaching, shaving, plucking, waxing, depilating, and electrolysis are effective measures that can be used alone or in combination with the previously described treatments. They remove terminal hair that is already present while the patient waits for medications to decrease new growth and rate of transformation to terminal hair.
Laser-assisted hair removal is an effective treatment for hirsutism. It is an outpatient procedure that uses ruby, alexandrite, diode, or yttrium aluminum garnet lasers, or intense pulsed light therapy, all of which cause thermal injury to the hair follicle. At least three to six treatments about 2 to 2.5 months apart are required. The techniques result in removal of hair, and a period of 2 to 6 months before the regrowth of hair, which is thinner and lighter. Alexandrite and diode lasers appear to be the most effective. Patients with light skin and dark hair have the best results with the fewest side effects. The side effects include minimal discomfort, local edema and erythema lasting 24 to 48 hours, rare petechiae, and infrequent hyperpigmentation lasting less than 6 months.

31. **How do you choose the appropriate therapy for the patient's hirsutism?**
Most patients are given a trial of OCPs, with or without spironolactone, and are advised to use cosmetic measures while waiting for the medications to work. The new topical cream eflornithine HCl may be used alone or in combination with other measures. Because of their more serious side effects and higher cost, the other medications are reserved for the most severe cases in which OCPs and spironolactone fail. No matter what therapy is chosen, the patient must be made aware that results will not be seen for at least 3 to 6 months. Although many medications and combinations have been used, only topical eflornithine HCl is currently approved by the Food and Drug Administration for treatment of hirsutism. Unfortunately, most patients will have a relapse of hirsutism approximately 12 months after discontinuation of medical therapy.

WEBSITES

1. Atlas of Dermatology. Available at: http://www.dermis.net/dermisroot/en/35888/diagnose.htm
2. eMedicine. Available at: http://www.emedicine.com/med/topic1017.htm

BIBLIOGRAPHY

1. Blank SK, McCartney CR, Marshall JC: The origins and sequelae of abnormal neuroendocrine function in polycystic ovary syndrome. Hum Reprod Update 12:351–361, 2006.
2. Lowenstein EJ: Diagnosis and management of the dermatologic manifestations of the polycystic ovary syndrome. Dermatol Ther 19:210–223, 2006.
3. Moghetti P, Tosi F, Tosti A, et al: Comparison of spironolactone, flutamide, and finasteride efficacy in the treatment of hirsutism: a randomized, double blind, placebo-controlled trial. J Clin Endocrinol Metab 85:89–94, 2000.
4. Ortega-González C, Luna S, Hernández L, et al: Responses of serum androgen and insulin resistance to metformin and pioglitazone in obese, insulin-resistant women with polycystic ovary syndrome. J Clin Endocrinol Metab. 90:1360–1365, 2005.

5. Pasquali R, Gambineri A: Insulin-sensitizing agents in polycystic ovary syndrome. Eur J Endocrinol 154:763–775, 2006.

6. Randall VA, Lanigan S, Hamzavi I, Chamberlain JL: New dimensions in hirsutism. Lasers Med Sci 21:126–133, 2006.

7. Rosenfield R: Hirsutism. N Engl J Med 353:2578–2588, 2005.

8. Speroff L, Fritz M: *Clinical gynecologic endocrinology and infertility*, ed 7, Baltimore, 2004, Lippincott Williams & Wilkins.

9. Smith SR, Piacquadio DJ, Beger B, Littler C: Eflornithine cream combined with laser therapy in the management of unwanted facial hair growth in women: a randomized trial. Dermatol Surg 32:1237–1243, 2006.

10. Wolf JE Jr, Shander D, Huber F, et al: Randomized, double-blind clinical evaluation of the efficacy and safety of topical eflornithine HCl 13.9% cream in the treatment of women with facial hair. Int J Dermatol 46:94–98, 2007.

CHAPTER 50

MENOPAUSE

William J. Georgitis

1. **Define menopause.**

   Menopause is the cessation of normal cyclic ovarian function. Menopause encompasses approximately one third of a woman's life span beginning with the transition phase spanning the latter reproductive years up to the final menstruation and then extends for the remainder of life. The final menstruation marks menopause for each woman and therefore can only be established retrospectively.

2. **When do ovulatory cycles decrease in frequency?**

   Ovulatory cycles usually decrease in frequency around age 38 to 42 years.

3. **When does menopause usually occur?**

   The median age for the last menses is 51.4 years. The range for menopause is broad. Ninety percent of women cease menstruating by age 55.

4. **What determines the timing of menopause?**

   Menses cease when the supply of ovarian oocytes is exhausted. Oocyte numbers peak in utero then decline in number rapidly. Approximately 80% of the oocytes vanish before birth. It is a curious fact that atresia rather than ovulation is the destiny of most oocytes (Fig. 50-1).

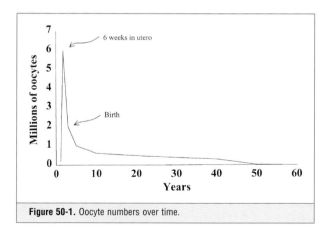

Figure 50-1. Oocyte numbers over time.

5. **What is premature ovarian failure? What causes it?**

   Cessation of cyclic ovarian function before age 35 years is considered premature. Either an inadequate complement of follicles from birth or accelerated follicular attrition results in premature menopause. Causes for premature ovarian failure include mumps oophoritis, irradiation, chemotherapy, autoimmune destruction, and genetic defects. The incidence of premature ovarian failure in women in the United States is about 0.3%. Approximately 146,000 cases occurred in 2000.

6. **Does the age of menopause vary with race, body size, age of menarche, geography, or socioeconomic conditions?**
No. Although the evidence against these factors being significant factors in the timing of menopause continues to be sparse. It is known that menopause occurs about 2 years earlier in cigarette smokers and that nulliparous women tend to experience an earlier menopause than multiparous women. Presumably, the months spent in the gravid state increase the duration of a multiparous woman's reproductive function. The severity of menopausal hot flashes does seem to vary somewhat with race.

7. **Does the appearance of the ovaries change with menopause?**
Yes, each ovary shrinks, and its surface becomes wrinkled. Transvaginal ultrasounds in 58,673 women demonstrated the mean ovarian volume was 4.9 cm^3 in premenopausal women and 2.2 cm^3 in postmenopausal women. Cortical width diminishes, whereas interstitial and hilar cells become more prominent, giving the stroma a hyperplastic appearance.

8. **What is the predominant circulating estrogen in menopause?**
Estradiol is the most abundant serum estrogen during the reproductive years. In menopause, estrone becomes the principal estrogen. Estrone is predominantly derived from adipose tissue conversion of adrenal androstenedione. Estrone is less biologically potent than estradiol. Atrophic changes after menopause affecting breast, vaginal mucosa, and pelvic musculature especially in leaner women with low adipose tissue mass can prompt woman to seek assistance for symptoms related to these changes including dyspareunia, urinary incontinence, and adjustment to changes in body configuration.

9. **What is a hot flash? Should it be called a flush?**
These terms refer to menopausal spells lasting seconds to minutes or rarely as long as an hour. Symptoms include a sudden reddening of the skin accompanied by a sensation of warmth. In some women, this is followed by profuse sweating. Body surface temperature rises, and core temperature falls mediated by hypothalamic-directed, vasomotor dilatation of surface blood vessels. The physiology of the flush or flash is complex. Catecholamines, prostaglandins, endorphins, and other neuropeptides all seem to participate.
   Both terms flash and flush, appear in the medical literature. Each is appropriately descriptive with flush apt y emphasizing vasodilatation and flash signifying the abrupt onset and brief duration of the spells. Many menopausal women also describe prodromal auras.

10. **Hot flushes are accompanied by surges in luteinizing hormone. Does excess luteinizing hormone trigger the spells?**
No. The luteinizing hormone (LH) surge is an epiphenomenon. Hypophysectomized women lacking LH pulsatility still may experience menopausal hot flushes. Furthermore, women with gonadal dysgenesis have highly elevated levels of gonadotropins but may fail to manifest hot flushes until after estrogen treatment and subsequent withdrawal. The hypothalamus appears to require priming with estrogens before later demonstrating episodic vasomotor instability in response to deficient levels of estrogen.

11. **Do all women develop menopausal vasomotor hot flushes? Do they last indefinitely?**
Approximately 85% of women experience vasomotor symptoms after menopause. The severity of the symptoms seems somewhat related to the rate of decline in estrogen levels. Women with abrupt decreases in estrogen levels following ovariectomy are often bothered the most. Left untreated, hot flushes tend to diminish.

12. **Are all menopausal symptoms clearly related to estrogen deficiency?**
No. Many symptoms are clearly nonspecific and could have other etiologies. Consider fatigue, nervousness, headache, insomnia, depression, irritability, joint pain, muscle pain, dizziness,

palpitations, and formication. Formication is a paresthesia resembling the sensation of ants crawling over the skin.

13. **What important physiologic changes accompany menopause?**
Hot flushes, urogenital atrophy, loss of bone calcium, increased rates of coronary heart disease, and alterations in serum lipids, including rises in low-density lipoprotein cholesterol and triglycerides with declines in high-density lipoprotein cholesterol, all occur during menopause.

14. **What is the principal cause of death in postmenopausal women?**
Cardiovascular disease. One in two women will die of heart disease or stroke, whereas only 1 in 25 will die of breast cancer.

15. **Does male menopause exist?**
Not really. Although hypogonadal men may suffer spells and accelerated loss of bone mineral similar to hypogonadal women, such symptoms do not represent a physiologically programmed event. A man complaining of hot flushes should first prompt testing to confirm hypogonadism. After a diagnosis of male hypogonadism is confirmed, it should be followed by a careful investigation for the cause.

16. **Historical records indicate the age of menarche has decreased over the centuries, perhaps as a result of improved nutrition and general health. Is this also true for the timing of menopause?**
No. Although the average age for first menstruation may have become lower as a result of improved nutrition and general health, a downward shift in the average age of menopause has not been recorded. Perhaps ongoing studies will confirm such changes in the future.

17. **How does one establish a diagnosis of menopause?**
In a woman more than 45 years old, 12 months of secondary amenorrhea suffices to diagnose menopause. Pelvic examination might confirm the impression by showing signs of atrophic vaginal mucosa. Often the pelvic exam may be unremarkable.
Laboratory tests alone also are not reliable for diagnosis. Toward the end of a woman's fertile years, serum levels of follicle-stimulating hormone (FSH) gradually rise. Anovulatory periods occur and may be accompanied by menorrhagia. After amenorrhea is well established, gonadotropins may become tonically elevated. FSH rises 10- to 20-fold, whereas elevations in LH are more modest in the range of 3-fold elevations. Levels of FSH above 40 IU/L are generally considered diagnostic of menopause or ovarian failure. However, hot flashes and gondatropin elevations may not be present in menopause especially in the presence of obesity. However, elevated gonadotropin levels alone may be misleading because the midcycle surge in gonadotropins before ovulation can give rise to LH and FSH levels that reach into the menopausal range.

18. **What routes of administration can be used for menopausal hormone replacement, and how effective are estrogens in relieving hot flushes?**
Routes of administration include oral, topical, and vaginal. All are effective with a dose-related response. Schemes for delivering the hormones include sequential dosing of estrogen and progestogen to mimic the normal hormone level variations through the menstrual cycle, continuous combined administration of estrogen and progestogen, and long cycle therapy in which the progestogen is administered a few times each year rather than on a repeating monthly schedule. Randomized trials with estrogen therapy show treatment reduces the severity of hot flushes from 80% to 95%.

19. **What are the most common indications for menopausal hormone replacement therapy?**
The most common indications are for relief of vasomotor symptoms or symptoms associated with urogenital atrophy. Short courses of treatment are now more often recommended over lifelong replacement.

KEY POINTS: MENOPAUSE

1. Menopause encompasses approximately one third of a woman's life.

2. The mean ovarian volume determined by transvaginal ultrasound of 2.2 cm^3 for postmenopausal women is less than half the mean ovarian volume found for premenopausal women.

3. Hormone replacement after menopause still may be used for relief of menopausal hot flushes.

4. Androgen replacement therapy for postmenopausal women is controversial.

5. The menopausal transition phase with accompanying symptoms or subtle changes in menstrual parameters and hormone levels precedes the final menstruation used to define menopause by several years.

20. **What levels of estradiol and estrone are achieved with replacement?**
Oral conjugated equine estrogens (0.625 mg), micronized estradiol (1.0 mg), and estrone sulfate (1.25 mg) deliver peak estradiol levels of 30 to 40 pg/mL and peak estrone levels of 150 to 250 pg/mL. Intravaginal estrogens yield levels approximately one fourth those achieved with oral regimens.

21. **Can gonadotropin levels be used to monitor adequacy or safety of replacement?**
No. Unlike primary hypothyroidism, in which the serum TSH can be used to individualize requirements for thyroxine replacement, gonadotropin levels remain elevated despite sex steroid replacement in many postmenopausal women. This elevation may result from a deficiency in inhibin, a polypeptide hormone normally produced by ovarian granulosa cells to inhibit secretion of FSH. If estrogen therapy is used for relief of menopausal symptoms, the therapy must be gauged by the response in symptoms and signs, not by gonadotropin levels.

22. **A major shift away from the use of estrogen replacement resulted from results of trials sponsored by the Women's Health Initiative. What were those trials and results that so dramatically shifted medical and public opinion away from the use of hormone replacement for menopause?**
In 2002, the Women's Health Initiative (WHI) published the results of hormone therapy trials investigating cardiovascular disease and the risks for thrombotic events associated with the use of estrogen alone and estrogen plus progesterone in 27,347 postmenopausal women. Risks outweighed benefits.
Both the estrogen alone and estrogen combined with progesterone replacement regimens increased the risk of stroke and blood clots while failing to prevent heart disease.
A survey before the WHI showed that only 3% to 10% of women stayed on hormone replacement for more than 5 years.

23. **What happened to sales of premarin?**

Premarin derives both the conjugated estrogens it contains and its name from pregnant mares urine. Sales had two major declines in sales over the past 50 years. Sales nearly doubled from 1960 to 1975 when the treatment of estrogen deficiency was widely promulgated by lay literature. Clinical trials published in 1975 reporting the increased risk of endometrial cancer from estrogen treatment provoked the first major sales decline. The addition of progesterone and rejuvenated enthusiasm for menopausal replacement therapy to prevent osteoporosis and improve lipid profiles in hopes of preventing cardiovascular disease led to a recovery in sales. By 1992, Premarin became the most frequently prescribed drug in the United States. A second major decline in Premarin sales followed the WHI publication in 2002 reporting increased cardiovascular and breast cancer risk. Sales decreased abruptly by 50%.

More recent publications from the WHI suggest that that short-term use of replacement hormones in menopause is not associated with increased risk of breast cancer, heart attack or stroke. Therefore hormone replacement to improve the quality of life by relieving menopausal vasomotor symptoms may increase once again. Low doses and short-term use is now recommended. Its use in older women should be determined on a case-by-case basis, factoring in individual cardiovascular disease risk factors.

24. **What alternative therapies may be used for the menopausal woman in lieu of estrogen replacement?**

Clonidine may be tried at bedtime for the relief of hot flushes, but side effects, including dry mouth and hypotension, limit its use. Medroxyprogesterone in a daily pill or as a depot injection every 3 months may also relieve hot flushes. Side effects are common. Some patients respond favorably to the antidepressant fluoxetine, but randomized trials of both selective serotonin-reuptake inhibitors and serotonin-norepinephrine reuptake inhibitors have not always confirmed their efficacy. Gabapentin shows modest ability to reduce hot flushes but also has side effects. Herbal preparations and dietary supplements are not regulated by the U.S. Food and Drug Administration (FDA), and safety and efficacy data are lacking. Widely used alternatives to prescribed hormones for hot flushes include black cohosh and soy, which have benefits attributed to phytoestrogens and side effects that have prompted regulatory agencies of some countries to recommend use for no longer than 6 months. Designer estrogen regimens, although widely advertised, also are not regulated, and so are lacking in standards for composition comparable to FDA-approved hormone prescription medications. These preparations contain estrogens that likely carry risks similar to other prescription estrogens.

25. **What about the diagnosis of androgen deficiency and its treatment in menopause?**

The endocrine society published a consensus statement recommending against making a diagnosis of androgen deficiency in women due to the lack of a well-defined clinical syndrome and the lack of normative data on testosterone levels across the life span to define androgen deficiency. Short-term treatment with testosterone in selected conditions such as surgical menopause can be efficacious, but the generalized use of testosterone by women was not recommended because the indications for treatment are currently inadequate and evidence of safety in long-term studies is still lacking.

26. **What web textbook might you recommend for providers seeking information about menopause?**

Endotext.com has a section titled "Female Reproductive Endocrinology," Robert W. Rebar, Editor; Chapter 11 is devoted to "Menopause and Hormone Replacement" by Michelle P. Warren and Jennifer E. Dominguez.

27. **What websites have good materials on menopause for patients?**
Two places to start include acog.org and menopause.org, representing the American College of Obstetricians and Gynecologists and the North American Menopause Society, respectively.

TOP SECRETS

1. Menopause occurs about 2 years earlier in cigarette smokers.

2. Nulliparous women experience menopause earlier than multiparous women.

3. The median age for the last menses is 51.4 years.

4. Premature ovarian failure is indicated by cessation of cyclic ovarian function before 35 years of age.

KEY POINTS: KEY WORDS

- Flush and flash
- Premature ovarian failure
- Gonadotropin
- Oocyte

WEBSITES

1. http://www.Endotext.com
2. http://www.acog.org
3. http://www.menopause.org

BIBLIOGRAPHY

1. Amundsen, DW, Diers CJ: The age of menopause in medieval Europe. Hum Biol 45:605–612, 1973.

2. Daly E, Gray A, Barlow D, et al: Measuring the impact of menopausal symptoms on the quality of life. BMJ 307:836–840, 1993.

3. Grady, D: Clinical practice. Management of menopausal symptoms. N Engl J Med 355:2338–2347, 2006.

4. McKinlay SM, Brambilla DJ, Posner JG: The normal menopause transition. Maturitas 14:103–115, 1992.

5. Pavlik EJ, DePriest PD, Gallion HH, et al: Ovarian volume related to age. Gynecol Oncol 77:410–412, 2000.

6. Rossouw JE, Anderson GL, Prentice RL, et al: Risks and benefits of estrogen plus progestin in healthy postmenopausal women: principal results from the Women's Health Initiative randomized controlled trial. JAMA 228:321–333, 2002.

7. Walsh BW, Ginsburg ES: Menopause. In Ryan KJ, editor, *Kistner's gynecology & women's health*, ed 7, St. Louis, 1999, Mosby. pp. 540–569.

8. Wierman, ME, Basson R, Davis SR, et al: Androgen therapy in women: an Endocrine Society clinical practice guideline. J Clin Endocrinol Metab 91:3697–3710, 2006.

CHAPTER 51

USE AND ABUSE OF ANABOLIC-ANDROGENIC STEROIDS AND ANDROGEN PRECURSORS

Kurt J. Reyes and Homer J. LeMar, Jr.

1. What are anabolic-androgenic steroids?

Anabolic-androgenic steroids (AASs) are a group of steroid hormones derived from chemical modification of testosterone. Their name is often shortened to anabolic steroids. The term "anabolic" refers to their ability to promote positive nitrogen balance and accretion of lean body mass. Androgenic refers to masculinization induced by these hormones. Although potency varies among various AASs, all possess both androgenic and anabolic properties.

2. Summarize the biological effects of AASs.

Endogenous AASs have diverse effects. The most prominent are effects on male sexual differentiation and secondary sexual characteristics, including growth and development of the prostate, seminal vesicles, penis and scrotum, beard, pubic, chest, and axillary hair; thickening of the vocal cords and enlargement of the larynx. AASs promote nitrogen retention, increase lean body mass, and alter fat distribution. They also stimulate release of clotting factors and erythropoietin with a secondary increase in hematocrit.

3. How do AASs exert their effects?

AASs act by binding to a specific receptor known as the androgen receptor. Both androgenic and anabolic effects appear to be mediated through the same receptor. Testosterone may bind directly to the androgen receptor or be converted by 5-alpha reductase to dihydrotestosterone, which binds to the receptor more tightly than does testosterone. Some testosterone is converted to estradiol by an enzyme in peripheral tissues called aromatase. Estradiol can then bind to the estrogen receptor.

4. Where are androgen receptors located?

Androgen receptors are present in many tissues, including the reproductive organs, skeletal muscle, bone, kidney, liver, brain, cardiac muscle, skin, fat, hematopoietic tissue, larynx, and thymus.

5. Why is it necessary to modify testosterone to make clinically useful AASs?

When administered orally, testosterone is rapidly metabolized by the first-pass effect through the gut and liver. The first-pass effect prevents any significant rise in plasma testosterone levels with oral intake of unmodified testosterone. Intramuscular injection of unmodified testosterone is also not useful because absorption is too rapid and duration of action is too short.

6. How is testosterone modified to make AASs?

Alkylation of testosterone at the 17-alpha position confers resistance to hepatic metabolism and results in AASs that can be administered orally. Esterification of testosterone at the 17-b-hydroxy position results in a hydrophobic molecule, which allows testosterone to be mixed with a fatty vehicle (sesame oil) and given by intramuscular injection. Also, the addition of carbon chains to the ring structure of testosterone increases fat solubility and extends the duration of action.

7. **What routes of administration are available?**
    Testosterone comes in oral, parenteral, patch, and gel forms. Sublingual and transbuccal preparations are also now available.

8. **What are the indications for AAS therapy?**
    AASs are indicated for use in male hypogonadism, constitutional delay of growth and puberty, hereditary angioneurotic edema, endometriosis, and fibrocystic breast disease; they also can benefit patients with aplastic or hypoplastic anemias. Androgens are useful in the anemia of end-stage renal disease but have been largely replaced by recombinant erythropoietin. Indications of specific agents are listed in Table 51-1.

9. **Are there any other potential uses for AASs?**
    AASs may help elderly men by increasing body weight and muscle mass, preventing bone loss, and improving the hematocrit. They also may be useful as male contraceptives. Both areas are under investigation. AASs are potentially useful in many other disorders, including severe chronic obstructive pulmonary disease and other wasting syndromes, autoimmune disorders, other hematologic disorders, alcoholic hepatitis, Turner's syndrome (by improving height), and osteoporosis

10. **Which of the indications in question 8 is the most common use of AASs?**
    Most likely none. The illegal use of AASs to enhance sports performance or physical appearance probably represents the single most common use. Abuse is widespread based on the belief that their anabolic properties will enhance the response to physical training, especially weight training.

KEY POINTS: INDICATIONS FOR ANABOLIC-ANDROGENIC STEROIDS

1. Male hypogonadism

2. Constitutional delay of growth and puberty

3. Hereditary angioneurotic edema

4. Endometriosis

5. Fibrocystic breast disease

6. Aplastic or hypoplastic anemias

11. **How common is abuse of AASs?**
    The true prevalence of AAS abuse is not known. An estimated 2 to 3 million American athletes have used AASs. Approximately 50% to 80% of body builders, weight lifters, and power lifters may use AASs.

12. **Who is at risk for using illegal AASs?**
    Use is highest among body builders and participants in sports favoring larger or stronger athletes. Because AASs increase the hematocrit through enhanced erythropoietin production, they may also be used by athletes participating in endurance-oriented sports. Nonathletes may use AASs solely to improve appearance. Surveys have shown a 5% to 11% prevalence of use among high school students. Most users are men, although up to 2% may be women. Other risk factors include involvement in school sports and the use of other illicit drugs, alcohol, or tobacco.

TABLE 51-1. ANABOLIC-ANDROGENIC STEROIDS AVAILABLE IN THE UNITED STATES

AAS	Use
Parenteral Agents	
Testosterone cypionate	Male hypogonadism
Testosterone enanthate	Male hypogonadism; delayed puberty; metastatic breast cancer (skeletal) 1-5 years after menopause
Testosterone propionate	Male hypogonadism; delayed puberty
Transdermal testosterone patches	Male hypogonadism; delayed puberty
Transdermal testosterone gel	Male hypogonadism; delayed puberty; concerns for transmission to female partners unlikely but of theoretical risk
Oral Agents (17-a-methylated)	
Methyl testosterone	Male hypogonadism; delayed puberty; combined with estrogen for menopausal vasomotor symptoms; metastatic breast cancer (skeletal) 1-5 years after menopause
Oxandrolone	Promotes weight gain after extensive surgery, trauma, chronic infections, prolonged corticosteroid therapy; bone pain in osteoporosis
Stanozolol	Hereditary angioedema
Danazol	Endometriosis; fibrocystic breast disease; hereditary angioedema
Fluoxymesterone	Male hypogonadism; delayed puberty; androgen-responsive breast cancer (recurrent) 1-5 years after menopause
Sublingual Agent	
Testosterone cyclodextrin	Male hypogonadism
Buccal Agent	
Testosterone buccal system	Male hypogonadism
Under Investigation	
Testosterone buciclate	Sustained-released preparation with action up to 12 weeks
Testosterone undecenoate	Sustained-released preparation with action up to 8 weeks

13. **Do AASs truly help athletes?**

Both athletes and coaches are likely to answer unequivocally, "Yes." AASs used in conjunction with adequate protein and carbohydrate intake, and proper training in experienced athletes seems to induce greater and more rapid gains than training and diet alone. In the past, studies were unable to show consistent gains in size and strength from AAS use in eugonadal men. However, a study comparing supraphysiological doses of testosterone enanthate with placebo in eugonadal men found clear increases in muscle size and strength, with or without weight-training exercise.

14. **How do AASs help athletes?**
Proposed mechanisms for increased size, strength, and performance include the anabolic effects of enhanced nitrogen retention and protein synthesis, anticatabolic effects of blocking cortisol at its receptor, and the psychological effect of increased motivation.

15. **What doses of AASs are used in attempts to enhance sports performance and appearance?**
Doses used for illicit purposes are markedly higher (10-fold or more) than therapeutic doses. Furthermore, multiple agents are often used in so-called stacking regimens or arrays. The drugs are often taken in 6- to 12-week cycles with variable periods off the drugs, but some athletes may use them as long as 1 year or more. Human chorionic gonadotropin may be used at the end of a cycle to stimulate gonadal function. Little is known about precise doses or stacking regimens; however, some anecdotal information is available, and examples of dosages are given in Table 51-2 in comparison to the usual therapeutic doses.

TABLE 51-2. COMPARISON OF DOSES IN THERAPEUTIC USE VERSUS ABUSE OF AASs*

AAS	Therapeutic Dose	Abuse
Testosterone cypionate	200 mg every 2 weeks	200-800 mg/week
Testosterone enanthate	200 mg every 2 weeks	200-800 mg/week
Oxandrolone	2.5 mg 2-4 times/day	2.5-8 mg/day or more
Stanozolol	2 mg 3 times/day, then once daily on alternate days	8-12 mg/day

AASs, anabolic-androgenic steroids.
*The doses for abuse are estimates from anecdotal data and may vary considerably in individual users. Two to five or more AASs are often combined at these or higher doses, yielding even higher total doses.

16. **How do athletes get AASs?**
AASs may be smuggled into the United States from countries where they are easily purchased without prescription. Some physicians may also prescribe them, and some AASs may be obtained from veterinarians. A significant black market exists, in which some of the preparations are fraudulent and potentially dangerous. A simple Internet search yields several companies outside the United States that do not require a presciption for AASs. Furthermore, websites also suggest various strategies to help avoid or reduce the side effects of AASs.

17. **What are the potential adverse effects of AAS use?**
A wide range of side effects have occurred with AAS use and abuse. See Table 51-3.

18. **What about side effects in women and children?**
All of the adverse effects mentioned earlier may occur in women and children. Women may experience oligomenorrhea or amenorrhea with inhibition of gonadotropin secretion. Such effects may reverse with cessation of AAS use. Virilizing effects, including hirsutism, clitoromegaly, and deepening of the voice, may not be reversible. Premature epiphyseal closure with a reduction in final adult height is an additional concern in adolescents using AASs.

TABLE 51–3. POTENTIAL ADVERSE EFFECTS OF AAS USE AND ABUSE

System Affected	Adverse Effects
Reproductive	Testicular atrophy, oligospermia, azoospermia, and priapism
Hepatotoxicity	Cholestatic hepatitis, peliosis hepatis (hemorrhagic liver cysts), and both benign and malignant hepatic tumors; predominantly with the 17-alkylated oral agents
Cardiovascular	Stroke and myocardial infarction reported in weight lifters
Hematologic	Increases in platelet count and aggregation; ventricular thrombosis and systemic embolism have been reported
Psychological	Aggressive behavior, psychotic symptoms, dependence and withdrawal
Lipid profile	Reduced high-density lipoprotein and higher low-density lipoprotein cholesterol levels
Skin	Increase sebum production and acne, male pattern baldness
Infectious	Local infections at injection site, septic arthritis, and HIV/hepatitis from needle sharing
Gynecomastia	Caused from aromatization to estradiol; not present with modified androgens that cannot be aromatized (5-a-reduced androgens)
Other effects	Weight gain from fluid retention and increased lean body mass

19. **Which AASs have the least potential to cause adverse effects?**
All AASs can cause significant adverse effects. However, hepatic toxicity and lipid derangements are seen predominantly with the oral alkylated AASs. The parenteral esters, patches, and gels are safer in this respect.

20. **What has been done on a national and worldwide level to prevent AAS abuse?**
Under Sections 351, 352, 353, and 355 of the Food, Drug, and Cosmetic Act 21 USCA, these substances came under Food and Drug Administration regulation, requiring a prescription from a licensed physician. The Anabolic Steroids Control Act of 1990 made AAS schedule III controlled substances. Possession with an intent-to-sell constitutes a federal felony. Most recently, the World Anti-Doping Agency was established in an effort to coordinate a worldwide strategy for detection of illegal ergogenic aids used by competing athletes. The Anabolic Steroids Control Act of 2004 has made prohormones schedule III controlled substance despite the fact that prohormones have not been shown to be anabolic.

21. **What has been done on an individual level to prevent AASs abuse?**
With regard to their use by athletes, routine and random drug screening has been implemented. As professional and serious amateur athletes spend vast amounts of energy, time, and resources in preparing for and competing in their sport, it is believed that the fear of being precluded from competition will serve as an effective deterrent.

KEY POINTS: EFFECTS AND SIDE EFFECTS OF ANABOLIC-ANDROGENIC STEROIDS

1. Biological effects include growth and development of the prostate, seminal vesicles, penis and scrotum, beard, pubic, chest, and axillary hair and thickening of the vocal cords and enlargement of the larynx.

2. Common side effects of anabolic-androgenic steroids (AAS) abuse include fluid retention, testicular atrophy, oligospermia, azoospermia, gynecomastia, cholestatic hepatitis, pelioses hepatis, both benign and malignant hepatic tumors, and reduced high-density lipoprotein and higher low-density lipoprotein cholesterol levels.

3. The illegal use of AASs to enhance sports performance or physical appearance probably represents the single most common use.

22. **What screening tests are used to detect AASs in athletes?**
Mass spectroscopy and gas chromatography can detect androgens other than testosterone when being used at the time of testing. To detect the use of exogenous testosterone, an increased ratio of urine testosterone to epitestosterone (greater than 6:1) can be confirmatory. Furthermore, urine samples with a high ratio of testosterone to leuteinizing hormone (LH; >30) suggests AAS abuse because LH secretion is suppressed in subjects using testosterone.

23. **What are the so-called androgen precursors or prohormones?**
These are compounds marketed and advertised to be metabolized to testosterone or other active metabolites. The current literature to substantiate these claims is sparse and the results are mixed.

24. **What are the effects if any of androgen precursors?**
The answer is mixed (see Table 51-4). Studies show that young men and untrained and trained athletes do not show an increase in serum testosterone at low to moderate doses. There is some evidence at larger doses of androstenedione or sublingual androstenediol, some young men may see a rise in serum testosterone levels acutely (within hours). Other studies show older men (>30 years of age), who already have low serum testosterone level, do show a dose responsive increase in serum testosterone with certain prohormones.

25. **Have androgen precursors, such as androstenedione and dehydroepiandrosterone, been shown to raise serum testosterone levels in women?**
Yes. Unlike men, the use of these precursors/prohormones have shown increases in serum testosterone without significant increases in estradiol in women. See Table 51-5.

26. **Have androgen precursors been shown to be anabolic in men or women?**
No. The data are currently lacking to show any anabolic effects of androgen precursors.

TABLE 51-4. SUMMARY OF ANDROGEN PRECURSORS: ACUTE AND CHRONIC SERUM CHANGES IN MEN

Precursor	Acute Serum Testosterone Change	Acute Serum Estrogen Change	Chronic Serum Testosterone Change	Chronic Serum Estrogen Change	Anabolic Effects
Androstenedione	100-200 mg: no change; 300 mg: increase in some: 2ith aromatase inhibitor and/or 5-a-reductase inhibitor: no increase	Dose-dependent increase	No change	Increased	Yes in hypogonadal men
Androstenediol	Oral: no change; Sublingual: increase (by passing first pass)	Increase	No change	Increased	None but evidence lacking
DHEA	No change	Increase	No change	No Data	No benefit

DHEA, dehydroepiandrosterone.

TABLE 51-5. SUMMARY OF ANDROGEN PRECURSORS: ACUTE AND CHRONIC SERUM CHANGES IN WOMEN

Precursor	Acute Serum Testosterone Change	Acute Serum Estrogen Change	Chronic Serum Testosterone Change	Chronic Serum Estrogen Change	Anabolic Effects
Androstenedione	50–100 mg: increase	None at 50–100 mg doses; increase at 300 mg	No Data		

WEBSITES

1. Anabolic Steroid Abuse. Available at: http://www.steroicabuse.org/
2. National Institute of Drug Abuse. Available at: http://www.nida.nih.gov/infofacts/steroids. html
3. NFL Players Association website about banned substances. Available at: http://www.nflpa. org/RulesAndRegs/RulesAndRegulations.aspx

BIBLIOGRAPHY

1. Bahrke M, Yesalis C, Kopstein A, et al: Risk factors associated with anabolic-androgenic steroid use among adolescents. Sports Med 29:397–405, 2000.
2. Basaria S, Wahlstrom J, Dobs A: Clinical review 138: anabolic-androgenic steroid therapy in the treatment of chronic diseases. J Clin Endocrinol Metab 86:5108–1517, 2001.
3. Bhasin S, Storer TW, Berman N, el al: The effects of supraphysiologic doses of testosterone on muscle size and strength in normal men. N Engl J Med 335:1–7, 1996.
4. Catlin DH: Anabolic steroids. In DeGroot LJ, et al, editors: *Endocrinology*, ed. 3, Philadelphia, 1995, W.B. Saunders, pp. 2362–2376.
5. Dickerman RD, McConathy WJ, Zachariah NY: Testosterone, sex-hormone binding globulin, lipoproteins, and vascular disease risk. J Cardiovasc Risk 4:363–366, 1997.
6. Fudala P, Weinrieb R, Calarco J, et al: An evaluation of anabolic-androgenic steroid abusers over a period of 1 year: seven case studies. Ann Clin Psych 15:121–30, 2003.
7. Griffin J, Wilson J: Disorders of the testes and the male reproductive tract. In William RH, Larsen PR, Kronenberg HM, et al, editors, *Williams textbook of endocrinology*, ed. 10, Philadelphia, 2003, W.B. Saunders, pp. 747–751.
8. Hameed A, Brothwood T, Bouloux P: Delivery of testosterone replacement therapy. Curr Opin Invest Drugs 4:1213–1219, 2003.
9. Kouri EM, Pope HG Jr, Oliva PS: Changes in lipoprotein-lipid levels in normal men following administration of increasing doses of testosterone cypionate. Clin J Sports Med 6:152–157, 1996.
10. Ravaglia G, Forti P, Maioli F, et al: Body composition, sex steroids, IGF-1, and bone mineral status in aging men. J Gerontol A Biol Sci Med Sci 55:516–521, 2000.
11. Rhoden EL, Morgentaler A: Risks of testosterone replacement therapy and recommendations for monitoring. N Engl J Med 350:482–492, 2004.
12. Storer TW, Magliano L, Woodhouse L, et al: Testosterone dose-dependently increases maximal voluntary strength and leg power, but does not affect fatigability or specific tension. J Clin Endocrinol Metab 88:1478–1485, 2003.
13. Foster ZJ, Housner JA: Anabolic-androgenic steroids and testosterone precursors: ergogenic aids and sport. Curr Sports Med Rep 3:234–241, 2004.

MULTIPLE ENDOCRINE NEOPLASIA

Arnold A. Asp

CHAPTER 52

1. **What are the multiple endocrine neoplasia (MEN) syndromes?**
   There are three well-characterized, inherited pluriglandular disorders in which several endocrine glands simultaneously undergo neoplastic transformation and become hyperfunctional. All of these disorders are genetically transmitted in an autosomal dominant fashion. These disorders include MEN-I, MEN-IIa, and MEN-IIb.

2. **Define MEN-I.**
   MEN-I consists of hyperplasia or neoplastic transformation of the parathyroids, pancreatic islets, and pituitary.

3. **Define MEN-IIa.**
   MEN-IIa consists of hyperplasia or neoplastic transformation of the thyroid parafollicular cells (medullary carcinoma of the thyroid [MTC]), parathyroid glands, and adrenal medulla (pheochromocytoma).

4. **Define MEN-IIb.**
   MEN-IIb consists of hyperplasia or neoplastic transformation of the thyroid parafollicular cells (MTC) and adrenal medulla (pheochromocytoma) with concomitant development of mucosal neuromas.

5. **How can so many various endocrine organs be affected in these syndromes?**
   This question is a matter of controversy and ongoing research. The cells that comprise many endocrine organs are able to decarboxylate various amino acids and convert the molecules to amines or peptides that act as hormones or neurotransmitters. These cells have been classified as amine precursor uptake and decarboxylation (APUD) cells and are considered to be embryologically of neuroectodermal origin. APUD cells contain markers of their common neuroendocrine origin, including neuron-specific enolase and chromogranin A. Neoplastic transformation of APUD cells long after organogenesis is complete appears to be due to a germline mutation (loss of a tumor suppressor gene in MEN-I or mutation of a protooncogene to an oncogene in MEN-IIa and MEN-IIb) in a gene that is expressed only in neuroectodermal cells. When neuroectodermal cells later migrate to specific developing organs, the genetic mutation likewise is distributed to those organs. This may explain the eventual development of tumors in so many diverse tissues.

6. **What is Wermer's syndrome?**
   This is the eponym for the MEN-I syndrome. Wermer first recognized the association of parathyroid hyperplasia, multicentric pituitary tumors, and pancreatic islet cell tumors in several kindreds and described the syndrome in 1954. Although neoplastic transformation occurs most commonly in the parathyroids, pituitary, and pancreas, hyperplastic adrenal cortical and nodular thyroid disorders have been described. Carcinoid tumors, especially involving the foregut (thymus, lung, stomach, and duodenum), are uncommon but also have been reported in MEN-I syndrome.

7. **How common is Werner's syndrome?**
   Wermer's syndrome is the most common form of MEN. Its prevalence is estimated to vary between 2 and 20 per 100,000 population. The syndrome is characterized by a high degree of penetrance; expression increases with age.

8. **Is hyperparathyroidism in MEN-I similar to sporadic primary hyperparathyroidism?**
   No. Hyperparathyroidism associated with MEN-I results from hyperplasia of all four glands, whereas sporadic primary hyperparathyroidism is usually characterized by adenomatous change in a single gland. Hyperparathyroidism is the most common and earliest manifestation of MEN-I, occurring in 80% to 95% of cases. It has been described in patients as young as 17 years and develops in nearly all patients with MEN-I by age 40.

9. **What causes the hyperplasia of parathyroid glands affected by MEN-I?**
   Hyperplasia of parathyroid glands affected by MEN-I results from expansion of multiple cell clones, whereas sporadic parathyroid adenomas result from activation of a single cell clone. Several groups have described a mitogenic factor (probably basic fibroblast growth factor) in the sera of patients with MEN-I. This factor potentiates the hyperplastic growth of parathyroid tissue. Complications of MEN-I hyperparathyroidism are similar to those of sporadic hyperparathyroidism; they include nephrolithiasis, osteoporosis, mental status changes, and muscular weakness.

10. **Summarize the therapy for hypoplastic parathyroid glands.**
    Therapy of both sporadic adenomas and MEN-I-associated hyperplastic glands depends on surgical resection. In sporadic primary hyperparathyroidism, removal of the solitary adenoma is curative in 95% of cases. In MEN-I-associated hyperplasia, at least 3.5 hyperplastic glands must be resected to restore normocalcemia. Only 75% of patients are normocalcemic postoperatively; 10% to 25% are rendered hypoparathyroid. Unfortunately, the parathyroid remnants in the patient with MEN-I have a great propensity to regenerate; 50% of cases become hypercalcemic again within 10 years of surgery. This recurrence rate dictates that surgery be delayed until complications of hypercalcemia are imminent or gastrin levels are elevated, as discussed in the following.

11. **How common is neoplastic transformation of pancreatic islet cells in MEN-I?**
    Neoplastic transformation of the pancreatic islet cells is the second most common manifestation of MEN-I, occurring in approximately 66% to 80% of cases.

12. **What types of pancreatic tumors are found in MEN-I syndrome?**
    Pancreatic tumors in MEN-I syndrome are usually multicentric and are often capable of elaborating several peptides and biogenic amines. They are, by convention, classified on the basis of the clinical syndrome produced by the predominant secretory product. This group of tumors characteristically progresses from hyperplasia to malignancy with metastases, making curative resection unlikely. Tumors of the pancreas may arise from normal islet cells (eutopic) or cells that are not normal constituents of the adult pancreas (ectopic).

13. **What is the most common type of pancreatic tumor in MEN-I?**
    Gastrinomas are the most common pancreatic tumors in MEN-I syndrome (47%–78% of cases). They are ectopic tumors; G cells are normally present in the fetal pancreas only. Gastrinomas also may occur independently of MEN-I (only 15%–48% of all patients with a gastrinoma are later found to have MEN-I). Gastrinomas associated with MEN-I are multiple and often extrapancreatic, occurring in the duodenal wall and retroperitoneal lymphatics.

14. **Describe the symptoms of gastrinomas associated with MEN-I.**
Excessive gastrin secretion by these tumors causes prolific production of gastric acid with resultant duodenal and jejunal ulcers and diarrhea. Basal acid output exceeds 15 mmol/h, and basal fasting serum gastrin levels usually exceed 300 pg/mL.

15. **What other conditions may cause hypergastrinemia?**
Hypergastrinemia also may result from any condition that stimulates normal gastrin secretion (hypercalcemia) or that interferes with normal gastric acid production and feedback to the ***G cells (achlorhydria, gastric outlet obstruction, retained antrum with a Billroth II procedure, vagotomy, and the use of histamine-2 [H_2] blockers and proton pump inhibitors). Hyperparathyroidism (see questions 8 and 9) can therefore falsely elevate serum gastrin levels.

16. **How are gastrinomas distinguished from other causes of hypergastrinemia?**
A secretin stimulation test may aid in the differentiation of gastrinomas from other hypergastrinemic states; serum gastrin levels in patients with gastrinomas increase by at least 200 pg/mL. More information about gastrinomas is included in Chapter 54.

17. **What is the second most common type of pancreatic tumor in MEN-I?**
Insulinomas are the second most common pancreatic islet-cell tumor in the MEN-I syndrome (12%–36% of islet-cell tumors) and the most common eutopic type. Persistent or disordered insulin secretion causes severe hypoglycemia; inappropriately elevated concentrations of insulin, proinsulin, and C-peptide are present in the serum. Insulinomas associated with MEN-I syndrome are more frequently multicentric and malignant than are the sporadic tumors. Approximately 1% to 5% of all patients with an insulinoma are eventually discovered to have MEN-I. An excellent discussion of the diagnosis and therapy of insulinomas is found in Chapter 54.

18. **What other pancreatic tumors may be seen in MEN-I?**
Pancreatic tumors less frequently associated with MEN-I include glucagonomas, somatostatinomas, and vasoactive intestinal polypeptide-secreting tumors (VIPomas). Associated syndromes and therapy are also described in Chapter 54.

19. **How are the most common pancreatic tumors of MEN-I Treated?**
Multicentric gastrinomas are rarely cured surgically (10%–15% of cases). Fortunately, symptoms of hypergastrinemia can be pharmacologically controlled with administration of an H_2 blocker, proton-pump inhibitor, or octreotide. Metastases to the liver become increasingly common when gastrinomas exceed 3 cm in diameter, prompting most surgeons to reserve excision for tumors larger than 3 cm. Gastrinomas express surface receptors for somatostatin, potentiating the use of somatostatin-receptor scintigraphy in combination with annual magnetic resonance imaging (MRI)/computed tomography (CT) surveillance to monitor tumor progression.

20. **Summarize the approach to treatment of hypoglycemia associated with insulinomas.**
Insulinomas, unlike gastrinomas, produce devastating hypoglycemia, which is difficult to counteract medically. Without effective long-term pharmacotherapy, surgical resection of the tumor(s) is required in most patients. Fortunately, when the largest tumor is excised, many of the patient's symptoms are ameliorated. Localization is accomplished preoperatively with endoscopic ultrasonography, MRI/CT, or by comparison of insulin levels in the right hepatic vein following selective infusion of the intrapancreatic arteries with calcium gluconate. Intraoperative ultrasonography may also assist precise localization at the time of surgery.

21. **Which pituitary tumors are associated with MEN-I?**
    Pituitary tumors occur in 50% to 71% of cases of MEN-I. They may result either from neoplastic transformation of anterior pituitary cells with clonal expansion to a tumor or from excessive stimulation of the pituitary by ectopically produced hypothalamic releasing factors elaborated by carcinoids or pancreatic islet cells.

22. **What pituitary tumors are most commonly associated with MEN-I?**
    Prolactinomas are the most common pituitary tumors associated with MEN-I, constituting 60% of the total. The symptoms of hyperprolactinemia (galactorrhea and amenorrhea in women; impotence in men) are the third most common manifestation of MEN-I. The tumors are typically multicentric and large but respond to dopamine agonists, such as bromocriptine. In earlier series, many pituitary tumors described as chromophobe adenomas were, in reality, prolactinomas that contained sparse, poorly staining secretory granules. These tumors are also discussed in Chapter 20.

23. **What is the second most common pituitary tumor in MEN-I?**
    The second most commonly encountered pituitary tumor type is the growth hormone-producing tumor, which is reported in 10% to 25% of patients. Overproduction of growth hormone results in gigantism in children and acromegaly in adults. The tumors are often multicentric and may result from secretion of growth hormone-releasing hormone by pancreatic or carcinoid tumors. Diagnosis and therapy is described in Chapter 21.

24. **What other pituitary tumors may be seen in MEN-I?**
    Corticotropin (adrenocorticotropin [ACTH])-producing tumors that cause Cushing's syndrome may be associated with MEN-I. Such tumors result from neoplastic transformation of the pituitary or elaboration of corticotropin-releasing hormone by pancreatic or carcinoid tumors. Diagnosis and therapy are described in Chapter 23.

25. **What causes MEN-I?**
    The gene predisposing to the development of MEN-I (MEN-I susceptibility gene) is located on the long arm of chromosome 11 (11q13) and encodes a protein known as menin, which functions as a tumor suppressor. The proband inherits an allele predisposing to MEN-I from the affected parent, whereas a normal allele is passed down from the unaffected parent. The gene for this tumor suppressor is unusually susceptible to mutation. When a somatic mutation later inactivates the normal allele, suppressor function is lost, permitting hyperplasia of the gland to occur.

26. **How should a kindred be screened after the proband is identified?**
    Carriers of the genetic defect must first be identified, the extent of their organ involvement determined, and their family screened for additional carriers of the susceptibility gene. As mentioned earlier, mutations in the gene coding for the tumor suppressor, menin, are apparent in patients with MEN-I and may be used to identify carriers of the disorder in the near future. Although mutational analysis using polymerase chain reaction techniques were previously restricted to research laboratories, clinical testing for mutations in the MEN-I gene is now available to detect disease within affected kindreds.

27. **At what age should screening begin?**
    Manifestations of MEN-I syndrome rarely occur before age 15; therefore, people at risk should not undergo endocrine screening before that time. Nearly all people at risk develop the disorder by the age of 40 years; screening may be unnecessary in members older than 50 who are proved to be disease-free.

28. **Summarize the tests used for screening of MEN-I individuals.**
Because hyperparathyroidism is temporally the first manifestation of MEN-I syndrome, serum calcium concentrations constitute the best screening test to identify carriers. Biochemical evidence of hyperparathyroidism in a member of MEN-I kindred establishes a presumptive carrier state. Evaluation then should focus on delineation of pancreatic and pituitary involvement. Serum levels of gastrin disclose the presence of a gastrinoma, whereas levels of prolactin most often reveal the presence of pituitary disease (especially in women). The latter two tests are cost-effective only in established disease and should not be used for preliminary screening of the kindred (unless symptoms of hypergastrinemia or prolactinoma are present). The frequency of screening has not been prospectively studied but recommended intervals range from 2 to 5 years.

KEY POINTS: MEN-I

1. MEN-I consists of neoplastic transformation in at least two of these three glands: parathyroids, pancreas, and pituitary.

2. MEN-I results from a mutation inactivating the menin tumor suppressor on chromosome 11. Routine clinical testing for the mutation is currently available.

3. Therapy for MEN-I includes surgical resection of hyperplastic parathyroid tissue and pituitary adenomas; surgical cure for the associated pancreatic tumors is not usually possible.

---

29. **What is Sipple's syndrome?**
This is the eponym for MEN-IIa. In 1961, Sipple recognized and described a patient who expired with an intracerebral aneurysm and was found at autopsy to have MTC, pheochromocytomas, and hyperparathyroidism. This disorder is inherited in an autosomal dominant fashion and exhibits a high degree of penetrance and variable expressivity. It is less common than MEN-1 syndrome.

30. **Is the form of MTC associated with MEN-IIa similar to the sporadic form of MTC?**
No. MTC results from malignant transformation of the parafollicular cells (or C cells) that normally elaborate calcitonin and are scattered throughout the gland. MTC accounts for 2% to 10% of all thyroid malignancies. The sporadic form of MTC, as described in Chapter 37, is more common (75% of all MTC), occurs in a solitary form (<20% multicentric), and metastasizes to local lymphatics, lung, bone, and liver early in the course of disease (metastasis may occur with primary tumors less than 1 cm in diameter). Sporadic MTC occurs more commonly in an older population (peak age: 40–60 years) and is usually located in the upper two thirds of the gland.

31. **Summarize the essential characteristics of MTC associated with MEN-IIa.**
MTC associated with MEN-IIa is multicentric (90% at the time of diagnosis), occurs at a younger age than sporadic MTC (as young as 2 years), and generally has a better prognosis than the sporadic form. MTC occurs in nearly 95% of all cases of MEN-IIa and is usually the first tumor to appear.

32. **How common is diarrhea in MTC associated with MEN-IIa?**
Calcitonin or other peptides elaborated by the tumor may cause a secretory diarrhea that is present in 4% to 7% of patients at the time of diagnosis but develops in 25% to 30% during the course of the disease.

33. How is MEN-II-associated MTC treated?

Parafollicular cells in patients with MEN-IIa characteristically progress through a state of C-cell hyperplasia to nodular hyperplasia to malignant degeneration over a variable period. It is imperative that patients at risk be diagnosed while still in the C-cell hyperplasia stage; total thyroidectomy precludes malignant degeneration and metastases.

34. How is C-cell hyperplasia detected?

Detection of C-cell hyperplasia is facilitated by the pentagastrin stimulation test. MTC also expresses peptides and hormones not commonly elaborated by parafollicular cells, including somatostatin, thyrotropin-releasing hormone, vasoactive intestinal peptide, proopiomelanocortin, carcinoembryonic antigen, and neurotensin.

35. What is the second most common neoplasm associated with MEN-IIa?

Pheochromocytomas occur in 50% to 70% of cases of MEN-IIa and are bilateral in up to 84% of patients. Compared with the sporadic form, pheochromocytomas associated with MEN-IIa secrete greater amounts of epinephrine. Hypertension is therefore less common, and urinary excretion of catecholamines may become supranormal later in the course of the disease.

36. Summarize the treatment of pheochromocytomas associated with MEN-IIa.

Surgical resection is indicated, but controversy surrounds the need for prophylactic resection of contralateral uninvolved adrenals, 50% of which develop pheochromocytomas within 10 years of the original surgery. The diagnosis and management of pheochromocytomas are discussed in Chapter 28.

37. Is hyperparathyroidism associated with MEN-IIa similar to that found in MEN-I?

Yes, but it is encountered much less commonly, involving only 40% of cases. No mitogenic factor (as in MEN-I) has been described in the sera of these patients.

38. What is the genetic basis for the MEN-IIa syndrome?

MEN-IIa is caused by an activating mutation of the RET protooncogene located on chromosome 10q11.2. The gene codes for a receptor tyrosine kinase that phosphorylates and activates enzymes critical to cellular development. The ligand that normally activates the tyrosine kinase is glial cell–derived neurotropic factor (GDNF). When GDNF binds, two receptors bind together (homodimerization), and phosphorylation of enzymes occurs downstream. Mutation of the RET protooncogene to an oncogene results in constitutive activation of the enzyme, causing unregulated phosphorylation of other critical enzymes. Inheritance of one RET oncogene from one affected parent is sufficient to cause MEN-IIa syndrome in offspring. Five distinct mutations involving exons 10 and 11 have been described in 98% of 203 kindreds with the disorder.

39. How should a kindred be screened after the proband with MEN-IIa is identified?

As explained in question 26, screening initially entails the differentiation of gene carriers from uninvolved family members and the subsequent delineation of organ involvement in the affected members. However, unlike MEN-I, direct DNA sequencing of the RET oncogene causing MEN-IIa is clinically available. With appropriate repeat analysis of positive and negative test results, the assay offers near 100% accuracy in identification of affected individuals. Genetic analysis of the kindred should be performed to identify the specific RET oncogene mutation; characterization of the familial oncogene precludes the need for repetitive biochemical screening of noncarriers in subsequent generations.

40. How is MEN-IIa treated?

Because C-cell hyperplasia has been described in gene carriers as young as 2 years, total thyroidectomy is suggested in affected individuals before age 5. An alternative to preemptive thyroidectomy is to perform annual pentagastrin stimulation tests and withhold surgery until a positive result is obtained. Because MEN-IIa–associated pheochromocytoma may produce large amounts of epinephrine that do not cause hypertension, annual timed urine collections for catecholamines should be obtained in all gene carriers. Serum levels of calcium should be assessed every 2 years. After the presence of the syndrome has been established, screening for adrenal and parathyroid involvement should continue through life.

41. What comprises the MEN-IIb syndrome?
MEN-IIb syndrome is the association of MTC and pheochromocytoma with multiple mucosal neuromas in an affected individual or kindred. Hyperparathyroidism is not associated with MEN-IIb. This syndrome is less common than the MEN-IIa and is more commonly sporadic than familial, but if inherited, it is transmitted in an autosomal dominant fashion.

42. What findings raise the suspicion of MEN-IIb syndrome?
The occurrence of multiple mucosal neuromas on the distal tongue, lips, and along the gastrointestinal tract should always raise the possibility of MEN-IIb. Other manifestations of MEN-IIb include marfanoid habitus (without ectopia lentis or aortic aneurysms), hypertrophic corneal nerves, and slipped femoral epiphysis.

43. How should MEN-IIb be treated?
The MTC associated with this syndrome is more aggressive than other forms; metastatic lesions have been described in infancy. Because of the propensity toward early metastasis, many advocate that children with the syndrome should undergo total thyroidectomy as soon as surgery can be tolerated. Pheochromocytomas occur in nearly half of all patients and follow a clinical course similar to those in the MEN-IIa syndrome.

44. What is the overall mortality rate associated with MEN-IIb?
Overall mortality in MEN-IIb is more severe; the average age of death for patients with MEN-IIa is 60 years, whereas in patients with MEN-IIb the average age of death is 30 years.

45. Summarize the screening recommendations for MEN-IIb.
Screening of family members with pentagastrin stimulation for MTC should begin at birth and continue through life if thyroidectomy is deferred. Screening for pheochromocytoma should begin at 5 years and continue for life.

46. What causes MEN-IIb?
More than 95% of the kindreds with MEN-IIb have been found to carry a mutation of the RET protooncogene at codon 918 (exon 16). This oncogene codes for a methionine-to-threonine substitution, resulting in activation of the innermost tyrosine kinase moiety of the same receptor associated with MEN-IIa.

47. Have the clinical presentations and prognoses of the MEN syndromes changed since the time of their original descriptions?
Yes. When the MEN syndromes were initially described, most patients presented with involvement of all of the aforementioned organ systems because diagnostic capabilities were limited. At present, early diagnosis of the proband and aggressive screening of the kindred may permit detection of hyperplasia and prompt prophylactic surgery or medical therapy that limits morbidity and mortality.

KEY POINTS: MEN-IIA AND MEN-IIB

1. MEN-IIa consists of neoplastic transformation of parathyroids, thyroid parafollicular C cells, and adrenal medulla.

2. MEN-IIb consists of neoplastic transformation of thyroid parafollicular C cells, and adrenal medulla, with mucosal neuromas.
3. Genetic testing for the RET mutation causing MEN-II syndromes is now clinically available.

BIBLIOGRAPHY

1. Benson L, Ljunghall S, Akerstrom G, et al: Hyperparathyroidism presenting as the first lesion in multiple endocrine neoplasia type 1. Am J Med 82:731–737, 1987.

2. Brandi ML, Auerbach GD, Fitzpatrick LA, et al: Parathyroid mitogenic activity in plasma from patients with familial multiple endocrine neoplasia type 1. N Engl J Med 314:1287–1293, 1986.

3. Brandi ML, Gagel RF, Angeli A, et al: Guidelines for diagnosis and therapy of MEN type 1 and type 2. J Clin Endocrinol Metab 86:5658–5671, 2001.

4. Cadiot G, Laurent-Piug P, Thuille B, et al: Is the multiple endocrine neoplasia type 1 gene a suppressor for fundic argyrophil tumors in Zollinger-Ellison syndrome? Gastroenterology 105:579–582, 1993.

5. Chandrasekharappa SCV, Guru SC, Manickam P, et al: Positional cloning of the gene for multiple endocrine neoplasia type 1. Science 276:404–407, 1997.

6. Eng C: The RET proto-oncogene in multiple endocrine neoplasia type 2 and Hirschsprung's disease. N Engl J Med 335:943–951, 1996.

7. Eng C, Clayton D, Schuffenecker I, et al: The relationship between specific RET proto-oncogene mutations and disease phenotype in multiple endocrine neoplasia type 2. JAMA 276:1575–1579, 1996.

8. Gagel RF: Multiple endocrine neoplasia. In Wilson JD, Foster DW, editors, *Williams' Textbook of Endocrinology*, 9th ed. Philadelphia, W.B. Saunders, 1998, pp. 1637–1649.

9. Gicquel C, Bertherat J, Le Bouc Y, et al: The pathogenesis of adrenocortical incidentalomas and genetic syndromes associated with adrenocortical neoplasms. Endocrinol Metab Clin North Am 29:1–13, 2000.

10. Grauer A, Raue F, Gagel RF: Changing concepts in the management of hereditary and sporadic medullary thyroid carcinoma. Endocrinol Metab Clin North Am 19:613–635, 1990.

11. Herman V, Draznin NZ, Gonsky R, Melmed S: Molecular screening of pituitary adenomas for gene mutations and rearrangements. J Clin Endocrinol Metab 77:50–55, 1993.

12. Kopp P. Applications of molecular biology and genetics in endocrinology. Endocr Pract 13:534–541, 2007.

13. Marx SJ (moderator): Multiple endocrine neoplasia type 1: clinical and genetic topics. Ann Intern Med 129:484–494, 1998.

14. Marx SJ, Vinik AI Santen RJ, et al: Multiple endocrine neoplasia type 1: assessment of laboratory tests to screen for the gene in a large kindred. Medicine 65:2226–2241, 1986.

15. Phay JE, Moley JF, Lairmore TL: Multiple endocrine neoplasias. Semin Surg Oncol 18:324–332, 2000.

16. Saad MF, Ordenez NG, Rashid RK, et al: Medullary carcinoma of the thyroid. Medicine 63:319–342, 1984.

17. Santoro M, Carlomagno F, Romano A, et al: Activation of RET as a dominant transforming gene by germline mutations of MEN-IIa and MEN-IIb. Science 267:381–383, 1995.

18. Tham E, Grandell U, Lindgren E, et al: Clinical testing for mutations in the MEN-I gene in Sweden: a report of 200 unrelated cases. J Clin Endocrinol Metab 92: 3389–3395, 2007.

19. Veldius JD, Norton JA, Wells SA, et al: Surgical versus medical management of multiple endocrine neoplasia (MEN) type 1. J Clin Endocrinol Metab 82:357–364, 1997.

CHAPTER 53

AUTOIMMUNE POLYENDOCRINE SYNDROMES

Arnold A. Asp

1. **Define the autoimmune polyendocrine syndromes. How many clinical forms are there?**

   The autoimmune polyendocrine syndromes (APSs) are disorders in which two or more endocrine glands are simultaneously hypofunctional or hyperfunctional as the result of autoimmune dysfunction. It is theorized that a defect in the T-suppressor cell subset inadvertently permits activation of the cellular and humoral arms of the immune system. The nature of this dysfunction is unknown. The two widely recognized clinical forms are appropriately designated APS type 1 and APS type 2. The common clinical link between the syndromes is adrenal insufficiency.

2. **Is evidence of nonendocrine autoimmune dysfunction associated with APSs?**

   Yes. Connective tissue diseases and hematologic and gastrointestinal autoimmune disorders are commonly associated with the APSs.

3. **What constitutes APS type 1?**

   APS type 1 is a pediatric disorder manifested by the presence of a combination of two of the following three disorders: hypoparathyroidism, adrenal insufficiency, and chronic mucocutaneous candidiasis. Usually hypoparathyroidism and candidiasis present by age 5 years. Adrenal insufficiency occurs by age 12 years, and all manifestations are present by age 15 years. Some affected individuals develop only one manifestation. Other endocrine conditions may also occur; the largest series of patients have noted the following endocrine manifestations:
   - Hypoparathyroidism: 89%
   - Thyroid disease: 12%
   - Adrenal insufficiency: 60%
   - Diabetes mellitus type 1: 1% to 4%
   - Gonadal failure: 45%

4. **Are nonendocrine manifestations associated with APS type 1?**

   Yes. Chronic mucocutaneous candidiasis occurs in 75% of patients, celiac disease in 25%, alopecia in 20%, pernicious anemia in 16%, and chronic autoimmune hepatitis in 9%. Dystrophy of the dental enamel, vitiligo, keratopathy, and hypoplasia of the teeth and nails also may occur, prompting the alternative designation for APS type 1: autoimmune polyendocrinopathy-candidiasis-ectodermal dystrophy.

5. **Explain the etiology of APS type 1.**

   Mutations of the autoimmune regulator (AIRE) gene on chromosome 21 cause APS type 1, which is inherited in an autosomal recessive pattern. There appears to be no human leukocyte antigen (HLA) association. The cause of the candidiasis is not known, although delayed hypersensitivity is defective in affected patients. Antibodies to adrenal enzymes (21-hydroxylase, an enzyme in the biosynthetic pathway for aldosterone and cortisol) and to poorly characterized parathyroid antigens have been described by some groups.

6. **What therapy can be offered?**
   Annual screening of levels of serum calcium, cosyntropin-stimulated cortisol, and liver-associated enzymes is performed in affected sibships until age 15 years. Adrenal insufficiency and hypoparathyroidism are treated with glucocorticoids and oral calcium/vitamin D supplementation, respectively. Mucocutaneous candidiasis is treated with fluconazole. Use of prophylactic immunosuppressives, such as cyclosporine, is not recommended.

7. **What disorders are associated with APS type 2?**
   APS type 2 occurs in adulthood and consists of autoimmune adrenal insufficiency with autoimmune thyroid disease and/or diabetes mellitus, type 1. The age of onset tends to be between 20 and 30 years; one half of the cases are sporadic and one half are familial. Endocrine organ involvement is as follows:
   - Adrenal insufficiency: 100%
   - Diabetes mellitus type 1: 50%
   - Autoimmune thyroid disease: 70%
   - Gonadal failure: 5% to 50%

   Very rarely geriatric hypoparathyroidism may be encountered in elderly patients with APS type 2.

8. **What is most common presenting disorder in APS type 2?**
   Adrenal insufficiency is the presenting disorder in 50% of cases, whereas adrenal insufficiency with diabetes mellitus or thyroid disease is present at the time of diagnosis in 20% of cases. In the remaining 30%, adrenal insufficiency occurs after other endocrine dysfunction. Between 69% and 90% of patients have circulating antibodies to 21-hydroxylase.

9. **What thyroid disorders are associated with APS type 2?**
   Thyroid disorders associated with APS type 2 include Graves' disease (50%) and Hashimoto's disease or atrophic thyroiditis (50%). As expected, thyroid-stimulating immunoglobulins (TSI) are present in cases of hyperthyroidism, whereas antibodies to thyroid peroxidase or thyroglobulin are present in cases of hypothyroidism.

10. **Summarize the significance of cytoplasmic islet-cell antibodies (ICAs) in APS type 2.**
    Cytoplasmic ICAs are present in patients with APS type 2 and diabetes mellitus; however, the significance of these antibodies is questionable. APS type 2 patients who have ICAs but not diabetes may have no compromise of beta-cell function and subsequently develop diabetes at a rate of 2% per year, whereas ICA-positive first-degree relatives of non-APS, type 1 diabetic individuals develop diabetes at a rate of 8% per year.

11. **How common is gonadal failure in APS type 2?**
    Gonadal failure is more common in women than in men and is associated with antibodies to gonadal tissue.

12. **Are nonendocrine abnormalities described in APS type 2?**
    Yes. In about 5% of cases, other autoimmune disorders are found, including vitiligo, pernicious anemia, alopecia, myasthenia gravis, celiac disease, Sjögren's syndrome, and rheumatoid arthritis.

13. **How should kindreds with suspected APS type 2 be screened?**
    Because APS type 2 appears in multiple generations and because 20 years may lapse between the development of various endocrine organ failures, affected patients should be screened by assessing levels of serum glucose, thyrotropin (TSH), and vitamin B12 every 3 to 5 years. Symptoms of adrenal insufficiency should be investigated by assessing levels of

cosyntropin-stimulated cortisol. First-degree relatives of the proband should be educated about the syndrome and advised to undergo screening every 3 to 5 years. Antibodies to thyroid peroxidase or thyroglobulin are so common in the general population as to preclude their use as a screening test.

14. **Explain the etiology of APS type 2.**
The genetic basis of APS type 2 is uncertain, although it appears to be associated with an HLA-DR3 phenotype that may be permissive for the development of autoimmunity. Organ-specific antibodies may cause organ dysfunction; for example, TSI may cause Graves' disease, and antiacetylcholine receptor antibodies may cause myasthenia gravis, or, like antithyroglobulin antibodies, they may be epiphenomena of disease. The only consistent abnormality noted in affected patients is decreased function of T-suppressor cells.

15. **What is POEMS syndrome?**
POEMS syndrome is a disorder of unknown etiology, unrelated to either APS type 1 or APS type 2, that appears to have an immunologic basis. The acronym highlights the cardinal features of the syndrome: polyneuropathy, organomegaly, endocrinopathy, monoclonal component, and skin changes. All of the symptoms are considered to be secondary to a plasma cell dyscrasia (monoclonal gammopathies of undetermined significance; plasmacytoma, osteosclerotic, osteolytic, or mixed myeloma) that produces the monoclonal gammopathy.

KEY POINTS: AUTOIMMUNE POLYENDOCRINE SYNDROMES

1. Autoimmune polyendocrine syndrome (APS) type 1 is a pediatric syndrome marked by hypoparathyroidism, adrenal insufficiency, and mucocutaneous candidiasis.

2. APS type 1 is inherited in an autosomal recessive manner and is clinically apparent by 15 years of age.

3. APS type 2 consists of adrenal insufficiency, thyroid dysfunction, and diabetes mellitus type 1.

4. APS type 2 associated organ failure progresses over many years during adulthood and effects multiple generations.

5. Both APS type 1 and APS type 2 manifest nonendocrine organ dysfunction, primarily gastrointestinal and dermatologic diseases.

16. **What eponym is associated with POEMS?**
Another name for the disorder is Crow-Fukase syndrome.

17. **How does POEMS usually present?**
The majority of patients are Asian males aged 45 to 55 years, but any ethnic group of either sex is susceptible. The most common presentation is that of a distal, symmetric peripheral sensorimotor neuropathy. There is usually loss of pin-prick and vibratory sense and decreased deep tendon reflexes predominantly in the lower extremities. The neuropathy is slowly progressive. Electromyograms and nerve biopsies are most consistent with both demyelination and axonal degeneration. Autonomic neuropathy has not been observed. Papilledema is present in 40% to 80% of cases. Nerve damage may result from myelin cross-reactivity with monoclonal immunoglobulin A (IgA) or IgG M proteins produced by plasmacytomas in sclerotic bone lesions, but evidence of intraneural immunoglobulin deposition has not been found in all series.

18. **How does the organomegaly manifest?**
Hepatomegaly (uncommon in multiple myeloma), splenomegaly, or both are noted in approximately two thirds of POEMS cases. The hepatomegaly may be associated with fibrosis and liver dysfunction.

19. **Which endocrine systems are involved?**
Diabetes mellitus type 2 is commonly encountered in either sex (28%–48%), as is primary hypothyroidism (45%–59%) or, rarely, adrenal insufficiency. Both males and females manifest elevated serum estrogen levels, which may promote hyperprolactinemia with galactorrhea and amenorrhea or impotence. Antibodies to the thyroid or adrenal glands have not been consistently detected.

20. **What skin changes have been encountered?**
Skin changes include sclerosis, hypertrichosis, hyperpigmentation, and hyperhidrosis.

21. **How is POEMS treated?**
Treatment of POEMS is based on elimination of plasmacytomas with radiation or chemotherapy, which, if successful, results in amelioration of the polyneuropathy and reduction in organomegaly. Endocrine deficiencies are treated with replacement hormones.

BIBLIOGRAPHY

1. Ahonen P, Myllarniemi S, Sipila I, et al: Clinical variation of autoimmune polyendocrinopathy-candidiasis-ectodermal dystrophy (APECED) in a series of 68 patients. N Engl J Med 322:1829–1836, 1990.

2. Betterle C, Grehhio NA, Volpato M: Autoimmune polyglandular syndrome type 1. J Clin Endocrinol Metab 83:1049–1055, 1998.

3. Consortium TF-GA: An autoimmune disease, APECED, caused by mutations in a novel gene featuring two PHD-type zinc finger domains. The Finnish-German APECED Consortium. Autoimmune Polyendocrinopathy Candidiasis Ectodermal Dystrophy. Nat Genet 17:399–403, 1997.

4. Eisenbarth GS, Verge CF: The immunoendocrinopathy syndromes. In Wilson JD, Foster DW, editors, *Williams' textbook of endocrinology*, ed 9, Philadelphia, 1998, W.B. Saunders, pp. 1651–1662.

5. Gavalas NG, Kemp EH, Krohn KJ, et al: The calcium-sensing receptor is a target of autoantibodies in patients with autoimmune polyendocrine syndrome type 1. J Clin Endocrinol Metab 92:2107–2114, 2007.

6. Gianani R, Eisenbarth GS: Autoimmunity to gastrointestinal endocrine cells in autoimmune polyendocrine syndrome type 1 [editorial]. J Clin Endocrinol Metab 88:1442–1444, 2003.

7. Kutteh WH: Immunology of multiple endocrinopathies associated with premature ovarian failure. Endocrinologist 6:462–466, 1996.

8. Leshin M: Polyglandular autoimmune syndromes. Am J Med Sci 290:77–88, 1985.

9. Perheentupa J: Autoimmune polyendocrinopathy-candidiasis-ectodermal dystrophy. J Clin Endocrinol Metab 91:2843–2850, 2006.

10. Mhyre AG, Halonen M, Eskelin P, et al: Autoimmune polyendocrine syndrome. Clin Endocrinol 45:211–217, 2001.

11. Soubrier M, Dubost JJ, Sauvezie B: POEMS syndrome: a study of 25 cases and a review of the literature. Am J Med 97:543–553, 1994.

12. Soubrier M, Sauron C, Souweine B, et al: Growth factors and proinflammatory cytokines in the renal involvement of POEMS syndrome. Am J Kid Dis 34:633–638, 1999.

CHAPTER 54

PANCREATIC ENDOCRINE TUMORS

Michael T. McDermott

1. **What are the pancreatic endocrine tumors?**
   These tumors arise from the islet cells of the pancreas and are generally named for the hormones that they secrete. They include tumors that secrete insulin (insulinomas), gastrin (gastrinomas), vasoactive intestinal polypeptide (VIPomas), glucagon (glucagonomas), somatostatin (somatostatinomas), corticotropin-releasing factor (CRFomas), adrenocorticotropic hormone (ACTHomas), growth hormone-releasing factor (GRFomas), and pancreatic polypeptide (PPomas) (Fig. 54-1).

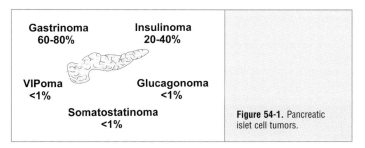

Gastrinoma   **Insulinoma**
60-80%   **20-40%**

VIPoma   **Glucagonoma**
<1%   **<1%**

Somatostatinoma
<1%

Figure 54-1. Pancreatic islet cell tumors.

2. **Are pancreatic endocrine tumors usually benign or malignant?**
   Insulinomas are usually benign (80%–90%); other pancreatic endocrine tumors are frequently malignant (50%–80%).

3. **Are pancreatic endocrine tumors associated with other endocrine disorders?**
   Up to 10% of pancreatic endocrine tumors occur as part of the multiple endocrine neoplasia type 1 (MEN-I) syndrome. This inherited disorder consists of pituitary tumors, pancreatic endocrine tumors, and hyperparathyroidism. Hyperparathyroidism usually precedes the pituitary and pancreatic tumors. The condition is caused by an inherited mutation in the menin gene.

4. **What are insulinomas?**
   Insulinomas are discrete insulin-producing tumors within the pancreas. They belong to a larger group of hyperinsulinemic pancreatic beta-cell disorders that include insulinomas, islet cell hyperplasia, and nesidioblastosis (neo-proliferation of beta cells along the pancreatic ducts).

5. **What is Whipple's triad?**
   - Hypoglycemia
   - Symptoms during hypoglycemia
   - Relief of symptoms with correction of hypoglycemia

6. **What glucose levels are considered to be hypoglycemia?**
   Glucose levels under 45 mg/dL are commonly considered to be hypoglycemic, but the best criteria for hypoglycemia continue to be controversial.

7. **What are the symptoms of hypoglycemia?**
   Hypoglycemic symptoms are classified according to the their type and their timing in relation to meals. Symptoms, such as confusion, slurred speech, blurred vision, seizures, and coma, result from inadequate delivery of glucose to the brain (neuroglycopenia). Symptoms, such as tremors, sweating, palpitations, and nausea, result from a counterregulatory discharge of catecholamines (adrenergic). When symptoms occur within 5 hours of the previous meal, they are considered to be "postprandial"; if they occur more than 5 hours after a meal they are considered to be "fasting." Insulinomas most commonly cause fasting neuroglycopenic symptoms, although postprandial and adrenergic symptoms may also occur.

8. **How is the diagnosis of an insulinoma made?**
   The diagnosis requires documentation of symptomatic hypoglycemia with endogenous hyperinsulinemia. Hyperinsulinemic hypoglycemia is defined as hypoglycemia with a serum insulin level 3 uU/mL or more, C-peptide 0.2 nmol/L or more, and proinsulin 5 pmol/L or more. If the patient does not present during a symptomatic episode, the physician must attempt to provoke hypoglycemia to make the diagnosis. This often requires a prolonged fast (up to 72 hours) with blood sampling for glucose, insulin, C-peptide, proinsulin, and beta-hydroxybutyrate levels every 6 hours until the glucose is less than 60 mg/dL and then every 1 to 2 hours, as well as during any symptoms that occur. C-peptide and proinsulin are markers of endogenous insulin secretion. A drug screen for sulfonylureas use is also recommended.

9. **How can insulinomas be distinguished from other causes of hyperinsulinemic hypoglycemia?**
   Hyperinsulinemic hypoglycemia can be due to insulinomas, surreptitious insulin administration, and medication use. Table 54-1 illustrates how these entities can be distinguished.

TABLE 54-1. INSULINOMAS VERSUS OTHER CAUSES OF HYPERINSULINEMIC HYPOGLYCEMIA

Test	Insulinoma	Surreptitious Insulin Use	Sulfonylurea or Meglitinide Use
Insulin	↑	↑	↑
C-peptide	↑	↓	↑
Proinsulin	↑	↓	NI
Drug screen	Neg	Neg	Pos

10. **How can an insulinoma be localized?**
    A computed tomography (CT) scan or magnetic resonance imaging (MRI) is usually the first localization procedure; the reported sensitivity of these techniques has varied anywhere from 15% to 90% in recent studies. Endoscopic ultrasound of the pancreas has higher sensitivity (56%–93%) and can detect tumors as small as 2 to 3 mm in size. Intra-arterial pancreatic calcium infusions with measurement of insulin changes in the right hepatic vein yields similar or superior results. Fluorine-18-L-dihydroxyphenylalanine positron emission tomography may also be useful if the above studies fail to identify a tumor. Intra-operative ultrasound is highly accurate and useful for finding small tumors that could not be localized preoperatively.

11. **What is the treatment for an insulinoma?**
    Surgery is the treatment of choice. When surgery is not desired, or when tumors are unresectable, medical therapy consists of multiple (usually six or more) small meals per day and the use of medications that inhibit insulin secretion. The most effective medication for this

purpose is oral diazoxide; other drugs that may be useful include propranolol, calcium channel blockers, thiazide diuretics, and phenytoin. Octreotide is rarely beneficial. Chemotherapy using streptozotocin with doxorubicin or with 5-fluorouracil reduces symptoms and improves survival in patients with malignant insulinomas.

12. **What are the clinical manifestations of gastrinomas?**
Gastrinomas secrete excessive gastrin, which stimulates prolific gastric acid secretion. Patients develop severe peptic ulcer disease, often associated with secretory diarrhea. This disorder is also known as the Zollinger-Ellison syndrome.

13. **Do gastrinomas always arise from pancreatic islet cells?**
Gastrinomas may arise from the pancreatic islets but also can occur in the duodenum and stomach.

14. **How is the diagnosis of gastrinoma made?**
The diagnosis is made by demonstrating the presence of high gastric acidity (pH <3.0) in association with a fasting serum gastrin level greater than 1000 pg/mL or a moderately elevated gastrin that increases by more than 200 pg/mL within 15 minutes after the intravenous administration of secretin.

15. **What is the best way to localize a gastrinoma?**
Localization of the tumor may be pursued with various techniques, including CT scan, MRI, endoscopic ultrasonography, octreotide scanning, transhepatic portal venous sampling, and selective arterial secretin infusions with right hepatic vein gastrin measurements.

16. **How are gastrinomas managed?**
Most benign and some malignant gastrinomas can be cured by surgery. Otherwise, attention should be directed toward reduction of gastric acid overproduction. Proton pump inhibitors are the drugs of choice for this purpose. Octreotide (Sandostatin, 50–500 mcg 2 or 3 times/day subcutaneously) or long-acting octreotide (Sandostatin LAR, 10–30 mg every month, intragluteally) are also highly effective agents for this condition. High-dose histamine-2 blockers may also be useful but are rarely adequate by themselves. Refractory patients may require total gastrectomy and vagotomy for symptom relief.

17. **How do you treat a malignant gastrinoma?**
Because most gastrinomas are malignant, chemotherapy is often necessary. The most effective chemotherapy combinations include the following: streptozotocin, 5-fluorouracil, and leucovorin; lomustine and 5-fluorouracil; etoposide, doxorubicin, and 5-fluorouracil; cisplatin, dacarbazine, and alpha-interferon. Finally, tumor embolization in conjunction with direct intra-arterial infusions of chemotherapy agents has shown additional promise as a palliative procedure.

18. **What are the characteristics of glucagonomas?**
Glucagon antagonizes the effects of insulin in the liver by stimulating glycogenolysis and gluconeogenesis. Glucagonomas, which secrete excessive glucagon, cause diabetes mellitus, weight loss, anemia, and a characteristic skin rash, necrolytic migratory erythema. Affected patients also have a thromboembolic diathesis. The diagnosis depends on finding an elevated level of serum glucagon (>500 pg/mL). Techniques similar to those used for gastrinomas are useful for localizing these tumors.

19. **How are glucagonomas treated?**
Treatment options include surgery for localized disease, octreotide to reduce glucagon secretion, and chemotherapy regimens similar to those used for gastrinomas. Chronic

anticoagulation to reduce the risk of thromboembolic events should also be considered. Finally, zinc supplements and intermittent amino acid infusions may help to reduce the skin rash and to improve the patient's overall sense of well-being.

20. **What are the characteristics of somatostatinomas?**
Among its multiple systemic effects, somatostatin inhibits secretion of insulin and pancreatic enzymes, production of gastric acid, and gallbladder contraction. Somatostatinomas secrete excess somatostatin, causing diabetes mellitus, weight loss, steatorrhea, hypochlorhydria, and cholelithiasis. The diagnosis is made by finding a significantly elevated serum somatostatin level.

KEY POINTS: PANCREATIC ENDOCRINE TUMORS

1. Insulinomas most often cause fasting hypoglycemia with neuroglycopenic symptoms but sometimes cause mainly postprandial symptoms.

2. Suspected insulinomas are investigated by measuring serum glucose, insulin, C-peptide, and proinsulin and screening for sulfonylureas during a symptomatic episode or a 72-hour supervised fast.

3. The treatment for an insulinoma is surgery, when possible, or multiple frequent feedings or the use of medications, such as diazoxide.

4. Gastrinomas (Zollinger-Ellison syndrome) cause aggressive peptic ulcer disease, which is sometimes with associated secretory diarrhea.

5. Gastrinomas are diagnosed by finding a markedly elevated serum gastrin or a prominent increase in serum gastrin after intravenous secretin administration in a patient with significant gastric acidity.

6. The treatment for a gastrinoma is surgery, when possible, or reduction of gastric acid production by high-dose proton pump inhibitors or a gastrectomy, if necessary.

21. **What is the treatment for somatostatinoma?**
Surgery is the treatment of choice. When surgery is not possible, somatostatin secretion and tumor size may be reduced by the same chemotherapy regimens used for other pancreatic endocrine tumors.

22. **What are the characteristics of VIPomas?**
VIPomas cause watery diarrhea, hypokalemia, and achlorhydria (WDHA syndrome, pancreatic cholera). This is also known as the Verner-Morrison syndrome. The diagnosis is made by finding an elevated level of serum VIP.

23. **How are VIPomas treated?**
Surgery is the treatment of choice. Octreotide effectively reduces diarrhea in most patients. Radiation therapy and chemotherapy also may effectively reduce diarrhea and tumor size.

24. **Briefly discuss the remaining pancreatic endocrine tumors.**
The remaining pancreatic endocrine tumors are rare. CRFomas and ACTHomas lead to the development of Cushing's syndrome, and GRFomas cause acromegaly. PPomas are initially

asymptomatic but may eventually enlarge to produce mass effects without a recognizable hormone hypersecretion syndrome. Localization procedures and treatments are similar to those described earlier for other pancreatic endocrine tumors.

BIBLIOGRAPHY

1. Arnold R, Simon B, Wied M: Treatment of neuroendocrine GEP tumors with somatostatin analogues. Review. Digestion 62(Suppl S1):84–91, 2000.

2. Baudin E: Gastroenteropancreatic endocrine tumors: clinical characterization before therapy. Nat Clin Pract Endocrinol Metab 3:228–238, 2007.

3. Boukhman MP, Karam JM, Shaver J, et al: Localization of insulinomas. Arch Surg 134:818–822, 1999 (discussion 822–823).

4. Doppman JL, Chang R, Fraker DL, et al: Localization of insulinomas to regions of the pancreas by intra-arterial stimulation with calcium. Ann Intern Med 123:269–273, 1995.

5. Hirshberg B, Livi A, Bartlett DL, et al: Forty-eight hour fast: the diagnostic test for insulinoma. J Clin Endocrinol Metab 85:3222–3226, 2000.

6. Jaffe BM: Current issues in the management of Zollinger-Ellison syndrome. Surgery 111:241–243, 1992.

7. Jensen RT: Pancreatic endocrine tumors: recent advances. Ann Oncol 10(Suppl 4)160–170, 1999.

8. Kar P, Price P, Sawers S, et al: Insulinomas may present with normoglycemia after prolonged fasting but glucose-stimulated hypoglycemia. J Clin Endocrinol Metab 91:4733–4736, 2006.

9. Kauhanen S, Sappanen M, Minn H, et al: Fluorine-18-L-dihydroxyphenylalanine (F18DOPA) positron emission tomography as a tool to localize an insulinoma or B-cell hyperplasia in adult patients. J Clin Endocrinol Metab 92:1237–1244, 2007.

10. Krejs GJ, Orci L, Conlon M, et al: Somatostatinoma syndrome: biochemical, morphologic and clinical features. N Engl J Med 301:283–292, 1979.

11. Leichter SB: Clinical and metabolic aspects of glucagonoma. Medicine 59:100–113, 1980.

12. Moertel CG, Johnson CM, McKusick MA, et al: The management of patients with advanced carcinoid tumors and islet cell carcinomas. Ann Intern Med 120:302–309, 1994.

13. Perry RR, Vinik AI: Diagnosis and management of functioning islet cell tumors. J Clin Endocrinol Metab 80:2273–2278, 1995.

14. Ricke J, Klose K: Imaging procedures in neuroendocrine tumors. Digestion 62(Suppl S1):39–44, 2000.

15. Service FJ: Classification of hypoglycemic disorders. Endocrinol Metab Clin North Am 28:501–517, 1999.

16. Service FJ: Recurrent hyperinsulinemic hypoglycemia caused by an insulin-secreting insulinoma. Nat Clin Pract Endocrinol Metab 2:467–470, 2006.

17. Service FJ, McMahon MM, O'Brien PC, et al: Functioning insulinomas—incidence, recurrence, and long-term survival of patients: a 60-year study. Mayo Clin Proc 66:711–719, 1991.

18. Wermers RA, Fatourechi V, Krols LK: Clinical spectrum of hyperglucagonemia associated with malignant neuroendocrine tumors. Mayo Clin Proc 71:1030–1038, 1996.

CHAPTER 55

CARCINOID SYNDROME

Michael T. McDermott

1. **What are carcinoid tumors? How are they classified?**
   Carcinoid tumors are neoplasms that arise from enterochromaffin or Kulchitsky cells. They are classified according to their site of origin as foregut (bronchus, stomach, duodenum, bile ducts, pancreas), midgut (jejunum, ileum, appendix, ascending colon), or hindgut (transverse and descending colon, rectum) carcinoids. They also occasionally occur in the ovaries, testes, prostate, kidney, breast, thymus, or skin.

2. **Define carcinoid syndrome.**
   The carcinoid syndrome is a humorally mediated disorder that consists of cutaneous flushing (90%), diarrhea (75%), bronchospasm (20%), endocardial fibrosis (33%), right-heart valvular lesions, and occasionally pleural, peritoneal, or retroperitoneal fibrosis.

3. **What are the biochemical mediators of the carcinoid syndrome?**
   Carcinoid tumors produce a variety of humoral mediators, including serotonin, chromogranin A, histamine, prostaglandins, bradykinin, tachykinins, neurotensin, motilin, and substance P. Diarrhea and fibrous tissue formation may be caused by serotonin, whereas flushing and wheezing are likely due to histamine, prostaglandins, or kinins (Fig. 55-1).

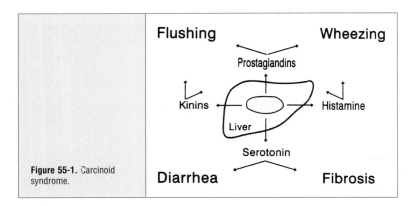

Figure 55-1. Carcinoid syndrome.

4. **Why does pellagra sometimes accompany the carcinoid syndrome?**
   Pellagra is due to niacin deficiency that results when the tumor diverts large amounts of tryptophan from niacin synthesis to produce serotonin.

5. **Why do intestinal carcinoid tumors so infrequently cause carcinoid syndrome?**
   The carcinoid syndrome occurs when humoral mediators enter the systemic circulation in large quantities. Solitary intestinal carcinoids secrete mediators into the portal circulation, where they are almost totally metabolized by the liver and never reach the systemic circulation. Carcinoid syndrome does not usually occur with these tumors unless there are hepatic metastases that

impair mediator metabolism or that secrete mediators directly into the hepatic vein. Extra-intestinal carcinoids, however, may cause carcinoid syndrome in the absence of metastases since they secrete mediators into venous systems that do not first pass through the liver.

6. **Do carcinoid tumors cause any other humoral syndromes?**
Carcinoids may also secrete corticotropin releasing factor (CRF) or corticotropin (adrenocorticotropin [ACTH]), causing Cushing's syndrome, or growth hormone-releasing factor (GRF), causing acromegaly. These syndromes have been reported mainly with bronchial and pancreatic carcinoid tumors.

KEY POINTS: CARCINOID SYNDROME

1. The carcinoid syndrome results from tumor production of humoral mediators that cause flushing, bronchospasm, diarrhea, and fibrous tissue formation.

2. Most patients with carcinoid syndrome have extensive liver metastases that either impair the metabolic clearance of mediators secreted by the primary tumor or that secrete the mediators directly into the hepatic vein.

3. Carcinoid syndrome is diagnosed by demonstrating markedly increased urinary excretion of 5-hydroxyindoleacetic acid (5-HIAA) or elevated serum levels of serotonin or chromogranin A.

4. The treatment for carcinoid syndrome is surgery, when possible, or palliation of symptoms by giving medications that reduce secretion of the humoral mediators or antagonize their effects.

5. A carcinoid crisis can be precipitated when a patient with a carcinoid tumor is given an adrenergic or sympathomimetic medication or a monoamine oxidase (MAO) inhibitor.

6. A carcinoid crisis is best treated with intravenous octreotide and hydrocortisone and avoiding the use of adrenergic and sympathomimetic agents.

7. **How is the diagnosis of carcinoid syndrome made?**
The diagnosis is made by finding markedly increased urinary excretion of 5-hydroxyindoleacetic acid, a breakdown product of serotonin, or increased serum concentrations of serotonin or chromogranin A. Although a nonspecific marker of neuroendocrine tumors, serum chromogranin A is one of the most sensitive markers of carcinoid and other gastroenteropancreatic endocrine tumors, including those that arise in the foregut.

8. **What is the treatment for carcinoid syndrome?**
Surgery can be curative when the carcinoid syndrome results from an extraintestinal carcinoid tumor that has not metastasized. Most patients with the carcinoid syndrome, however, have extensive metastases at the time of diagnosis. The goal of therapy is therefore usually not to cure but to provide palliation and to prolong survival. Medications to control symptoms (flushing, diarrhea, bronchospasm) and chemotherapy to reduce the tumor burden are the most effective general management strategies.

9. **How does one control the symptoms of carcinoid syndrome?**
The most troublesome symptoms patients with carcinoid syndrome experience are intense flushing and frequent diarrhea. Octreotide, a somatostatin analog, is highly effective in controlling most carcinoid symptoms. Table 55-1 lists the various medications or combinations that may be tried for symptom relief.

TABLE 55-1. MEDICATIONS FOR RELIEF OF SYMPTOMS RELATED TO CARCINOID SYNDROME

Medications to Control Carcinoid Flushing

Octreotide (Sandostatin)	50–150 mcg 2 or 3 times/day subcutaneously
Octreotide, long acting (Sandostatin LAR)	10–30 mg every month intragluteally
Phentolamine (Regitine)	25–50 mg 1–3 times/day
Phenoxybenzamine (Dibenzyline)	30 mg/day
Cyproheptadine (Periactin)	2–4 mg 3 or 4 times/day
Methysergide (Sansert)	2 mg 3 times/day
Prochlorperazine (Compazine)	5–10 mg every 4–6 hours
Chlorpromazine (Thorazine)	10–25 mg every 4–6 hours
Clonidine (Catapres)	0.1–0.2 mg 2 times/day
Methyldopa (Aldomet)	250 mg 3 times/day
Cimetidine (Tagamet), plus:	300 mg 3 times/day
Diphenhydramine (Benadryl)	50 mg 4 times/day
Glucocorticoids	

Medications to Control Carcinoid Diarrhea

Standard antidiarrheal measures, plus:

Octreotide (Sandostatin)	50–150 mcg 2 or 3 times/day subcutaneously
Octreotide, long acting (Sandostatin LAR)	10–30 mg every month intragluteally
Clonidine (Catapres)	0.1–0.2 mg 2 times/day
Cyproheptadine (Periactin)	2–4 mg 3 or 4 times/day
Methysergide (Sansert)	2 mg 3 times/day
Ondansetron (Zofran)	8 mg 3 times/day

---

10. **What chemotherapy regimens are most effective in carcinoid tumors?**
    Although not generally curative, chemotherapy may reduce the total tumor burden sufficiently to reduce carcinoid symptoms. The following chemotherapy regimens have thus far shown the greatest efficacy in these patients: streptozotocin, 5-fluorouracil and leucovorin; lomustine and 5-fluorouracil; etoposide, doxorubicin, and 5-fluorouracil; cisplatin, dacarbazine, and α-interferon. Another promising approach for hepatic tumor debulking has been hepatic artery embolization along with direct intra-arterial chemotherapy infusions.

11. **What is a carcinoid crisis?**
    A carcinoid crisis is an acute episode of severe flushing, bronchospasm, and hypotension. These episodes are most commonly provoked by the administration of adrenergic agents, such as epinephrine and sympathomimetic amines, or monoamine oxidase (MAO) inhibitors in patients with underlying carcinoid tumors. Patients need not have previously experienced symptoms of the carcinoid syndrome to have a carcinoid crisis.

12. **How can a carcinoid crisis be prevented?**
    Patients with known carcinoid syndrome should not be given epinephrine, sympathomimetic amines or MAO inhibitors. When these patients require a surgical procedure, they should be pretreated with octreotide (Sandostatin) 100 mcg subcutaneously 30 to 60 minutes before the

operation. Anesthesiologists should be specifically notified that the patient has carcinoid syndrome.

13. **Can a carcinoid crisis be predicted?**
   Patients with carcinoid tumors who have not developed carcinoid syndrome can be tested for their potential to have a carcinoid crisis. This is most commonly accomplished with an epinephrine provocation test; patients are given progressive intravenous (IV) boluses of epinephrine every 5 minutes, starting with a dose of 1 μg and increasing, if necessary, to 10 μg , while monitoring heart rate and blood pressure every 60 seconds. A positive response consists of flushing or a blood pressure drop of 20 mm systolic or 10 mm diastolic 45 to 120 minutes after an injection. All patients undergoing this test must have venous catheters and be monitored carefully throughout the test; IV phentolamine (Regitine) 5-mg and methoxamine (Vasoxyl) 3-mg preparations must also be available to reverse a crisis should it occur.

14. **Describe the management of a carcinoid crisis.**
   An effective treatment for an acute carcinoid crisis is the administration of IV octreotide and hydrocortisone. If this does not successfully abort the episode, other options include methotrimeprazine (an antiserotonin agent), methoxamine (a direct vasoconstrictor), phentolamine (an alpha-adrenergic blocker), ondansetron (a serotonin receptor antagonist), and glucagon. It is critical to avoid the use of adrenergic and sympathomimetic agents in patients with suspected carcinoid crisis because these drugs can significantly worsen the condition. Effective medication dose regimens for this condition are listed in Table 55-2.

TABLE 55-2. MANAGEMENT OF CARCINOID CRISIS

Medication	Dose Regimen
Octreotide (Sandostatin)	50 mcg IV over 1 min, then 50 mg IV over 15 min
Hydrocortisone (Solu-Cortef)	100 mg IV over 15 min
Methotrimeprazine (Levoprome)	2.5–5.0 mg slow IV push
Methoxamine (Vasoxyl)	3–5 mg slow IV push, followed by an infusion
Phentolamine (Regitine)	5 mg slow IV push
Ondansetron (Zofran)	20 mg IV over 15 min
Glucagon	0.5–1.5 mg slow IV push

IV, intravenous.
From Warner RRP: Gut neuroendocrine tumors. In Bardin CW, editor, *Current Therapy in Endocrinology and Metabolism,* ed 6, St. Louis, 1997, Mosby, pp. 606–614.

BIBLIOGRAPHY

1. Baudin E. Gastroenteropancreatic endocrine tumors: clinical characterization before therapy. Nat Clin Pract Endocrinol Metab 3:228–238, 2007.
2. Fehmann HC, Wulbrand U, Arnold R: Treatment of endocrine gastroenteropancreatic tumors with somatostatin analogues. Recent results. Cancer Res 153:15–22, 2000.
3. Feldman JM: The carcinoid syndrome. Endocrinologist 3:129–135, 1993.
4. Galanis E, Kvols LK, Rubin J: Carcinoid syndrome. J Clin Oncol 16:796–798, 1998.
5. Halford S, Waxman J: The management of carcinoid tumors. Q J Med 91:795–798, 1998.

6. Janmohamed S, Bloom SR: Review: Carcinoid tumours. Postgrad Med J 73:207–214, 1997.

7. Kulke MH, Mayer RJ: Review: Carcinoid tumors. N Engl J Med 340:858–868, 1999.

8. Oberg K: Carcinoid tumors: current concepts in diagnosis and treatment. Oncologist 3:339–345, 1998.

9. O'Toole D, Ducreaux M, Bommelaer G, et al: Treatment of carcinoid syndrome: a prospective crossover evaluation of lanreotide versus octreotide in terms of efficacy, patient acceptability, and tolerance. Cancer 88:770–776, 2000.

10. Soga J, Yakuwa Y, Osaka M: Carcinoid syndrome: a statistical evaluation of 748 reported cases. J Exp Clin Cancer Res 18:133–141, 1999.

11. Stuart K, Levy DE, Anderson T, et al: Phase II study of interferon gamma in malignant carcinoid tumors (E9292): a trial of the Eastern Oncology Group. Invest New Drugs 22:75–81, 2004.

CHAPTER 56

CUTANEOUS MANIFESTATIONS OF DIABETES MELLITUS AND THYROID DISEASE

Gary Goldenberg and James E. Fitzpatrick

1. **How often do patients with diabetes mellitus demonstrate an associated skin disorder?**

   Most published studies report that 30% to 50% of patients with diabetes mellitus ultimately develop a skin disorder attributable to their primary disease. However, if one includes subtle findings such as nail changes, vascular changes, and alteration of the cutaneous connective tissue, the incidence approaches 100%. Skin disorders most often present in patients with known diabetes mellitus, but cutaneous manifestations also may be an early sign of undiagnosed diabetes.

KEY POINTS: CUTANEOUS MANIFESTATIONS

1. Patients with diabetes mellitus demonstrate cutaneous findings attributable to diabetes in almost 100% of cases.

2. The most common cause of acanthosis nigricans is diabetes associated with insulin resistance and obesity.

3. Necrobiosis lipoidica is a granulomatous dermatitis that is typically associated with diabetes mellitus in almost two thirds of cases.

4. Scleredema adultorum, a disorder characterized by accumulation of collagen and mucin in the skin is most commonly associated with diabetes mellitus.

5. Generalized myxedema is the most characteristic cutaneous sign of hypothyroidism.

---

2. **Are any skin disorders pathognomonic of diabetes mellitus?**

   Yes. Bullous diabeticorum (bullous eruption of diabetes, diabetic bullae) is specific for diabetes mellitus, but it is uncommon. Bullous diabeticorum most often occurs in patients with severe diabetes, particularly those with associated peripheral neuropathy. In general, all other reported skin findings may be found to some extent in normal individuals. However, some cutaneous conditions (e.g., necrobiosis lipoidica diabeticorum) demonstrate strong associations with diabetes.

3. **What is bullous diabeticorum?**

   Bullous diabeticorum is a a a blistering disorder that primarily occurs on the distal extremities of diabetics. They typically appear as spontaneous tense blisters that are asymptomatic except for a burning sensation. The exact mechanism is not understood, but a high percentage of patients have peripheral neuropathy, retinopathy, or nephropathy.

4. **What are the skin disorders most likely to be encountered in diabetics?**
   See Table 56-1. The most common skin disorders are finger pebbles, nail bed telangiectasia, red face (rubeosis), skin tags (acrochordons), diabetic dermopathy, yellow skin, yellow nails, and pedal petechial purpura. Less common cutaneous disorders that are closely associated with diabetes mellitus include necrobiosis lipoidica diabeticorum, bullous eruption of diabetes, acanthosis nigricans, and scleredema adultorum.

TABLE 56-1. COMMON CUTANEOUS FINDINGS IN DIABETES MELLITUS		
Cutaneous Finding	Incidence in Controls (%)	Incidence in Diabetics (%)
Finger pebbles	21	75
Nail bed telangiectasia	12	65
Rubeosis (red face)	18	59
Skin tags	3	55
Diabetic dermopathy	Uncommon	54
Yellow skin	24	51
Yellow nails	Uncommon	50
Erythrasma	Uncommon	47
Diabetic thick skin	Uncommon	30

5. **What are finger pebbles?**
   Finger pebbles are multiple, grouped minute papules that tend to affect the extensor surfaces of the fingers, particularly near the knuckles. They are asymptomatic and may be extremely subtle in appearance. Histologically finger pebbles are due to increased collagen in the dermal papillae. The pathogenesis is not understood.

6. **What is acanthosis nigricans?**
   Acanthosis nigricans is a skin condition due to papillomatous (wartlike) hyperplasia of the skin. It is associated with various conditions, including diabetes mellitus, obesity, acromegaly, Cushing's syndrome, certain medications, and underlying malignancies. In acanthosis nigricans associated with insulin-dependent diabetes, it has been linked to insulin resistance by three mechanisms: type A (receptor defect), type B (antireceptor antibodies), and type C (postreceptor defect). It is proposed that in insulin-resistant states, there is hyperinsulinemia that competes for the insulin-like growth factor receptors on keratinocytes and thus stimulates epidermal growth. In the case of hypercortisolism as seen in Cushing's disease, there is induced insulin resistance, which is believed to induce epidermal growth.

7. **What does acanthosis nigricans look like?**
   It is most noticeable in axillary, inframammary, and neck creases where it appears as hyperpigmented velvety skin that has the appearance of being "dirty" (Fig. 56-1). The tops of knuckles may also demonstrate small papules that resemble finger pebbles except that they are more pronounced (Fig. 56-2).

8. **What is diabetic dermopathy?**
   Diabetic dermopathy (shin spots or pretibial pigmented patches) is a common affliction of diabetics that initially presents as erythematous to brown to browish-red macules that typically measure 0.5 to 1.5 cm in size with variable scale on the pretibial surface (Fig. 56-3). The lesions are typically asymptomatic but are occasionally pruritc or are associated with a burning

Figure 56-1. Acanthosis nigricans. Characteristic velvety hyperpigmentation of flexural areas.

Figure 56-2. Acanthosis nigricans. Typical papillomatous lesions over the knuckles.

Figure 56-3. Diabetic dermopathy. Characteristic brown macules over pretibial areas.

sensation. Patients with diabetic dermopathy are more likely to have retinopathy, nephropathy, and neuropathy. They heal with varying degress of atrophy and hyperpigmentation over 1 to 2 years. The pathogenesis is unknown, but skin biopsies from the lesions demonstrate diabetic microangiopathy characterized by a proliferation of endothelial cells and thickening of the basement membranes of arterioles, capillaries, and venules. Although many physicians attribute these lesions to trauma, this is not supported by an unusual study in which patients with diabetes mellitus did not develop lesions after being struck on the pretibial surface with a hard rubber hammer! There is no known effective treatment.

9. **What is necrobiosis lipoidica diabeticorum?**
Necrobiosis lipoidica diabeticorum is a disease that most commonly occurs on the pretibial areas, although it may occur at other sites. Early lesions present as nondiagnostic erythematous papules or plaques that evolve into annular lesions characterized by a yellowish or yellowish-brown color, dilatated blood vessels, and central epidermal atrophy. Developed lesions are characteristic and usually can be diagnosed by clinical appearance. Less commonly, ulcers may develop. Biopsies are usually diagnostic and demonstrate palisaded granulomas that surround large zones of necrotic and sclerotic collagen. Additional findings include dilatated vascular spaces, plasma cells, and increased dermal fat. The pathogenesis is not known, but proposed causes include an immune complex vasculitis and a platelet aggregation defect.

10. **What is the relationship of necrobiosis lipoidica diabeticorum to diabetes mellitus?**
In a major study of patients with necrobiosis lipoidica diabeticorum, 62% had diabetes. Approximately one half of the nondiabetic patients had abnormal glucose tolerance tests, and almost one half of the nondiabetics gave a family history of diabetes. However, necrobiosis lipoidica diabeticorum is present in only 0.3% of patients with diabetes. The term "necrobiosis lipoidica" is used for patients who have the disorder without associated diabetes. Because of the strong association between these conditions, patients who present with necrobiosis lipoidica should be screened for diabetes; patients who test negative should be reevaluated periodically.

11. **How should necrobiosis lipoidica diabeticorum be treated?**
Necrobiosis lipoidica occasionally may resolve without treatment. It does not seem to respond to treatment of diabetes in new cases or to tighter control of established diabetes. Early lesions may respond to treatment with potent topical or intralesional corticosteroids. More severe cases may respond to oral treatment with stanozolol, niacinamide, pentoxyfylline, mycophenolate mofetil, or cyclosporine. Severe cases with recalcitrant ulcers may require surgical grafting.

12. **Are skin infections more common in diabetics than in control populations?**
Yes, but skin infections are probably not as common as most medical personnel believe. Studies show that an increased incidence of skin infections strongly correlates with elevated levels of mean plasma glucose.

13. **What are the most common bacterial skin infections associated with diabetes mellitus?**
The most common serious skin infections associated with diabetes mellitus are related to diabetic foot and amputation ulcers. One autopsy study revealed that 2.4% of all diabetics had infectious skin ulcerations of the extremities compared with 0.5% of a control population. Even though there are no well-controlled studies, it is felt that staphylococcal skin infections, including furunculosis and staphylococcal wound infections, are more common and serious in diabetics. Erythrasma, a benign superficial bacterial infection caused by *Corynebacterium minutissimum,* was present in 47% of adult diabetics in one study. Clinically it presents as tan to reddish-brown macular lesions with slight scale in intertriginous areas such as the groin.

Because the organisms produce porphyrins, the diagnosis can be made by demonstrating a spectacular coral red fluorescence with a Wood's lamp.

14. **What is the most common fungal mucocutaneous infection associated with diabetes mellitus?**
The most common mucocutaneous fungal infection associated with diabetes is candidiasis, usually caused by *Candida albicans*. Women are particularly prone to get vulvovaginitis. One study demonstrated that two thirds of all diabetics have positive cultures for *Candida albicans*. In women with signs and symptoms of vulvitis, the incidence of positive cultures approaches 99%. Similarly, positive cultures are extremely common in diabetic men and women who complain of anal pruritus. Other mucocutaneous forms of candidiasis include thrush, perleche (angular cheilitis), intertrigo, erosio interdigitalis blastomycetica chronica (Fig. 56-4), paronychia (infection of the soft tissue around the nail plate), and onychomycosis (infection of the nail). The mechanism appears to be due to increased levels of glucose that serve as a substrate for *Candida* species to proliferate. Patients with recurrent cutaneous candidiasis of any form should be screened for diabetes.

Figure 56-4. Erosio interdigitalis blastomycetic chronica. *Candida* infection in the interdigital spaces in a diabetic patient. A very long name for a very small infection!

15. **Why are diabetics in ketoacidosis especially prone to mucormycosis?**
Some zygomycetes, including *Mucor, Mortierella, Rhizopus,* and *Absidia* species, are thermotolerant, prefer an acid pH, grow rapidly in the presence of high levels of glucose, and are among the few fungi that utilize ketones as a growth substrate. Thus diabetics in ketoacidosis provide an ideal environment for the proliferation of these fungi. Fortunately, these fulminant and often fatal fungal infections are rare.

16. **Are any skin complications associated with the treatment of diabetes mellitus?**
Yes. Adverse reactions to injected insulin are relatively common. The reported incidence varies from 10% to 56%, depending on the study. In general these complications may be divided into three categories: reactions due to faulty injections (e.g., intradermal injection), idiosyncratic reactions, and allergic reactions. Several types of allergic reactions have been described, including localized and generalized urticaria, Arthus reactions, and localized delayed hypersensitivity. Oral hypoglycemic agents occasionally may produce adverse cutaneous reactions, including photosensitivity, urticaria, erythema multiforme, and erythema nodosum. Chlorpropamide in particular may produce a flushing reaction when consumed with alcohol.

17. **What is scleredema adultorum?**
Scleredema adultorum is a woody induration that most commonly presents on the posterior neck, upper back, and shoulders. Less commonly it may be more extensive and involve the face, abdomen, and extremities. It is most commonly associated with insulin-dependent diabetes and

less commonly associated with monoclonal gammopathies and following streptococcal infections. Biopsies demonstrate increased dermal collagen and hyaluronic acid (dermal mucin). The pathogenesis is not understood. When associated with insulin-dependent diabetes, scleredema adultorum is chronic and recalcitrant to therapy.

18. **What are the most important cutaneous manifestations of the hypothyroid state?**

Generalized myxedema is the most characteristic cutaneous sign of hypothyroidism. Other skin findings include xerosis (dry skin), follicular hyperkeratosis (Fig. 56-5), diffuse hair loss (especially the outer one third of the eyebrows), dry and brittle nails, yellowish discoloration of the skin, and thyroid acropachy (thickening of the distal fingers). These skin changes are all reversible with appropriate thyroid replacement.

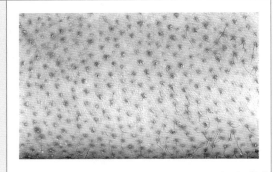

Figure 56-5. Hypothyroidism. Marked follicular hyperkeratosis that quickly disappeared with thyroid replacement.

19. **Why do hypothyroid patients often have yellow skin?**

The yellow color is due to the accumulation of carotene (carotenoderma) in the top layer of the epidermis (stratum corneum). Carotene is excreted by both the sweat and the sebaceous glands and tends to concentrate on the palms, soles, and face. The increased levels of carotene are probably secondary to impaired hepatic conversion of beta-carotene to vitamin A.

20. **What are the clinical findings in generalized myxedema?**

Generalized myxedema is characterized by pale, waxy, edematous skin that does not demonstrate pitting. These changes are most noticeable in the periorbital area but may also be observed in the distal extremities, lips, and tongue (Fig. 56-6).

Figure 56-6. Generalized myxedema. Pale, waxy skin of upper eyelids associated with marked pendulous edema of lower eyelids. These changes quickly disappeared with thyroid replacement.

21. What is the pathogenesis of generalized myxedema?

The skin demonstrates an increased accumulation of dermal acid mucopolysaccharides, of which hyaluronic acid (ground substance) is the most important. Studies also have demonstrated that an increased transcapillary escape of serum albumin into the dermis adds to the edematous appearance. Neither of these changes are permanent; both are reversible with replacement therapy.

22. What is the difference between generalized myxedema and pretibial myxedema?

Generalized myxedema is associated with only the hypothyroid state, whereas pretibial myxedema is characteristically associated with Graves' disease. Patients with pretibial myxedema may be hypothyroid, hyperthyroid, or euthyroid when the skin disorder appears. The pathogenesis has not been proved but it has been demonstrated that serum from patients with pretibial myxedema will stimulate the production of acid mucopolysaccharides of fibroblasts. Fibroblasts from the pretibial area are more sensitive to stimulation than fibroblasts from other areas, which would account for the tendency for these lesions to occur in pretibial areas. The nature of this circulating factor is unknown but antithyroid immunoglobulins that bind to fibroblasts may be the cause. It has also been postulated that activated T cells induce fibroblast proliferation and induce the production of acid mucopolysaccharides.

23. What are the clinical manifestations of pretibial myxedema?

Pretibial myxedema occurs in approximately 3% to 5% of patients with Graves' disease. The majority of patients have associated exophthalmos. Thyroid acropachy is also present in 1% of patients with Graves' disease (Fig. 56-7). Clinically pretibial myxedema is characterized by edematous, indurated plaques over the pretibial areas, although other sites of the body also may be involved. The plaques are usually sharply demarcated, but diffuse variants are also reported. The overlying skin surface is usually normal, although it may be studded with smaller papules. The color varies from skin-colored to brownish-red (Fig. 56-8). Overlying hypertrichosis may be present on rare occasions. Histologically, pretibial myxedema demonstrates massive accumulation of dermal hyaluronic acid.

Figure 56-7. Thyroid acropachy. Patient with Graves' disease demonstrating swelling of soft tissue and increased curvature of the nail plate.

24. How is pretibial myxedema treated?

Studies comparing different treatment modalities have not been performed. Because the condition is not harmful to patients and because it may resolve spontaneously, treatment is not always indicated. Many cases respond to potent topical corticosteroids under occlusion or intralesional corticosteroids. More extensive cases may be treated with oral systemic corticosteroids. Treatment of the thyroid disease does not affect the cutaneous findings.

Figure 56-8. Pretibial myxedema. Indurated brownish-red plaque of the pretibial area.

25. **What are the skin manifestations of hyperthyroidism?**

    Studies have shown that as many as 97% of all patients with hyperthyroidism develop skin manifestations. Common cutaneous findings include cutaneous erythema, evanescent flushing, excoriations, smooth skin, hyperpigmentation, moist skin (due to increased sweating), pretibial myxedema, pruritus (itching), and warm skin. Nails are often brittle and may separate from the underlying bed (onycholysis). The hair also may be thinner than normal.

26. **What effect does obesity have on skin function and physiology?**

    Obesity effects skin function and physiology in many ways. The skin barrier function is altered in obese individuals, who show a significantly increased transepidermal water loss. The elevation of androgens, insulin, growth hormone, and insulin-like growth factor seen in obese patients is related to an increase in sebaceous gland function and sebum production, exacerbating diseases such as acne vulgaris. The activity of apocrine and eccrine sweat glands is also increased in obese patients. Lymphatic flow is impeded in obese individuals, leading to accumulation of protein-rich lymphatic fluid in the subcutaneous tissue, which in turn leads to lymphedema. In animal studies, obesity is associated with altered collagen structure and function and impaired wound healing.

27. **What are some of the cutaneous manifestations of obesity?**

    Obese patients have myriad cutaneous manifestations, including changes related to insulin resistance, as well as infectious, mechanical, inflammatory conditions. These include acanthosis nigricans (discussed earlier), acrochordons (skin tags), keratosis pilaris, striae distensae, and hidradenitis suppurativa.

28. **Does obesity aggravate any skin diseases?**

    Yes. Obesity aggravates multiple skin diseases, including intertrigo, hidradenitis suppurativa, cellulite, psoriasis, and chronic venous insufficiency. Bacterial skin infections are also aggravated by obesity. These range from superficial infections, such as folliculitis, to deep infections, such as cellulitis and necrotizing fasciitis.

TOP SECRETS

1. Bullous diabeticorum is the only cutaneous finding that is pathognomonic of diabetes mellitus.

2. Acanthosis nigricans is associated with several endocrinopathies including diabetes mellitus (most common), acromegaly, and Cushing's syndrome, in addition to several genetic disorders, medications, and malignancies.

3. Mucomycosis is more common in diabetics in ketoacidosis because the fungi are thermotolerant, grow well in an acid pH, grow rapidly in the presence of high glucose, and are one of the few types of fungi that can utilize ketones as a food substrate.

4. Loss of the lateral one third of a the eyebrows is a classic cutaneous finding associated with hypothyroidism.

5. Hypothyroid patients have yellowish skin because of carotenodermia, which is due to the accumulation of carotene in the top layer of the epidermis.

BIBLIOGRAPHY

1. Anderson CK, Miller OF III: Triad of exophthalmos, pretibial myxedema, and acropachy in a patient with Graves' disease. J Am Acad Dermatol 48:970–972, 2003.

2. Bello YM, Phillips TJ: Necrobiosis lipoidica. Indolent plaques may signal diabetes. Postgrad Med 109:93–94, 2001.

3. Ferringer T, Miller FIII: Cutaneous manifestations of diabetes mellitus. Dermatol Clin 20:483–492, 2002.

4. Hollister DS, Brodell RT: Finger "pebbles." A dermatologic sign of diabetes mellitus. Postgrad Med 107:209–210, 2000.

5. Jabbour SA: Cutaneous manifestations of endocrine disorders: a guide for dermatologists. Am J Clin Dermatol 4:315–331, 2003.

6. Lipsky BA, Berendt AR: Principles and practice of antibiotic therapy of diabetic foot infections. Diabetes Metab Res Rev 16(Suppl 1):S42–S46, 2000.

7. Niepomniszcze H, Amad RH: Skin disorders and thyroid diseases. J Endocrinol Invest 24:628–638, 2001.

8. Pirotta SS, Johnson JD, Young G, Bezzant J: Bullosis diabeticorum. J Am Podiatr Assoc 85:169–171, 1995.

9. Shemer A, Bergman R, Linn S, et al: Diabetic dermopathy and internal complications in diabetes mellitus. Int J Dermatol 37:113–115, 1998.

10. Stoddard ML, Blevins KS, Lee ET, et al: Association of acanthosis nigricans with hyperinsulinemia compared with other selected risk factors for type 2 diabetes in Cherokee Indians: the Cherokee Diabetes Study. Diabetes Care 25:1009–1014, 2002.

11. Yosipovitch G, DeVore A, Dawn A: Obesity and the skin: skin physiology and skin manifestations of obesity. J Am Acad Dermatol. 56:901–916, 2007.

CHAPTER 57

AGING AND ENDOCRINOLOGY

Heather E. Brooks, Wendy M. Kohrt, and Robert S. Schwartz

1. **What effect does aging have on body weight?**
   Aging is associated with important changes in body composition that may be influenced by the endocrine milieu and that in return can have important endocrine/metabolic consequences. In cross-sectional studies, body weight increases until about age 55 years and then declines. This may be due to a "die-off" effect in the heaviest patients during middle age. Prospective studies suggest that weight does begin to decline after age 65 to 70 years. This reduction in body weight, whether intentional or unintentional, appears to be associated with an increase in mortality, morbidity, and disability. The explanation for this is not clear, but it is possible that any sustained weight loss may, in fact, be truly unintentional because intentional weight loss is exceptionally difficult to maintain. Weight loss in the face of illness or disease that raises cytokine levels may predispose to a disproportionate loss of weight as lean mass (muscle mass), thereby exacerbating age-related sarcopenia and leading to a catabolic state.

2. **What changes in lean body mass occur with aging?**
   There is an inevitable loss of lean body mass, mostly skeletal muscle mass, with aging. This aging-associated loss of muscle has been termed sarcopenia and has been blamed for much, but not all, of the age-related decline in muscle strength and power. In cross-sectional studies, a 20% to 30% loss of lean mass has been detected between ages 30 and 80 years. The decline in strength is even greater, with longitudinal studies finding up to a 60% loss from age 30 to 80 years. Furthermore the loss of strength and power are not as linear as the loss of muscle mass and seems to progress more rapidly at older ages. A 25% decline in strength has been detected just between 70 and 75 years. Power (work per unit time) may decline at even double the rate of strength. These changes in lean mass, muscle mass, strength, and power have complex but important functional consequences for older people.

   A recent concept, termed sarcopenic obesity, considers the degree of adiposity relative to lean mass. Currently, because a consensus on how sarcopenic obesity should be defined is lacking, the prevalence and clinical relevance has not been clearly established.

3. **What changes in bone mass and density occur with aging?**
   Prospective data indicate that peak bone mass occurs during the late teenage years in women and about a decade later in men. Because of the intimate structural and functional link between muscle and bone, the occurrence of peak bone mass likely corresponds with peak skeletal muscle development. It is generally thought that bone mass is maintained, or decreases slowly (<0.2% per year), at least through age 40 years in women and age 50 years in men. Intuitively, a decline in physical activity during middle age might be expected to induce an even faster rate of bone loss. However, the increase in body weight that typically also occurs during middle age may counter this to a large extent by increasing mechanical loading forces acting on the skeleton during weight-bearing activity. There also appears to be an inevitable loss of bone mass in old age that increases risk for osteoporosis in elderly men and augments risk for osteoporosis in postmenopausal women. In both elderly women and men, the decrease in bone mineral at the hip appears to be accelerated ($\approx$1% per year) relative to the changes at the spine, which may increase in advanced age. Vertebral compression fractures and the development of

extravertebral osteophytes lead to an increase in bone mineral density (BMD) that is not reflected in increased vertebral bone strength. The utility of spine BMD for the diagnosis of osteoporosis is therefore compromised in this most important situation.

4. **Does menopause have an independent effect on bone mass?**
There is undoubtedly an accelerated decline in BMD around the time of menopause in women. What remains somewhat controversial is whether the menopause-induced increase in bone resorption diminishes after a few years or persists further into old age. In this regard, observational studies of women aged 65 years and older indicate that the rate of bone loss continues to increase with age, particularly in the hip region. This is corroborated by observations that serum markers of bone turnover increase at the menopause and remain elevated into old age.

5. **Can weight-bearing exercise prevent the menopause-related loss of bone mineral in women?**
It is unlikely that even vigorous weight-bearing exercise can effectively counteract the deleterious effects of estrogen deficiency on BMD. Older female athletes not on hormone replacement therapy have lower BMD than premenopausal athletes. Moreover, young female athletes with menstrual cycle dysfunction can have BMD levels in the osteopenic (1.0–2.5 SD below the average peak BMD) and even the osteoporotic range (>2.5 SD below the average peak BMD), despite their participation in sports that involve high levels of mechanical loading (e.g., gymnastics, distance running).

6. **Do sex hormones influence the skeletal response to exercise?**
Although the direct effects of estrogens on bone metabolism are well known, increasing evidence indicates that the responses of bone cells to mechanical stress involve the activation of estrogen receptor alpha. The effects of age-related sex hormone deficiency on receptor density and function in bone remain unknown. In animal models, the effects of mechanical stress in the presence of estrogens (in females) or androgens (in males) on the bone proliferative response have been found to be additive or possibly synergistic (i.e., more than additive). There is also evidence for additive or synergistic effects of exercise and estrogens on BMD in postmenopausal women.

7. **Does fat mass increase or redistribute with aging?**
There is an increase in total adiposity and shift toward more abdominal fat distribution with advancing age. The increase in central adiposity begins in young men after puberty, but this does not appear to occur in women until around the time of the menopausal transition. Although the loss of lean mass was once thought to be the primary determinant of physical disability in old age, recent studies indicate that increased adiposity is an independent, and perhaps stronger, predictor of disability in older individuals. The increase in abdominal visceral adiposity (along with the decline in physical activity) plays an important role in the age-associated increase in insulin resistance and probably contributes to the high incidence and prevalence of type 2 diabetes mellitus and metabolic syndrome in old age.

8. **Does menopause trigger an increase in abdominal obesity in women?**
Cross-sectional comparisons of women across the age spectrum suggest that waist size increases more rapidly in women aged 50 years and older than in younger women. Prospective studies indicate that increases in waist circumference are related to both chronologic and ovarian age, with the most rapid increases in waist girth occurring in perimenopausal women. Premenopausal women treated with gonadotropin-releasing hormone agonists to suppress sex hormones gain 1 to 2 kg of fat mass in 4 to 6 months, with a disproportionate increase in central body regions. Several randomized, controlled trials have provided evidence that postmenopausal women on hormone therapy gain less weight and have less increase in waist

size than the placebo-treated women. The effects seem to be slightly larger with unopposed estrogens. It has not yet been determined whether estrogens specifically prevent or attenuate intra-abdominal fat accumulation.

9. **What are the results of prospective studies of voluntary weight loss in the elderly?**
There are few studies of intentional weight loss in the elderly. Hypocaloric diets have been effective in reducing cardiovascular risk factors with better glucose tolerance, increased insulin sensitivity, decreased visceral fat, decreased blood pressure, and increased pulmonary function. Diet and exercise improve pain, disability, and physical function in patients with osteoarthritis. However, intentional weight loss is also associated with a loss of lean mass (muscle and bone), which may exacerbate sarcopenia and risk for osteoporosis. There is some evidence that combining exercise with diet for weight loss better preserves lean mass than diet alone, and improves frailty and cardiovascular risk factors (e.g., lower glucose, triglycerides (TG), fatty acids, blood pressure, and waist circumference). It is recommended that diet-induced weight loss should be attempted in combination with exercise to help maintain muscle and adequate calcium and vitamin D to help maintain bone.

10. **Why is vitamin D status important in older adults?**
Vitamin D supplementation has been found to reduce the incidence of osteoporotic fractures in the elderly. This may occur through increased bone mineralization and improved muscle function and reduction in falls. Vitamin D deficiency is defined as a 25-hydroxyvitamin D (25-OHD) evel of less than 20 ng/mL (50 nmol/L). It has been estimated that more than 40% of community-dwelling older women and men in the United States are vitamin D deficient, and the prevalence is even higher in nursing home residents. There are multiple causes of vitamin D deficiency in older adults, including decreased skin synthesis; decreased sun exposure; decreased intake; impaired absorption, transport, or liver hydroxylation of oral vitamin D; medications altering vitamin D metabolism; chronic illnesses associated with malabsorption; and liver and kidney disease. Supplementation with vitamin D3 (cholecalciferol) is roughly 3 times more effective in increasing serum 25-OHD acutely when compared with the more widely available vitamin D2 (ergocalciferol) and thus is the preferred type of replacement.
  BMD is adversely affected when serum 25-OHD is less than 40 ng/mL. Vitamin D3 supplementation of 700 to 800 IU/day or 100,000 IU every 3 months has been found to reduce the incidence of fractures. There is currently no evidence for antifracture efficacy of D2 supplementation, although because of lower cost, this is the most common type of replacement available.
  Vitamin D deficiency also causes muscle weakness. Proximal muscle strength is linearly related to serum 25-OH D when levels are less than 40 ng/mL. Vitamin D supplementation has been associated with a 22% reduction in falls. Nursing home residents randomized to receive 800 IU/day of vitamin D2 plus calcium had a 72% reduction in falls.
  In addition to its important role in muscle and bone metabolism, vitamin D deficiency is postulated to influence immune function, cancer risk, parathyroid hormone and renin production, and insulin secretion.

11. **What are the recommendations for vitamin D daily intake in older adults?**
Many experts believe that the current recommendations from the institute of Medicine for vitamin D intake of 400 IU/day for 51 to 70 year olds and 600 IU/day for 70+ year olds remain inadequate. It has been suggested that 800-1000 IU/day is a more appropriate target in this population. A cost-effective strategy for correcting vitamin D deficiency and maintaining adequate levels in older adults is a 50,000 IU vitamin D2 tablet once per week for 8 weeks, followed by 50,000 IU vitamin D2 once every 2 to 4 weeks or 1000 IU vitamin D3 daily thereafter.

12. **What interventions have been associated with increased longevity, and have they been shown to work in humans?**
Studies of yeast, worms, flies, rodents, and mammals have demonstrated that caloric restriction (CR; 30%–40% reduction in daily energy intake) increases mean (i.e., average life expectancy) and maximal life span. Interestingly, generating a negative energy balance in rodents through increased energy expenditure (exercise) results in similar improvements in mean life span as CR but does not increase maximal life span. Long-term studies of CR in humans and other primates are underway, but short-term studies suggest that CR produces physiological, metabolic, and hormonal effects that parallel many of the positive effects found in other species.

It is estimated that one quarter to one third of the differences in life expectancy in humans are explained by genetic factors, but there are currently no definitive biomarkers or genes associated with longevity in humans. Large-scale collaborations, such as the pan-European Genetics of Healthy Aging consortium and the United States Longevity Consortium, are studying different populations to address this issue.

13. **What happens to testosterone and estradiol levels with aging in men?**
Total testosterone (TT) concentrations decline with age. Additionally sex hormone–binding globulin (SHBG) levels increase with age, which results in an even greater relative reduction in calculated bioavailable and free testosterone (FT) with age (declines of −14.5% for TT vs. −27% FT per decade of aging).

Total plasma estradiol levels in adult men do not change significantly with age, but bioavailable and free estradiol levels decrease due to the increase in SHBG with aging (estradiol binds to SHBG with half the affinity of testosterone). In absolute terms, serum estrogen levels of elderly males are somewhat higher than those of postmenopausal women (average of 33 pg/mL vs. 21 pg/mL).

14. **What is the cause of decreases in male testosterone levels with aging?**
In addition to an age-related decline, changes in health and lifestyle factors, such as weight gain, illness, smoking cessation, polypharmacy, and widowhood, can reduce TT. For instance, the decline in TT associated with becoming obese (−12%) is comparable to that associated with 10 years of aging among subjects whose obesity status is stable (−13%). Low endogenous testosterone levels are predictive of future development of metabolic syndrome, cardiovascular, respiratory, all-cause mortality, and cognitive decline. It is as yet not known whether raising testosterone levels by supplementation translates into decreased mortality.

There also appears to be an independent secular decline in total testosterone levels (i.e., decreasing age-specific testosterone levels in recent birth cohorts compared with earlier birth cohorts), observed in U.S. and Danish cohorts. However, whereas there was a concomitant decrease in bioavailable testosterone in the U.S. cohort, there was no secular decrease in calculated free T in the Danish cohort as a result of lower SHBG. Whether these changes in total or bioavailable T are related to the observed secular decreases in male fertility and sperm counts is an area of current investigation. The causes of these secular trends are unknown but have been attributed to differences in assay techniques, health and lifestyle changes (e.g., increasing levels of obesity), or as yet unidentified environmental exposures.

15. **What is the prevalence of hypogonadism in older men?**
The exact prevalence is not known because of the lack of consensus on the definition of hypogonadism with aging. The development of a consensus definition is complicated by a number of factors: (1) whether there should be age-specific reference ranges or testosterone levels in all men should be compared with young male levels; (2) whether the definition should be based on total (SHBG bound + albumin bound + free), bioavailable (albumin bound + free), or free testosterone levels; (3) concern regarding the reliability and variability immunoassays versus mass spectroscopy; (4) formulas for calculating bioavailable and free testosterone may

not be valid in some or all older populations; (5) whether the definition of hypogonadism should relate only to a serum concentration, a concentration plus symptoms, or just symptoms alone. When defined as TT less than 300 ng/dL and FT less than 5 ng/dL, almost 50% of men aged 50+ years with hypogonadism were asymptomatic, and 65% of men with symptoms had normal testosterone levels. The prevalence of symptomatic androgen deficiency is estimated to be at least 5% in men aged 50 to 70 years and 18% in older men.

16. **Are there benefits of testosterone supplementation for older men?**
Of the few randomized controlled trials that have been conducted in healthy, older men, most found an increase or stabilization of fat-free mass (bone and muscle) and a decrease in fat mass (including abdominal visceral) in response to testosterone. Whether such physiological effects translate into functional and strength improvements are equivocal. Furthermore, improvements in sexual function and sense of well-being have been inconsistent.

The lack of consistent findings among trials of testosterone supplementation is likely related to variability in study cohorts (e.g., baseline testosterone levels, symptoms, body composition, comorbidities, physical function), the type of testosterone supplementation therapy (e.g., oral, transdermal, intramuscular, dosage, and average testosterone concentration achieved), and duration of intervention (e.g., months vs. years).

17. **Is there evidence for adverse effects of testosterone supplementation?**
Supraphysiological replacement of eugonadal men appears to have harmful effects, both on liver function and cognition. A consistent side effect of testosterone replacement is an increase in hemoglobin. Surprisingly, adverse prostate effects have not been consistently observed. Testosterone replacement in hypogonadal men can result in a small initial increase in prostate-specific antigen (PSA), but most interventional studies of men with low to normal testosterone levels have not found a persistent increase in PSA, symptoms of benign prostatic hypertrophy (BPH), or incidence of prostate cancer. Other potential side effects include worsening of edema and acne. There are only a few studies that have commented on the effects of testosterone supplementation or replacement on obstructive sleep apnea, and these have not been consistent.

18. **Should healthy older men receive testosterone supplementation?**
Low testosterone may be a cause or consequence of the metabolic syndrome and is predictive of mortality. Additionally, higher endogenous testosterone concentrations are associated with lower mortality. Whether this is because low testosterone is a biomarker for or a cause of underlying disease is unknown.

It is not clear whether the decline of testosterone levels with aging is physiological or pathological. In either case, an important question is whether testosterone supplementation attenuates physiological decline or leads to improvements in body composition, physical function, cognition, and mortality. Current clinical practice guidelines are based on low-quality evidence and expert opinion. The current research evidence does not clearly define (1) who should be supplemented, (2) what formulation is preferred, (3) what is the best replacement/supplementation dosage to maximize anabolic effects and minimize side effects, (4) what the target testosterone level should be, (5) how long individuals should be replaced/supplemented, (6) at what age to begin any replacement/supplementation, and (7) what are expected beneficial effects (primary vs. secondary prevention and/or treatment) or expected side effects. At this time, testosterone supplementation should be reserved for the minority of men with frankly low serum testosterone levels and clear clinical symptoms of hypogonadism who do not have an existing clear contraindication for androgen therapy (prostate cancer, severe obstructive uropathy, liver disease, and polycythemia).

19. **Should estrogen therapy be given to postmenopausal women?**
This has been an area of terrific controversy since the completion of the Women's Health Initiative (WHI) trials. Similar to debates about testosterone replacement, controversy exists

regarding who should be treated (age, years menopausal, symptomatic), by what formulation (conjugated estrogens vs. estradiol, progesterone vs. medroxyprogesterone acetate [MPA], continuous vs. intermittent progestins), at what dose (fixed vs. target serum estradiol level), what route (oral, transdermal, transvaginal), and for what length of time. The WHI trials generated important results but raised equally important questions. Oral conjugated estrogens with or without MPA may not have the same effects (good or bad) as transdermal estradiol with or without intermittent progesterone. The WHI trials appeared to support the "timing hypothesis," that cardiovascular benefits may occur when therapy is initiated near to the time of menopause. However, initiating hormone treatment after 10 or more years of estrogen deficiency may increase risk for cardiovascular events.

The loss of estrogen with menopause appears to be linked with deleterious changes in body composition, including increased central fat accumulation and decreased BMD, which translates long-term into increased risk for cardiovascular disease and fractures. Additionally the loss of estrogen is associated with hot flashes, decreased sleep quality, vaginal dryness, and worsening of mood disturbances, the sum of which equals a decreased quality of life for many women.

Currently, estrogen therapy is indicated for relief of menopausal symptoms not relieved by other methods, using the lowest dosage for the shortest time possible. Transdermal estradiol appears to be associated with less thromboembolic events than oral estrogens. Because continuous conjugated estrogens plus MPA was associated with increased incidence of invasive breast CA in the WHI (whereas conjugated estrogens alone was not), intermittent progesterone may be a better alternative for endometrial protection.

20. **How does dehydroepiandrosterone concentration change with aging?**
Dehydroepiandrosterone (DHEA) and its sulfate (DHEAS), collectively referred to as DHEA/S, are the most abundant steroid hormones in humans, with approximately 95% coming from the adrenal glands. DHEAS is considered one of the best biological markers of human aging. Peak serum DHEAS levels are reached early in the third decade and then decline steadily. By age 60 to 70 years, circulating levels are only about 20% of peak levels. The decrease in DHEA/S with aging does not represent a general decline in adrenal function, because similar changes in other adrenal hormones do not occur.

21. **What are the biological effects of DHEA/S?**
Despite the abundance of DHEA/S and the distinctive age-related changes, little is known about the real biological effects of DHEA/S in humans. The actions of DHEA/S in humans are thought to be mediated primarily through conversion to sex hormones, and thus it may function as a large storage pool of prehormone. DHEA is the precursor for 30% to 50% of androgens in older men and more than 70% of androgens in older women; it is also a major source of estrogens in men and postmenopausal women. The decline in DHEA/S with aging may contribute to physiological changes that occur as a result of sex hormone deficiency (e.g., the loss of bone and muscle mass). Other proposed biologic effects of DHEA/S include increased insulin-like growth factor type 1 (IGF-1), antiglucocorticoid effects, and anti-inflammatory effects through peroxisome proliferator-activated receptor alpha (PPARa) agonism.

22. **What are the hormonal effects of DHEA supplementation?**
The United States, DHEA is considered a dietary supplement, and therefore it is not a Food and Drug Administration–regulated drug. Hence, over-the-counter products vary greatly in the amounts of bioactive hormone that they contain (if any) and may have quite different pharmacokinetic profiles. Even batch-to-batch variability within a brand can be great. Despite being labeled a "dietary supplement," DHEA has measurable effects on concentrations of hormones. In older adults, DHEA 50 mg of bioactive hormone per day results in 300% to 600% increases in plasma DHEAS concentration in men and women; a 100% increase in plasma testosterone in women with nonsignificant changes in men; a 70% to 300% rise in plasma estradiol in women and 30% to 200% in men; and increases in IGF-1 of 25% to 30% in women

and 5% to 10% in men. However, the physiological effects of DHEA supplementation in humans appear quite variable.

23. **Summarize the controlled studies of DHEA administration to older adults.**

In recent randomized, placebo-controlled trials of 1 to 2 years, DHEA replacement alone in older adults did not result in significant changes in fat or muscle mass or metabolic improvements. Studies of DHEA plus an exercise stimulus (either endurance, resistance, or both) have shown mixed effects. In postmenopausal women, 12 weeks of DHEA was not more effective than placebo at potentiating effects of endurance and resistance exercise on body composition, glucose, and lipid metabolism. In contrast, 16 weeks of DHEA improved muscle volume and strength tests compared with placebo when combined with high-intensity resistance exercise in older women and men.

Studies of DHEA on BMD have shown consistent trends for increases in indices at the hip, but improvements at other sites appear to be more study- and sex-specific. None of the studies to date has been powered to demonstrate antifracture efficacy. Although the increases in BMD in response to short-term DHEA replacement therapy have been small (1% to 2%), the effects of longer therapy (more than 1–2 years) on attenuation of the age-related decline in BMD are not known.

DHEA replacement trials have not shown significant adverse events (such as increases in PSA), but much larger trials would be necessary to establish its safety and efficacy.

24. **Describe the changes in the growth hormone/IGF-1 axis with aging.**

Aging is associated with a significant decline in the growth hormone (GH) area under the curve (AUC), as well as the number and amplitude of GH peaks. These changes in GH secretion are associated with a steady decline in IGF-1 after age 30 years. By age 65, most individuals have an IGF-1 concentration that is near or below the lower limit of normal for young healthy individuals. The observed decline in the GH/IGF-1 axis appears to occur above the level of the pituitary because chronic treatment with growth hormone releasing hormone (GHRH) or other GH secretagogues (GHS) mitigates much of the decline. The cause of the fall-off in axis activity is not clear but could be explained by age-related changes in GHRH, somatostatin, or ghrelin tone. Ghrelin appears to be the natural ligand for the GH receptor. Although there is a close physiological relationship between GH secretion and slow-wave sleep, it is unclear whether the altered GH/IGF-1 axis is the consequence or cause of profound aging-related changes in sleep architecture.

25. **Is the decline in the GH/IGF-1 axis related to age-related changes in body composition and function?**

Many of the body composition changes that occur with aging seem consistent with a GH/IGF-1-deficient state. Indeed, GH-deficient adults have many of the same physiological abnormalities as older individuals, including:

- Reduced lean body and muscle mass
- Reduced strength and aerobic capacity
- Excess total, central, and intra-abdominal fat
- High incidence of metabolic syndrome
- Reduced bone mass and density
- Reduced or absent slow-wave sleep
- High incidence of mood disturbance (depression)

26. **Is GH replacement recommended for the healthy elderly?**

Although GH therapy improves body composition, bone density, and cholesterol levels and may decrease death in younger patients who are clearly GH deficient, the efficacy and safety of therapy for the otherwise "healthy" elderly is controversial. A recent systematic review of clinical trials of GH in the healthy elderly concluded that therapy does increase IGF-1 concentrations, although women may require higher doses of GH for longer periods than men to achieve physiological replacement levels. Despite higher doses per kg body weight, women do not consistently demonstrate the increase in lean body mass or decrease in fat mass that occur in men. Further, translation into clinically significant changes in strength, function, bone density, and improved metabolic parameters has been difficult to demonstrate. GH treatment is associated with several important adverse events, such as a significant additional incidence compared with placebo in soft tissue edema (42%), arthralgias (16%), carpal tunnel syndrome (15%), gynecomastia (6%), new impaired fasting glucose (IFG) or impaired glucose tolerance (IGT) (4%), and new onset of diabetes (4%).

The scant clinical experience of GH treatment for the healthy elderly suggests that although GH may minimally improve body composition, it does not improve other clinically relevant outcomes such as strength or function, and it is associated with high rates of adverse events. Furthermore, invertebrate and rodent models suggest that lower GH axis activity may be protective for longevity. On the basis of available evidence, GH cannot be recommended for use among the healthy elderly. Large randomized controlled trials are necessary to determine the safety and efficacy of GH combined with an exercise intervention, combined with sex hormones, effects in nonhealthy frail populations, and other replacement strategies such as GHRH.

27. Does GHRH supplementation affect GH secretion, sleep, and cognition?
The elderly often experience lack of sleep and feeling tired during the day. This may be because of the almost total loss of slow-wave sleep (stages 3 and 4). Of interest, the periods of slow-wave sleep in younger individuals coincide exactly with the nighttime peaks of GH secretion. Indeed, there are animal and some human data suggesting that appropriately timed GHRH supplementation may restart pulsatile GH secretion and stimulate slow-wave sleep. There is also limited evidence that suggests that chronic GHRH supplementation may improve cognitive function, specifically psychomotor and perceptual processing speed, as well as fluid memory.

28. What happens to the hypothalamic-pituitary-adrenal (HPA) axis with aging?
As is the case for most hormones, distinguishing between the independent effects of age-related and body-composition-related changes in the HPA axis is challenging. For example, morning cortisol levels tend to be lower and stress-induced HPA axis responsiveness tends to be greater in older compared with young adults, but such findings are also associated with central obesity (commonly found with aging; see earlier discussion). However, several characteristics appear to be unique to aging. First, there is evidence for a phase advance characterized by an earlier morning cortisol peak. Second, the evening cortisol nadir appears to be higher in older persons, resulting in a compression of the diurnal amplitude. Third, glucocorticoid-mediated negative feedback is decreased. In total, mean 24-hour serum cortisol concentrations are 20% to 50% higher in both older women and men, likely reflecting the sum of alterations in glucocorticoid clearance, HPA axis responsiveness to stress, and central glucocorticoid-mediated negative feedback.

Whether an increase in the exposure to systemic or local (through 11-beta hydroxysteroid dehydrogenase-1) glucocorticoids in the elderly contributes to such age-related changes as central obesity, insulin resistance, decreased lean body mass, increased risk for fractures, decreased sleep quality, and poor memory (all common symptoms of cortisol excess) are areas of ongoing investigation.

29. What is a normal thyroid-stimulating hormone (TSH) level in older adults?
This is an area of debate. The conventional thinking has been that both secretion and clearance of thyroid hormones decrease with advancing age, with the net effect, in healthy individuals free of thyroid dysfunction or thyroid antibodies, being thyroid-stimulating hormone (TSH) concentrations similar to those of young adults. However, recent National Health and Nutrition Examination Survey (NHANES) epidemiological studies suggest that the distribution and peak frequency of TSH increases with age, even after excluding individuals with thyroid dysfunction or antibodies. Recognition of age-specific reference ranges would have important implications for defining subclinical hypothyroidism in the elderly and treatment targets for thyroid hormone replacement.

30. **What thyroid conditions are more prevalent with aging?**

Thyroid nodules increase with age, with an estimated prevalence of 37% to 57%. The risk of malignancy in a nodule also increases with age. The rate of carcinoma in a follicular nodule is increased in adults aged over 60 years old and is higher in men than in women.

The most frequent cause of hyperthyroidism in older adults is toxic multinodular goiter rather than Graves' disease. Presenting symptoms of hyperthyroidism may be more atypical, with apathetic symptoms being more common compared with younger patients.

Hypothyroidism increases significantly with age due to multiple conditions, including autoimmune thyroid dysfunction, use of medications, and nonthyroidal illness, which can lead to low serum thyroid hormone concentrations. The incidence of myxedema coma is also higher in older adults.

Subclinical hypothyroidism increases with age, but the actual incidence depends on the definition of upper limits of normal for TSH. For instance, 15% of disease-free U.S. people over age 80 have TSH levels greater than 4.5 mIU/L, but if the definition were to change to TSH greater than 2.5, the incidence would be as high as 40%.

31. **Should subclinical hypothyroidism be treated in the elderly?**

As opposed to agreement for treatment of subclinical hyperthyroidism, which can lead to risk for atrial fibrillation and osteoporosis, the treatment of subclinical hypothyroidism remains an area of debate. One reason is an unclear definition of the "normal range" for TSH with aging. Additionally, there is lack of definitive evidence in favor of routine therapy of patients with a TSH less than 10 mIU/L on outcomes such as cardiac function and hyperlipidemia.

32. **What implications could prescribing generic thyroid hormones have in the elderly?**

One important point to remember is that even at the same dosage, different brands of the hormone may vary in hormone bioavailability and potency from various batches of hormone. The difference may be small, but in older patients with a slower metabolism, this could have significant effects.

33. **What factors are necessary to take into account when determining treatment goals for the management of type 2 diabetes in older patients?**

At least 20% of patients over the age of 65 years have diabetes, and that number is expected to grow rapidly in the coming decades. In patients under age 65, intensive blood pressure control and lipid therapy improve macrovascular end points within 2 to 3 years; whereas tight glycemic control does not improve microvascular outcomes until after approximately 8 years. There are no clinical trials data on macrovascular or microvascular consequences of intensive glycemic control specifically in elderly adults. However, the risks of intensive glycemic control (hypoglycemia, polypharmacy, and drug-drug and drug-disease interactions) are likely to be greater in the elderly than in younger adults because of the high prevalence of common geriatric syndromes, including polypharmacy, depression, cognitive impairment, and injurious falls.

The American Diabetes Association and American Geriatrics Society recommend that a reasonable goal for Hb_{A1C} in relatively healthy older adults with good functional status is 7% or lower. For older adults who are frail, have a life expectancy of less than 5 years, or for whom the risks of intensive glycemic control appear to outweigh the benefits, a less stringent target, such as 8%, may be more appropriate.

34. **What medications should be considered for the treatment of diabetes in older adults?**

Special care is required in prescribing and monitoring drug therapy for the older patient with diabetes. Metformin is often contraindicated because of renal insufficiency. It should be remembered that serum creatinine alone is often not an adequate reflection of glomerular filtration rate in older patients; age and body weight must be taken into consideration.

Thiazolidinediones should not be used in patients with congestive heart failure (New York Heart Association grade III and IV), and recent evidence suggests they may contribute to osteoporosis. Insulin secretagogues, such as sulfonylureas, can cause hypoglycemia, and the elderly may be particularly predisposed. Insulin therapy requires good visual and motor skills and cognitive ability of the patient or a caregiver and can cause hypoglycemia. Hypoglycemia in older subjects maybe particularly hard to identify and may be incorrectly diagnosed as irreversible cognitive impairment. Diabetes treatment can be improved in patients with visual impairments through the use such devices as glucometers with large, easier-to-read screens, audio glucometers, magnifying glasses to help see syringes, or preloaded insulin pens.

Most older patients with diabetes will also be on other medications for comorbid cardiovascular diseases. When treating hypertension, angiotensin-converting enzyme inhibitors and angiotensin receptor blockers have an increased risk of decreased renal function and hyperkalemia, and hydrochlorothiazide/loop diuretics are associated with an increased risk of hypokalemia, arrhythmia, polyuria, urinary incontinence, dehydration, and falls. 3-Hydroxy-3-methyl-glutaryl-CoA reductase inhibitors (statins), especially in setting of polypharmacy, can lead to drug-drug interactions based on liver metabolism and increased risk of rhabdomyolysis. Finally, aspirin increases risk of gastrointestinal bleeding in older adults.

KEY POINTS: HORMONES AND AGING

1. Weight loss in the obese elderly is associated with improvements in cardiovascular risk factors, but exercise may be necessary to attenuate loss of muscle and bone mass during weight loss and mitigate against frailty.

2. Adequate calcium and vitamin D are essential for fall and fracture prevention.

3. Most hormonal axes are associated with a gradual decline over time, beginning at about age 30, with the exception of the relatively rapid decline in estrogen associated with the female menopause.

4. Serum total testosterone decreases with time in men, but there are numerous other independent health, lifestyle, and secular trends that can accelerate the decline.

5. Age-specific reference ranges for thyroid-stimulating hormone may be appropriate and have important implications in defining subclinical hypothyroidism in older adults.

6. Clinicians caring for older adults with diabetes must take into consideration the clinical and functional heterogeneity of their patients when setting and prioritizing an individual's treatment goals and drug regimen.

TAKE HOME MESSAGE: NO MAGIC HORMONAL FOUNTAIN OF YOUTH

1. Physical activity and long-term caloric restriction have the best evidence for ameliorating aging-related increases in adiposity and cardiovascular risk factors.

2. Estrogen therapy is controversial other than for treatment of severe postmenopausal symptoms, but there may be cardiovascular benefits if therapy is initiated early (near menopause).

3. Testosterone therapy for older hypogonadal men is generally associated with improvements in body composition (decreased fat and increased fat free mass), but it remains uncertain whether there are true metabolic or functional benefits.

4. Dehydroepiandrosterone replacement therapy increases levels of estradiol, testosterone (women only), insulin-like growth factor type 1, and bone mineral density but does not appear to be associated with clear improvements in metabolism or body composition in older humans.

5. Growth hormone supplementation appears to be more effective at increasing lean body mass in older men than women. These changes have not been demonstrated to translate into functional improvements, and treatment is associated with high rates of adverse events.

BIBLIOGRAPHY

1. American Diabetes Association: Standards of Medical Care in Diabetes 2008. Diabetes Care 31:S12–S54, 2008.
2. Araujo AB, Esche GR, Kupelian V, et al: Prevalence of symptomatic androgen deficiency in men. J Clin Endocrinol Metab 92:4241–4247, 2007.
3. Gozansky WS, Van Pelt RE, Jankowski CM, et al: Protection of bone mass by estrogens and raloxifene during exercise-induced weight loss. J Clin Endocrinol Metab 90:52–59, 2005.
4. Holick MF: Vitamin D deficiency. N Engl J Med 357:266–281, 2007.
5. Jankowski CM, Gozansky WS, Schwartz RS, et al: Effects of dehydroepiandrosterone replacement therapy on bone mineral density in older adults: a randomized, controlled trial. J Clin Endocrinol Metab 91:2986–2993, 2006.
6. Kaufman JM, Vermeulen A: The decline of androgen levels in elderly men and its clinical and therapeutic implications. Endocr Rev 26:833–876, 2005.
7. Kennedy BK, Steffen KK, Kaeberlein M: Ruminations on dietary restriction and aging. Cell Mol Life Sci 64:1323–1328, 2007.
8. Laron Z: Do deficiencies in growth hormone and insulin-like growth factor-1 (IGF-1) shorten or prolong longevity? Mech Ageing Dev 126:305–307, 2005.
9. Liu H, Bravata DM, Olkin I, et al: Systematic review: the safety and efficacy of growth hormone in the healthy elderly. Ann Intern Med 146:104–115, 2007.
10. Miner MM, Seftel AD: Testosterone and ageing: what have we learned since the Institute of medicine report and what lies ahead? Int J Clin Pract 61:622–632, 2007.
11. Sherlock M, Toogood AA: Aging and the growth hormone/insulin like growth factor-I axis. Pituitary 10:189–203, 2007.
12. Sowers M, Zheng H, Tomey K, et al: Changes in body composition in women over six years at midlife: ovarian and chronological aging. J Clin Endocrinol Metab 92:895–901, 2007.
13. Surks MI, Hollowell JG: Age-specific distribution of serum thyrotropin and antithyroid antibodies in the U.S. population: implications for the prevalence of subclinical hypothyroidism. J Clin Endocrinol Metab 92:4575–4582, 2007.
14. Travison TG, Araujo AB, Kupelian V, et al: The relative contributions of aging, health, and lifestyle factors to serum testosterone decline in men. J Clin Endocrinol Metab 92:549–555, 2007.
15. Vanderschueren D, Venken K, Ophoff J, et al: Clinical review: sex steroids and the periosteum—reconsidering the roles of androgens and estrogens in periosteal expansion. J Clin Endocrinol Metab 91:378–382, 2006.
16. Villareal DT, Banks M, Sinacore DR, et al: Effect of weight loss and exercise on frailty in obese older adults. Arch Intern Med 166:860–866, 2006.
17. Villareal DT, Holloszy JO: DHEA enhances effects of weight training on muscle mass and strength in elderly women and men. Am J Physiol Endocrinol Metab 291:E1003–E1008.
18. Villareal DT, Miller BV III, Banks M, et al: Effect of lifestyle intervention on metabolic coronary heart disease risk factors in obese older adults. Am J Clin Nutr 84:1317–1323, 2006.
19. Wierman ME, Kohrt WM: Vascular and metabolic effects of sex steroids: new insights into clinical trials. Reprod Sci 14:300–314, 2007.

CHAPTER 58

ENDOCRINE SURGERY

Christopher D. Raeburn, Jonathan A. Schoen, and Robert C. McIntyre, Jr.

THYROID

1. **List the possible results of fine-needle aspiration of thyroid nodules and describe the appropriate surgical intervention.**
   - Nondiagnostic: Repeat once using ultrasound guidance. Perform thyroid lobectomy if still nondiagnostic.
   - Benign: The false-negative rate for fine-needle aspiration (FNA) is less than 5%. An asymptomatic thyroid nodule can be safely followed if the FNA is benign.
   - Malignant: Patients with FNA findings of cancer can undergo a definitive cancer operation. The false-positive rate for FNA is less than 5%.
   - Suspicious: An FNA result of "suspicious for thyroid cancer" is associated with up to a 75% risk of being malignant. Patients can be given the option of thyroid lobectomy or thyroidectomy; however, patients with large nodules (>4 cm), family history of thyroid cancer, exposure to neck radiation or bilateral nodular disease should undergo thyroidectomy. If a lobectomy is performed and the final pathology is cancer, most patients will require a second operation for completion thyroidectomy. An intraoperative frozen section is sometimes used to determine whether lobectomy or thyroidectomy is appropriate; however, the accuracy of frozen section for thyroid nodules is not much better than FNA and is therefore not routinely used.
   - Follicular: An FNA result of follicular neoplasm is treated similar to that of a suspicious result; however, the diagnosis of follicular cancer requires the finding of capsular, vascular, or lymphatic invasion on permanent section, so intraoperative frozen section is not useful. The patient has the option of thyroid lobectomy or thyroidectomy. If the final pathology is consistent with follicular carcinoma (15%–20%), then completion thyroidectomy is usually required.

2. **Should ultrasound guidance be used for all FNAs of thyroid nodules?**
   Ultrasound guidance for FNA of easily palpable thyroid nodules increases cost without improving diagnostic accuracy and should not be used routinely. However, it is recommended that all patients with a palpable thyroid nodule undergo thyroid ultrasound. This will frequently detect additional nonpalpable nodules, solid components in primarily cystic nodules, and posteriorly positioned nodules, all of which might require ultrasound guidance.

3. **What are the differences between total, near-total, and subtotal thyroidectomy?**
   A total thyroidectomy removes all grossly visible thyroid tissue. A near-total thyroidectomy removes all grossly visible thyroid tissue except for a small amount (<1 g) adjacent to where the recurrent laryngeal nerve enters the larynx. A total and near-total thyroidectomy have equivalent oncologic outcomes and are often considered synonymous. A subtotal thyroidectomy leaves more than 1 g of thyroid tissue and is not an appropriate cancer operation. It is used occasionally in patients with benign multinodular goiter or hyperthyroidism in an attempt to

leave enough thyroid so that thyroid hormone replacement is not required. However, doing so increases the risk of recurrent disease compared with near-total thyroidectomy

4. **What is the appropriate extent of thyroidectomy for differentiated thyroid carcinoma?**
Most patients with differentiated thyroid carcinoma (papillary, follicular, Hürthle cell) should undergo a total or near-total thyroidectomy. Several studies have shown that for larger tumors, total or near-total thyroidectomy compared with lesser resections results in lower recurrence rates and improved survival. A recent study reviewed data from the National Cancer Data Base and found that there was no difference in outcome (recurrence or survival) between patients who underwent lobectomy versus near-total or total thyroidectomy when the size of the tumor was less than 1 cm. However, near-total or total thyroidectomy for tumors larger than 1 cm resulted in lower recurrence and improved survival compared with patients who underwent lobectomy. This improved outcome was seen even in the subset of patients with tumors 1 to 2 cm in size. Therefore the majority of patients should undergo total or near-total thyroidectomy. In addition, near-total or total thyroidectomy facilitates postoperative treatment with radioiodine and permits accurate long-term surveillance for disease recurrence by thyroglobulin measurement.

5. **A patient underwent a thyroid lobectomy for a suspicious thyroid nodule, and the final pathology revealed papillary carcinoma. How do you decide whether completion thyroidectomy is necessary?**
In most cases, a completion thyroidectomy would be indicated; however, patients with differentiated thyroid cancer can be stratified into low-, intermediate-, and high-risk populations. The main determinants that increase risk are age (>45), tumor size (>2 cm), local invasion, and distant metastases. A lobectomy may be sufficient treatment for low risk patients who meet the following criteria: young age (<45), tumor less than 1 cm, no nodules in the residual thyroid, no regional or distant metastases, no history of neck radiation exposure, and no family history of thyroid cancer.

6. **Is the risk of complication higher in patients treated with lobectomy followed by completion thyroidectomy compared with those who undergo total thyroidectomy at the initial operation?**
No. In experienced hands, a completion thyroidectomy is a safe operation. The rates of temporary and permanent recurrent laryngeal nerve injury and temporary and permanent hypocalcemia are equivalent when thyroidectomy is performed in one stage versus two stages.

7. **Describe the appropriate surgical management for medullary thyroid carcinoma.**
Medullary thyroid carcinoma is not sensitive to radioiodine or thyroid-stimulating hormone (TSH) suppression; therefore total thyroidectomy is the only treatment. Because of the high incidence of regional lymph node involvement, a central neck dissection is performed at the time of thyroidectomy. Some surgeons also advocate routine bilateral modified neck dissection at the initial surgery because of the risk of lateral nodal metastases (approximately 75% ipsilateral and 50% contralateral to the thyroid tumor). Despite this aggressive approach, normalization of calcitonin occurs in only about 50% of patients. Another approach is to perform lateral neck dissection selectively on the basis of clinically or ultrasonographically abnormal nodes.

8. **Discuss the role of surgery in anaplastic carcinoma of the thyroid.**
Anaplastic carcinoma of the thyroid is one of the most aggressive solid tumors known and is rarely curable. At the time of diagnosis, 50% of patients harbor distant metastases, and 95% have local invasion precluding a curative resection. Surgery is usually restricted to a diagnostic or palliative role. Palliative surgical debulking and tracheostomy should be reserved for symptoms of dysphagia or airway compromise, respectively, because they do not prolong survival. An attempt at a curative resection should be reserved for younger patients, without

distant disease and only when all gross cervical and mediastinal disease can be resected without excessive morbidity. In this select subgroup of patients, curative-intent surgery combined with adjuvant external beam radiation, chemotherapy, or both has been shown to prolong survival compared with patients treated with adjuvant therapy alone.

9. What is a central and modified radical neck dissection?

A central neck dissection removes all the perithyroidal and tracheoesophageal groove nodes (level VI) from the hyoid bone superiorly down to the thoracic inlet. Laterally, the dissection extends from carotid to carotid artery. The lateral spread of disease usually involves high, middle, and low jugular lymph nodes (levels II–IV) and rarely posterior (level V) nodes. A modified radical neck dissection, sometimes referred to as a functional dissection, removes all lymphatic tissue from levels II through IV (and sometimes V) and spares the internal jugular vein, sternocleidomastoid muscle, and spinal accessory nerve, because sacrificing these structures (radical neck dissection) does not improve outcome.

10. What is the incidence of lymph node metastasis in well-differentiated thyroid cancer, and when is a neck dissection indicated?

Differentiated thyroid cancer (predominantly papillary) involves cervical lymph nodes in 30% to 80% of cases. Unlike many other malignancies, the presence of lymph node metastases does not worsen the outcome for most patients with differentiated thyroid cancer, and routine neck dissection does not clearly improve outcome except for patients in the high-risk group. For these reasons, the decision to perform a neck dissection for differentiated thyroid cancer is somewhat controversial. The following are some general guidelines:

- All patients with clinically palpable nodes require a compartment (central and/or lateral) dissection.
- Preoperative full neck ultrasound in patients with malignant FNA cytology should be performed. Any suspicious lateral nodes should have FNA biopsy and, if positive, should be removed through formal neck dissection at the same time as thyroidectomy.
- The American Thyroid Association Guidelines Taskforce recommends that routine central neck dissection should be considered at the time of thyroidectomy for all patients undergoing surgery for papillary carcinoma. This recommendation is based on the observation that central neck dissection may improve survival (compared with historic controls) and reduce the risk for nodal recurrence requiring further surgery in the central neck.

11. When is surgery indicated for recurrent thyroid cancer?

Suspected recurrent disease in the neck consisting of either palpable nodes or sonographically suspicious nodes should have FNA biopsy. Confirmed nodal recurrence should be treated with neck dissection. A recurrence in an area already subjected to formal neck dissection can be challenging. After a neck dissection has been performed, repeat neck dissection is virtually impossible because of tissue plane scarring. If the recurrence is palpable, then local excision can often be performed. If not palpable, intraoperative ultrasound can sometimes be used to localize the lesion and guide the surgeon. For patients who are poor surgical candidates or have had multiple neck operations, percutaneous ethanol injection of cervical nodal metastases is an alternative. Radioiodine is the standard therapy for distant metastatic disease, but isolated metastases can be surgically resected or treated with external beam radiation.

12. How many times should a thyroid cyst be aspirated if it reaccumulates fluid? Should the cyst fluid be sent for cytology?

Thyroid cysts are most often benign. The initial diagnostic and therapeutic procedure is aspiration. The complete disappearance of a palpable lesion is adequate therapy for thyroid cysts; however, about 50% will reaccumulate fluid. If the cyst recurs after a second aspiration, it should be considered for surgical excision. Fluid cytology results are typically nonspecific;

however, it may be prudent to perform cytology on cysts that reaccumulate fluid. If the nodule does not completely disappear after aspiration, it may be a complex cyst, which is associated with higher malignant potential. Therefore FNA of the solid component should be performed.

13. **List the indications for thyroidectomy in hyperthyroidism.**
In the United States, thyroidectomy is not commonly performed for hyperthyroidism unless secondary to a single hyperfunctioning adenoma or because of a toxic multinodular goiter containing a suspicious nodule. Despite the excellent success, low recurrence rate, safety, and more rapid return to a euthyroid state, fewer than 10% of patients with hyperthyroidism undergo thyroidectomy.

14. **List possible indications for thyroidectomy in patients with hyperthyroidism.**
   - Failure of antithyroid medications
   - Large goiter and low iodine uptake
   - Compression symptoms, such as dysphagia, stridor, or hoarseness
   - Nodules suspicious for cancer
   - Children
   - Pregnant patient who is difficult to treat medically
   - Young female who wants to become pregnant in the near future
   - Noncompliance
   - Cosmetic concerns
   - Severe Graves' ophthalmopathy

15. **How should patients with hyperthyroidism be prepared for surgery?**
It is important to render patients euthyroid before surgery for hyperthyroidism to avoid perioperative thyroid storm. Antithyroid medications administered for 4 weeks before surgery are usually adequate. Some surgeons use saturated solution of potassium iodide (SSKI or Lugol's solution 3–5 drops 3 times a day) for 3 to 5 days before surgery to decrease the vascularity of the goiter and reduce the risk of bleeding. Patients who are very symptomatic may benefit from preoperative beta-blockade. For more rapid induction of a euthyroid state, patients may also be given dexamethasone, which can return T4 and T3 to within the normal range in less than 7 days.

16. **What is the extent of thyroidectomy for hyperthyroidism?**
The controversy over the appropriate extent of thyroidectomy for hyperthyroidism resides in the desire to render the patient euthyroid without inducing hypothyroidism while balancing the risk of recurrence. Many surgeons prefer to perform near-total thyroidectomy, which successfully cures hyperthyroidism in nearly 100% of patients; however, it does so with the drawback of uniform hypothyroidism. Patients willing to accept the risk of recurrent hyperthyroidism may undergo subtotal thyroidectomy, which leaves approximately 4 to 8 g of visible thyroid tissue with an adequate blood supply. Subtotal thyroidectomy results in a euthyroid state (no need for postoperative thyroid replacement therapy) in approximately 60% of patients, but it has a 5% to 10% incidence of persistent or recurrent hyperthyroidism.

17. **What are the complications of thyroidectomy?**
Thyroidectomy is a safe procedure with a mean length of hospitalization in large series of less than 1.5 days. The incidence rates of specific complications after thyroidectomy are as follows:
   - Cervical hematoma: 1%
   - Recurrent laryngeal nerve injury: 1%
   - Superior laryngeal nerve injury: 1%
   - Temporary hypocalcemia: 10% to 15%
   - Permanent hypoparathyroidism: 1% to 5%
   - Mortality: 0.3%

18. **What is the significance of an incidentally noted thyroid hot spot on positron emission tomography scan?**
   Fluorodeoxyglucose (FDG) whole-body positron emission tomography (PET) scan is increasingly being used in the diagnostic workup or follow-up of patients with various types of cancer. A focal area of increased FDG uptake within the thyroid is incidentally noted in up to 4% of PET scans. The risk of malignancy in these lesions ranges from 25% to 50%. Thus thyroid incidentalomas noted on PET scans have a high rate of malignancy and warrant appropriate diagnostic evaluation.

19. **What is the appropriate therapy for an intrathoracic goiter?**
   Intrathoracic goiters are typically cervical goiters with mediastinal extension, although primary intrathoracic goiters do occur secondary to abnormal descent of the thyroid during development. The incidence of carcinoma residing in intrathoracic goiters is reported as high as 17%; moreover, approximately 40% of patients present with compressive symptoms resulting from impingement on the airway, esophagus, vascular structures, or nerves. Radioiodine ablation is not typically recommended because of the risk of transient enlargement of the goiter during initiation of therapy, potentially resulting in life-threatening airway compromise. Thus the presence of an intrathoracic goiter is generally accepted as an indication for thyroidectomy. Because the arterial supply of intrathoracic goiters originates in the neck, the vast majority of these tumors can be resected through a cervical approach. Extension into the posterior mediastinum, malignancy, or compression of the vena cava may necessitate a combined cervical and sternotomy approach, although this is required in less than 5% of cases.

20. **When should thyroglossal duct cysts be removed? Describe the operation.**
   During the embryologic development of the thyroid, a diverticulum forms from the foramen cecum at the base of the tongue and descends as the thyroglossal duct to the future anatomical position of the thyroid overlying the anterolateral surface of the upper tracheal rings. The thyroglossal duct normally disappears during further development but in rare cases will persist as a patent duct or as a thyroglossal duct cyst. Patients may complain of infection, pain, or compressive symptoms, or they may have cosmetic concerns. Because of the risk of infection, thyroglossal duct cysts should be removed; this requires excision of the entire cyst and cyst tract from the origin at the foramen cecum down to the cyst itself. Because the tract nearly always passes through the hyoid bone, the center of the hyoid should be resected to lower the risk of recurrence; this causes no disability and requires no repair.

KEY POINTS: THYROID SURGERY

1. All patients with a palpable thyroid nodule should undergo thyroid ultrasound.

2. Fine-needle aspiration (FNA) is the single most important diagnostic test in the evaluation of a thyroid nodule.

3. Near-total or total thyroidectomy (as opposed to thyroid lobectomy) is indicated for all differentiated thyroid cancers 1 cm or larger.

4. Lymph node involvement in thyroid cancer should be treated with a systematic compartment node dissection.

5. A thyroid-stimulating hormone stimulated serum thyroglobulin level is the preferred test to detect clinically inapparent recurrence of papillary thyroid cancer.

6. Incidental thyroid hot spots discovered on positron emission tomography scans have a high rate of malignancy and should be evaluated by ultrasound-guided FNA.

PARATHYROID

21. **Discuss the indications for parathyroidectomy.**

Patients with classic symptoms of hyperparathyroidism (nephrolithiasis, severe bone disease or fractures, or overt neuromuscular syndrome) should undergo parathyroidectomy; however, the majority of patients with hyperparathyroidism (HPT) do not have the classic symptoms. The National Institutes of Health (NIH) established criteria to assist clinicians in determining which asymptomatic patients with HPT should undergo surgery:

- Calcium greater than 1.0 mg/dL above normal
- 24-hour urine calcium greater than 400 mg
- Creatinine clearance reduced by greater than 30%
- Bone mineral density reduced greater than 2.5 standard deviations below mean peak adult value (T score)
- Age less than 50 years
- Patients who do not desire or cannot undergo surveillance

Nonspecific symptoms, such as fatigue, mental slowing, musculoskeletal aches and pains, and depression, were not included in the NIH indications for surgery but are commonly reported by patients. Compared with controls (patients undergoing thyroid surgery), patients with HPT score significantly lower on preoperative quality of life questionnaires. Several studies indicate improvement in these patient-reported outcomes following parathyroidectomy. One such study compared a group of patients who met NIH criteria and underwent parathyroidectomy with another group who did not meet NIH criteria but still underwent surgery. The preoperative degree of impairment in quality of life and the postoperative improvement was equivalent between groups. Thus many patients with "asymptomatic" HPT who do not meet any of the NIH criteria still undergo parathyroidectomy.

22. **When should preoperative parathyroid localization studies be performed?**

An experienced parathyroid surgeon does not require preoperative localization before an initial bilateral neck exploration. However, preoperative localization enables minimally invasive parathyroidectomy. Patients with a prior history of neck surgery and certainly all patients with persistent or recurrent hyperparathyroidism should undergo preoperative localization studies before planned reexploration. The best localization study available is the 99m technetium sestamibi scan, although ultrasound, computed tomography (CT) scan, magnetic resonance imaging (MR), and arteriography with or without venous sampling may all be useful in certain situations, especially persistent or recurrent hyperparathyroidism.

23. **Define minimally invasive parathyroidectomy.**

A conventional parathyroidectomy entails bilateral neck exploration, identification of all four glands, and removal of the grossly enlarged gland(s). The development of accurate preoperative localization studies and a rapid intraoperative parathyroid hormone (ioPTH) assay has fostered the development of minimally invasive approaches to parathyroidectomy. A directed unilateral approach utilizes preoperative imaging to limit the dissection to one side. The abnormal gland is found and removed, and after 10 to 15 minutes, a postexcision blood sample is drawn; the PTH level is then compared with a preexcision blood sample. A reduction of the PTH to 50% of the preoperative level and into the normal range predicts successful removal of all abnormal glands, and the surgery is terminated. If the PTH does not drop appropriately, then all four glands must be identified because the patient likely has multiglandular disease.

24. **What is minimally invasive radio-guided parathyroidectomy?**

Minimally invasive radio-guided parathyroidectomy (MIRP) is a second alternative to conventional parathyroidectomy and involves a 99m technetium sestamibi scan the morning of the surgery. A small, handheld gamma probe is used intraoperatively to localize the abnormal gland. A directed incision is performed, and the gland is removed. An intraoperative PTH assay is frequently used to further exclude the small number of patients with multiglandular disease (5%).

25. **Summarize the advantages of minimally invasive approaches.**
Multiple studies have shown the minimally invasive approaches to be as safe and effective as conventional parathyroidectomy. Some studies have found the minimally invasive approaches to be more time- and cost-efficient because they limit the amount of dissection required and can be performed without hospitalization. Because the minimally invasive approach is typically performed through a smaller incision, cosmesis is improved.

26. **Describe when an ioPTH assay should be used.**
A rapid assay for intraoperative PTH (ioPTH) allows intraoperative assessment of the functional success of the operation. This test is performed by drawing a sample of blood before the operation and 10 minutes after the suspected abnormal gland(s) has/have been removed. A reduction of the ioPTH to 50% of the preoperative level and into the normal range predicts successful removal of all abnormal glands, and the surgery is terminated. ioPTH is most useful in patients with hyperplasia, those undergoing reoperation, and during minimally invasive parathyroidectomy. The rate of multiglandular disease is approximately 5% when ioPTH is used to determine the completeness of resection, whereas the rate is 10% to 35% when conventional parathyroidectomy is performed (i.e., bilateral neck exploration and removal of grossly enlarged parathyroids). Therefore the use of ioPTH may prevent the unnecessary removal of glands that appear enlarged but are not hyperfunctional.

27. **What is the expected success of surgery for primary hyperparathyroidism?**
Parathyroidectomy is highly successful for primary hyperparathyroidism, correcting hypercalcemia in more than 95% of patients when performed by an experienced surgeon. Bone density increases in the vast majority of patients. Successful parathyroidectomy significantly decreases the risk of kidney stone recurrence. Nearly all patients experience improvement in the vague, nonspecific symptoms of hyperparathyroidism.

28. **Describe the appropriate management of a "missing" parathyroid.**
Despite meticulous operative technique during conventional parathyroidectomy (identification of all four glands), the surgeon occasionally encounters a "missing gland." Up to 20% of parathyroid glands are ectopic. A systematic search of the most common ectopic locations is required for successful outcome in these patients. When three normal glands have been identified and the fourth gland is not in a normal position, the most likely ectopic location depends on whether it is a missing upper or lower gland.

29. **List the likely locations for an ectopic inferior parathyroid gland.**
   ▪ Thyrothymic ligament
   ▪ Thymus
   ▪ Mediastinum outside thymus
   ▪ Undescended gland

30. **List the likely locations for an ectopic superior parathyroid gland.**
   ▪ Posterior to thyroid
   ▪ Tracheoesophageal groove
   ▪ Retroesophageal
   ▪ Posterosuperior mediastinum
   ▪ Intrathyroid

31. **What if a patient has multiglandular parathyroid disease?**
A single adenoma is by far the most common cause of primary hyperparathyroidism; however, 10% to 15% of patients have multiglandular disease. This may be secondary to either multiple

adenomas or four-gland hyperplasia. Hyperplasia may be sporadic or secondary to a multiple endocrine neoplasia (MEN) syndrome or may be due to secondary or tertiary hyperparathyroidism. When four glands are hyperplastic, the patient must undergo either subtotal (removal of 3.5 glands [SPTx]) or total parathyroidectomy with autotransplantation of parathyroid tissue (TPTx + AT). The success of either approach depends on finding all four glands. Most patients (95%) will have normal calcium and low or normal parathyroid hormone levels in the early postoperative period; however, recurrent hyperparathyroidism occurs in 10% to 30% of patients.

32. **Discuss the advantages and disadvantages of SPTx versus TPTx + AT.**
It is generally thought that SPTx has a lower incidence of temporary postoperative hypocalcemia; however, the rate of permanent hypoparathyroidism is similar with either approach (10%–15%). The advantage of TPTx + AT is that persistent or recurrent hypercalcemia (10%–15%) can be treated by partially or completely removing the grafts (usually placed in a forearm muscle) under local anesthesia, whereas the same complication occurring after SPTx requires repeat neck operation with higher morbidity. One small prospective, randomized trial demonstrated a clear benefit of TPTx + AT for secondary hyperparathyroidism in renal failure patients; in those it resulted in a more rapid return of normal calcium homeostasis and relief of symptoms.

33. **How is autotransplantation performed?**
Autotransplantation is performed by placing 10 to 15 grafts of 1-mm pieces of parathyroid into two or three separate pockets formed in either the sternocleidomastoid muscle or a forearm muscle and marked with a nonabsorbable suture and metallic clips for easy identification. Placement of the graft to the forearm facilitates subsequent surgery should the patient develop recurrent hyperparathyroidism due to graft hyperplasia.

34. **List the complications of parathyroidectomy and their prevalence.**
   - Persistent or recurrent hyperparathyroidism: 1% to 12%
   - Transient hypocalcemia: 10% to 25%
   - Permanent hypoparathyroidism: 2% to 5%
   - Permanent recurrent laryngeal nerve injury: less than 1%
   - Temporary recurrent laryngeal nerve injury: 3%
   - Mortality: less than 0.5%

35. **Define persistent or recurrent hyperparathyroidism.**
Persistent hyperparathyroidism is defined as failure of calcium and PTH levels to normalize or remain normal in the initial 6 months after operation, whereas recurrent hyperparathyroidism is defined by recurrence of hypercalcemia after 6 months.

36. **Discuss the approach to patients with persistent or recurrent hyperparathyroidism.**
The approach to patients with persistent or recurrent hyperparathyroidism requires confirmation of the diagnosis (exclude familial hypocalciuric hypercalcemia, vitamin D deficiency, etc.), estimation of disease severity, careful review of the operative and pathology reports, and preoperative localization. Causes of failure include missed adenoma in a normal location, ectopic glands, inadequate resection in multiglandular disease, and supernumerary glands.

37. **Discuss the options for treatment of persistent or recurrent hyperparathyroidism.**
Preoperative localization is usually achieved by 99m technetium sestamibi scan. Repeat cervical exploration is successful in normalizing PTH levels in about 85% of patients and may be aided

by intraoperative ultrasound and ioPTH assay. Mediastinal parathyroid tissue is most often removed through the transcervical approach, but thoracoscopy or median sternotomy may be required 1% to 2% of the time. Angiographic ablation of mediastinal parathyroid tissue using high doses of ionic contrast may be successful in selected patients with high surgical risk.

38. **How does one recognize parathyroid cancer?**
Parathyroid cancer is the rarest of all endocrine tumors, with a reported incidence of less than 1% in patients with primary hyperparathyroidism. It is difficult to distinguish parathyroid cancer from the more common benign causes of hyperparathyroidism, and the diagnosis is frequently not suspected preoperatively. Parathyroid cancer should be suspected preoperatively when patients present with rapid onset, severe, symptomatic hypercalcemia (>14 mg/dL), very high PTH levels (>5 times normal), a palpable neck mass, or hoarseness. It should be suspected intraoperatively when the tumor is large, firm, fibrotic or invading the thyroid or other surrounding structures. Successful outcome requires early recognition and complete resection of the tumor and any involved structures.

39. **Describe the management of parathyroid cancer.**
Surgery is the mainstay of treatment for parathyroid cancer because radiation and chemotherapy have shown little benefit. Local invasion and pathological nodes should be assumed to represent cancer. Any suspicious parathyroid lesions should be carefully removed without disrupting the parathyroid capsule, because this may result in tumor spillage and local recurrence. If a parathyroid gland is obviously abnormal and infiltrating other tissues, those tissues should be resected en bloc with the tumor whenever possible, including the ipsilateral thyroid lobe when necessary. Removal of the central nodes on the side of the tumor is indicated at the initial operation. Any obviously enlarged lateral nodes should be resected in an appropriate neck dissection. Prophylactic neck dissections have shown no benefit. The histopathological diagnosis of this cancer is also difficult; thus intraoperative frozen section is rarely useful other than to confirm parathyroid tissue.

40. **Give the recurrence and survival rates for parathyroid cancer.**
Recurrence rates are high and depend on whether the patient underwent a routine parathyroidectomy for presumed benign disease (>50% recurrence) or an en bloc resection for suspicion of cancer (10%–33%). Despite this high recurrence rate, prolonged survival is still possible. The National Cancer Data Base reports 5- and 10-year survival rates of 85.5% and 49.1%, respectively.

KEY POINTS: PARATHYROID

1. Indications for parathyroidectomy in primary hyperparathyroidism include the classic symptoms of nephrolithiasis and overt bone or neuromuscular syndrome.

2. Indications in asymptomatic patients include high serum calcium (>1.0 mg/dL above normal), age under 50 years, osteoporosis, high urinary calcium (>400 mg/day), and reduced creatinine clearance.

3. Surgery for primary hyperparathyroidism results in normocalcemia in more than 95% of patients when performed by an experienced parathyroid surgeon.

4. Parathyroid cancer is rare but should be suspected in patients with a palpable mass and symptomatic hypercalcemia that is severe and of rapid onset.

ADRENAL GLANDS

41. **Should all incidentally discovered adrenal masses be resected?**
    No. Clinically inapparent adrenal masses are common (6% in autopsy series, 4% in abdominal CT series), and most are benign, nonsecreting adenomas that require no treatment. The decision to surgically remove an adrenal incidentaloma is based on tumor size, imaging characteristics, and biochemical activity.

42. **Summarize the appropriate laboratory evaluation of an adrenal mass.**
    Hormonally active adrenal tumors should be resected and up to 20% of adrenal incidentalomas are found to have subclinical hormonal dysfunction. Therefore patients should be screened for subclinical Cushing's syndrome, silent pheochromocytoma, and, if hypertensive, hyperaldosteronism by the following tests:
    - 24-hour urinary free cortisol and/or 1 mg overnight dexamethasone suppression test
    - 24-hour urinary fractionated metanephrines and catecholamines
    - In hypertensive patients: a morning plasma aldosterone-plasma renin activity ratio
    Routine screening for excess androgens or estrogens is not warranted because sex hormone–secreting adrenal tumors are rare and typically occur in the presence of clinical manifestations.

43. **What imaging studies are available for evaluating adrenal pathology?**
    The appropriate imaging study for adrenal lesions depends on the diagnosis. For incidentally discovered, hormonally inactive adrenal tumors, an "adrenal protocol" CT scan is an appropriate choice. This involves thin-cut imaging through the adrenals with and without intravenous contrast and delayed images to assess how quickly the contrast washes out. For cortisol-producing adenomas and most pheochromocytomas, CT scans are accurate because the tumors are usually larger than 2 cm by the time they are diagnosed. MRI is essentially equivalent to CT for adrenal tumors; however, it may be superior in recurrent or metastatic disease and for pheochromocytomas. Meta-iodobenzylguanidine (MIBG) scans are best for recurrent or nonadrenal pheochromocytomas. Aldosteronomas are typically less than 2 cm in diameter, and therefore the sensitivity of CT scans is only 85%. When CT scanning fails to demonstrate an adenoma, adrenal venous sampling is useful to differentiate small adenomas from bilateral hyperplasia.

44. **What findings on CT or MRI help to distinguish between benign and malignant tumors?**
    Although most adrenal incidentalomas are benign, a series of more than 2000 patients found that adrenocortical carcinoma accounted for 4.7% of tumors and metastatic cancer another 2.5%. The size of the mass and its appearance on imaging are the two major predictors of malignancy. Adrenocortical carcinoma accounts for 2% of tumors less than 4 cm but up to 25% of tumors greater than 6 cm. The lipid content of the adrenal mass and rapidity of the washout of contrast are also important CT characteristics in differentiating benign tumors from adrenal cancer, pheochromocytoma and metastatic disease. Benign adenomas typically have high lipid content (low attenuation) and rapid contrast washout (>50% washout at 10 minutes after contrast). The following imaging characteristics are used to estimate malignant potential of adrenal incidentalomas.
    - Benign tumors are typically less than 4 cm, homogeneous with smooth borders, and have low attenuation (<10 Hounsfield units [HU]) and rapid contrast washout.
    - Malignant tumors are typically >6 cm, heterogeneous with irregular borders, and have increased attenuation (>10 HU) and slower contrast washout.

45. **Discuss the role of percutaneous biopsy in the evaluation of an adrenal mass.**
    Percutaneous biopsy is rarely indicated; however, metastases are the cause of adrenal incidentaloma in approximately half of patients who have a prior history of malignant disease.

Therefore percutaneous biopsy is reserved for patients with a history of cancer to evaluate for metastasis and is performed only if the result will influence therapy. It is always necessary to exclude pheochromocytoma first. The complication rate is 3% with bleeding, pain, infection, and malignant seeding of biopsy tract most commonly reported.

46. **List the indications for surgery.**
    - Unilateral tumor with signs or symptoms of hormonal dysfunction
    - Subclinical hormone dysfunction
    - Size greater than 6 cm (some sources recommend a threshold of >4 cm)
    - Size less than 6 cm with worrisome radiographic signs (rapid growth, heterogeneous appearance, irregular borders, high attenuation (>10–20 HU), or delayed washout of contrast

47. **Describe the open technique for adrenalectomy.**
    There are many surgical approaches to the adrenal glands. Conventional open adrenalectomy can be performed through an anterior (transperitoneal), an anterolateral (extraperitoneal), or a posterior (retroperitoneal) approach. Rarely, a combined thoracoabdominal approach is required for extremely large or malignant lesions.

48. **Discuss the role of laparoscopic surgery.**
    Advances in laparoscopic surgical techniques have been applied to adrenalectomy; currently most endocrine surgeons agree that laparoscopic adrenalectomy is the procedure of choice for benign adrenal tumors, with open adrenalectomy reserved for malignant tumors. Laparoscopic adrenalectomy has been associated with decreased hospital stay, less postoperative pain, less blood loss, shorter recovery, and overall increased patient satisfaction compared with the open techniques.

49. **What approaches are used for laparoscopic surgery?**
    Just as with open adrenalectomy, several laparoscopic approaches are available. The most common technique is via an anterolateral approach, which provides excellent exposure but does not allow removal of both glands without repositioning the patient. An anterior approach provides access to both adrenal glands, but exposure is more difficult. A posterior endoscopic approach avoids entering the peritoneal cavity altogether; however, this approach provides a limited working space and may hinder removal of larger lesions.

50. **Summarize the long-term success of adrenalectomy for functional tumors.**
    Following adrenalectomy for aldosteronomas, blood pressure is improved in 60% to 70%; however, only 33% require no antihypertensive therapy. The aldosterone level normalizes and hypokalemia is corrected in at least 95%; however, the long-term effect on hypertension is variable. The factors that predict postoperative normotension are younger age (<40), short duration of hypertension (<6 years), 2 or fewer antihypertensives, and no family history of hypertension. In older patients with severe, long-standing hypertension associated with renal dysfunction, adrenalectomy may not normalize the blood pressure but often results in easier control of hypertension with fewer or lower-dose medications. Unilateral adrenalectomy is 95% effective in treating cortisol-producing adenomas; bilateral adrenalectomy, in patients failing hypophysectomy for ACTH-dependent Cushing's syndrome, is slightly less effective, with approximately 25% of patients having persistent symptoms, hypertension, or diabetes. For patients undergoing unilateral adrenalectomy for Cushing's syndrome, the hypothalamic-pituitary-adrenal axis recovers in a mean time of 9 months. Patients who undergo bilateral adrenalectomy require lifelong hormone replacement. Adrenalectomy for nonfamilial benign pheochromocytomas is curative in most cases; however, a 5% to 10% late recurrence rate has been reported, and therefore these patients should undergo lifelong surveillance with annual 24-hour urinary catecholamine and metanephrine measurements.

51. Describe the appropriate management of adrenal malignancy.

Adrenocortical carcinoma is a rare (1–2 per million) and aggressive cancer that is frequently metastatic by the time of diagnosis. Approximately 60% of adrenocortical carcinomas are functioning tumors, and the mean size of tumors at the time of diagnosis is greater than 10 cm. The overall 5-year survival rate is approximately 25% and depends largely on the stage at diagnosis. Patients undergoing complete resection of small tumors (<5 cm) without local invasion (stage 1) have a 5-year survival of 60%, whereas patients with metastases or invasion into other organs (stage 4) have a median survival less than 12 months. The only chance for cure is surgery, which should be offered to all patients without metastases with a reasonable surgical risk. Surgery should also be considered for young patients with an isolated, easily resectable metastasis. Despite limited response rates, patients with stage 3 or 4 disease are frequently offered adjuvant therapy with mitotane ($\pm$ cytotoxic chemotherapy), radiotherapy, or both because of the high recurrence rate (up to 85%).

52. Describe the appropriate management of pheochromocytoma.

Most pheochromocytomas are benign, sporadic tumors, and adrenalectomy is curative in nearly all patients. However, approximately 10% of pheochromocytomas are malignant, and the differentiation of benign and malignant lesions is difficult histopathologically. Surgical resection offers the only chance for cure; therefore care must be taken not to disrupt the tumor during resection and en bloc resection of any structure invaded by the tumor should be performed when feasible. Five-year survival is approximately 40% and depends on the completeness of the resection and whether distant metastases are present.

53. What is a cortical-sparing adrenalectomy, and when is it indicated?

Approximately 20% to 30% of pheochromocytomas occur in patients with a hereditary predisposition such as multiple endocrine neoplasia type-2, von Hippel-Lindau syndrome, neurofibromatosis type I, or defects in the genes encoding succinate dehydrogenase subunits D and B. This subset of patients is at increased risk of developing bilateral and recurrent pheochromocytoma. To prevent adrenocortical insufficiency, these patients may undergo a cortical-sparing adrenalectomy. This is actually a partial adrenalectomy in which the tumor and a margin of normal adrenal is resected. Tumors that occur in the medial or lateral portions of the adrenal are more amenable to this approach. This approach balances the benefit of avoiding hormone replacement with a slightly higher risk of recurrent pheochromocytoma in the adrenal remnant.

54. How should patients with pheochromocytoma be prepared for surgery?

The stress of anesthesia or manipulation of the tumor during surgery can result in a rapid increase in circulating catecholamine levels and precipitate a hypertensive crisis or arrhythmia even in patients who have not had significant preoperative hypertension. Thus all patients should undergo preoperative alpha-adrenergic blockade using either phenoxybenzamine or another selective alpha-antagonist. The addition of a beta-blocker can be used to control tachycardia if necessary but only after initiation of an alpha-blocker. Beta blockade should never be started first because the unopposed alpha-adrenergic effect can cause a hypertensive crisis. Calcium channel blockers have been shown to be a safe alternative to adrenergic antagonists. Because of the hyperadrenergic state, patients with pheochromocytoma are typically volume contracted and can become orthostatic on initiation of alpha-blockade. Volume expansion is accomplished by instructing patients to increase their salt intake (>5 g/day) after starting alpha-blockers. Intraoperatively, the patient's blood pressure can change dramatically during manipulation of the tumor and ligation of the adrenal vein. An experienced anesthesiologist who is prepared for these hemodynamic changes is critical to a safe operation.

KEY POINTS: ADRENAL GLANDS

1. Adrenal tumors smaller than 4 cm are rarely malignant; however, 25% of tumors larger than 6 cm are malignant.

2. Cortisol-producing adenoma is the most common functional adrenal tumor.

3. Patients with incidentally discovered adrenal tumors should be evaluated by 1-mg overnight dexamethasone suppression test, 24-hour urinary fractionated metanephrines and catecholamines and, in hypertensive patients, a plasma aldosterone-plasma renin activity ratio.

4. Laparoscopic adrenalectomy is now the preferred approach for most adrenal tumors; however, recurrence rates may be higher than the open approach if the tumor is malignant.

NEUROENDOCRINE TUMORS OF THE PANCREAS AND GASTROINTESTINAL TRACT

55. How common are pancreatic endocrine tumors?

Pancreatic endocrine tumors (PETs) are the most common neuroendocrine tumor occurring in the abdomen but are much less common than pancreatic adenocarcinoma, accounting for only 7% of pancreatic malignancies.

56. Are most PETs functional?

Approximately half of PETs are nonfunctional; however, up to 80% will secrete biologically inactive peptides such as chromogranins, neuron specific enolase, and pancreatic polypeptide. Nonfunctional PETs typically present similarly to pancreatic adenocarcinoma with abdominal pain and biliopancreatic duct obstruction or are found incidentally. The definitive diagnosis of a nonfunctional PET is often not made until final histopathology is performed. Compared with pancreatic adenocarcinoma, patients undergoing resection for malignant PETs have improved median survival (13 months vs. 60 months).

57. What are the types of functional PETs?

Insulinoma is the most common functional PET (60%–70%), and more than 90% are benign. Gastrinoma is the second most common functional PET (20%–30%), and approximately 50% are malignant. Glucagonoma is the next most common, of which 80% are malignant. Vasoactive intestinal peptide secreting tumors (VIPoma) and somatostatinomas are even more rare.

58. How should functional PETs be imaged?

When a hormonally active tumor is suspected, the diagnosis should be confirmed biochemically before any imaging is undertaken. This is important not only for reasons of cost-effectiveness but also for patient safety because some localization studies are invasive. Because of the small size of many PETs, preoperative localization is often difficult, and the extent of preoperative imaging that is necessary is controversial. Ultrasound, CT, MRI, and angiography have reported sensitivities around 60%. Octreotide scans are highly sensitive (85%), especially for metastases, in locating most PETs, with the exception of insulinomas (50% sensitivity). Provocative arterial stimulation (secretin for gastrinomas and calcium for insulinomas) and hepatic venous sampling have a higher sensitivity and have replaced portal vein sampling, but their invasiveness and ability only to regionalize a tumor make them less desirable. Recent reports have shown endoscopic ultrasound to be the most sensitive preoperative test for localizing PETs, although it is invasive and highly operator dependent.

59. **How important is it to localize functional PETs before surgery?**
When performed by an experienced surgeon, intraoperative palpation with intraoperative ultrasound will localize nearly 100% of PETs. Therefore many surgeons believe that exhaustive efforts to localize islet cell tumors preoperatively are unwarranted. They prefer to obtain a preoperative ultrasound or CT scan to identify obviously invasive or metastatic tumors and then rely on intraoperative palpation and ultrasound for tumor localization. All patients undergoing reexploration for PETs should undergo thorough preoperative localization studies.

60. **What is the appropriate surgical approach for insulinomas?**
Insulinomas account for approximately 90% of nonfamilial PETs. The small size of these tumors and the rarity of malignancy allow simple enucleation (60% of cases) or distal pancreatectomy (35% of cases) in the vast majority of cases. Rarely, formal pancreaticoduodenectomy is required (<5% of cases), most typically for malignant tumors. Laparoscopy for enucleation or distal pancreatectomy is used selectively in some centers.

61. **Describe the surgical approach to gastrinomas.**
The surgical approach to gastrinomas is more complex because these tumors are more frequently malignant and occur outside the pancreas in up to 50% of cases. Tumors occurring distal to the pancreatic neck should be removed by formal pancreatic resection because of the high incidence of malignancy. Tumors in the pancreatic head can often be enucleated, reserving formal pancreaticoduodenectomy for more invasive tumors or those in close proximity to the pancreatic duct. Careful evaluation of the duodenum by palpation, endoscopic transillumination, or duodenotomy is necessary to identify tumors within the duodenal wall, which occur commonly and can be quite small. Small submucosal lesions can be enucleated, but a full-thickness resection of the duodenal wall may be necessary. The propensity for these tumors to metastasize to lymph nodes necessitates a regional lymph node dissection in all patients.

62. **How should other sporadically occurring islet cell tumors be managed?**
Other sporadically occurring islet cell tumors are typically large, and 50% are malignant, requiring an individualized surgical approach in these rare cases.

63. **Should PETs occurring in patients with MEN 1 be approached differently than those occurring sporadically?**
Yes. Approximately 70% of patients with MEN 1 develop pancreatic islet cell tumors, with gastrinoma being most common. Because of the multifocal nature and diffuse islet cell dysplasia seen in these patients, aggressive surgery rarely results in biochemical cure. The morbidity and mortality rates of aggressive surgical resection combined with low cure rate and the availability of effective palliative treatment options for symptomatic patients sway many clinicians to treat patients medically unless there is suspicion of malignancy. Other surgeons take a more aggressive approach, citing recent studies that demonstrate decreased development of liver metastases and improved survival in those undergoing surgery. Further, the larger tumors seen on preoperative imaging (>2 cm) often account for symptoms, and therefore surgical extirpation of these tumors may be beneficial. Formal resection of the distal pancreas accompanied by enucleation of tumors in the pancreatic head is necessary. Search for duodenal tumors and resection of the lymph nodes must accompany resection of pancreatic tumors.

64. **Discuss the role of surgery for liver metastases from neuroendocrine tumors.**
Patients who undergo resection of isolated liver metastases from neuroendocrine tumors experience symptomatic improvement in 95% of cases and have prolonged survival (60%–75%

vs. 25%–30% 5-year survival rates) compared with patients with similar tumor burdens not undergoing hepatic resection. Patients with unresectable liver metastases or those with prohibitive surgical risks may benefit from either cryosurgical or radiofrequency thermal ablation.

65. **Describe the presentation of nonpancreatic neuroendocrine tumors (carcinoid tumors).**

Bronchial carcinoids may present with hemoptysis or carcinoid syndrome. Gastric carcinoids are frequently found incidentally on endoscopy but may also cause symptoms such as pain or bleeding. Neuroendocrine tumors of the small intestine are the most likely to result in carcinoid syndrome, which typically does not occur until the patient has developed metastases to the liver. These tumors frequently result in a desmoplastic (fibrotic) reaction of the adjacent mesentery resulting in bowel obstruction. Hindgut carcinoids do not usually produce active hormones and are typically found incidentally during endoscopy performed for other reasons.

66. **Describe the carcinoid syndrome.**

Carcinoid syndrome results from the production and release of serotonin from neuroendocrine tumors, most commonly those of the small intestine. The liver metabolizes serotonin to inactive products, so most patients do not develop carcinoid syndrome until they have developed liver metastases, which permits serotonin to enter the systemic circulation. Patients frequently experience intermittent abdominal pain, brief flushing episodes, and diarrhea. Asthmalike symptoms, hypotension, and heart failure (marantic endocarditis) can also occur.

67. **After a patient is diagnosed with carcinoid syndrome, what is the next step?**

The tumor must then be localized. This goal may be difficult because of the small size of most carcinoid tumors. Tumors arise in the small bowel and appendix in nearly 70% of patients, and therefore a small bowel contrast study or abdominal CT scan is often the initial study performed. If these tests fail to localize the tumor, a chest x-ray or chest CT scan (or both) should be obtained to exclude a bronchial carcinoid. Metaiodobenzylguanidine or octreotide scintigraphy is sometimes able to localize tumors not found by conventional methods.

68. **Describe the appropriate surgical management for carcinoid tumors.**

Bronchial carcinoids tend to spread locoregionally and therefore should be resected by formal lobectomy when possible. Gastric and small intestinal carcinoids without metastases should be excised by segmental resection and lymph node dissection. Appendiceal carcinoids are typically incidentally discovered and occur most commonly at the appendiceal tip. Distal lesions of less than 2 cm are adequately treated by appendectomy. The presence of a carcinoid near the appendiceal base, carcinoid size greater than 2 cm, or grossly involved lymph nodes require formal right hemicolectomy. Rectal carcinoids often present with bleeding or are incidentally found on endoscopy. Extensive surgery for rectal carcinoids offers no survival advantage over local excision.

69. **Discuss the role of surgery in carcinoid syndrome.**

Patients with surgically resectable hepatic tumors experience improvement in symptoms and survival comparable to that for pancreatic endocrine tumors metastatic to the liver. The development of somatostatin analogs has allowed successful control of symptoms in most patients with carcinoid syndrome and diffuse hepatic metastases. Systemic chemotherapy and hepatic artery embolization have not been effective in palliating these patients; however, selective hepatic artery chemoembolization has been successful in decreasing tumor burden and alleviating symptoms in up to 80% of patients. Patients who do not respond to medical palliation may benefit from aggressive tumor debulking by resecting the primary tumor and as many of the liver metastases as feasible.

KEY POINTS: NEUROENDOCRINE TUMORS OF THE PANCREAS AND GASTROINTESTINAL TRACT

1. Insulinoma is the most common pancreatic endocrine tumor, is usually benign, and can be treated by enucleation.

2. Gastrinoma is usually malignant and can occur in the pancreas, duodenum, and lymph nodes.

3. Octreotide scintigraphy and endoscopic ultrasound are the most useful preoperative imaging studies for gastrinoma.

4. Arterial stimulation with hepatic venous sampling has replaced portal venous sampling for localization of islet cell tumors.

5. Pancreatic endocrine tumors in patients with multiple endocrine neoplasia type 1 are frequently multifocal and usually treated medically because of the low cure rate following surgery.

6. Resection of isolated liver metastasis from neuroendocrine tumors improves symptoms and prolongs survival.

BARIATRIC SURGERY

70. **Define obesity. How common is it?**
Obesity is simply defined as the excess of body fat. The degree of body fat relative to weight is calculated by the body mass index (BMI; kg/m^2). Obesity is a BMI 30 or higher. Morbid obesity is a BMI $\geq$ 40 or higher. Increasing BMI correlates with increasing health issues including diabetes mellitus, hypertension, sleep apnea and Pickwickian syndromes, asthma, coronary artery disease, cardiomyopathy, gastroesophageal reflux disease, degenerative joint disease, hyperlipidemia, fatty liver, gout, urinary incontinence, gallbladder disease, psychological disorders, menstrual irregularities, and certain cancers (endometrial, colon, postmenopausal breast, and kidney). Most important, a BMI greater than 40 increases the risk of death from all causes by twofold. Sixty-four percent or 127 million adults in the United States are considered overweight, and 31% or 60 million adults are considered obese.

71. **What are the limitations of BMI?**
The BMI can be misleading in those with a higher proportion of fat relative to muscle (the elderly) or in those with an unusually high proportion of muscle (bodybuilders).

72. **How successful is nonsurgical treatment of obesity?**
Evidence suggests that nonsurgical treatment (diet/behavior modification, exercise programs, and psychological support) for morbid obesity has a more than 90% failure rate. Similarly, pharmacological therapy for morbid obesity has been hampered by serious side effects and, overall, has met with disappointing results.

73. **What are the indications for surgery for obesity?**
An NIH Consensus Conference held in 1991 recommended that the following patients be considered for bariatric surgery:
- BMI greater than 40
- BMI of 35 to 40 if associated with other severe medical problems that are likely to improve with weight reduction

Patients must be well informed and motivated and should have failed nonoperative attempts at weight loss before being considered for surgery.

74. **List the contraindications to bariatric operations.**
   - Endocrine disorders that cause morbid obesity
   - Psychological instability
   - Alcohol or drug abuse
   - Comorbidities resulting in prohibitive anesthetic risk
   - Binge-eating disorders

75. **Categorize the various surgical options for weight reduction.**
   Surgical options for weight reduction can be divided into either restrictive or malabsorptive; however, some procedures use a component of both.

76. **List the options for restrictive surgery.**
   Vertical-banded gastroplasty: A stapling device is used to divide the stomach vertically along the lesser curve starting at the angle of His to create a small (20-mL) pouch. A prosthetic device is then wrapped around the outlet of the pouch to prevent it from dilatating over time. This operation has fallen out of favor because of poor long-term success and is only rarely performed.

   Gastric banding (Fig. 58-1): This procedure is now commonly performed laparoscopically and involves placement of an adjustable band around the top of the stomach to create a small (20-mL) pouch. The band is connected to a reservoir placed in the subcutaneous tissue that enables band adjustment.

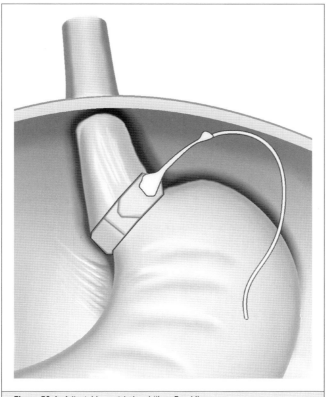

Figure 58-1. Adjustable gastric band "Lap-Band."

Sleeve gastrectomy (Fig 58-2): This procedure is gaining in popularity and involves stapling and removing the majority of the gastric body and fundus. This results in a long, tubelike stomach and an intact pylorus. Patients lose weight from the restrictive effect and because of a reduction in ghrelin, a hormone made in the stomach that helps to regulate food intake. This procedure is sometimes used as the initial operation for patients with very high BMI. After the patient has lost some of his or her excess weight, a second operation is performed, usually a bypass procedure, to achieve additional weight loss.

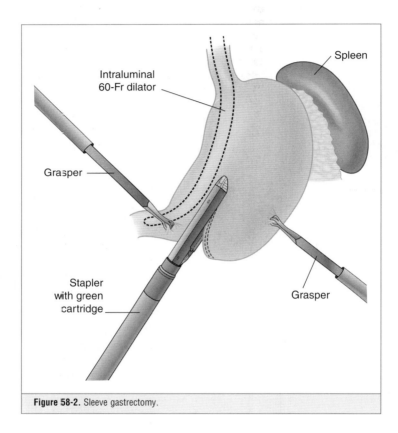

Figure 58-2. Sleeve gastrectomy.

77. **What is the option for malabsorptive surgery?**
    Biliopancreatic diversion with or without a duodenal switch. A subtotal gastrectomy is performed, leaving a gastric remnant of 250 to 500 mL. The small bowel is divided 200 to 300 cm proximal to the ileocecal valve, and the ileum is anastomosed to the stomach. The jejunum is connected to the side of the ileum approximately 50–100 cm from the ileocecal valve. A duodenal switch is similar, but instead of a subtotal gastrectomy, a sleeve gastrectomy is performed with anastomosis of the ileum to the duodenum just past the pylorus. Biliopancreatic diversion results in malabsorption by creating a short common channel for digestion and absorption of food. It is effective in weight reduction but is technically more challenging and has some increased risk of malnutrition, anemia, and diarrhea.

78. **Explain the combined option.**
Known as the Roux-en-Y gastric bypass (Fig. 58-3), the top of the stomach is stapled (and commonly divided) horizontally to create a small, 15- to 30-mL proximal stomach pouch. This small reservoir restricts the amount of food that can be ingested at one time. The jejunum is then divided just distal to the ligament of Treitz and the distal end anastomosed to the proximal stomach pouch. The proximal end of the jejunum is then anastomosed to the side of the jejunum 75 to 150 cm distal to the gastrojejunostomy. The length of this Roux limb determines the degree of malabsorption and is typically made longer for patients with very high BMIs. This procedure is now commonly performed using laparoscopic technique.

79. **How much weight do patients lose following bariatric surgery?**
Success following bariatric surgery is determined by both weight lost and improvement in obesity-related comorbidities. However, many surgical studies report outcome as percentage excess weight loss (EWL) and consider loss of at least 50% of excess weight as a minimum criterion for success. The lap band typically produces 40% to 60% EWL gradually over 2 to 3 years, but it has a 20% failure rate. The gastric bypass typically produces 60% to 80% EWL rapidly over 2 years but has some recidivism and an estimated 10% failure rate. The biliopancreatic diversion is arguably the most effective weight loss procedure and results in the loss of 80% of excess weight maintained over the long term. The sleeve gastrectomy is currently being studied for long-term success and so far mimics the gastric bypass in terms of weight loss efficacy.

80. **What are the effects of bariatric surgery on obesity-related comorbidities?**
Long-term weight loss following bariatric surgery has been shown to reduce obesity-related comorbidities significantly. Approximately 85% of patients with diabetes, hyperlipidemia, and obesity hypoventilation syndrome will be improved or cured at 2 years after surgery. In fact, the gastric bypass is now being studied as a surgical option for resolution of type 2 diabetes in those without severe obesity. Hypertension also improves or resolves in more than two thirds of patients after successful weight loss. Salutary effects on other comorbidities, such as asthma, depression, arthritic pain, and unemployment, are frequently observed following surgery.

81. **What are the complications of bariatric surgery?**
Perioperative mortality for the lap band is 0.1%, for the gastric bypass is 0.5% to 1% and for biliopancreatic diversion 1% to 3%. The laparoscopic technique has changed the pattern of perioperative complications. Although wound complications and postoperative cardiopulmonary complications are less frequent, anastomotic stenosis, gastrointestinal (GI) bleeding, and bowel obstruction occur more frequently with laparoscopic compared to open techniques. Mean hospital stay following laparoscopic bariatric surgery is 2 to 3 days, which is significantly shorter than after open surgery (5–7 days). The lap band is usually performed as either an outpatient procedure or 24-hour stay. Each procedure has its own unique risk of complications, with the lap band having the fewest serious complications and the biliopancreatic diversion having the greatest.

82. **Give the incidence of complications following laparoscopic bariatric procedures in general.**
   - Anastomotic leak (1%–2%)
   - Anastomotic stenosis (5%–10%)
   - Postoperative bowel obstruction (3%)
   - GI bleed (2%)
   - Gallstones (10%)
   - Protein-calorie malnutrition (3%–5%)
   - Anemia (30%)
   - Vitamin deficiency (30%)
   - Wound complication (infection, dehiscence, and hernia) (4%–5%)
   - Band slippage or erosion into stomach (1%–5%)

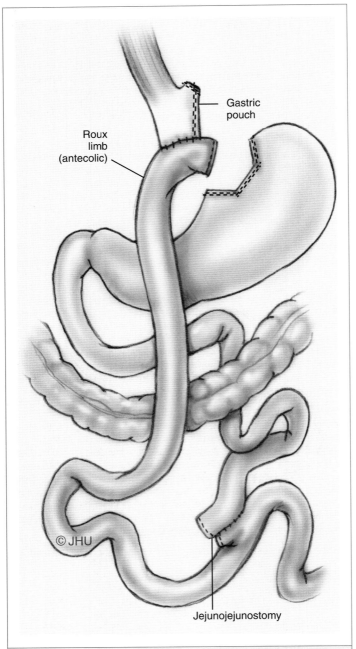

Figure 58-3. Roux-en-Y gastric bypass.

KEY POINTS: BARIATRIC SURGERY

1. Surgery is the only therapy that consistently results in significant, long-term weight loss in morbidly obese patients.

2. Laparoscopic Roux-en-Y gastric bypass is currently the most common bariatric operation performed in the United States and results in loss of 60% to 80% of excess weight.

3. Surgical weight loss significantly reduces obesity-related comorbidities and is a surgical cure for diabetes mellitus.

WEBSITE

http://endocrinesurgeons.org/home.html

BIBLIOGRAPHY

THYROID

1. Abraham-Nordling M, Törring O, Hamberger B, et al: Graves' disease: a long-term quality-of-life follow up of patients randomized to treatment with antithyroid drugs, radioiodine, or surgery. Thyroid 15:1279–1286, 2005.

2. Bilimoria KY, Bentrem DJ, Ko CY, et al: Extent of surgery affects survival for papillary thyroid cancer. Ann Surg 246:375–381, 2007.

3. Choi JY, Lee KS, Kim HJ, et al: Focal thyroid lesions incidentally identified by integrated 18F-FDG PET/CT: clinical significance and improved characterization. J Nucl Med 47:609–615, 2006.

4. Cooper DS, Doherty GM, Haugen BR, et al: Management guidelines for patients with thyroid nodules and differentiated thyroid cancer. Thyroid 16:109–142, 2006.

5. Fialkowski EA, Moley JF: Current approaches to medullary thyroid carcinoma, sporadic and familial. J Surg Oncol 94:737–747, 2006.

6. White ML, Gauger PG, Doherty GM: Central lymph node dissection in differentiated thyroid cancer. World J Surg 31:895–904, 2007.

7. Yang J, Schnadig V, Logrono R, Wasserman PG: Fine-needle aspiration of thyroid nodules: a study of 4703 patients with histologic and clinical correlations. Cancer 111:306–311, 2007.

PARATHYROID

8. Allendorf J, DiGorgi M, Spanknebel K, et al: 1112 consecutive bilateral neck explorations for primary hyperparathyroidism. World J Surg 31:2075–2080, 2007.

9. Bilezikian JP, Potts JT Jr, Fuleihan Gel-H, et al: Summary statement from a workshop on asymptomatic primary hyperparathyroidism: a perspective for the 21st century. J Clin Endocrinol Metab 87:5353–5361, 2002.

10. Eigelberger MS, Cheah WK, Ituarte PH, et al: The NIH criteria for parathyroidectomy in asymptomatic primary hyperparathyroidism: are they too limited? Ann Surg 239:528–535, 2004.

11. Mazzaglia PJ, Berber E, Kovach A, et al: The changing presentation of hyperparathyroidism over 3 decades. Arch Surg 143:260–266, 2008.

12. Richards ML, Wormuth J, Bingener J, Sirinek K: Parathyroidectomy in secondary hyperparathyroidism: is there an optimal operative management? Surgery 139:174–180, 2006.

13. Rodgers SE, Perrier ND: Parathyroid carcinoma. Curr Opin Oncol 18:16–22, 2006.

14. Sharma J, Mazzaglia P, Milas M, et al: Radionuclide imaging for hyperparathyroidism (HPT): which is the best technetium-99m sestamibi modality? Surgery 140:856–863, 2006.

15. Udelsman R, Donovan PI: Remedial parathyroid surgery: changing trends in 130 consecutive cases. Ann Surg 244:471–479, 2006.

16. Westerdahl J, Bergenfelz A: Unilateral versus bilateral neck exploration for primary hyperparathyroidism: five-year follow-up of a randomized controlled trial. Ann Surg 246:976–980, 2007.

ADRENAL GLANDS

17. Allolio B, Fassnacht M: Clinical review: adrenocortical carcinoma: clinical update. J Clin Endocrinol Metab 91:2027–2037, 2006.

18. Giacchetti G, Mulatero P, Mantero F, et al: Primary aldosteronism, a major form of low renin hypertension: from screening to diagnosis. Trends Endocrinol Metab 19:104–108, 2008.

19. Palazzo FF, Sebag F, Sierra M, et al: Long-term outcome following laparoscopic adrenalectomy for large solid adrenal cortex tumors. World J Surg 30:893–898, 2006.

20. Porterfield JR, Thompson GB, Young WF Jr, et al: Surgery for Cushing's syndrome: an historical review and recent ten-year experience. World J Surg 32:659–677, 2008.

21. Poulose BK, Holzman MD, Lao OB, et al: Laparoscopic adrenalectomy: 100 resections with clinical long-term follow-up. Surg Endosc 19:379–385, 2005.

22. Young WF Jr: Clinical practice. The incidentally discovered adrenal mass. N Engl J Med 356:601–610, 2007.

23. Zarnegar R, Lee J, Brunaud L, et al: Good blood pressure control on antihypertensives, not only response to spironolactone, predicts improved outcome after adrenalectomy for aldosteronoma. Surgery 142:921–929, 2007.

NEUROENDOCRINE TUMORS OF THE PANCREAS AND GASTROINTESTINAL TRACT

24. Alexakis N, Neoptolemos JP: Pancreatic neuroendocrine tumours. Best Pract Res Clin Gastroenterol 22:183–205, 2008.

25. Kouvaraki MA, Shapiro SE, Cote GJ, et al: Management of pancreatic endocrine tumors in multiple endocrine neoplasia type 1. World J Surg 30:643–653, 2006.

26. Musunuru S, Chen H, Rajpal S, et al: Metastatic neuroendocrine hepatic tumors: resection improves survival. Arch Surg 141:1000–1004, 2006.

27. Nikfarjam M, Warshaw AL, Axelrod L, et al: Improved contemporary surgical management of insulinomas: a 25-year experience at the Massachusetts General Hospital. Ann Surg 247:165–172, 2008.

28. Norton JA, Fraker DL, Alexander HR, et al: Surgery increases survival in patients with gastrinoma. Ann Surg 244:410–419, 2006.

29. Perez EA, Koniaris LG, Snell SE, et al: 7201 carcinoids: increasing incidence overall and disproportionate mortality in the elderly. World J Surg 31:1022–1030, 2007.

BARIATRIC SURGERY

30. Anthone GJ, Lord RV, DeMeester TR, Crookes PF: The duodenal switch operation for the treatment of morbid obesity. Ann Surg 238:618–627, 2003.

31. Biertho L, Steffen R, Ricklin T, et al: Laparoscopic gastric bypass versus laparoscopic adjustable gastric banding: a comparative study of 1,200 cases. J Am Coll Surg 197:536–544, 2003.

32. Brolin RE: Bariatric surgery and long-term control of morbid obesity. JAMA 288:2793–2796, 2002.

33. Lee WJ, Lee YC, Ser KH, et al: NIH Consensus Conference. Gastrointestinal surgery for severe obesity. Ann Int Med 115:956–961, 1991.

34. Podnos Y, Jimenez JC, Wilson SE, et al: Complications after laparoscopic gastric bypass. Arch Surg 138:957–961, 2003.

35. Schauer PR, Burguera B, Ikramuddin S, et al: Effect of laparoscopic Roux-en Y gastric bypass on type 2 diabetes mellitus. Ann Surg 238:467–484, 2003.

36. Sjöström L, Narbro K, Sjöström CD, et al: Effects of bariatric surgery on mortality in Swedish obese subjects. N Engl J Med 357:741–752, 2007.

CHAPTER 59

ENDOCRINOLOGY IN THE MANAGED CARE ENVIRONMENT

Elliot G. Levy

1. **Define managed care.**

   The American College of Physicians/American Society of Internal Medicine has defined managed care as "a system of health-care delivery provided by contracted providers in which the entities responsible for financing the cost of health care exert influence on the clinical decision-making of those who provide the health care in an attempt to provide health care that is cost effective, accessible, and of acceptable quality."

2. **Is there only one type of managed care?**

   Managed care is actually a spectrum of health care delivery systems ranging from managed indemnity insurance through preferred provider organizations (PPOs) and point-of-service (POS) plans to various types of health maintenance organizations (HMOs). Collectively, these organizations are called managed care organizations (MCOs). To a greater or lesser extent, all managed care systems attempt to shift financial risk in one way or another to the providers of care.

3. **Who is the patient's initial contact in a managed care environment?**

   In most cases, the patient's initial contact is with a health care provider, conveniently called a "primary care provider" (PCP). This person is usually a physician, such as a family medicine, family practice, or general practice physician, but often may be a physician who has specialized in internal medicine or an internist with a subspecialty (such as endocrinology) who enjoys practicing primary care in addition to his or her subspecialty or does not have enough subspecialty work to fill his or her schedule. The PCP can also be a physician extender, such as a nurse practitioner or a physician assistant. Some MCOs use physicians in large clinic type settings in an effort to control costs. In other situations, PCPs function out of their usual private practice offices—in a sense, mixing their private (or non-MCO) patients with their HMO or PPO patients.

4. **Do pediatricians and gynecologists function as PCPs?**

   There has been a movement over the past few years to allow pediatricians to become PCPs for children and for obstetrics and gynecology specialists to become PCPs for women of childbearing years, who often have no need to see other types of physicians.

5. **How does the patient make contact with a subspecialist?**

   A patient is allowed to see a subspecialist, such as an endocrinologist, only with the recommendation of a PCP. Usually, an endocrinologist is not allowed to function as both a PCP and a subspecialist within a given HMO. In these situations, when a fully trained endocrinologist is serving as a PCP, he or she cannot even perform specialty-type procedures and must refer them to another endocrinologist.

6. **What is a meant by the MCO's "panel" of providers?**

   After an MCO has established itself in a community, it begins to develop a "panel" of all the providers it requires, including PCPs, medical subspecialists, surgeons and surgical subspecialists, pediatricians, obstetricians-gynecologists, and dermatologists. Simultaneously, the MCO contracts with hospitals (strategically located around the community that it wants to "penetrate '), nursing homes, home health agencies, physical therapy centers, dialysis centers, outpatient diagnostic centers, clinical (commercial) laboratories, and, sometimes, even outpatient diabetes education centers or dietitians.

7. **Explain the MCO directory.**

The panel of providers is published yearly in a directory that goes by a variety of names (e.g., preferred provider list) and is distributed to all participants of the MCO. This directory is sometimes called the "list." It is used by patients to determine which PCP is available for them to use (although in some HMOs, the new patients are immediately assigned to a PCP of the HMO's choice). It is used by a PCP to know which subspecialists, diagnostic center, and laboratory to use. It is also used by the MCO itself as a marketing tool to solicit business for itself by proudly showing which subspecialists belong to its panel of providers. It is therefore necessary to be on "the list" to receive referrals from this HMO. However, your presence on the list as a subspecialist does not mean that you will ever receive referrals. The health care for the MCO is then provided by this entire group of health care providers, all of whom are under contracts with the HMO to provide the care in the manner and for the price that is negotiated. Thus the MCO has managed to do what the health care system was never able to do by itself—organize all the health care into one unit.

8. **Explain the POS option.**

In some cases, the POS option allows the patient to see any specialist, although the reimbursement schedule is different. In addition, the patient's out-of-pocket expenses (copayment) are often much larger. The POS option differs greatly among insurance companies that offer it.

9. **How do MCOs compare with other business units?**

When one looks at the managed care system from afar, it is not so different from any other business unit that has to negotiate with vendors to provide services that it cannot provide on its own. Think of a business unit as the cruise ship industry, which negotiates with its own employees, as well as entertainers, doctors, food suppliers, fuel suppliers, ports, and travel agents, to provide for its customers (passengers) a total package for their enjoyment. So have the MCOs attempted to organize the United States health care system. It is clearly a private, non-government-regulated, for-profit (in most cases) system with the primary goal of earning a profit for its shareholders while attempting to contain costs for the entire health care system. Not-for-profit MCOs are not necessarily any more efficient in providing the care to its members and often have the same fiscal problems as for-profit MCOs.

10. **What is the difference between a PPO and an HMO?**

A preferred provider organization (PPO) is a plan, as originally conceived 10–20 years ago, which contracts with independent providers at a discounted fee for service. When the PPO systems first started, their representatives would approach a PCP or a specialist and offer a discounted fee schedule to a physician in exchange for the potential of being specifically referred a group of patients who otherwise would not be able to see that physician. There developed the concept of "panels" (i.e., the "lists" discussed earlier), in which a list of accepted providers would be given to patients covered by the plan, who must agree to use only the physicians on such a panel in order for their care to be covered by the plan. This concept has been modified many times (see question 12).

HMO was originally defined as a prepaid organization that provided comprehensive health care services to voluntarily enrolled members in return for a prepaid fixed amount of money. Nowadays, an HMO can be a health plan that places some providers at risk for medical expenses or a health plan that uses PCPs as gatekeepers.

11. **Are there other types of MCO plans?**

As pressure was placed on businesses with large numbers of employees who were not happy with the original types of plans and the costs involved with the yearly premiums of certain plans, many other insurance options were created.

12. **What are blended policies?**

Blended policies include PPO with an assigned PCP and full coverage for specialty referral within the network of contracted providers but partial payment for use of specialists outside the network. Plans can have different deductibles for office visits, hospitalizations, and brand-name versus generic medications. In some HMOs, an entire clinic provides all of the health care, and referrals must be made internally. Other HMOs may contract with certain physicians within a community to be PCPs and with other physicians to be the specialists. Referrals may be scrutinized carefully, and PCPs may be indirectly penalized by withholding bonuses or even reprimanded when they refer too many patients to specialists. There are many more plans as insurance companies try to provide options to employers that meet the needs of the employees but keep the cost down to the employer. In many MCOs, a physician must provide care for both HMO and PPO patients, although some times with different fee schedules. Some MCOs allow physicians to participate in one or the other.

13. **How does an endocrinologist join an HMO?**

As many options are there for a physician to practice, such are the options for joining MCOs. In some cases, an endocrinologist is employed by a faculty group practice of a large medical center or a large group practice, in which all members are participants in the specific plan. He or she is most likely to become a provider as soon as his or her credentials are approved by the MCO. In areas of the country with a shortage of endocrinologists, you will be approached by many MCOs to participate immediately. For the most part, if an endocrinologist decides to practice solo or joins a group practice in an area where the MCO is satisfied with the doctors already on the panel, joining the HMO can be difficult; in some cases, it may be impossible. Trying to open a solo office for general endocrinology in an area of great HMO penetration may be extremely difficult and frustrating. Sometimes, however, the MCO is under pressure to increase the number of endocrinologists, especially in certain geographic areas, and welcomes the applications of new doctors. At other times, MCOs receive specific requests from patients or employers to include in their panels certain groups of doctors who were not previously participants. In general, the process of application, review of application, and final approval for participation can be quite long, maybe even more than 6 months. During this time, a physician cannot see patients for the MCO.

14. **How does an HMO patient get to your office?**

After a PCP determines that he or she does not have the experience or expertise to treat a certain endocrine problem, the patient is referred to your office. Sometimes the referral is made by the patient's HMO or "center," as it is often called. The patient must have in hand some kind of a referral form, either an authorization form or a special slip of paper giving you the specific authority to evaluate and treat the patient. Without the referral form or some kind of definite referral from the center, you will not be compensated for the consultation visit. Each subsequent visit must also be authorized in the same manner, or payment will be withheld. It can be frustrating when a patient arrives for follow-up at the physician's office without the authorization form. Naturally the doctor wants to see the patient and has blocked out the time in his or her schedule for the visit. Nonetheless, the HMO will definitely refuse to back-issue a referral form, and, most likely, the doctor will receive no compensation for the visit.

15. **What can you expect to be able to do for the patient at the initial consultation or at subsequent follow-up visits?**
In general, you will be allowed to perform a history and physical examination and order simple diagnostic tests without hassle. Blood tests should be allowed, although the samples usually have to be sent to the laboratory with which the MCO has contracted (see question 17). Other tests have to be approved in writing by the HMO center or by the main HMO office, depending on the individual company's policy. Approval for simple procedures, such as thyroid scans, ultrasound studies, radioactive iodine treatment, and even fine-needle aspiration (FNA) biopsies can take from hours to days. Some HMOs require that PCPs schedule all tests, which can be a problem because you may not know when or where the study is scheduled or when to have the patient return to discuss the results. The more expensive a test is (such as an MRI), the more difficult it is to arrange.

16. **Can you use your own physician office laboratory (POL) for HMO patients?**
Although many endocrinologists have their own laboratories, accredited to perform certain endocrine tests, you usually cannot use them for HMO patients. Often the HMO has arranged special fees with commercial labs. This situation can create logistical problems in your office if you work for several HMOs, all of which use different commercial labs. Your laboratory technicians must keep straight which specimens go where. In addition, some HMOs require that the patients have all blood tests drawn at the office of the PCP. This requirement is especially a problem because sometimes you will not know whether your patient went to the PCP's office to have the blood drawn, and the test results may not be returned to you until the patient returns for a follow-up visit. You may have to call the PCP's office to have the results given to you over the phone or by fax.

17. **What potentially serious problem may arise in regard to pathology services?**
Endocrinologists often perform FNA biopsy of a thyroid nodule. Most endocrinologists trust the interpretations by one particular laboratory, often at a university setting. The MCO may not have a contract with that laboratory and may require you to use a totally different laboratory for FNA cytology interpretation. Sometimes the pathologists at that laboratory may not be used to interpreting thyroid FNAs, and the results you receive may not be as accurate. This particular problem is being addressed at present by the American Thyroid Association and the College of American Pathologists.

18. **What happens if your patient changes jobs and receives health insurance from a company for which you are not providing services, or if the patient's employer switches insurance because the price of the original plan was too high?**
Obviously, this problem is highly frustrating for both patient and physician. The concept of long-term loyalty has been changed. Occasionally a POS option may be available in the new plan, but often the patient gets tired of paying the extra copayment. Sometimes a physician will give the patient a discount to continue their professional relationship. At other times, patients feel so strongly about the opinion of their doctor that they pay the fee out of pocket to the doctor, especially if the patient only has to be seen once or twice a year. There are movements in Congress to allow the continuation of the patient–physician relationship. Until such time, the physician has to understand that losing patients in this way may be unavoidable. He or she should always welcome the patient back to his or her practice if the insurance situation changes.

19. **Describe the process by which the endocrinologist submits the bill for patient services.**
After endocrinologists finish seeing the patient, they usually complete a "superbill" by entering the type of office visit performed, any diagnostic tests ordered that are performed in house, and the proper diagnosis code covering the patient's medical condition. The doctor then turns the chart and superbill over to a clerical person, thus ending the patient–physician interaction of the

day. What happens thereafter is usually a total mystery to most doctors. A secretary or administrative assistant usually enters the charges and the diagnosis into some type of physician management system, where an insurance claim is generated and sent electronically or by paper to the insurance carrier. The carrier examines the claim, and eventually a check is cut covering what the carrier feels is appropriate. The check returns to the physician's office after some period of time, and a clerical person posts the payment received in the patient's account. There was somewhat of an "honor system" in the past, whereby the insurance company trusted the physician explicitly. This is no longer the case.

20. **Why are payments often delayed?**
    MCOs are notorious for holding back payments. There are all kinds of excuses:
    - Deliberate down-coding (i.e., stating that the service provided was really a level 3 service, even though the claim was submitted at level 4)
    - Bundling (e.g., including the charges for the physician component of treatment for a hyperthyroid patient with the cost of the radiopharmaceutical)
    - Delayed payments (holding on to the claim for 6–8 rather than 2–3 weeks)
    - Wrongful denial of claims (such as stating, inappropriately, that there is no coverage, no authorization, a nonexistent preexisting condition, or improper completion of the insurance form).

21. **What problems may result from such practices?**
    These problems result in inappropriate payments (always less than expected), prolonged time before the claims are finally resolved, and endless amounts of paperwork, administrative time, and loss of income. In fact, there was a recently settled lawsuit against five MCOs, filed on behalf of the Florida Medical Association, California Medical Association, Texas Medical Association, and Medical Association of Georgia, for using such practices. For this reason, physicians must understand all of the potential problems before they enter into contract to see patients for a specific HMO or continue seeing their patients without checking with their billing offices to find out what kinds of problems may exist.

22. **Is it advisable to continue seeing patients for MCOs if such problems exist?**
    This becomes a personal and financial decision that each physician or group practice has to make. Some doctors work for a company strictly on a salary basis. Seeing all patients is just part of what they have to do. Physicians who are in solo practice or small groups must be aware of all the problems so that the decision to begin or continue seeing patients is made for the right economic reasons. Many doctors react out of fear and anger, the worst emotions to invoke when an economic decision has to be made.

23. **Explain why doctors must be involved in all aspects of the MCO relationship.**
    Doctors must be involved in all aspects of the MCO relationship, from contract negotiation to ongoing monitoring of day-to-day problems in seeing patients for the particular MCO and awareness of reimbursement problems. The practice must monitor collections, be on top of claims, and resubmit claims that were rejected, down-coded, or held for a long time without payment. The doctor must make sure that the collection of claims is not forgotten and that all claims are actively pursued, especially when third-party payment (i.e., from an insurance company) is involved. Doctors or their staff must have a policy in force to ensure that referrals are obtained, claims submitted on time, and proper payments received.

24. **What special concerns apply to doctors in small groups?**
    Doctors in small groups must make sure that the MCO in question is contributing a significant amount to the gross revenue of the practice to be worth the "hassle" involved in seeing its patients. As a particular doctor gets busier and busier, it might be more worthwhile to replace patients from an HMO with a low reimbursement schedule with patients from HMOs with higher

schedules. Perhaps the doctor can see only patients covered by higher-paying PPOs or choose not to be involved in MCOs at all, if there are enough patients to fill his or her schedule. For those new in practice, it may be worthwhile to see more and more patients, despite the associated problems.

25. **What pitfalls should doctors avoid in making decisions about participation in MCOs?**

The decision to join MCO panels or to resign from a particular panel should not be an emotional one, such as fear that if you do not accept a contract with what you consider an inadequate reimbursement schedule, another endocrinologist will do so. In addition, do not make a decision in anger, when a company denies payment or down-codes a series of claims without good reason. Work out the economics associated with leaving rather than resign out of anger. In fact, first try to work it out with the MCO, then look at all these issues and decide whether resignation is appropriate for economic reasons, not emotional ones.

26. **What factors should be taken into account in deciding whether to renew a specific MCO contract?**

Contracts for most HMOs come up for renewal each year. Doctors have a chance to decide whether the contract should be continued. The decision to continue should be based on facts rather than feelings: revenue tracking, handling of claims, and fee schedule.

27. **Explain revenue tracking.**

Doctors should track their revenue during each year from all payers to make sure that no single MCO becomes such a large percentage of their practice that dropping the company or, even worse, being dropped by the company may result in a gigantic loss of revenue. No one can say for sure what the ideal percentage should be, but some physicians use 10% to 15% as the ceiling for the cutoff. A doctor must be careful, however, in turning away new referrals from that HMO, because there might be some contractual obligations that must be followed.

28. **What factors are relevant to handling of claims?**

Practice management software should be able to provide information, such as how many claims for each MCO were down-coded, bundled, or denied. How many claims were delayed in payment for more than 3 weeks? How many times did a billing clerk have to call the company before payment was finally received? Each time a claim is not paid properly or promptly, administrative costs are associated with collecting these fees. These extra costs effectively reduce the expected amount of reimbursement. In addition, talk to the secretaries to find out what kinds of hassles are encountered in receiving referrals, scheduling procedures, and getting laboratory tests done promptly. They can guide you in your decision.

29. **How do you evaluate the fee schedule?**

After the decision is made to continue seeing the patients for an MCO, the physician must look at the fee schedule. Try not to sign a document that expresses reimbursement in terms of a percentage of Medicare or some other baseline. Try to be specific in providing a list of office visit codes that will be used and agree on a criteria for judging what documentation is required for each level. Also provide the company with a list of procedures and tests that you perform in your office and agree on a fee schedule. Make sure that the company signs off on the reimbursement expected for each item. This strategy will save a major hassle later when down-coding or denials appear.

30. **Should doctors consult a lawyer before signing an MCO contract?**

Yes. Do not expect to understand the contract that is provided to you. Have an attorney, especially one well versed in health care law, review it, and point out the potential problems. Many physicians are reluctant to spend the money to do so, but this reluctance is shortsighted.

31. **Can doctors negotiate the terms of MCO contracts?**
Contracts are always up for discussion. Do not feel that you cannot negotiate for terms other than those initially provided.

32. **Does the physician have to be a good businessperson to survive in the managed care environment?**
Unfortunately, yes. Most physicians go to medical school to learn how to become a good doctor. They work hard during their residency and fellowship to learn as much internal medicine and then endocrinology as they can. Most likely, nothing is taught about practice management, contract negotiation skills, and cost-effective medical care. In addition, the traditional role of a physician as a healer of the sick without concern for compensation because doctors "always made a good living" is no longer applicable. It is becoming too expensive to run an office without being aware of the costs of every aspect of the practice, the revenue stream, and the "bottom line." Some doctors sell their practices in order not to deal with these problems, only to find out that working for a physician management company or a hospital that acquires practices, or very large groups creates an entirely different set of problems that they never expected.
To have a financially successful practice, the doctor must have a totally different attitude from that of physicians of a generation ago. The doctor has to view practice as a business, with the provision of health care as only one part of the practice. It takes time, effort, experiential learning, and even mistakes to be successful. Doctors have high intellectual abilities. They must apply these abilities to learning the business aspects of their practices. Combining a career in clinical endocrinology with a successful income stream is certainly possible and should be the goal of all practicing endocrinologists.

BIBLIOGRAPHY

1. Levy EG: On entering private practice: a personal perspective. A guide for the young endocrinologist about to embark on a career in private practice. Endocrinologist 9:119, 1999.
2. Levy EG: *Private practice—what you don't learn as a resident*, Endocrine Society Press, Chevy Chase, MD, 2007.

CHAPTER 60

SLEEP AND ENDOCRINOLOGY

Roger A. Piepenbrink, Brian T. Allenbrand, and William C. Frey

Sleep medicine is a relatively new frontier, especially when intersected with endocrinology. This chapter covers normal human sleep and endocrine system involvement, developing the endocrine aspects of sleep deprivation and obstructive sleep apnea. It focuses on the health consequences of disruptive sleep and the improvements that result from successfully treating sleep abnormalities.

1. **Do sleep disorders cause endocrine disease or does endocrine disease cause sleep disorders?**
   Sleep disorders are common in many endocrine conditions, and endocrine diseases can have associated sleep disorders. For example, acromegalic patients are at risk for sleep apnea. Excessive androgens can worsen obstructive sleep apnea (OSA), as can hypothyroidism. Thyrotoxicosis can contribute to insomnia. Disruptive sleep is now known to be associated with increased risk for diabetes and obesity.

2. **What are the stages of sleep?**
   Sleep is organized into non-rapid eye movement (NREM) sleep and rapid eye movement (REM) sleep (Table 60-1). In classic teaching, NREM was organized into four stages. Typically, adults enter sleep through Stage 1 which is characterized on electroencephalogram (EEG) by low

TABLE 60-1. COMPARISON OF SLEEP STAGES		
Characteristics	NREM	REM
Responsiveness to Stimuli	Reduced	Reduced to Absent
Sympathetic Activity	Reduced	Reduced or Variable
Parasympathetic Activity	Increased	Markedly Increased
Eye Movements	SEMs	REMs
Heart Rate	Bradycardia	Tachy/Brady
Respiratory Rate	Decreased	Variable; apneas can occur
Muscle Tone	Reduced	Markedly decreased
Upper Airway Muscle Tone	Reduced	Moderately decreased to absent
Cerebral Blood Flow	Reduced	Markedly Increased
Other Characteristics	Sleep Walks	Dreams
	Night Terrors	

Modified from: Chokroverty, S: Disorders of Sleep. In: NEUROLOGY Chapter XIII; American College of Physicians Medicine November 2006 WebMD Inc.
REMs, rapid eye movements; SEMs, slow eye movements.

amplitude mixed frequency waves. As one enters Stage 2, the EEG displays predominately sleep spindles, and K complexes. The 2007 American Academy of Sleep Medicine (AASM) Manual combines Stages 3 and 4 into one stage, N3, or slow wave sleep (SWS). In SWS, the EEG slows and is associated with a progressive increase in number of delta waves, which are characterized by increased amplitude and slowed frequency. It may take up to 100 minutes for first NREM sleep cycle to finish, but once completed, it heralds the first REM period. Although REM is not defined by characteristic EEG patterns, the EEG can look like that of Stage 1. The true hallmark of REM sleep, however, is rapid movement of the eyes in all directions compared to the slow eye movements (SEM) in Stage 1 sleep on the electrooculography (EOG). Also defining REM is muscle atonia, usually manifested in low electromyography (EMG) tone and absence of chin muscle movement. The only somatic muscles working in REM are the extraocular muscles and diaphragm!

3. **What is the progression of sleep stages in a usual night of sleep?**
    In the human, NREM and REM sleep typically alternate in 90 to 120 minute cycles (Fig. 60-1). Four to six cycles occur during a normal sleep period depending on the length of sleep. Each cycle is similar, with sleep onset initiating in Stage 1, progressing to Stage 2, then to SWS, and without significant arousal back to Stage 2. In a typical night of adult sleep, Stage 1 will comprise up to 5% of total sleep, Stage 2 up to 50%, SWS up to 20%, and REM up to 25%.

Figure 60-1. Stages of sleep. From Kales AM, Kales JD: Sleep disorders. N Engl J Med 1974; 290(9): 487-499. Used with permission, Copyright 1974 Massachusetts Medical Society. All rights reserved.

SWS is predominately experienced in the first third of sleep and REM in the last half of sleep. Achieving SWS has neuroendocrine significance.

4. **What are the fundamental changes in the nervous system in NREM versus REM sleep, and what other differences are noted between the phases of NREM and REM (See Table 60-1)?**
   Sleep is characterized by reversible unconsciousness and variable responsiveness to stimuli. There is a shift in the autonomic nervous system (ANS) in sleep, with parasympathetic nervous system (PNS) predominance in NREM and especially in REM. There is decrease in sympathetic nervous system (SNS) tone in NREM which is also usually the case in REM, but sympathetic tone in REM can be variable. In NREM, there are decreases in respiratory rate (RR), heart rate (HR), blood pressure (BP), and cardiac output. Normal REM is characterized by fluctuations in BP, HR, and RR. Dreaming and somatic muscle hypotonia to atonia (which includes reduced to absent upper airway muscle tone) are also REM events. REM can have a few periods of decreased or absent breathing. Cerebral metabolic rates for glucose and oxygen decrease during NREM but increase to above waking levels in REM.

5. **What are the two brain mechanisms responsible for anterior pituitary hormone cycling in a 24-hour period?**
   There are two separate but interrelated brain processes governing sleep and hormone release in a 24-hour period. The first process is the brain's master 24-hour clock, called Process-C, for circadian process. The other is sleep-wake homeostasis (SWH), also known as Process-S. SWH is dependent on Process-C but the circadian process in not dependent on SWH. Process-C is regulated in the hypothalamic suprachiasmatic nuclei (SCN). It receives a variety of input and works with the pineal gland melatonin from the pineal. Additionally, Process-C receives input from environmental cues, the strongest of which is light. The SCN uses autonomous, intrinsic electrical and molecular mechanisms to maintain a near 24-hour rhythm. The SWH process relates the amount and intensity of sleep to the duration of prior wakefulness. So, if one has 24 hours with no sleep, then there is increased pressure to sleep. The pressure to sleep is least when most rested. This pressure increases during the day and peaks just before midnight. The interaction of these two processes, Process-C and Process-S, influences the hypothalamic generators of releasing or inhibiting hormones that influence anterior pituitary function.

6. **How do the sleep stages change during one's life span?**
   As we age, total sleep time decreases and sleep begins to fragment (See Fig. 60-1). The time in sleep declines with age from 16 to 18 hours a day in a newborn to 9 to 10 hours in a 10 year old to 7 ½ to 8 hours in the average adult, to 6 hours in an 80 year old. A newborn's sleep is up to 50% REM sleep and declines to 25% of sleep by the time he/she is one year old (25% is usual REM percent for an adult). There is also a progressive decrease in SWS with aging. This loss of SWS also has endocrine repercussions since there is anterior pituitary hormone release associated with SWS. This fact challenges the assertion that hormone release is solely based on a feedback loop.

7. **Name the two hormones that are elevated early in sleep and the two hormones that are elevated late in sleep.**
   Recall that SWS predominates in the first third of sleep, and that REM predominates in the last half of sleep. Growth hormone (GH) and prolactin (PRL) are entrained to SWS (Table 60-2). The nighttime GH and PRL surges are associated with the first period of SWS. Females have a GH surge midday as well. The surge of PRL and GH is lost if the patient goes sleepless and returns if the patient gets recovery sleep. It is the onset of sleep and not the time of day that triggers the release of these hormones. The hormones that increase later in sleep are cortisol and testosterone. Testosterone rises just after midnight and cortisol begins its rise at 2 a.m., peaking between 6 and 9 am. The timing and amount of REM sleep are related to the late-sleep

TABLE 60-2. PRIMARY INFLUENCE ON 24 HOUR VARIATION		
Hormone	Sleep Wake Homeostasis	Circadian
GH	+++	+
PRL	+++	++
TSH	++	+++
Testosterone	−	+++
Cortisol	+	+++

rise of these two hormones in men. But the 24-hour rhythm for both testosterone and cortisol is primarily controlled by circadian rhythmicity (Process-C) and not sleep-wake homeostasis (Process-S).

8. **How do the gonadotropins levels vary with sleep?**
They vary with sleep according to gender and stage of maturity. Prior to puberty, there is daytime pulsatile gonadotropin release, which is augmented with sleep onset. One of the hallmarks of puberty for the child is increased nocturnal amplitude of LH and FSH. Both Process-S and Process-C contribute to this nocturnal surge in pubertal children. As the pubescent male enters adulthood, there is increased daytime LH as well, so the variation on a 24-hour cycle is less apparent. In adult men, LH has a low amplitude but testosterone is markedly increased. This suggests the SWH process is involved. Indeed, plasma levels of free testosterone are increased until the first REM occurs.

9. **Is the LH pattern the same in women?**
In women, plasma LH is significantly influenced by the menstrual cycle. There is, however, some modulation of LH levels, as the LH pulse frequency slows during sleep. In early follicular and early luteal phases, the amplitude of LH pulses actually increases. The frequency, however, decreases and the nocturnal LH pulse frequency slowing becomes evident. In mid and late follicular and luteal phases, this slowing is less apparent to absent. In the postmenopausal women there are elevated FSH and LH levels without circadian variation.

10. **Do the gonadal steroid hormones follow the LH and FSH changes mentioned in the question above?**
Gonadotropins have pulse amplitude and frequency, which are not reflected in the gonadal steroids (i.e., the gonadal steroids do not have pulsations). For pubertal girls, there is a daytime estradiol elevation. For pubescent boys, the testosterone increase coincides with elevation of the gonadotropins, as described, with minimal testosterone levels in the late evening and highest levels in early am. In post menopausal women, the gonadotropins increase in an attempt to stimulate estradiol production, and there is no consistent circadian gonadotropin pattern.

11. **What factors influence thyroid stimulating hormone (TSH) release?**
TSH release is primarily related to the circadian rhythm, though there is Process-S influence. TSH release in young healthy males shows a decline by late afternoon, an early evening circadian elevation, then a decline in levels shortly after sleep onset. The inhibitory influence of sleep on TSH is thought to be SWS, as it continues to chart a nocturnal decline to reach daytime values. With acute sleep loss, TSH takes its usual early evening upturn at approximately 6 pm, but then continues to rise to nearly twice normal maximum through the middle of the usual sleep period. The loss of inhibitory effect of sleep on the circadian TSH elevation may contribute to the elevated TSH values seen in acutely ill hospitalized patients.

12. **Since TSH and cortisol release are circadian, are their levels parallel through the night and day?**

TSH is influenced by Process-C and, to a lesser extent, influenced by the SWH process. Cortisol is primarily influenced by the circadian process with some influence from Process-S (see Table 60-2). So a change to one's sleep-wake cycle influences the release of these hormones but to different extents. In general, TSH fluctuations precede cortisol, with cortisol peaking later and staying up longer. TSH begins to rise under circadian rhythm, reaches maximum levels around mid-sleep (midnight to 2 a.m.), and nadirs 1.5 microIU/milliliter by mid-afternoon. TSH then levels off stopping a would-be ascent after sleep onset, reflecting sleep suppression of TSH. In a study of healthy young man during nocturnal sleep deprivation between 10 p.m. to 6 a.m. (SWS suppression removed) TSH more than doubled. That is, TSH went from its afternoon nadir of approximately 1.5 microIU/ml to a new peak of approximately 3.8 microIU/ml at 2 a.m. In the follow-on recovery sleep (10 a.m.– 6 p.m.) TSH returned to a mean of 1.25 microIU/ml. Cortisol, on the other hand, rises abruptly after midnight, peaks around 6-9 am, then declines throughout the day (reaching a nadir at midnight). It is well documented that interruptions to nocturnal sleep are associated with short-term TSH elevations. TSH levels normalize when normal nocturnal sleep is resumed. Repeated and prolonged nocturnal interruptions of sleep result in an elevation of cortisol.

13. **What changes in sleep will influence cortisol levels?**

Insomniacs, whose total time asleep/total time in bed is less than 70% of normal, have significantly higher evening and early sleep cortisol levels. In a study of young adults whose circadian rhythms were perturbed by a flight from Europe to US, GH secretory patterns adjusted within a few days to the new sleep-wake cycle but the cortisol levels remained disassociated for two weeks. This dissociation is thought to contribute to the symptoms of jet lag syndrome.

14. **How do circadian and sleep-wake processes influence glucose and insulin levels?**

Glucose and insulin levels are influenced by both processes. Studies in normal adults have demonstrated a 30% increase in glucose and a 60% increase in insulin levels during nocturnal sleep. In sleep deprivation, glucose and insulin secretion rates increase at habitual sleep time, though to a much lesser degree, suggesting circadian modulation. In recovery sleep, however, secretion of both insulin and glucose rates markedly increase, suggesting modulation by sleep itself.

15. **How does aging change hormonal release?**

Changes to sleep architecture with aging lead to hormonal change. Recall that GH and PRL rise primarily in relation to the SWS of NREM, whereas TSH, cortisol, and testosterone have increases that are primarily circadian. Since there is less SWS with aging (see Fig. 60-1), there are decreases in nocturnal GH and PRL secretion. In general, the extent of hormone release decreases from young to old. The extent of circadian changes in cortisol and TSH are less dramatic with aging. Day-night TSH fluctuations also dampen with age.

16. **What is the definition of sleep disordered breathing (SDB) and how does this differ from obstructive sleep apnea (OSA)?**

Confusion arises when the terms sleep related breathing disorders (SRBD), SDB, and OSA are used interchangeably in the literature and in sleep lab reports. SRBD and SDB are disease headings under which other diseases are arranged (much like COPD comprises a general reference for other specific disease entities). SRBD on the one hand contains for example adult and pediatric central apnea syndromes and obstructive sleep apnea syndromes. OSA on the other hand is a specific disorder that is diagnosed with polysomnography (PSG). It can be suspected on the basis of patient or bed partner complaints. Such complaints include: unintentional sleep episodes during wakefulness, daytime sleepiness, unrefreshing sleep, fatigue or insomnia, waking from sleep with breath holding, gasping or choking, loud snoring, and breathing interruptions. The PSG criteria are not as stringent if associated with patient or bed partner complaints. Accompanied by complaints, the PSG must have five or more respiratory events per hour of sleep associated with increased respiratory effort. Without a history of complaints, the PSG instead must contain 15 or more such respiratory events. In either case, rendering the diagnosis of OSA includes ruling out current medical, neurological, and/or substance abuse disorders. Of note, some prescribed medications can also increase risk for OSA.

17. What are respiratory events?

Respiratory events are apneas, hypopneas and respiratory effort-related arousals (RERA). An apneic episode is an airflow decrease of at least 90% from baseline which lasts at least 10 seconds (Try holding your own breath for 10 seconds!). Hypopnea is defined as 10 seconds of at least a 30% decrease in airflow which results in 4% or more of desaturation on pulse oximetry. On the other hand, RERA criteria should be sought if an observed event does not meet apnea or hypopnea criteria. RERA is defined as a sequence of breaths greater than 10 seconds in duration that is associated with increased respiratory effort and results in an arousal from sleep. AASM directs apneas, hyopopneas and RERAs, if present, to be scored in the routine PSG interpretation. The average number of apneas and hypopneas in one hour is referred to as the apnea-hypopnea index (AHI). But if RERAs are present then the average number of apneas, hyopopneas and RERAs should be calculated. This is called respiratory disturbance index (RDI). Note AHI does not equal RDI, but one does see these used interchangeably—such an interchange could create confusion.

18. What is the prevalence of OSA?

The prevalence is dependent on the definition of OSA. Earliest epidemiological investigations, primarily of white men, estimated that up to 4% had OSA (60-90% were obese). The classic prevalence of OSA for adults aged 30–60 is 24% in men and 9% in women. In non-obese patients, genetic craniofacial features like retrognathy are correlated with OSA. As OSA data matures, prevalence may become unique to populations or ethnicities. In Asian non-obese male office workers, BMI and age were positively correlated with OSA, but weight was less so than in white, non-Asian subjects. Risk factors for OSA other than adiposity, such as pharyngeal narrowing, retrognathia or micrognathia, and pharyngeal collapsibility, are thought to assume greater pathologic significance in Chinese subjects.

19. Define sleep deprivation. How common is it?

Sleep deprivation can be acute or chronic. By definition, going without sleep for 24 hours is acute sleep loss, whereas sleeping less than six hours a night for six nights or greater is considered chronic sleep deprivation. Patients in industrialized nations are sleeping less. In the United States, for example, over 30% of adults less than 64 years of age report sleeping less than six hours per night, leaving no doubt that many patients are accumulating chronic sleep deprivation.

20. What are the key features of sleep deprivation versus sleep apnea?

In sleep deprivation, one doesn't sleep but breaths normally. In OSA, one sleeps but doesn't breathe well during sleep. The AASM classifies volitional sleep deprivation as Behaviorally Induced Insufficient Sleep Syndrome as long as it is associated with daytime sleepiness. One can objectively measure excessive daytime sleepiness (EDS) with a standardized tool (Table 60-3), such as the Epworth Sleepiness Scale (ESS). An ESS score of greater than 9 is consistent with EDS. Patients with acute or chronic shortening of sleep resist the drive to sleep with no impairment of gas exchange. In OSA, there is a repetitive collapse of the upper airway, which induces apneic and hypopneic episodes despite persistent thoracic and abdominal respiratory effort. This leads to increased mechanical load on the upper airway, chest wall, and diaphragm. What follows are hypoxia, hypercarbia, and a marked increase in adrenergic tone. OSA often leads to a disruption or fragmentation of the usual sleep wake cycle and endocrine responsiveness. Both can contribute to fatigue and daytime sleepiness. If EDS is secondary to sleep deprivation, the

TABLE 60-3. EPWORTH SLEEPINESS SCALE

How likely are you to doze off or fall asleep in the following situations? This refers to your usual way of life in recent times. Use the following scale to choose the most appropriate number for each situation:
 	
0 = no chance of dozing
 	
1 = slight chance of dozing
 	
2 = moderate chance of dozing
 	
3 = high chance of dozing
 	
Situation
 	
Sitting and reading
 	
Watching TV
 	
Sitting inactive in a public place (e.g a theater or a meeting)
 	
As a passenger in a car for an hour without a break
 	
Lying down to rest in the afternoon when circumstances permit
 	
Sitting and talking to someone
 	
Sitting quietly after a lunch without alcohol
 	
In a car while stopped for a few minutes in traffic
 	
Interpretation is the sum of scores assigned to each situation
 	
   ■ 0–6 you are getting sufficient sleep
 	
   ■ 6–8 average score, normal population
 	
   ■ >9 seek medical advice
 	
The Epworth Sleepiness Scale has been validated primarily in obstructive sleep apnea. It is used to measure excessive daytime sleepiness, and is repeated after the administration of treatment (e.g. CPAP) to document improvement of symptoms.

patient's sleep continuity is normal and is often associated with an increase in SWS. Recall the inhibitory influence of daytime recovery sleep (TDRS) on TSH, which occurred if TDRS followed nocturnal sleep deprivation (see question 12).

21. **In view of increased SNS tone in OSA, (see question 4), does the co-morbidity of OSA interfere with the assessment of metanephrines and catecholamines when screening for pheochromocytoma?**
Yes. OSA results in an appropriate release of catecholamines in response to physiologic stress or disease, just as a myocardial infarctions, cerebral vascular accidents, and acute heart failure are associated with appropriate catecholamine increases. If a 24-hour urinary collection is performed in the setting of undiagnosed or poorly treated OSA, it would likely contain elevated levels of metanephrines and catecholamines. This may falsely suggest a diagnosis of pheochromocytoma.

22. **What endocrine diseases are associated with OSA?**
The most common diseases are hypothyroidism, acromegaly and polycystic ovary syndrome (PCOS). Although it was once thought that all OSA patients have subclinical hypothyroidism, this

has now been shown not to be the case. Evidence in the past four years suggests that the prevalence of OSA in hypothyroid patients is about 30%. OSA is reversible in the majority of such patients once they are treated appropriately with thyroid hormone replacement. In one prospective study of nonobese, middle-aged men and women with newly-diagnosed symptomatic hypothyroidism, 30% had OSA by PSG at study onset. Eight-four percent of these subjects had reversal of OSA with normalization of TSH. Finally, insulin levels and measures of glucose tolerance in PCOS were strongly correlated with the risk and severity of OSA. Additionally, among those PCOS women with normal glucose tolerance, insulin levels were significantly higher in those at high versus low OSA risk, independent of body mass index.

23. **How is the sleep apnea of GH excess different from the sleep apnea of thyroid hormone deficiency?**
GH excess is associated with a high proportion of central sleep apnea, while hypothyroidism is almost uniformly associated with obstructive sleep apnea. Up to 60% of acromegalics are eventually found to have sleep apnea by PSG studies. In one series, over 30% had central sleep apnea. This is not from macroglossia, as endoscopy revealed little occlusive posterior tongue movement during sleep. This assertion is further supported by the observation that these patients have lower arterial carbon dioxide levels while awake and have increased ventilatory responsiveness when compared to those with OSA. The mechanism for central sleep apnea in these patients is not clear.

24. **How does sleep deprivation influence glucose tolerance?**
In one study, after one week of sleeping 4 hour per night, there were increases in post-breakfast insulin resistance. During sleep restriction, glucose tolerance is nearly 40% worse than when compared to a group with sleep extension. Interestingly, it was the first phase of insulin release that was found to be markedly reduced. When the sleep deprived individuals go into recovery sleep (sleeping during the day due to their sleep deprivation), there are marked elevations of glucose and insulin levels, indicating that sleep also exerts modulatory influences on glucose regulation independent of the circadian rhythm.

25. **What is the evidence linking OSA to abnormal glucose metabolism?**
Snoring, sleep deprivation, and OSA have all been linked to type 2 diabetes mellitus (DM2) risk. Data gathered from diverse patient populations suggest that OSA severity is a risk for DM2 development. At present, available data does not definitively prove direct causation. Snoring, in the nonobese Asian and especially in the obese, has been independently associated with abnormal oral glucose tolerance tests and higher HbA1c percentages. In epidemiologic studies, sleep quality has been positively correlated with the risk of developing DM2. Observational studies have shown that patients who report less than 6 hours of sleep per night have an increased prevalence of glucose intolerance and DM2. Very recently, it was found that the duration of sleep (<6 and >8 hours per night) was predictive of an increased incidence of DM2. OSA, as diagnosed by PSG, is independently associated with abnormal glucose metabolism. Another recent paper extends this independent association through rigorous assessment of the potential confounders of overweight/obesity. In this cross-sectional analysis of 2,588 patients, it was shown that impaired fasting glucose (IFG), impaired glucose tolerance (IGT), and occult diabetes are associated (but to different degrees) with OSA in both the normal-weight (BMI < 25 kg/m^2) and overweight/obese subgroups. This suggests that individuals with OSA are at special risk for diabetes and its cardiovascular complications.

26. **What are the two main mechanisms underlying the development abnormal glucose metabolism in sleep apnea patients?**
The hallmark of OSA is airflow reduction, which is typically associated with intermittent hypoxemia and sleep fragmentation. In animal studies, insulin sensitivity has been shown to vary with intermittent hypoxemia, independent of activation of the SNS. Additionally, it has been

shown that in the non-diabetic overweight to mildly obese male, every 4% decrease in oxygen saturation is associated with an odds ratio that approaches 2 for worsened glucose tolerance. Sleep fragmentation has also been associated with abnormal glucose metabolism. In one study of healthy adults, selective suppression of SWS (without decreasing total sleep time) was associated with decreases in insulin sensitivity by nearly 25%. This suggests the low levels of SWS in the elderly and obese may contribute to the increased incidence of DM2.

27. **With respect to causality, does the use of CPAP improve abnormal glucose metabolism?**
Yes. Trials reporting CPAP adherence definitions and the trials demonstrating no change in BMI during the study period do show improvement. A study of nondiabetic patients with moderate to severe OSA reported that CPAP significantly improved insulin sensitivity after only 2 days of treatment and that the improvement persisted at the three-month follow-up with no significant changes in body weight. Interestingly, this influence was most pronounced in the non-obese population. In contrast, this same lab showed no improvement in insulin sensitivity in the obese DM2 patients.

28. **Does the effective use of CPAP in the OSA patient lead to weight loss?**
Yes it does apparently working through two distinct mechanisms. First, the patient with treated sleep apnea usually wakes more rested and with a sense of improved vitality or energy. Once on treatment, patients with treated OSA have even been shown to exercise more. Secondly, treatment of sleep apnea results in normalization of leptin, the so-called satiety hormone. As will be elaborated below, leptin is suppressed during sleep deprivation and untreated sleep apnea.

29. **What are the effects of sleep deprivation on leptin (the satiety hormone) and ghrelin (hunger hormone)?**
With sleep deprivation, leptin (from the Greek word *leptos*, meaning "thin") decreases and ghrelin (from the original root *ghre* meaning "to grow") increases. In longer than average sleep, leptin increases and ghrelin decreases. It has been documented that leptin release is blunted in the sleep deprived patient such that over a six month period of time the patient with sleep deprivation gains an average of 10 pounds more than rested patients.

30. **Is the testosterone decline observed with aging related to the changes associated with sleep pattern of aging?**
As discussed previously, aging is associated with less time in sleep and less time in slow wave sleep. In older men, the amplitude of LH pulses are less but the frequency is increased. The sleep-related rise of testosterone is still seen, though the amplitude is less. The rise of nocturnal testosterone leading up to the first REM, however, is no longer seen in the elderly patient. Furthermore, the relationship of LH levels with latency to the first REM period is less prominent with aging.

31. **How does androgen influence sleep?**
Exogenous testosterone may worsen existing OSA or lead to changes associated with sleep apnea. One randomized controlled trial revealed that high dose testosterone administration in hypogonadal, otherwise healthy, elderly men shortened total sleep time and worsened coexisting undiagnosed sleep apnea. Though there have been no substantiated reports of decreased cognition and impaired driving ability with hypogonadism, it is incumbent on the prescriber to screen the patient for the possibility of undiagnosed OSA.

32. **How does the testosterone panel change with OSA and does OSA treatment influence the panel?**
The androgen changes of OSA are distinct from those seen in aging and obesity (Table 60-4). In OSA, there are decreases in the sex hormone binding globulin and free and total testosterone

TABLE 60-4. ANDROGEN CHANGES IN COMMON CIRCUMSTANCES			
Condition	SHBG	Total Testosterone	Free Testosterone
Aging	↑	↓	↓
Obesity	↓	↓	normal
OSA	↓	↓	↓

without concomitant increases in gonadotropins. In fact, one study showed LH pulse disturbances with untreated OSA. Interestingly, testosterone levels improve with OSA treatment, whether by CPAP or with UPPP. These findings point to a hypothalamic abnormality related to the low testosterone levels of untreated OSA.

33. **How well are providers in diabetes clinics screening their patients for OSA? What are good tools for screening historically and on physical exam?**
A study of diabetic patients, using a validated clinical measurement and questionnaire to quantify OSA risk and sleepiness, revealed that 56% of patients reported snoring, 29% had fatigue upon awakening, and 34% reported feeling tired during wake time. The authors of the study concluded that 56% of those questioned were at high risk of OSA. This finding supports a call for greater vigilance in screening for OSA in diabetics given the high prevalence of SDB found in that patient population. Certain screening tools may be helpful towards this end. BMI is proportional to OSA, and neck size greater than 17 inches is the most sensitive physical finding. Some craniofacial changes, such as retrognathia, also place a patient at high-risk. Keep in mind that a patient with OSA is often unaware of the neurocognitive changes that have developed slowly over time, and thus he or she may not volunteer history consistent with OSA unless directly queried.

KEY POINTS: SLEEP AND ENDOCRINOLOGY

1. Endocrine diseases associated with abnormal sleep include acromegaly, hyperthyroidism, hypothyroidism, and polycystic ovarian syndrome.

2. Normal sleep preserves normal 24-hour hormone cycling. Sleep deprivation and obstructive sleep apnea can impair hormone cycling.

3. Mechanisms responsible for 24-hour hormone cycling are circadian, sleep-wake homeostatic, or both. These sleep mechanisms are distinct and superimposed on classic feedback loop mechanisms responsible for hormone levels.

4. Sleep architecture changes with aging include less total sleep time and less SWS.

5. OSA requires PSG for diagnosis.

6. Acute sleep loss eliminates the nocturnal TSH suppression.

7. Sleep deprivation disrupts SWS which is associated with decreases in hormone levels entrained to SWS (GH and PRL).

8. Short-term sleep deprivation increases cortisol levels, suppresses insulin secretion and diminishes glucose tolerance. Leptin increases and ghrelin decreases and such patients gain weight compared to non sleep deprived patients.

9. OSA results in less predictable hormone changes depending on the extent of sleep fragmentation, elevation of adrenergic tone, and hypoxia. It is associated with decreased insulin sensitivity and worsening glucose tolerance proportional to severity of OSA.

10. Effective treatment of OSA improves sleep architecture, normalizes hormone release, improves abnormal glucose metabolism.

WEBSITES

1. Sleep Research Society
   http://www.sleepresearchsociety.org/

2. NIH, NHLBI, National Center on Sleep Disorders Research
   http://www.nhlbi.nih.gov/about/ncsdr/index.htm

3. American Academy of Sleep Medicine
   http://www.aasmnet.org

BIBLIOGRAPHY

1. Aurora RN, Punjabi, NM: Sleep apnea and metabolic dysfunction: cause or correlation? Sleep Medicine Clinic 2:237–250, 2007.

2. Chokroverty, S: Disorders of Sleep. In: NEUROLOGY Chapter XIII; American College of Physicians Medicine. November 2006 WebMD Inc.

3. Grunstein, R. Chapter 105: Endocrine Disorders. In: Kryger, MH et al: Principles and Practice of Sleep Medicine, 4th edition. Elsevier Saunders. 2005.

4. Iber C, et al: The American Academy of Sleep Medicine Manual for the Scoring of Sleep and Associated Events: Rules, Terminology and Technical Specifications, 1st ed. Westchester, Illinois: American Academy of Sleep Medicine, 2007.

5. Ip MS, et al: A community study of sleep disordered breathing in middle-aged Chinese men in Hong Kong. Chest 119: 62–69, 2001.

6. Jha A, Surendra KS, et al: Thyroxine replacement therapy reverses sleep disordered breathing patients with primary hypothyroidism. Sleep Medicine 7:55–61, 2006.

7. Jun J, Polotsky VY: Sleep disordered breathing and metabolic effects: evidence from animal models. Sleep Medicine Clinic 2:263–277, 2007.

8. Kales A, Kales JD: Sleep disorders: Recent findings in the diagnosis and treatment of disturbed sleep. N Engl J Med 290 (9):487–499, 1974.

9. Kelly E, et al: Are we missing OSAS in the diabetic clinic? European Journal of Internal Medicine 19 e13, 2008.

10. Knutson KL, et al: The metabolic consequences of sleep deprivation. Sleep Medicine Reviews 11:163–178, 2007.

11. Liu PY, et al: Androgens, obesity and sleep-disordered breathing in men. Endocrinology and Metabolism Clinics of North America 36:349–363, 2007.

12. Punjabi NM, et al: Sleep-disordered breathing and insulin resistance in middle-aged and overweight men. Am J Respir Crit Care Med 165:677–682, 2002.

13. Seicean S, et al: Sleep disordered breathing and impaired glucose metabolism in normal-weight and overweight/obese individuals: The Sleep Heart Health Study. Diabetes Care 31(5):1001–1006, 2008.

14. Spiegel K, Leproult R, et al: Leptin levels are dependent on sleep duration: relationships of sympathovagal balance, carbohydrate regulation, cortisol, and thyrotropin. JCEM 89:5762–5771, 2004.

15. Spiegel K, et al: Impact of sleep debt on metabolic and endocrine function. The Lancet 354:1435–1439, 1999.

16. Tasali E, et al: Obstructive Sleep Apnea and Type 2 Diabetes: Interacting Epidemics. Chest 133:496–506, 2008.

17. Tasali E, et al: Slow wave sleep and the risk of type 2 diabetes in humans. Proceedings of the National Academy of Science USA 105(3):1044–1049, 2008.

18. Tasali E, et al: Relationships between sleep disordered breathing in glucose metabolism in polycystic ovarian syndrome. JCEM 91(1):36–42, 2006.

19. Tuomilehto H, et al: Sleep duration is associated with an increased risk for prevalence of type 2 diabetes in middle-aged women–The FIN-D2D survey. Sleep Medicine 9:221–227, 2008.

20. Young WF, Jr: Chapter 15 Endocrine Hypertension. In: Kronenberg HM, et al (ed) Williams Textbook of Endocrinology 11th edition Saunders, 2008.

21. Zee PC, Manthena, P: The brain's master circadian clock: implications and opportunity for therapy of sleep disorders. Sleep Medicine Reviews 11:59–70, 2007.

CHAPTER 61

ENDOCRINE CASE STUDIES

Michael T. McDermott

1. **A 34-year-old woman has new-onset hypertension. Her serum potassium level is 2.7 mEq/L. Initial hormone screening shows a plasma aldosterone (PA) of 55 ng/dL (normal (nl), 1–16) and a plasma renin (PR) of 0.1 ng/mL/h (nl, 0.15–2.33). Subsequent testing reveals a PA after a 2 liter saline infusion of 54 ng/dL (nl, 1–8). What is the probable diagnosis?**
The presence of hypertension and hypokalemia suggests primary aldosteronism (Conn's syndrome). The PA level is elevated, the PR is suppressed, and the PA/PR ratio is greater than 20, supporting this diagnosis. It is confirmed by the failure of PA to suppress after volume expansion with saline. The next step is to determine whether the cause is an aldosterone-producing adenoma or bilateral adrenal hyperplasia. An abdominal computed tomography (CT) scan should be performed next. Because of her young age and very low serum potassium level, an aldosterone producing adrenal adenoma is the most likely cause. The treatment for an aldosterone-producing adrenal adenoma is surgery. Spironolactone should be given to control blood pressure and to normalize the serum potassium preoperatively (see Chapter 27).

2. **A 32-year-old business executive develops amenorrhea. She has not recently lost weight but states that her job is very stressful. Evaluation reveals the following laboratory results: serum estradiol = 14 pg/mL (nl, 23–145), luteinizing hormone (LH) = 1.2 mLU/mL (nl, 2–15), follicle-stimulating hormone (FSH) = 1.5 mIU/mL (nl, 2–20), prolactin = 6.2 ng/mL (nl, 2–25), thyroid-stimulating hormone (TSH) = 1.2 mU/L (nl, 0.5–5.0), and a serum pregnancy test is negative. A magnetic resonance imaging (MRI) scan of her pituitary gland is normal. What is the probable diagnosis?**
The patient has secondary amenorrhea with low levels of estradiol and gonadotropins. This clinical picture is most consistent with hypothalamic amenorrhea, which sometimes occurs in women who exercise excessively or who have stressful jobs. The disorder results from reduced frequency of gonadotropin-releasing hormone (GnRH) pulses in the hypothalamus. Treatment consists of stress management and, if menses do not resume, estrogen replacement therapy (see Chapter 47).

3. **A nulliparous 48-year-old woman presents with symptoms of thyrotoxicosis. She has a modest, nontender goiter and no exophthalmos. She takes no medications and has had no recent radiology procedures. The following results are found on thyroid evaluation: free T_4 = 3.5 ng/dL (nl, 0.7–2.7), TSH <0.1 mU/L, 24-hour radioactive iodine uptake (RAIU) = 1% (nl, 20%–35%), thyroglobulin = 35 ng/mL (nl, 2–20), and sedimentation rate = 10 mm/h. What is the likely diagnosis?**
The patient has clinical and biochemical thyrotoxicosis, but the RAIU is low. The differential diagnosis includes postpartum thyroiditis, silent thyroiditis, subacute thyroiditis, factitious thyrotoxicosis, and iodine-induced thyrotoxicosis. She has never been pregnant and denies medication use and recent iodine exposure. The nontender gland, elevated thyroglobulin, and normal sedimentation rate are most consistent with silent thyroiditis. A transient (1–3 months)

thyrotoxic phase followed by a transient (1–3 months) hypothyroid phase is expected before the condition resolves; 20% of patients, however, remain hypothyroid. If symptomatic, the thyrotoxic phase is best treated with beta-blockers, and the hypothyroid phase can be managed, if necessary, with levothyroxine (see Chapters 33 and 35).

4. **A 38-year-old man has coronary artery disease, xanthomas of the Achilles tendons, and the following serum lipid profile: cholesterol = 482 mg/dL, triglycerides (TG) = 152 mg/dL, high-density lipoprotein (HDL) cholesterol = 42 mg/dL, and low-density lipoprotein (LDL) cholesterol = 410 mg/dL. What is the probable diagnosis?**
Significant elevations of total cholesterol and LDL cholesterol, normal TG, tendon xanthomas, and premature coronary artery disease are most consistent with a diagnosis of heterozygous familial hypercholesterolemia. This disorder is usually due to deficient or abnormal LDL receptors or an abnormal apoprotein B-100 molecule. Aggressive lipid lowering with combinations of statins, ezetimibe, bile acid resins, niacin, and occasionally plasmapheresis or LDI pheresis, is indicated (see Chapter 6).

5. **A 28-year-old man presents because of infertility. He is found to have small, firm testes and gynecomastia. Laboratory testing shows the following abnormalities: testosterone = 260 ng/dL (nl, 300–1000), LH = 88 mIU/mL (nl, 2–12), and FSH = 95 mIU/mL (nl, 2–12). What is the likely diagnosis?**
The patient has hypergonadotropic hypogonadism with small firm testes and gynecomastia, which is most consistent with a diagnosis of Klinefelter's syndrome. Such patients usually have a 47XXY karyotype. Androgen replacement therapy is the treatment of choice (see Chapter 44).

6. **A 38-year-old nurse presents in a stuporous state; the blood glucose level is 14 mg/dL. Additional blood is drawn, and the patient is quickly resuscitated with intravenous glucose. Further testing on the saved serum reveals the following: serum insulin = 45 mU/mL (normal <22), C-peptide = 4.2 ng/mL (nl, 0.5–2.0), and proinsulin = 0.6 ng/mL (nl, 0–0.2). A sulfonylurea screen is negative. What is the probable diagnosis?**
The patient has hyperinsulinemic hypoglycemia. The differential diagnosis includes insulinoma, surreptitious insulin injection, and oral sulfonylurea ingestion. The elevated serum C-peptide and proinsulin levels are most consistent with an insulinoma. After an appropriate localizing procedure, surgical removal is the treatment of choice (see Chapter 54).

7. **A 28-year-old woman with type 1 diabetes develops amenorrhea. Further testing reveals the following serum hormone values: estradiol = 15 pg/mL (nl, 23–145), LH = 78 mIU/mL (nl, 2–15), FSH = 92 mIU/mL (nl, 2–20), prolactin = 12 ng/mL (nl, 2–25), TSH = 1.1 mU/L; a pregnancy test is negative. What is the most likely diagnosis?**
The patient has secondary amenorrhea with low levels of estradiol and elevated gonadotropins. The differential diagnosis includes premature ovarian failure and the resistant ovary syndrome. In a patient with another autoimmune disease (type 1 diabetes mellitus), the most likely diagnosis is premature ovarian failure. Hormone replacement therapy is the treatment of choice (see Chapter 47).

8. **A 34-year-old woman presents with galactorrhea, amenorrhea, headaches, fatigue, and weight gain. Laboratory evaluation reveals the following: prolactin = 58 ng/mL (nl, 2–25), free T_4 = 0.2 ng/dL (nl, 4.5–12), and TSH >60 mU/L (nl, 0.5–5.0). She has an enlarged pituitary gland on MRI scan. What is the probable diagnosis?**
The patient has moderately increased serum prolactin levels, pituitary enlargement, and severe primary hypothyroidism. Her entire clinical picture is most likely explained solely by the

hypothyroidism, which is well known to cause secondary hypersecretion of prolactin and pituitary enlargement due to thyrotroph hyperplasia. All abnormalities should resolve after adequate thyroid hormone replacement is established (see Chapters 20 and 48).

9. **A 6-year-old girl has recently developed breast enlargement and some pubic hair. She has not complained of headaches and has had good health otherwise. Her older sister entered puberty at approximately 8 years of age. Her height is at the 90th percentile for her age, and her physical examination reveals Tanner stage III breast development and stage II pubic hair growth. Abdominal and pelvic examinations are normal. Laboratory tests show the following results: LH = 7 mIU/mL (nl, 2–15), FSH = 8 mIU/mL (nl, 2–20), prolactin = 6 ng/mL (nl, 2–25), TSH = 1.9 mU/L (nl, 0.5–5.0), and a normal pituitary MRI scan. Her bone age is 1.8 years ahead of the chronologic age. What is the probable diagnosis?**
The patient has gonadotropin-dependent true precocious puberty. The etiology includes pituitary and hypothalamic tumors, but most cases in girls are idiopathic. The normal pituitary MRI points to a diagnosis of idiopathic precocious puberty. A long-acting GnRH analog should successfully arrest her premature development and allow her to enter puberty at a later, more appropriate time (see Chapter 43).

10. **A 19-year-old man presents with excessive thirst and urination. Laboratory evaluation shows the following: serum glucose = 88 mg/dL, serum sodium = 146 mEq/L, serum osmolality = 298 mOsm/kg, and urine volume = 8800 mL/24 h. A water deprivation test is performed, and it shows a urine osmolality of 90 mOsm/kg with no response to water deprivation and an increase in urine osmolality to 180 mOsm/kg after the administration of vasopressin. What is the likely diagnosis?**
The patient has polyuria and polydipsia with maximally dilute urine. The differential diagnosis includes central diabetes insipidus, nephrogenic diabetes insipidus, and primary polydipsia. The lack of response to water deprivation and the more than 50% increase in urine osmolality after administration of vasopressin are most consistent with central diabetes insipidus. This may be caused by inflammatory or mass lesions in the hypothalamus but is often idiopathic. An MRI of the pituitary-hypothalamic region should be performed. The treatment of choice is intranasal or oral desmopressin (see Chapters 18 and 24).

11. **A 25-year-old woman presents with a cushingoid appearance. The results of hormone testing are as follows: 24-hour urine cortisol = 318 μg (nl, 20–90), morning serum cortisol = 28 μg/dL (nl, 5–25), and morning plasma adrenocorticotropic hormone (ACTH) = 65 pg/mL (nl, 10–80). After an 8-mg oral bedtime dose of dexamethasone, the morning serum cortisol = 3 μg/dL. What is the probable diagnosis?**
Cushingoid features and elevated urinary excretion of cortisol confirm the diagnosis of Cushing's syndrome. The cause is usually an ACTH-secreting pituitary adenoma (65%–80%), ectopic production of ACTH (10%–15%), or a cortisol-producing adrenal adenoma (10%–15%). The normal plasma level of ACTH, which is inappropriate for the elevated serum cortisol level, and suppression of serum cortisol with high-dose dexamethasone are most consistent with a pituitary adenoma (Cushing's disease). This should be confirmed with an MRI of the pituitary gland and possibly inferior petrosal sinus sampling. Transsphenoidal surgical removal is the treatment of choice (see Chapter 23).

12. **An 8-year-old boy with known adrenal insufficiency complains of paresthesias of the lips, hands, and feet and intermittent muscle cramps. He has a positive Chvostek's and Trousseau's sign on examination. Results of blood testing are as follows: calcium = 6.2 mg/dL (nl, 8.5–10.2), phosphorous = 5.8 mg/dL (nl, 2.5–4.5), intact parathyroid hormone (PTH) = 6 pg/mL (nl, 10–65), and 25-hydroxyvitamin D = 42 ng/mL (nl, 30–100). What is the most likely diagnosis?**
    Hypocalcemia, hyperphosphatemia, and a low serum PTH level are diagnostic of primary hypoparathyroidism. This disorder, which is often autoimmune in nature, may occur in association with adrenal insufficiency as part of the autoimmune polyendocrine syndrome type I (APS I). The treatment of this condition is calcium supplementation along with calcitriol administration. Calcitriol is necessary because the lack of PTH makes these patients unable to convert 25 hydroxyvitamin D into 1,25 dihydroxyvitamin D in the kidneys, and the latter vitamin D metabolite is necessary for normal intestinal calcium absorption (see Chapters 16 and 53).

13. **A 52-year-old man has a personal and family history of early coronary artery disease, minimal alcohol consumption, and no xanthomas on examination. He has the following results on serum testing: cholesterol = 328 mg/dL, TG = 322 mg/dL, HDL = 35 mg/dL, LDL = 229 mg/dL, apoprotein B = 178 mg/dL (nl, 60–130), apoprotein E phenotype = E3/E3, TSH = 2.1 mU/L (nl, 0.1–4.5), and glucose = 85 mg/dL. What is the probable diagnosis?**
    The patient has elevations of both serum cholesterol and TG and no detected disorders that cause secondary dyslipidemia. The differential diagnosis includes familial combined hyperlipidemia and familial dysbetalipoproteinemia. The elevated level of apoprotein B and the normal apoprotein E phenotype are most consistent with familial combined hyperlipidemia. The top treatment priority is LDL reduction with a statin. After LDL cholesterol is under the National Cholesterol Education Program (NCEP) goal, persistent TG elevations should be addressed with the possible addition of a fibrate, niacin, or fish oils (see Chapter 6).

14. **A 58-year-old man has recently developed diabetes mellitus, weight loss, and a skin rash that is most prominent on the buttocks; a dermatologist diagnoses this as necrolytic migratory erythema. What is the probable underlying diagnosis?**
    Diabetes mellitus, weight loss, and necrolytic migratory erythema are virtually diagnostic of a glucagon-secreting pancreatic endocrine tumor (glucagonoma). The diagnosis can be confirmed by finding an elevated serum level of glucagon. After appropriate localizing procedures, surgery is the treatment of choice, if possible. Chemotherapy should be considered for unresectable malignant tumors or tumor remnants (see Chapter 54).

15. **A 29-year-old woman has asymptomatic hypercalcemia. Her mother and a sister also have hypercalcemia and have had failed neck explorations for presumed parathyroid tumors. Further testing results: serum calcium = 11.0 mg/dL (nl, 8.5–10.2), phosphorous = 3.0 mg/dL (nl, 2.4–4.5), creatinine = 0.9 mg/dL, intact PTH = 66 pg/mL (nl, 10–65), 25-hydroxyvitamin D = 42 ng/mL (nl, 30–100), 24-hour urine calcium = 13 mg (nl, 100–300), and creatinine =1100 mg. What is the probable diagnosis?**
    The vast majority of patients with hypercalcemia and a mildly elevated serum PTH level have hyperparathyroidism. However, in this case, the very low urinary calcium excretion and family history of unsuccessful parathyroidectomies point to a likely diagnosis of familial hypocalciuric hypercalcemia. The diagnosis is confirmed by finding a calcium/creatinine clearance ratio (urine calcium × serum creatinine/serum calcium × urine creatinine) of less than 0.01. This autosomal dominant disorder results from a heterozygous inactivating mutation in the gene that encodes the calcium receptor. The mutant receptors, present in parathyroid and renal tubular cells, have

a raised threshold for calcium recognition. The result is a physiological equilibrium, in which hypercalcemia coexists with mild elevations of PTH and low urinary calcium excretion. The disorder causes no morbidity and does not require treatment (see Chapters 13 and 14).

16. **A 39-year-old HIV-positive man with *Pneumocystis carinii* pneumonia has the following serum thyroid hormone values: $T_4 = 4.0$ mg/dL (nl, 4.5–12.0), $T_3 = 22$ ng/dL (nl, 90–200), T_3 resin uptake $= 48\%$ (nl, 35%–45%), and TSH $= 1.3$ mU/L (nl, 0.5–5.0). What is the most likely endocrine diagnosis?**
   The very low T_3, mildly low T_4, elevated T_3 resin uptake, and normal TSH are most consistent with the euthyroid sick syndrome. This is not a primary thyroid disorder but is instead a set of circulating thyroid hormone abnormalities that occur in the presence of nonthyroidal illnesses; it corrects when the underlying illness resolves. Treatment of the condition with thyroid hormone administration is not currently recommended, although this remains controversial (see Chapter 39).

17. **An 18-year-old girl has not yet begun menstruating. She has a height of 56 inches, a small uterus, and no breast development. The results of hormone tests are as follows: estradiol $= 8$ pg/mL (nl, 23–145), LH $= 105$ mIU/mL (nl, 2–15), FSH $= 120$ mIU/mL (nl, 2–20), prolactin $= 14$ ng/mL (nl, 2–15), and TSH $= 1.8$ mU/L (nl, 0.5–5.0). What is the probable diagnosis?**
   Primary amenorrhea, short stature, a low serum estradiol level, and elevated gonadotropins are most consistent with a diagnosis of Turner's syndrome. This disorder, characterized by ovarian dysgenesis, is associated with a 45XO karyotype. These patients should be given hormone replacement therapy with estrogen and progesterone. Growth hormone (GH) therapy should be considered because it has been shown to improve longitudinal growth and final height (see Chapter 47).

18. **A 62-year-old woman presents for evaluation of recent nephrolithiasis and low back pain. Her estimated calcium intake is 800 mg/day, and she takes no vitamins. Her physical examination is unremarkable. Spinal x-rays reveal osteopenia and a compression fracture the second lumbar vertebra (L2). Laboratory evaluation shows the following: serum calcium $= 13.0$ mg/dL (nl, 8.5–10.5), phosphorus $= 2.3$ mg/dL (nl, 2.5–4.5), albumin $= 4.4$ g/dL (nl, 3.2–5.5), intact PTH $= 72$ pg/mL (nl, 11–54), and 24-hour urine calcium $= 312$ mg (nl, 100–300). What is the most likely diagnosis?**
   Hypercalcemia, hypophosphatemia, and elevated serum PTH levels are characteristic of primary hyperparathyroidism. The only other cause of hypercalcemia with increased serum PTH levels is familial hypocalciuric hypercalcemia. Hyperparathyroidism is usually due to a solitary parathyroid adenoma, but familial cases and those associated with multiple endocrine neoplasia (MEN) syndromes more often have four-gland hyperplasia. Surgical indications include serum calcium levels greater than 1 mg/dL above the normal range, urine calcium greater than 400 mg/ 24 h, kidney stones, renal impairment, osteoporosis, or symptoms related to hyperparathyroidism. Observation alone or bisphosphonate therapy may be appropriate for patients with mild, asymptomatic disease or only mild bone loss (see Chapter 14).

19. **A 32-year-old woman presents with the recent onset of fatigue, palpitations, profuse sweating, and emotional lability. She gave birth to her second child 8 weeks ago. Her pulse is 100/min, and she has mild lid retraction, a fine hand tremor, and a slightly enlarged, nontender thyroid gland. She is not breast feeding her child. Laboratory tests are as follows: TSH <0.03 mU/L (nl, 0.5–5.0), free $T_4 = 3.8$ ng/dL (nl, 0.7–2.7), and RAIU is $<1\%$ at 4 and 24 hours. What is the probable diagnosis?**
   Postpartum thyrotoxicosis is most often due to Graves' disease or postpartum thyroiditis. The RAIU will distinguish the two, being high in Graves' disease and very low in postpartum

thyroiditis. This patient has postpartum thyroiditis, a condition caused by lymphocytic inflammation with leakage of thyroid hormone from the inflamed gland. There is often a thyrotoxic phase (lasting 1–3 months) followed by a hypothyroid phase (lasting 1–3 months) and eventual return to euthyroidism, although nearly 20% remain permanently hypothyroid. Treatment consists of beta-blockers, if necessary, for symptom control in the thyrotoxic phase, and levothyroxine, if necessary, for symptom control in the hypothyroid phase and for those who remain permanently hypothyroid (see Chapters 33 and 35).

20. **A 70-year-old man complains of a 1-year history of weakness, weight loss, and hand tremors. He has been treated with amiodarone for nearly 3 years for a diagnosis of paroxysmal atrial flutter. Laboratory tests show the following: TSH <0.01 mU/L (nl, 0.5–5.0), free T_4 = 3.35 ng/dL (nl, 0.7–2.7), and the RAIU was 2.7% at 6 hours and 4.1% at 24 hours. Thyroid scan showed scant patchy tracer uptake. What is the likely diagnosis?**
This man most likely has amiodarone-induced thyrotoxicosis (AIT). This condition occurs in up to 10% of patients using amiodarone, which has very high iodine content. There are two subtypes: type 1 AIT results from iodine overload and occurs mainly in patients with underlying goiters; type 2 AIT results from drug-induced thyroid follicular damage. Both are associated with a low RAIU. There are no tests to distinguish the two subtypes reliably, although an underlying goiter and a detectable RAIU are more common in type 1 AIT. Treatment of type 1 AIT consists of administering thionamides with or without potassium perchlorate, whereas type 2 AIT may respond to steroid therapy. Difficult cases may require plasmapheresis, dialysis, or thyroidectomy (see Chapter 33).

21. **A 20-year-old man presents for failure to enter puberty. He has small, soft testes, no gynecomastia, normal visual fields, and decreased sense of smell. Laboratory evaluation is as follows: serum testosterone = 70 ng/dL (nl, 300–1000), LH = 2.0 mIU/mL (nl, 2–12), FSH = 1.6 mIU/mL (nl, 2–12), prolactin = 7 ng/mL (nl, 2–20), and TSH = 0.9 mU/L (nl, 0.5–5.0). An MRI of the pituitary gland is normal. What is the probable diagnosis?**
This picture is most consistent with idiopathic hypogonadotropic hypogonadism, also known as Kallmann's syndrome. This disorder is due to a deficiency of GnRH, resulting from failure of fetal migration of the GnRH secreting neurons from the olfactory placode to the hypothalamus. Mutations of the Kal gene have been detected in some patients. Maldevelopment of the olfactory lobe causes the associated anosmia. Androgen therapy is indicated to promote appropriate masculinization. When desired, these patients can also become fertile by receiving treatment with GnRH or gonadotropin preparations (see Chapters 43 and 44).

22. **A 32-year-old man complains of impotence and retro-orbital headaches intermittently for the past year. He is adopted and does not know his natural family history. He has bitemporal visual field loss, but his examination is otherwise normal. Laboratory tests reveal the following: serum calcium = 11.8 mg/dL (nl, 8.5–10.5), phosphorous = 2.5 mg/dL (nl, 2.5–4.5), albumin = 4.8 g/dL (nl, 3.2–5.5), intact PTH = 58 pg/mL (nl, 11–54), and prolactin = 2650 ng/mL (nl, 0–20). What is the likely diagnosis?**
This patient has a prolactinoma, manifested by impotence, headaches, bitemporal hemianopsia, and a significantly elevated serum prolactin level. Hypercalcemia with an elevated serum PTH level indicates that he also has hyperparathyroidism. The MEN type 1 syndrome (MEN 1), which consists of hyperparathyroidism, pituitary tumors, and pancreatic endocrine tumors, results from an inherited mutation in the menin gene. This patient should be screened for a gastrinoma and insulinoma by measuring serum gastrin, insulin, proinsulin, and glucose following an overnight fast. After pituitary imaging studies, he should be treated with a dopamine agonist,

transsphenoidal surgery, or both, and subsequently with parathyroid surgery (see Chapters 20 and 52).

23. **A 52-year-old woman complains of a 1-year history of progressive fatigue, puffy eyes, dry skin, and mild weight gain. She had acromegaly treated with transsphenoidal surgery and radiation therapy 10 years ago. Physical examination shows normal visual fields, mild periorbital edema, and dry skin. Laboratory testing reveals the following: GH = 1.2 ng/mL (nl, <2.0), insulin-like growth factor 1 (IGF-1) = 258 mg/mL (nl, 182–780), TSH = 0.2 mU/L (nl, 0.5–5.0), and free T_4 = 0.6 ng/dL (nl, 0.7–2.7). What is the most likely cause of this patient's symptoms?**

This patient has central hypothyroidism due to pituitary damage from the combined effects of surgery and radiation treatment of her pituitary tumor 10 years earlier. Such a lengthy delay in the development of this condition is not uncommon. The diagnosis of central hypothyroidism is based on the presence of symptoms of thyroid hormone deficiency, a low serum free T_4, and a low or low-normal serum TSH. Treatment consists of levothyroxine replacement in doses sufficient to relieve symptoms and to maintain the serum free T_4 level in the mid-normal or upper-normal range. Because TSH secretion is impaired, the serum TSH level cannot be used to monitor this patient's response to therapy. Assessment of her pituitary-adrenal axis is also indicated (see Chapters 18 and 34).

24. **A 32-year-old woman complains of deep pain in both thighs. She was diagnosed as having type 1 diabetes mellitus at age 20. She currently has 2 to 3 bowel movements each day. Her menses are regular. Her diet is well balanced with adequate calcium intake, and she takes a multivitamin. Physical examination is normal. Laboratory studies show the following: serum calcium = 8.2 mg/dL (nl, 8.5–10.5), phosphorous = 2.3 ng/dL (nl, 2.5–4.5), alkaline phosphatase = 312 U/L (nl, 25–125), PTH = 155 pg/mL (nl, 11–54), and 25 hydroxyvitamin D = 7 ng/mL (nl, 30–100). Explain the findings in this patient and suggest a probable underlying diagnosis.**

Her biochemical profile of hypocalcemia, hypophosphatemia, elevated alkaline phosphatase, and significant secondary hyperparathyroidism suggests vitamin D deficiency, which is confirmed by the low serum 25-hydroxyvitamin D level. Lactose intolerance can cause chronic diarrhea but seldom results in vitamin D and calcium malabsorption. Celiac disease (gluten sensitive enteropathy), which occurs with increased frequency in patients with type 1 diabetes mellitus, should be suspected. The diagnosis can be confirmed by the measurement of tissue transglutaminase antibodies, or by a small bowel biopsy. The treatment is elimination of gluten (wheat, rye, barley, and oats) from the diet and supplementation with calcium and vitamin D (see Chapter 11).

25. **A 42-year-old man presents for evaluation of a skin rash that has recently developed. He has known type 2 diabetes mellitus. He drinks 2 to 3 alcoholic beverages several nights each week. Physical examination shows eruptive xanthomas (red papules with golden crowns) all over his body, most prominently on the buttocks, thighs, and forearms. Laboratory studies reveal the following: glucose = 310 mg/dL, hemoglobin A_{1c} (HbA1C) = 12.9%, cholesterol = 1082 mg/dL, and TG = 8900 mg/dL. Discuss the cause and treatment of this lipid disorder.**

The patient has severely elevated serum TG. This condition usually results from combining a secondary cause of TG elevation (uncontrolled diabetes mellitus, excess alcohol use) with an inherited TG disorder (familial hypertriglyceridemia or familial combined hyperlipidemia). His LDL cholesterol cannot be assessed until the serum TG levels are less than 400 mg/dL. Because he is at high risk of developing acute pancreatitis, the priority is to quickly lower his serum TG level to less than 1000 mg/dL. This goal can be achieved most effectively with a temporary very low fat ($< 5\%$ fat) diet, blood glucose control, and discontinuation of alcohol. TG levels will fall by about 20% a day on this regimen. A fibrate or fish oil (or both) should then be added, and he should be switched to an American Heart Association diet. Diabetes control must be continued and further alcohol intake discouraged (see Chapter 6).

26. A 26-year-old woman requests to be tested for a type of thyroid cancer that has recently been found in her mother and two of five siblings. She notes that she has had intermittent headaches and palpitations for the past year. Her blood pressure is 164/102. She has a 1-cm, left-sided thyroid nodule without associated lymphadenopathy. Laboratory testing shows the following results: serum calcium = 11.2 mg/dL (nl, 8.5–10.5), phosphorus = 2.4 mg/dL (nl, 2.5–4.5), albumin = 4.5 g/dL (nl, 3.2–5.5), intact PTH = 55 pg/mL (nl, 11–54), calcitonin = 480 pg/mL (nl, 0–20), and 24-hour urine catecholamines = 1225 mg (nl, 0–200). Discuss her diagnosis and management.

The thyroid nodule, elevated serum calcitonin, and family history make medullary thyroid cancer (MCT) likely. Her hypertension, headaches, palpitations, and high urinary catecholamines indicate a probable pheochromocytoma. She also has hyperparathyroidism. MEN type 2A (MEN 2A) consists of MCT, pheochromocytoma, and hyperparathyroidism. It is an autosomal dominant syndrome that results from a germLine mutation in the Ret gene. After alpha-blocker administration and blood pressure control, treatment of this patient would consist of removal of the pheochromocytoma(s) followed by later removal of the abnormal thyroid and parathyroid glands. Screening at-risk family members for the Ret/MCT oncogene should also be performed (see Chapters 37 and 52).

27. A 68-year-old man complains of a 10-year history of progressive pain in the shins, knees, and left arm. He also notes progressive hearing loss. Physical examination reveals tenderness above the left elbow and enlarged, bowed shins. Bone scan shows intense uptake in both tibias and the left humerus. Skeletal x-rays show enlargement with multiple focal lytic and sclerotic areas in the tibias and the distal left humerus. Laboratory evaluation reveals: serum calcium = 9.8 mg/dL (nl, 8.5–10.5) and alkaline phosphatase = 966 U/L (nl, 25–125). What is the probable diagnosis?

Bone pain and deformity, reduced hearing, and markedly elevated serum alkaline phosphatase levels suggest a diagnosis of Paget's disease. Intense radioisotope uptake on bone scanning supports this diagnosis and the characteristic findings on skeletal radiographs confirm it. Treatment options include analgesics, intermittent oral or intravenous bisphosphonates, and calcitonin, all of which may control but will not cure the disease (see Chapter 12).

28. A 19-year-old man has experienced fatigue, muscle weakness, and dizziness for the past 3 weeks. This morning he fainted when he went outdoors to exercise. His blood pressure is 95/60, and his pulse is 110. His skin is cool, dry, and tanned. His thyroid feels normal. Laboratory testing shows the following: hematocrit = 36%, glucose = 62 mg/dL, sodium = 120 mEq/L, potassium = 6.7 mEq/L, creatinine = 1.4 mg/dL, and blood urea nitrogen (BUN) = 36 mg/dL. What endocrine disorder should be considered and evaluated?

Hyponatremia with hyperkalemia always suggests primary adrenal insufficiency (Addison's disease). Fatigue, weakness, hypotension, tanned skin, anemia, azotemia, and hypoglycemia are also consistent with this diagnosis. The most common cause is autoimmune destruction of the adrenal glands. The diagnosis is made by a Cosyntropin stimulation test that shows a low basal serum cortisol level that fails to increase after ACTH administration. During an adrenal crisis, however, one does not have time to wait for the test results. When this diagnosis is suspected, one should draw blood for a serum cortisol measurement and then start treatment with intravenous fluids and glucocorticoids (hydrocortisone, 100 mg every 6 hours). Precipitating conditions should be actively sought and treated. After the patient is stable, he can be switched to oral hydrocortisone and fludrocortisone for chronic maintenance. The diagnosis is likely if the serum cortisol measured during the crisis was low, but this should be confirmed by repeat Cosyntropin stimulation testing upon recovery from the acute event (see Chapter 30).

CHAPTER 62

FAMOUS PEOPLE WITH ENDOCRINE DISORDERS

Kenneth J. Simcic and Michael T. McDermott

1. **Name the former college basketball star from Gonzaga University who was diagnosed with type 1 diabetes at age 14.**
   Adam Morrison. After his final college season, Morrison shared college basketball's Player of the Year Award with J.J. Redick of Duke. He was then selected third overall in the 2006 National Basketball Association (NBA) draft by the Charlotte Bobcats.

2. **This female track star recovered from Graves disease and went on to win the title of "Fastest Woman in the World" at the 1992 Summer Olympics in Barcelona. Who is she?**
   Gail Devers. Devers repeated as champion in the women's 100 meters at the 1996 Olympics in Atlanta. She has enjoyed remarkable longevity in her sport. In February 2007, at age 40, she won the 60 meter hurdles at the Mellrose games with a time of 7.86 seconds.

3. **Name the dwarf actor who gained fame for his role as Tattoo on the television series *Fantasy Island* (1977–1984).**
   Herve Villechaize (1943–1993). Villechaize's short stature was due to achondroplasia. His adult height was only 3 feet, 2 inches.

4. **Television and film actress Mary Tyler Moore has what endocrine disorder?**
   Type 1 diabetes. Moore was diagnosed at age 33. Her diabetes has been complicated by retinopathy and recurrent foot infections.

5. **George Bush and his wife Barbara were both diagnosed with Graves disease during his presidency (1989–1993). How did the president's Graves disease present clinically?**
   Atrial fibrillation. (Mrs. Bush's Graves disease was also complicated by ophthalmopathy. In addition to radioactive iodine for her hyperthyroidism, she also required treatment with glucocorticoids and orbital radiation therapy for her eye disease.)

KEY POINTS:

1. Because many endocrine disorders are common, it is not surprising that famous people have or have had endocrine disorders.
2. Most endocrine disorders are either curable or treatable.
3. Many famous people have accomplished great things despite their endocrine disorders.
4. The lives of these famous people can serve as sources of encouragement to patients who suffer from similar endocrine conditions.

6. **Pulitzer Prize–winning film critic Roger Ebert was diagnosed with what endocrine disorder at age 59?**
   Papillary thyroid cancer (treated with thyroidectomy and radioactive iodine). Ebert has a major risk factor for papillary thyroid cancer. As a child, he was given radiation treatment for an ear infection.

7. **Name the acromegalic giant who played the character Jaws in the James Bond films *The Spy Who Loved Me* (1977) and Moonraker (1979).**
   Richard Kiel (Kiel is 7 feet, 2 inches tall).

8. **Name the 2 foot, 8 inch, dwarf actor best known for his role as Mini-Me in the film *Austin Powers: The Spy Who Shagged Me* (1999).**
   Vern Troyer. Troyer's dwarfism is secondary to chondrodysplasia. He has had acting roles in more than 15 feature films.

9. **What late actor, who appeared in the film Young Frankenstein (1974), had obvious Graves ophthalmopathy?**
   Marty Feldman (1933–1982).

10. **Ancient Egyptian sculptures and paintings suggest that Tutankhamen (1357–1339 b.c.) and other pharaohs of the Eighteenth Egyptian Dynasty had what endocrine disorder?**
    Gynecomastia. Familial aromatase excess syndrome is a possible explanation for this historical finding.

11. **What famous male ice skater overcame growth failure related to a childhood illness to win the gold medal at the 1984 Winter Olympics in Sarajevo?**
    Scott Hamilton. As a child, Hamilton suffered from Shwachman syndrome, a rare disorder of the pancreas. His adult height is 5 feet, 3 inches. Hamilton was also diagnosed with testicular cancer at age 38, and with a craniopharyngioma at age 46.

12. **How was Scott Hamilton's craniopharyngioma treated?**
    After a biopsy to confirm the diagnosis, Hamilton was treated with gamma knife radiosurgery.

13. **In 1999, Tipper Gore, the wife of former Vice President Al Gore, had surgery for what endocrine disorder?**
    Thyroid nodule (benign).

14. **Name the late professional wrestler (and actor) who was well known for his height and acromegalic facial features.**
    Andre "The Giant" Rousimoff (1947–1993).

15. **Charles Sherwood Stratton (1838–1883) reached an adult height of only 3 feet, 4 inches. what was his circus name?**
    General Tom Thumb. In 1863, Stratton married fellow diminutive circus performer Lavinia Warren, whose height was only 2 feet, 8 inches.

16. **Actress Catherine Bell, who starred as Lt. Col. Sarah "Mac" MacKenzie on the television series JAG (1995–2005), has been treated for what thyroid disorder?**
    Papillary thyroid cancer.

17. Oscar award–winning actress Halle Berry was diagnosed with what endocrine disorder at age 21?
   Diabetes (probably type 1).

18. After successful treatment for Graves disease, this professional golfer captained the United States team to the 1999 Ryder Cup in what has been called the greatest comeback in Ryder Cup history. Who is he?
   Ben Crenshaw.

19. Vocalist Rod Stewart has had surgery for what endocrine disorder?
   Thyroid cancer (most likely papillary). It took 9 months for Stewart's voice to recover from the surgery.

20. Ron Santo won six Golden Glove Awards and played in nine All Star games while playing third base for the Chicago Cubs. He was diagnosed with type 1 diabetes at what age?
   Eighteen years, just after signing his first contract to play major league baseball. Since his retirement from baseball, Santo has suffered the following macrovascular complications of his diabetes: coronary artery disease requiring a quadruple coronary artery bypass operation and implantation of an automatic cardiac defibrillator device; bilateral below the knee amputations for peripheral vascular disease.

21. Name the 3-foot, 7-inch, 65-pound midget who batted one time for the St. Louis Browns on August 19, 1951.
   Eddie Gaedel (1925–1961). Gaedel was walked on four pitches by Detroit Tigers' pitcher Bob Cain.

22. Gheorghe Muresan of the Washington Bullets is the tallest player in the history of the NBA (7 feet, 7 inches). What treatments has he received for his acromegaly and gigantism?
   Transsphenoidal pituitary surgery, pituitary radiation, and somatostatin analogue injections (Note: Shaquille O'Neal is 7 feet, 1 inch tall).

23. In his 6-year NBA career (Washington Bullets 1993–1997; New Jersey Nets 1998–2000), Muresan twice led the league in what category?
   Field goal percentage (1995–1996 season: .584; 1996–1997 season: .604).

24. Regardless of their acting ability, it seems like every famous giant gets an acting role in a movie. Gheorghe Muresan starred in what movie with Billy Crystal?
   My Giant (1998).

25. The late actor Rondo "The Creeper" Hatton had severe acromegalic facial features. He played the villain in numerous horror films such as the Pearl of Death (1944), House of Horrors (1946), and The Brute Man (1946). How old was Hatton at the time of his death?
   Hatton died of a myocardial infarction at age 51. At the time of his death, he also reportedly suffered from diabetes and loss of vision. All of these conditions were probably sequelae of his untreated acromegaly.

26. Nicole Johnson was 24 years old when she was crowned Miss America 1999. At age 19, she was diagnosed with what endocrine disorder?
   Type 1 diabetes.

27. **Name the former chief justice of the U.S. Supreme Court who died of anaplastic thyroid cancer at age 80.**
William Rehnquist. Rehnquist was diagnosed with anaplastic cancer in October 2004, and he died less than one year later in September 2005.

28. **Grammy award–winning vocalists Johnny Cash (1932–2003), Ella Fitzgerald (1917–1996), Waylon Jennings (1937–2002), and Luther Vandross (1951–2005) all died from complications of what endocrine disorder?**
Type 2 diabetes.

29. **Track star Carl Lewis competed in five consecutive Olympics. He is one of only three athletes who have won nine gold medals in an Olympic career. With what endocrine disorder was he diagnosed at age 35?**
Primary hypothyroidism (secondary to Hashimoto's thyroiditis).

30. **Name the American swimmer who was diagnosed with type 1 diabetes 18 months before he won two gold medals at the 2000 Olympics in Sydney, Australia.**
Gary Hall, Jr.

31. **Carla Overbeck, women's soccer star and captain of the 1996 U.S. gold medal Olympic team, was diagnosed with what endocrine disorder at age 32?**
Graves disease.

32. **Based on a true story, the film Lorenzo's Oil (1992) portrays a family's struggle with what rare adrenal disorder?**
Adrenoleukodystrophy. The film's main character, Lorenzo Odone, was diagnosed with this condition at age five.

33. **Despite his type 1 diabetes, this former National Hockey League star led the Philadelphia Flyers to back-to-back Stanley Cup championships in 1973–1974 and 1974–1975.**
Bobby Clarke. Clarke's diabetes was diagnosed at age 13.

34. **The demanding ironman Triathlon requires a 2.4-mile swim followed by a 112-mile bike ride and a 26.2-mile run. Name the three-time member of the U.S. National Team for Long Course Triathlon who was diagnosed with type 1 diabetes at age 24.**
Jay Hewitt. Hewitt began competing in the Triathlon after his diagnosis of diabetes.

TOP SECRETS

1. Although type 1 diabetes is a serious disease, athletes with this condition have been able to compete and succeed at the professional level in almost every sport.

2. The accomplishments of track star Gail Devers emphasize the excellent prognosis of properly treated Graves disease.

3. Perhaps the most fascinating of all endocrine disorders are the disorders of growth. This explains why dwarfs and giants have been so popular as circus performers and movie actors.

4. The curability of most thyroid cancers is illustrated by the lives of Rod Stewart, Catherine Bell, and Roger Ebert.

5. The high mortality of untreated acromegaly is illustrated by the short lives of wrestler Andre "The Giant" Rousimoff and actor Rondo Hatton.

BIBLIOGRAPHY

1. Dawson LY: Skating at the cutting edge: Bobby Clarke. Diab Forecast (March): 6–19, 1994.

2. Mandernach M: Short hitter, long memory. Sports Illustrated (September) 2:5, 1996.

3. Montville L: Giant. Sports Illustrated October 2:50–56, 1995.

4. Paulshock BZ: Tutankhamun and his brothers: familial gynecomastia in the eighteenth dynasty. JAMA 244:160–164, 1980.

5. Ford-Martin P. Famous people who have diabetes: http://diabetes.about.com//cs/diabetesfame/. Accessed November 23, 2003.

6. Famousheights.com: http://www.famousheights.com. Accessed November 23, 2003.

7. Shomon M: Famous People w/Thyroid Conditions: http://www.thyroid.about.com/cs/amouspeople/. Accessed November 23, 2003.

8. Mazur ML: Here she is Miss America. Diab Forecast (July):49–51, 1999.

9. Drimmer F: *Very special people*. New York, 1991, Carol Publishing Group.

10. Falcon M, Shoop SA: Roger Ebert reviews his thyroid cancer (April 5, 2002): http://www.usatoday.com/news/health/spotlight/2002/03/20-ebert.htm. Accessed November 23, 2003.

11. D'Arrigo T: Hot shot NBA rookie Adam Morrison scores with control. Diab Forecast (February):42–45, 2007.

12. Lerner BH: When illness goes public. Baltimore, 2006, Johns Hopkins University Press.

CHAPTER 63

INTERESTING ENDOCRINE FACTS AND FIGURES

Michael T. McDermott, MD

1. **Who is the tallest man on record?**
   The man with the greatest medically documented height was Robert Wadlow of Alton, Illinois. He was 8 feet, 11.1 inches tall and weighed 439 pounds when he died in 1940 at age 22 years; he was 7 feet, 1.75 inches at age 13 years. His condition was the result of a growth hormone–secreting pituitary tumor that developed before closure of the skeletal epiphyseal plates (gigantism). The tallest currently living man is Xi Shun of China, who stands 7 feet, 8.95 inches tall.

2. **Name the tallest woman on record.**
   Zeng Jinlian of Hunan Province, China, is the tallest woman on record. She was 8 feet, 1.75 inches just before her death at age 17 in 1982 and had been 7 feet, 1.5 inches tall at age 13 years. She also had a growth hormone–secreting tumor that developed during childhood.

3. **How tall was the shortest man on record?**
   Gul Mohammed of India was measured at 22.5 inches (57 cm) tall in 1990; he died in 1997. The shortest currently living man is Younis Edwan of Jordan, who is 25.5 inches (65 cm) tall.

4. **Who is the shortest woman on record?**
   The shortest adult woman on record was Pauline Musters of the Netherlands. She was 23.2 inches tall and weighed 9 pounds shortly before her death at age 19 years in 1895. Because of her relatively normal proportions, she is believed to have had pituitary growth hormone deficiency, although growth hormone assays were clearly not available in 1895.

5. **Who had the most variable adult stature?**
   Adam Rainer of Austria was a 3-feet, 10.45-inch dwarf at age 21 years but rapidly grew into a 7-foot, 1.75-inch, giant at age 32 years in 1931. He was 7 feet, 8 inches tall when he died in 1950 at age 51 years.

6. **Which is the tallest tribe in Africa?**
   The Watusi (or Tutsi) tribe of Sudan, Rwanda, Burundi, and Central African Republic are the tallest in the world. The men average 6 feet, 5 inches, and the women average 5 feet, 10 inches. Their tall stature is believed to be a genetic adaptation.

7. **Which is the shortest tribe?**
   The Mbuti pygmies of central Africa have the lowest mean height. The men average 4 feet, 6 inches, and the women 4 feet, 5 inches. Their short stature is thought to result from genetic resistance to growth hormone, possibly due to deficient growth hormone receptors.

8. **Who was the heaviest man on record?**
   Jon Brower Minnoch of Bainbridge Island, Washington, was 6 feet, 1 inch, tall and weighed approximately 1400 pounds when he was admitted to the hospital at age 37 years of congestive heart failure. He remained in the hospital for 2 years on a 1200-calorie diet and was discharged

at 476 pounds; his weight loss of 924 pounds is also a record. He weighed 798 pounds when he died at age 42 years in 1983. His wife weighed 110 pounds.

9. **How much did the heaviest woman on record weigh?**
The heaviest woman on record was Rosalie Bradford, who weighed 1199 pounds in 1987. She also holds the record for weight loss, having shed 917 pounds over the subsequent 7 years.

10. **What is the greatest rate of weight gain ever recorded?**
Arthur Knorr of the United States gained 294 pounds during the last 6 months of his life; this s an average weight gain of 1.6 pounds a day. Since a pound of fat has about 3500 kcal, this represents an excess intake (above caloric expenditures) of 5600 kcal a day. Doris James holds the record for women, having gained 328 pounds in the last year of her life (3150 kcal/day excess) before she died at age 38, weighing 675 pounds.

11. **What is the largest recorded waist size?**
Walter Hudson of New York, who stood 5 feet, 10 inches, had a peak weight of 1197 pounds and a waist size of 119 inches.

12. **Who are the heaviest twins on record?**
Billy McCrary and Benny McCrary of Hendersonville, North Carolina, weighed 743 and 723 pounds, respectively. Both had 84-inch waists. One brother died in a motorcycle accident, but the other is alive at the time of this printing.

13. **What is the longest anyone has ever survived without food or water?**
Andreas Mihavecz of Austria was put in jail in 1979. The guards forgot about him and gave him no food or water for 18 days, after which he was found still alive, but barely.

14. **What is the greatest known number of children born to one woman in a lifetime?**
A peasant woman from Shuya, east of Moscow, Russia, gave birth to 69 children from 1725 to 1765. She had 27 pregnancies, producing 16 pairs of twins, 7 sets of triplets, and 4 sets of quadruplets. Sixty-seven of the children survived infancy. Her husband had 18 more children with a second wife.

15. **Who is the oldest known woman to give birth?**
Adriana Emilia Illiescu of Romania gave birth to a daughter by Cesarean section in 2005, at age 66 years, 230 days. Donna Maas of California is the oldest woman to give birth to twins, having delivered twin boys by Cesarean section in 2004 at age 57 years, 286 days.

16. **What is the highest reported number of multiple births for a single gestation?**
Ten births (decaplets) were reported in Brazil (1946), China (1936), and Spain (1924). Nine births (nonuplets) were recorded in Australia (1971), Philadelphia (1972), and Bangladesh (1977). The largest number to survive a multiple gestation is seven (septuplets), which has happened on three occasions; the mothers were Bobby McCaughey of Nebraska (1997), N kem Chukwu of Texas (1998), and Hasna Mohammed Humair of Saudi Arabia (1998).

17. **What is the highest single birth weight ever recorded?**
Anna Bates, living in Seville, Ohio, gave birth to a 23 pound, 12 ounce (10.8 kg) baby boy who died 11 hours later in 1879. Anna was 7 feet, 5.5 inches tall. Carmelina Fedele of Italy gave birth in 1955 to the largest surviving baby, who weighed 22 pounds, 8 ounces (10.2 kg).

18. **What is the oldest age to which a human has been documented to live?**
Jeanne Louise Calment of Arles, France, lived to be 122 years, 164 days old. She died on August 4, 1997. The oldest man was Shigechiyo Izumi of Japan, who lived to be 120 years, 237 days old before he died in 1986.

19. **What is the highest blood glucose level ever reported?**
A 12-year-old boy with new-onset diabetes mellitus was still conscious when he was discovered to have a blood glucose level of 2350 mg/dL in 1995.

20. **What is the record for most kidney stones produced by one individual?**
Don Winfield of Canada passed 3711 kidney stones over a 15-year period (1986–2001).

21. **What is the largest tumor ever reported?**
A 328-lb ovarian cyst was removed from a woman in Texas in 1905.

22. **What is the longest hair ever recorded?**
Hoo Sateow of Thailand had his hair measured at 16 feet, 11 inches in 1997. He had not cut his hair for 70 years.

23. **What is the record distance walked by an individual in 24 hours?**
The record for men is 142.25 miles, by Jesse Castenda of the United States in 1976. The record for women is 131.27 miles by Annie Van der Meer-Timmerman of the Netherlands in 1986. The 24-hour record for an individual in a wheelchair is 77.58 miles by Nik Nikzaban of Canada in 2000.

24. **Did King David of Israel have an endocrine disorder?**
"When King David was old and advanced in years, though they spread covers over him, he could not keep warm. His servants therefore said to him, 'Let a young virgin be sought to attend you, lord king, and to nurse you. If she sleeps with your royal majesty, you will be kept warm'. . . . The maiden, who was very beautiful, nursed the king and cared for him, but the king did not have relations with her" (I Kings 1:1–4). Some speculate King David was afflicted with hypothyroidism.

25. **What endocrine disorder might Goliath of Gath have had?**
Goliath of Gath, who was killed by a stone from David's sling (I Samuel 17:1–51), probably stood about 6 feet, 10 inches. His tall stature may have resulted from a growth hormone–secreting pituitary tumor. Others add that the ease with which David's stone became embedded in Goliath's skull may have been due to hyperparathyroidism, and his bizarre behavior may have resulted from hypoglycemia due to an insulinoma. He may thus be the earliest known case of multiple endocrine neoplasia type 1 syndrome.

26. **What endocrine disorder did President John F. Kennedy have?**
Kennedy had primary adrenal insufficiency—Addison's disease. He was sustained throughout the later years of his life and his presidency by therapy with oral glucocorticoids.

WEBSITE

http://www.guinnessworldrecords.com

BIBLIOGRAPHY

1. Baumann G, Shaw MN, Merimee TJ: Low levels of high affinity growth hormone-binding protein in African Pygmies. N Engl J Med 320:1705–1709, 1989

2. Farlan D, editor *The Guinness book of world records*, New York, 1991, Bantam Books.

3. Folkard C, editor: *The Guinness book of world records*, New York, 2003, Bantam Books.

4. Glenday C, editor: *The Guinness book of world records*, New York, 2007, Bantam Books.

5. *The New American Bible*. Catholic Publishers, Thomas Nelson, Inc. (Camden, NJ) 1971.

INDEX

Page numbers followed by *t* indicate tables; *f*, figures. Page numbers in **boldface type** indicate complete chapters.